S0-CEE-515

ATLAS OF CANCER MORTALITY

IN THE

EUROPEAN ECONOMIC COMMUNITY

INTERNATIONAL AGENCY FOR RESEARCH ON CANCER

The International Agency for Research on Cancer (IARC) was established in 1965 by the World Health Assembly, as an independently financed organization within the framework of the World Health Organization. The headquarters of the Agency are at Lyon, France.

The Agency conducts a programme of research concentrating particularly on the epidemiology of cancer and the study of potential carcinogens in the human environment. Its field studies are supplemented by biological and chemical research carried out in the Agency's laboratories in Lyon and, through collaborative research agreements, in national research institutions in many countries. The Agency also conducts a programme for the education and training of personnel for cancer research.

The publications of the Agency are intended to contribute to the dissemination of authoritative information on different aspects of cancer research. A complete list is printed at the back of this book.

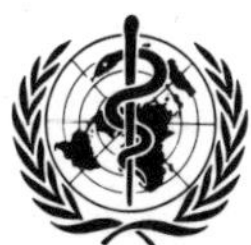

INTERNATIONAL AGENCY FOR RESEARCH ON CANCER
WORLD HEALTH ORGANIZATION

ATLAS OF CANCER MORTALITY IN THE EUROPEAN ECONOMIC COMMUNITY

Edited by

M. Smans, C.S. Muir and P. Boyle

in collaboration with

M.R. Alderson, L.H. Anderson, H. Bille, A. Doneux, P. Henkes,
W.J. Hunter, K. Kern, P. Morganti, M.H. Pejovic, A. Rezvani,
D. Salmond, J. Stephens and J.K.S. van Ginneken

IARC Scientific Publications No. 107

International Agency for Research on Cancer
Lyon, France
1992

Published by the International Agency for Research on Cancer,
150 cours Albert Thomas, 69372 Lyon Cedex 08, France

Distributed by Oxford University Press, Walton Street, Oxford OX2 6DP, UK

Distributed in the USA by Oxford University Press, New York

ISBN 92 832 2107 9

ISSN 0300-5085

Printed in France

Contents

Contents

FOREWORD

Epidemiology has been defined as use of knowledge on the occurrence and distribution of disease in the search of determinants. A map can convey the distribution in a way that pages of tables do not. This atlas, depicting the patterns of cancer mortality in the member states of the EEC, the second of a series of such atlases to be produced jointly by the International Agency for Research on Cancer and national bodies, illustrates once again the truism that a single picture is worth a thousand words.

The signal variations in mortality which exist within and between countries for some cancers such as those of the oesophagus contrast with other forms of malignant disease such as breast cancer for which, in contrast to international differences, death rates tend to be fairly uniform within a country. Such contrasts form the point of departure for further studies to uncover possible determinants of risk.

To set these findings in perspective, the editors have provided, on the basis of material contributed by national vital statistics offices and the statistical services of the EEC, information on death registration and selected characteristics of the countries concerned. Trying to introduce a measure of uniformity of content and presentation, together with delays in receipt of material, have meant that the data pertain to the latter half of the 1970s, and further do not cover all current EEC members. The next issue of this atlas will cover these lacunae.

The Editors have taken considerable care to discuss those aspects of data collection that may influence the interpretation of the results. The fascinating differences in the patterns of cancer mortality portrayed cry out for further investigations into cause, as without knowledge of etiology there can be no rational prevention.

This volume is the outcome of a collaborative project, largely funded by the Commission of the European Communities, between IARC and relevant authorities in each of the countries covered. We are grateful for the generous support and cooperation of all concerned.

L. Tomatis, M.D.
Director, IARC

CHAPTER 1

AIMS OF THE ATLAS

Maps may be topographic or thematic. The former display the physical features, the location of cities and towns, roads, railways, and the like—the latter concentrate on displaying the geographical occurrence and variation of a single phenomenon—the theme of the map. In this Atlas the theme is cancer mortality.

The geographical representation of cancer on maps describes the 'cancer scenery' of a country (Frenztel-Beyme *et al.*, 1979). As cancer occurs in people, not geographical areas, the real purpose of a cancer atlas lies in the identification of geographical areas that require more detailed study and, above all, the formulation of etiological hypotheses to account for observed differences. These hypotheses can then be pursued by appropriate analytical and environmental studies.

These aims are attainable. Over 2000 years ago Hippocrates listed the kinds of question which should be asked when relating disease to environment and geographical distribution. A classical, and frequently cited, example comes from an outbreak of cholera in London in 1854. John Snow, by recording and *mapping* the addresses of the victims of the epidemic, was able to show that the disease was much commoner in people drinking water supplied by the Southwark and Vauxhall Water Company and, more precisely, from a pump in Broad Street, than in those drinking water from other sources. Removing the handle from the Broad Street pump effectively stopped the epidemic.

The first map for cancer was apparently produced for females in England and Wales by Haviland in 1875. Haviland, who observed that 'by studying the geographical laws of disease we shall know where to find its exciting[1] as well as its predisposing causes and how to avoid it', was 'struck by the definite character of the arrangement that the mortality assumes throughout the country'. Stocks, who mapped cancer mortality in England and Wales in the 1930s, later attempted to correlate the distribution, as had Haviland (1875), with the mineral content, notably zinc and cadmium, of the soil (Stocks, 1928, 1936, 1937, 1939). Howe (1963, 1970) published national disease atlases in the United Kingdom, and described the mapping of disease in history.

There was a renaissance of cancer mapping when Burbank (1971) published computer-drawn maps of the distribution of cancer mortality for the 49 states which comprised the United States of America. The State was soon recognized as being too large an areal unit, which resulted in the publication of a County Cancer Atlas in two volumes, one for Whites and one for non-Whites (Mason *et al.*, 1975, 1976). Since then numerous cancer atlases have appeared (Table 1.1).

---
[1] Underlying

Table 1.1. List of national cancer atlases (incidence or mortality)

Country	Title	Editors	Publisher
Australia	Cancer in Australia 1982 Scientific Publication No. 1	Giles, G.G., Armstrong, B.K., Smith, L.R.	National Cancer Statistics Clearing House (1987)
Austria	Österreichichser Todesursachenatlas 1978/1984	Austrian Central Statistical Office	Austian Central Statistical Office, Vienna (1989)
Belgium	Atlas of Cancer Mortality in Belgium (1969–1976)	Ryckeboer, R., Janssens, G., Thiers, G.L.	Institute of Hygiene and Epidemiology, Ministry of Public Health and Environment, Brussels (1983)
Brazil	Cancer no Brasil: Dados Histopatológicos 1976–80	Brumini, R.	Campanha Nacional de Combate as Câncer, Ministerio de Saude, Rio de Janeiro, (1982)
Canada	Mortality Atlas of Canada. Vol. 1: Cancer	Health and Welfare Canada	Canadian Government Publishing Centre, Hull (1980)
China	Atlas of Cancer Mortality in the People's Republic of China	The Editorial Committee for the Atlas of Cancer Mortality in the People's Republic of China	China Map Press, Beijing (1979)
Denmark	Atlas over Kroeftforekomst i Denmark 1970–79	Carstensen, B., Møller Jensen, O.	Danish Cancer Society, Environmental Protection Agency (1986)
England and Wales	Atlas of Cancer Mortality in England and Wales 1968–78	Gardner, M.J., Winter, P.D., Taylor, C.P., Acheson, E.D.	John Wiley, Chichester (1983)
Finland	Atlas of Cancer Incidence in Finland	Pukkala, E., Gustavsson, N., Teppo, L.	Cancer Society of Finland, Helsinki, (1987)
France	Atlas de la Mortalité par Cancer en France (1971–1978)	Rezvani, A., Doyon, F., Flamant, R.	Les Editions INSERM, Paris (1985)
Germany, FR	Cancer Atlas of the Federal Republic of Germany	Frentzel-Beyme, R., Leutner, R., Wagner, G., Wiebelt, H.	Springer-Verlag, Berlin (1979)
Germany, FR	Atlas of Cancer Mortality in the Federal Republic of Germany	Becker, N., Frentzel-Beyme, R., Wagner, G.	Springer-Verlag, Berlin (1984)
Italy	Data, Statistics and Maps on Cancer Mortality, Italia, 1975/1977	Cislaghi, C., DeCarli, A., LaVecchia, C., Mezzanotte, G., Smans, M.	Pitagora Editrice, Bologna (1986)
Japan	Atlas of Cancer Mortality for Japan by Cities and Counties 1969–71	Segi, M.	DAIWA Health Foundation, Tokyo (1977)

Netherlands	Atlas of Cancer Mortality in the Netherlands 1969–1978	Netherlands Central Bureau of Statistics	Staatsuitgeverij, The Hague (1980)
New Zealand	A Cancer Mortality Atlas of New Zealand (Special Report No. 63)	Borman, B.	National Health Statistics Centre, Department of Health (1982)
Nordic Countries	Atlas of Cancer Incidence in the Nordic Countries	Møller Jensen, O., Carstensen, B., Glattre, E., Malker, B., Pukkala, E., Tulinius, H.	Nordic Cancer Union, Helsinki (1988)
Norway	Atlas over Kreftinsidens i Norge 1970–79	Glattre, E., Finne, T.E., Olesen, O., Langmark, F.	Norwegian Cancer Society, Oslo (1986)
Poland	Atlas of Cancer Mortality in Poland 1975–1979	Zatonski, W., Becker, N.	Springer-Verlag, Paris (1988)
Portugal	Atlas do Cancro em Portugal 1980–1982	DaMotta, L.C., Falcao, J.M.	Ministerio Da Saude, Departamento de Estudos e Planeamento da Saude, Lisbon (1987)
Scotland	Atlas of Cancer in Scotland: 1975–1980; Incidence and Epidemiological Perspective (IARC Scientific Publications No. 72)	Kemp, I., Boyle, P., Smans, M., Muir, C.	International Agency for Research on Cancer, Lyon (1985)
Spain	Atlas del Cáncer en Espana (1984)	López-Abente, G., Escolar, A., Errezola, M.	Gráficas Santamaria, Vitoria-Gasteiz
Switzerland	Géographie de la Mortalité Due au Cancer en Suisse 1969–71	Brooke, E.	Institut Universitaire de Médecine Sociale et Préventive, Bern (1976)
Switzerland	La Distribution Géographique de la Mortalité Cancéreuse en Suisse 1979/81	Office Féderal de la Statistique	Office Féderal de la Statistique, Bern, 1987
Taiwan	Color Atlas of Cancer Mortality by Administrative and Other Classified Districts in Taiwan Area: 1968–1976	Chen, K.-P., Wu, H.-Y., Yeh, C.-C., Cheng, Y.-J.	National Science Council, Taiwan Taipei (1979)
USA	Atlas of Cancer Mortality for US Counties: 1950–1969 DHEW Publication (NIH) 75–780	Mason, T.J., McKay, F.W., Hoover, R., Blot, W.T., Fraumeni, J.F., Jr	US Government Printing Office, Washington, DC (1976)
USA	U.S. Cancer Mortality Rates and Trends, 1950–1979. Volume IV: Maps	Riggan, W.B., Creason, J.P., Nelson, W.C. *et al.*	United States Environmental Protection Agency, Washington, DC (1987)
USA	Atlas of U.S. Cancer Mortality Among Whites, 1950–1980 DHHS Publication (NIH) 87–2900	Pickle, L.J., Mason, T.J., Howard, N., Hoover, R., Fraumeni, J.F., Jr	U.S. Government Printing Office, Washington, DC (1987)
Uruguay	Cáncer en el Uruguay	Vassallo, J.A., Registro Nacional de Cáncer del Uruguay	Dirección del Registro Nacional de Cáncer, Montevideo (1989)

The US cancer maps led to the identification of areas of unexpected high mortality. For example, the geographical distribution of oral cancer among females by US county showed a concentration of mortality in the south-east which led to field studies that identified the risk as arising among workers in the textile industry. Further investigation showed that the excess could not be directly attributed to occupation but was due to the fact that, following smoking restrictions at the workplace, the predominantly female workforce took to snuff-dipping instead of cigarette smoking (Winn *et al.*, 1981). Interesting variations in colon cancer were also uncovered, which was found to be surprisingly frequent in parts of Nebraska. This led to a case-control study which identified increased risk among farmers of Moravian descent who had a diet high in fat, consumed large quantities of beer and also had a higher than expected occurrence of familial polyposis.

As will become evident in Chapter 5, the present atlas, based on over 3.6 million deaths from cancer, reveals many distinctive patterns of cancer mortality distribution within the EEC[2] which clearly and urgently require further study from the standpoint of causation. The maps may also be used as an aid in planning the provision of the health services required to combat this disease.

The maps

The maps present age-standardized mortality rates by sex (see below) for 355 areas designated as being at levels II or III by the EEC statistical services[3]. These areas, identified by a three-character code, frequently have a national equivalent such as Département in France, County in England and Wales, or Regierungsbezirk in the Federal Republic of Germany[4]. The transparent overlays which accompany this Atlas can be used to locate these areas, the code numbers for which are also used by the country in question. Thus, B21 identifies the city of Brussels and the surrounding region; F69, the Département of Rhône in France, I12, Varese in Italy (for key see Table 1.2). For a given cancer the higher rates are in shades of orange/red, the median rates being yellow and the lower rates in shades of green (see Kemp *et al.*, 1985, for a fuller explanation). The distribution of the mortality rates is shown in the bottom left corner of each map. It should be borne in mind that a given colour will represent a different range of values according to the site of cancer. The exact value for the age-standardized mortality in a given district is given, with other statistical information, in the Tables in Annex 1 of this atlas.

The tables

The statistical tables, on which the maps are based, identify each area by a code number, the key for which appears in Table 1.2. These code numbers also appear on one of the transparent overlays. The first table lists the population data for each area, for males and females. In all the subsequent tables, the data are presented in six columns from left to right. The first column lists the three-character district codes mentioned above. Codes which have a 'dash' in the second position refer to a region at EEC level I. Thus, B-V gives data for the region of Flanders (Vlaanderen). A code with a 'stop' in the second position refers to a country, B.0 pertaining to Belgium. EEC-9 presents a grand total for the nine EEC countries. Column 2 gives the total number of cases, column 3 the crude rates, i.e. the total cases

[2]Although the European Economic Community currently comprises 12 nations, at the time work began on this Atlas, mortality data were readily available to the required level of detail for Belgium, the Federal Republic of Germany, Denmark, France, the United Kingdom of Great Britain and Northern Ireland, Italy, Ireland, Luxembourg and the Netherlands. Detailed data for Greece, Portugal and Spain will appear in a future edition of the Atlas.

[3]Luxembourg and Northern Ireland which appear as one unit at level II, have been divided into three districts and four planning regions.

[4] All data in this atlas from Germany relate to the Federal Republic as constituted before the reunification with the old Germany Democratic Republic in 1990.

divided by the person-years at risk. Column 4 gives the age-standardized rates (world standard) followed by the result of testing the rate for a given area for statistically significant differences from the rest of EEC-9 (for further details see Kemp *et al.*, 1985). The fifth column gives the standard error of the rate given in the fourth column, the sixth column gives the rank of the age-standardized mortality rate for an area (1 is the highest) among the 355 districts. Regional and national values are not included in the ranking.

Validity of the data in this atlas

Perhaps the most important requirement of a cancer atlas is that it should present cancer patterns with minimal distortion. Chapter 3 thus contains information which will alert readers to possible sources of bias: many of the factors influencing interpretation are also examined in much greater detail elsewhere in the Atlas (Chapter 5). The sources of the data and the methods of computation and technical details concerning the production of the maps are outlined in Chapter 2.

Table 1.2. Key to code numbers used for the areas mapped

BELGIE-BELGIQUE (1971-78)

BRUSSEL-BRUXELLES

B21 BRUSSEL-BRUXELLES

VLAANDEREN

B10 ANTWERPEN
B29 BRABANT (Halle & Leuven)
B30 WEST-VLAANDEREN
B40 OOST-VLAANDEREN
B70 LIMBURG

B-V + VLAANDEREN

WALLONIE

B25 BRABANT (Nivelles)
B50 HAINAUT
B60 LIEGE
B80 LUXEMBOURG
B90 NAMUR

B-W + WALLONIE

B.0 ++ BELGIE-BELGIQUE

BR DEUTSCHLAND (1976-80)

BADEN-WURTTEMBERG

D81 STUTTGART
D82 KARLSRUHE
D83 FREIBURG
D84 TUBINGEN

D-A + BADEN-WURTTEMBERG

BAYERN

D91 OBERBAYERN
D92 NIEDERBAYERN
D93 OBERPFALZ
D94 OBERFRANKEN
D95 MITTELFRANKEN
D96 UNTERFRANKEN
D97 SCHWABEN

D-B + BAYERN

BERLIN(WEST)

DB0 BERLIN(WEST)

BREMEN

D40 BREMEN

HAMBURG

D20 HAMBURG

HESSEN

D64 DARMSTADT
D66 KASSEL

D-F + HESSEN

NIEDERSACHSEN

D31 BRAUNSCHWEIG
D32 HANNOVER
D33 LUNEBURG
D34 WESER-EMS

D-G + NIEDERSACHSEN

NORDRHEIN-WESTFALEN

D51 DUSSELDORF
D53 KOLN
D55 MUNSTER
D57 DETMOLD
D59 ARNSBERG

D-H + NORDRHEIN-WESTFALEN

RHEINLAND-PFALZ

D71 KOBLENZ
D72 TRIER
D73 RHEINHESSEN-PFALZ

D-I + RHEINLAND-PFALZ

SAARLAND

DA0 SAARLAND

SCHLESWIG-HOLSTEIN

D10 SCHLESWIG-HOLSTEIN

D.0 ++ BR DEUTSCHLAND

DANMARK (1971-80)

K15 KOBENHAVN
K20 FREDERIKSBORG
K25 ROSKILDE
K30 VESTSJAELLAND
K35 STORSTROM
K40 BORNHOLM
K42 FYN
K50 SONDERJYLLAND
K55 RIBE
K60 VEJLE
K65 RINGKOBING
K70 ARHUS
K76 VIBORG
K80 NORDJYLLAND

K.0 ++ DANMARK

FRANCE (1971-78)

ALSACE

F67 BAS-RHIN
F68 HAUT-RHIN

F-A + ALSACE

AQUITAINE

F24 DORDOGNE
F33 GIRONDE
F40 LANDES
F47 LOT-ET-GARONNE
F64 PYRENEES-ATLANTIQUES

F-B + AQUITAINE

AUVERGNE

F03 ALLIER
F15 CANTAL
F43 HAUTE-LOIRE
F63 PUY-DE-DOME

F-C + AUVERGNE

BASSE-NORMANDIE

F14 CALVADOS
F50 MANCHE
F61 ORNE

F-D + BASSE-NORMANDIE

BOURGOGNE

F21 COTE-D'OR
F58 NIEVRE
F71 SAONE-ET-LOIRE
F89 YONNE

F-E + BOURGOGNE

BRETAGNE

F22 COTES-DU-NORD
F29 FINISTERE
F35 ILLE-ET-VILAINE
F56 MORBIHAN

F-F + BRETAGNE

CENTRE

F18 CHER
F28 EURE-ET-LOIRE
F36 INDRE
F37 INDRE-ET-LOIRE
F41 LOIR-ET-CHER
F45 LOIRET

F-G + CENTRE

CHAMPAGNE-ARDENNE

F08 ARDENNES
F10 AUBE
F51 MARNE
F52 HAUTE-MARNE

F-H + CHAMPAGNE-ARDENNE

CORSE

F20 CORSE

FRANCHE-COMTE

F25 DOUBS
F39 JURA
F70 HAUTE-SOANE
F90 TERRITOIRE-DE-BELFORT

F-J + FRANCHE-COMTE

HAUTE-NORMANDIE

F27 EURE
F76 SEINE-MARITIME

F-K + HAUTE-NORMANDIE

ILE-DE-FRANCE

F75 VILLE-DE-PARIS
F77 SEINE-ET-MARNE
F78 YVELINES
F91 ESSONE
F92 HAUTS-DE-SEINE
F93 SEINE-SAINT-DENIS
F94 VAL-DE-MARNE
F95 VAL-D'OISE

F-L + ILE-DE-FRANCE

LANGUEDOC-ROUSSILLON

F11 AUDE
F30 GARD
F34 HERAULT
F48 LOZERE
F66 PYRENEES-ORIENTALES

F-M + LANGUEDOC-ROUSSILLON

LIMOUSIN

F19 CORREZE
F23 CREUSE
F87 HAUTE-VIENNE

F-N + LIMOUSIN

LORRAINE

F54 MEURTHE-ET-MOSELLE
F55 MEUSE
F57 MOSELLE
F88 VOSGES

F-O + LORRAINE

MIDI-PYRENEES

F09 ARIEGE
F12 AVEYRON
F31 HAUTE-GARONNE
F32 GERS
F46 LOT
F65 HAUTES-PYRENEES
F81 TARN
F82 TARN-ET-GARONNE

F-P + MIDI-PYRENEES

NORD-PAS-DE-CALAIS

F59 NORD
F62 PAS-DE-CALAIS

F-Q + NORD-PAS-DE-CALAIS

PAYS DE LA LOIRE

F44 LOIRE-ATALNTIQUE
F49 MAINE-ET-LOIRE
F53 MAYENNE
F72 SARTHE
F85 VENDEE

F-R + PAYS DE LA LOIRE

PICARDIE

F02 AISNE
F60 OISE
F80 SOMME

F-S + PICARDIE

POITOU-CHARENTES

F16 CHARENTE
F17 CHARENTE-MARITIME
F79 DEUX-SEVRES
F86 VIENNE

F-T + POITOU-CHARENTES

PROVENCE-ALPES-COTE D'AZUR

F04 ALPES-DE-HAUTE-PROVENCE
F05 HAUTES-ALPES
F06 ALPES-MARITIMES
F13 BOUCHES-DU-RHONE
F83 VAR
F84 VAUCLUSE

F-U + PROVENCE-ALPES-COTE D'AZUR

RHONE-ALPES

F01 AIN
F07 ARDECHE
F26 DROME
F38 ISERE
F42 LOIRE
F69 RHONE
F73 SAVOIE
F74 HAUTE-SAVOIE

F-V + RHONE-ALPES

F.0 ++ FRANCE

UNITED KINGDOM (1976-80)

EAST ANGLIA

G25 CAMBRIDGESHIRE
G46 NORFOLK
G55 SUFFOLK

G-A + EAST ANGLIA

EAST MIDLANDS

G30 DERBYSHIRE
G44 LEICESTERSHIRE
G45 LINCOLNSHIRE
G47 NORTHAMPTONSHIRE
G50 NOTTINGHAMSHIRE

G-B + EAST MIDLANDS

NORTHERN

G14 TYNE&WEAR
G27 CLEVELAND
G29 CUMBRIA
G33 DURHAM
G48 NORTHUMBERLAND

G-C + NORTHERN

NORTH-WEST

G11 GREATER-MANCHESTER
G12 MERSEYSIDE
G26 CHESHIRE
G43 LANCASHIRE

G-D + NORTH-WEST

SOUTH-EAST

G01 GREATER-LONDON
G22 BEDFORDSHIRE
G23 BERKSHIRE
G24 BUCKINGHAMSHIRE
G34 EAST-SUSSEX
G35 ESSEX
G37 HAMPSHIRE
G39 HERTFORDSHIRE
G41 ISLE-OF-WIGHT
G42 KENT
G51 OXFORDSHIRE
G56 SURREY
G58 WEST-SUSSEX

G-E + SOUTH-EAST

SOUTH-WEST

G21 AVON
G28 CORNWALL
G31 DEVON
G32 DORSET
G36 GLOUCESTERSHIRE
G53 SOMERSET
G59 WILTSHIRE

G-F + SOUTH-WEST

WEST MIDLANDS

G15 WEST-MIDLANDS
G38 HEREFORD&WORCESTER
G52 SALOP
G54 STAFFORDSHIRE
G57 WARWICKSHIRE

G-G + WEST MIDLANDS

YORKSHIRE AND HUMBERSIDE

G13 SOUTH-YORKSHIRE
G16 WEST-YORKSHIRE
G40 HUMBERSIDE
G49 NORTH-YORKSHIRE

G-H + YORKSHIRE AND HUMBERSIDE

WALES

G61 CLWYD
G62 DYFED
G63 GWENT
G64 GWYNEDD
G65 MID-GLAMORGAN
G66 POWYS
G67 SOUTH-GLAMORGAN
G68 WEST-GLAMORGAN

G-I + WALES

SCOTLAND(1975-80)

S01 HIGHLAND
S02 GRAMPIAN
S03 TAYSIDE
S04 FIFE
S05 LOTHIAN
S06 BORDERS
S07 CENTRAL
S08 STRATHCLYDE
S09 DUMFRIES&GALLOWAY
S10 ORKNEY
S11 SHETLAND
S12 WESTERN-ISLES

G-J + SCOTLAND(1975-80)

NORTHERN IRELAND

JE EASTERN
JN NORTHERN
JS SOUTHERN
JW WESTERN

G-K + NORTHERN IRELAND

G.0 ++ UNITED KINGDOM

ITALIA (1975-79)

ABRUZZI

I66 L'AQUILA
I67 TERAMO
I68 PESCARA
I69 CHIETI

I-A + ABRUZZI

BASILICATA

I76 POTENZA
I77 MATERA

I-B + BASILICATA

CALABRIA

I78 COSENZA
I79 CATANZARO
I80 REGGIO-DI-CALABRIA

I-C + CALABRIA

CAMPANIA

I61 CASERTA
I62 BENEVENTO
I63 NAPOLI
I64 AVELLINO
I65 SALERNO

I-D + CAMPANIA

EMILIA-ROMAGNA

I33 PIACENZA
I34 PARMA
I35 REGGIO-NELL'EMILIA
I36 MODENA
I37 BOLOGNA
I38 FERRARA
I39 RAVENNA
I40 FORLI

I-E + EMILIA-ROMAGNA

FRIULI-VENEZIA GIULIA

I30 UDINE
I31 GORIZIA
I32 TRIESTE
I93 PORDENONE

I-F + FRIULI-VENEZIA GIULIA

LAZIO

I56 VITERBO
I57 RIETI
I58 ROMA
I59 LATINA
I60 FROSINONE

I-G + LAZIO

LIGURIA

I08 IMPERIA
I09 SAVONA
I10 GENOVA
I11 LA-SPEZIA

I-H + LIGURIA

LOMBARDIA

I12 VARESE
I13 COMO
I14 SONDRIO
I15 MILANO
I16 BERGAMO
I17 BRESCIA
I18 PAVIA
I19 CREMONA
I20 MANTOVA

I-I + LOMBARDIA

MARCHE

I41 PESARO-E-URBINO
I42 ANCONA
I43 MACERATA
I44 ASCOLI-PICENO

I-J + MARCHE

MOLISE

I70 CAMPO-BASSO
I94 ISERNIA

I-K + MOLISE

PIEMONTE

I01 TORINO
I02 VERCELLI
I03 NOVARA
I04 CUNEO
I05 ASTI
I06 ALESSANDRIA

I-L + PIEMONTE

PUGLIA

I71 FOGGIA
I72 BARI
I73 TARANTO
I74 BRINDISI
I75 LECCE

I-M + PUGLIA

SARDEGNA

I90 SASSARI
I91 NUORO
I92 CAGLIARI
I95 ORISTANO

I-N + SARDEGNA

SICILIA

I81 TRAPANI
I82 PALERMO
I83 MESSINA
I84 AGRIGENTO
I85 CALTANISSETTA
I86 ENNA
I87 CATANIA
I88 RAGUSA
I89 SIRACUSA

I-O + SICILIA

TOSCANA

I45 MASSA-CARRARA
I46 LUCCA
I47 PISTOIA
I48 FIRENZE
I49 LIVORNO
I50 PISA
I51 AREZZO
I52 SIENA
I53 GROSSETO

I-P + TOSCANA

TRENTINO-ALTO ADIGE

I21 BOLZANO-BOZEN
I22 TRENTO

I-Q + TRENTINO-ALTO ADIGE

UMBRIA

I54 PERUGIA
I55 TERNI

I-R + UMBRIA

VALLE D'AOSTA

I07 AOSTA

VENETO

I23 VERONA
I24 VICENZA
I25 BELLUNO
I26 TREVISO
I27 VENEZIA
I28 PADOVA
I29 ROVIGO

I-T + VENETO

I.0 ++ ITALIA

IRELAND (1976-80)

CONNAUGHT

R07 GALWAY
R12 LEITRIM
R16 MAYO
R20 ROSCOMMON
R21 SLIGO

R-A + CONNAUGHT

LEINSTER

R01 CARLOW
R06 DUBLIN
R09 KILDARE
R10 KILKENNY
R11 LAOIGHIS
R14 LONGFORD
R15 LOUTH
R17 MEATH
R19 OFFALY
R24 WESTMEATH
R25 WEXFORD
R26 WICKLOW

R-B + LEINSTER

MUNSTER

R03 CLARE
R04 CORK
R08 KERRY
R13 LIMERICK
R22 TIPPERARY
R23 WATERFORD

R-C + MUNSTER

ULSTER

R02 CAVAN
R05 DONEGAL
R18 MONAGHAN

R-D + ULSTER

R.0 ++ IRELAND

LUXEMBOURG (1971-80)

LE GREVENMACHER
LN DIEKIRCH
LS LUXEMBOURG

L.0 ++ LUXEMBOURG

NEDERLAND (1976-80)

N01 GRONINGEN
N02 FRIESLAND
N03 DRENTHE
N04 OVERIJSSEL
N05 GELDERLAND
N06 UTRECHT
N07 NOORDHOLLAND
N08 ZUIDHOLLAND
N09 ZEELAND
N10 NOORDBRABANT
N11 LIMBURG

N.0 ++ NEDERLAND

EEC-9

EEC ++ EEC-9

CHAPTER 2

MAPPING OF CANCER

Cancer

Cancer is a group of diseases which possess a common feature, viz., the uncontrolled growth of the cells that make up the part of the body affected (Cairns, 1977).

The cancers described in this atlas are defined by the 8th Revision of the International Classification of Diseases (WHO, 1967), hereafter referred to as ICD-8. The ICD-8 code numbers for the cancers arising in the various sites (organs) are used in the text, tables and maps.

Mortality

Mortality is the number of deaths from cases of cancer occurring in a given population in a particular time period, usually expressed as a rate per 100 000 population per annum.

Choice of area size

There are constraints on the choice of areal unit that are outside the control of the cancer mapper; the smallest usable unit is that for which population information is available. The intention was to choose the smallest administrative unit that could be expected to provide reliable rates over a period short enough for time trends to be unimportant.

The areas mapped in this atlas conform to at least level II of the EEC statistical services, with finer subdivision where population numbers are great enough. Population data for the areas used in this atlas are given in the first table of annex 1 (pp.130–131). Only seven of the 355 areas have less than 100 000 person years of risk, the smallest number, 56 000, occurring in the Orkney Islands, to the north of the mainland of Scotland (Area S10).

Use of age-standardized rates

As malignant disease becomes commoner as people grow older, valid comparison of the risk of dying from cancer between areas can be hampered if the age structures of the populations in areas differ. Taking median age as an indicator of differences in age-structure between regions, map 1 (males) and map 2 (females) demonstrate the variation which exists within Europe. These maps are prepared according to the same scheme as the cancer rate maps (see page 10).

To overcome this problem, age-standardization is undertaken. The resultant statistic—an age-standardized mortality rate per hundred thousand per annum—is taken to represent the risk of dying from cancer in a particular area. In this atlas all rates, unless otherwise stated, are average annual rates per 100 000 population, age-standardized to the world population (see below). For brevity they are presented in the text as figures only, e.g. "mortality from stomach cancer in females in Belgium was 9.8" rather than "the average annual age-standardized mortality from stomach cancer in females in Belgium was 9.8 per 100 000".

The age-standardized rate can be regarded as giving the magnitude of the risk in each of the areas and countries compared. The crude rate gives the burden of cancer in terms of the number of deaths from cancer per hundred thousand population in each area or country.

There are two widely used methods of standardization—the direct and indirect, each with its own advantages and disadvantages.

One advantage of using the direct method, as in this atlas, is that it then becomes possible to standardize to some universally accepted population, such as the world standard population originally described by Segi (1960) and used, after adaptation, in successive volumes of *Cancer Incidence in Five Continents* (Doll *et al.*, 1966).

There is a great temptation, when a series of maps is being produced for a country, to standardize to some local population, as this results in standardized rates which are close to the current crude mortality rates. However, for the present atlas this would have implied calculation of an EEC standard population based on EEC membership at the time of data collection. As the community has since increased in size and as the age-structure of its constituent populations changes, such a solution becomes less attractive. Hence the use of the world standard population in this atlas which permits comparison with a wide variety of published data. Further it is possible to compare not only the rate of one site of cancer in each of the areas mapped but also with that for another form of cancer directly, e.g., lung and kidney (see following paragraph). As the world standard population has a younger age structure than that of the EEC, the age-standardized rates are usually lower than the crude (non-standardized) rates.

Indirect standardization, as the name implies, also takes population age-structure into account. Here, the age-specific rates for a particular cancer for the EEC as a whole are applied to the population of each area mapped and the number of cancer deaths to be expected if that region had the same mortality as the EEC as a whole is computed. This number is compared with the number actually observed and the ratio of observed to expected is presented as a percentage. The EEC value is taken to be 100. The advantage of this method is that it reduces distortions associated with small numbers of cancers in small populations. However, as the populations for the area covered in this atlas yield a minimum of 50 000 person-years, this advantage is less important. The disadvantages are that it is not possible to compare rates for individual sites directly, all being related to 100, nor to follow trends over time, particularly when EEC membership changes.

Illustrating differences between areas

The maps indicate the level of age-standardized mortality in the 355 areas mapped. Colour has been used to distinguish between districts with high, medium and low mortality rates. To this end a relative scale using seven classes for each cancer was used, namely, the lowest 5% of the observed rates, the next 10%, the next 20%, the middle 30%, the next 20%, the next 10%, ending with the highest 5%. These classes are depicted by three shades of orange-red for the higher rates, yellow for the mid-range and three shades of green for the lower rates. The scale at the lower left-hand corner of each map shows the range of mortality rates for that site. While it would have been desirable to have maps with colours which represented the same range of mortality on each map, the mortality rates vary from zero to over 300. As the mortality for individual cancers may fall within only one segment of this wide range, e.g., thyroid cancer in females from 0.0 to 2.3, it would be impossible to separate clearly by shade and hue areal differences for each cancer site. The reader must thus, as previously mentioned, constantly bear in mind that a given colour will represent a different range of values according to the site of cancer.

Patterns of cancer distribution

As will become evident in the descriptions of the cancer patterns which follow in Chapter 5, emphasis has been placed on painting a broad canvas rather than picking out isolated areas of high mortality. While there is frequently a tendency to dismiss an isolated area of high mortality as being due to statistical chance, each such area should be examined critically to see whether any reasons for a high mortality are likely to exist. If a pattern for isolated areas becomes evident, then such close enquiry becomes all the more essential. For example, concentration of deaths from mesothelioma in towns with shipbuilding industries was eventually related to the industrial use of asbestos.

None the less, it is instructive to look at the spatial distribution of cancer of the liver (ICD-8 155) in males in the 40 areas of the Netherlands depicted in the Cancer Atlas for that country (Netherlands Central Bureau of Statistics, 1980). This shows one area with a standardized mortality ratio which is significantly above the national average at the 5% probability level and a further area significantly above the national average at the 10% level. Similarly, there are two areas which were significantly lower at the 10% and 5% levels. Such a finding is exactly what one would expect from the laws of statistical probability and this phenomenon must constantly be borne in mind. In this atlas 355 areas are compared: by chance alone, 17 could be expected to have rates significantly greater than the EEC-9 average and a similar number of rates significantly lower at the 5% level of statistical significance.

Presence of a group of areas with higher or lower than average cancer mortality which are contiguous or close at hand is always of interest as these suggest the presence or absence of risk factors common to these areas. For further discussion, see Kemp *et al.* (1985).

CHAPTER 3

SOURCES OF ERROR AND BIAS

Introduction

The validity of comparison of mortality rates between countries and their constituent areas is based on four implicit assumptions:

1. That death certification is uniformly complete in the countries considered;
2. That all the items of information such as age, sex, residence and cause of death are accurate;
3. That the appropriate denominators have been used;
4. That the data have been classified, coded and processed in the same way.

It is highly unlikely that these criteria, discussed further below, have been fully met. Indeed, only the first item, complete death certification, can be relied upon. For the period covered by this atlas, all deaths were recorded and the cause of death certified by a medical practitioner.

Validity of death certificates

Although age and sex are likely to be accurate, the precision of cause-of-death statements varies. The following quotation from Smithers (1960) should be constantly kept in mind:

> 'Cancer mortality statistics must be seen for what they are, which is a summary of what thousands of doctors of varying skill have, under very different conditions and opportunities for accurate diagnosis, seen fit to write as their opinion of the cause of death.'

The issues regarding the validity of cancer mortality statistics have been discussed, *inter alia*, by Boyle (1989) and are outlined below.

It has been repeatedly shown when death certificates are compared with autopsy findings that cancer death certification is subject to error (Heasman & Lipworth, 1968; Cameron & McCoogan, 1981), the level of error varying from one cancer site to another, although many of these errors have a tendency to cancel out so that the totals are much the same (Puffer & Wynn Griffith, 1967).

Further, it has been clearly shown that even when 'cancer' is recognized in life, it is not always correctly described (in anatomical or histological terms) or mentioned on the death certificate (Percy *et al.*, 1981) (see below).

Apart from the question of failure to recognize that a given death was due to cancer, or to record it accurately, there may be, within parts of the EEC, a further possible source of bias associated with a reluctance by medical practitioners to certify a death as being due to cancer as this diagnosis may, for cultural reasons, not be acceptable. Such factors were known to operate in the past for deaths due to syphilis and tuberculosis. Conversely, given the current awareness of the frequency of cancer, there may be in other areas a tendency to over-estimate cancer deaths. Without *ad hoc* study, there is no way in which the importance of such factors can be assessed. There is a further complication in that the same death certificate may be coded in more than one way by coders working in different national vital statistics offices, the major problem lying in the interpretation of the rules for deciding the underlying cause of death (see below).

In the countries where there are high autopsy rates, a certain number of hitherto unsuspected cancers are discovered and this finding may increase the number of certified cancer deaths at any age. Females are less likely to be autopsied than males and there are proportionately fewer autopsies of older persons than of the young. There is very little published information on national or regional variations in the frequency of autopsy by sex and age; that collated by WHO (1989) is given in Table 3.1. However, given the increasing rarity of autopsy in the EEC, this is not likely to be an important source of bias. Most countries have a mechanism for querying imprecise and illegible death certificates but in some this is rarely used (Table 3.1).

Table 3.1. Proportion of deaths occurring in a hospital or other medical establishment and proportion of deaths necropsied in EEC-9 countries

Country	Proportion of deaths		Follow-up in case of doubt about cause of death
	In hospital	Necropsied	
Belgium	59%	NI	Yes, in cases when the underlying cause of death is improbable or ill-defined
Denmark	56%	2%	Yes, about 8% of deaths
France	50%	NI	Yes
Germany	53%	8%	For some, but not systematically
Ireland	62%	7%	Yes, certifying doctor or coroner is queried for further information
Italy	37%	NI	Yes, in 1984 about 3500 certificates were queried
Luxembourg	69%	NI	Yes, if cause stated is imprecise or illegible
Netherlands	46%	10%	Yes, further information sought from certifying physician if necessary
United Kingdom:			
England & Wales	63%	27%	Yes, each year 2–3% of death certificates are followed up, typically when with unspecified or poorly specified codes
Northern Ireland	61%	11%	Yes, in case of doubt a query is sent to the coroner
Scotland	65%	15%	Yes, medical enquiry forms are sent out when further information is required.

Source: WHO (1989)
NI: no information

Loss of information and precision

Several of the publications quoted in the preceding paragraphs emphasize the difficulties that may arise in the diagnosis of cancer. However, even when such a diagnosis has been correctly made in the live patient and reported to a cancer registry, that diagnosis may not be recorded on the death certificate after the individual dies. Percy *et al.* (1981) examined the death certificates of 48 826 persons diagnosed as having cancer during the US Third National Cancer Survey (TNCS) which took place in 1969–1971. The death certificates in which cancer was not given as the underlying cause of death were excluded (e.g., deaths ascribed to heart disease). The study thus reported only deaths considered due to cancer in persons previously diagnosed as having cancer. There were substantial differences. Many of these arose from the use of less precise terms on the death certificate; thus an individual with rectal cancer (ICD-8 154) not infrequently had cancer of the large bowel on the death certificate and was assigned not to ICD-8 154 (rectal cancer) but to ICD-8 153.9 (colon cancer), the correct code number for this diagnosis. Similarly, leukaemia of precise cell type, e.g. myeloid leukaemia, appeared on the death certificate as leukaemia and hence was coded to ICD-8 208.9 (leukaemia NOS) rather than ICD-8 205.9 (myeloid leukaemia). The major sources of distortion are shown in Table 3.2.

Thus for cancer of the oesophagus, 921 persons were diagnosed as having this disease in life, but 997 of the 48 826 incident cases had this site on the death certificate, i.e. some 8% more. Only 858 of the 921 cases had oesophagus both in TNCS records and the death certificate. The two columns on the right-hand side of the table give the sensitivity and specificity. The sensitivity indicates that if an individual had a diagnosis of oesophageal cancer and subsequently died, there were 93 chances out of 100 that this would appear correctly on the death certificate. The specificity, somewhat lower at 86%, reflects the probability that a death certificate bearing mention of oesophageal cancer pertained to someone who had really had oesophageal cancer. While for most sites both sensitivity and specificity are close to or above 80%, there are significant exceptions for common cancers, such as the rectum, due to the tendency to write cancer of large bowel on death certificates. For primary liver cancers, there was only one chance in two that this diagnosis would appear on the death certificate. For primary cancer of the bone, there was over-reporting on death certificates: there was a 78% chance that such a diagnosis, if made in life, would appear on the death certificate but only half of the death certificates mentioning bone cancer as the underlying cause of death were truly primary bone cancers. The degree of concordance by site is given in Table 3.2.

Among the ten leading sites of cancer deaths, seven sites—lung, breast, prostate, pancreas, urinary bladder, ovary and leukaemia—had high rates for both detection and confirmation, and hence the mortality rates for these sites (at least in the USA) can be considered reliable. Further, these sites represent 65% of all cancer deaths in this atlas.

To the best of our knowledge, no similar study has been carried out in the countries represented in this atlas. Regrettably, until it is possible to accurately link cancer registry holdings with death certificates, these highly informative and relatively inexpensive studies will not be possible for many EEC countries.

National differences in coding of cancer deaths

In 1978, Percy and Dolman published a comparison of the coding of death certificates mentioning cancer in seven countries. In essence, 1246 US death certificates, each bearing a cancer-related diagnosis, were sent to the Vital Statistics Departments of seven countries which had agreed to participate in the study. The EEC

Table 3.2. Number of deceased cases of cancer diagnosed in Third National Cancer Survey (TNCS) with cancer as the underlying cause of death on the death certificate (DC), for selected sites

ICD-8 rubric		No. with site in TNCS	No. with this site as cause on DC	No. with same site on both TNCS and DC	Sensitivity (%)	Specificity (%)
140–207	All sites	48 826	48 826	40 379	89	83
140–149	Buccal cavity and pharynx	1397	1187	1098	79	93
150	Oesophagus	921	997	858	93	86
151	Stomach	2365	2321	2109	89	91
153–154	Colon and rectum	6644	6498	6171	93	95
153	Colon	4546	5131	4062	89	79
154	Rectum	2098	1367	1182	56	86
155	Liver etc.	536	347	266	50	77
162	Lung	10 059	10 178	9560	95	94
170	Bone	160	252	125	78	50
174	Breast (F)	4734	4583	4498	95	98
180	Cervix uteri	995	869	786	79	90
182	Corpus etc.	674	768	549	82	72
185	Prostate	2621	2579	2483	45	96
188	Bladder	1211	1179	1103	91	94
189	Kidney	984	930	865	88	93
191–192	Brain etc.	1074	1044	1044	97	89
195–199	Ill-defined	2320	2763	1231	53	45
200, 202	Non-Hodgkin lymphoma	1562	1470	1300	83	88
201	Hodgkin's disease	572	536	496	87	93
204–207	Leukaemia	2152	2140	2069	94	97
207	Unspecified leukaemia	204	434	149	73	34

Source: Percy *et al.* (1981)

countries involved were France, England and Wales and the Federal Republic of Germany

A portion of the findings is given in Table 3.3. It will be observed that, although there are very substantial differences in the interpretation of the underlying cause of death in these countries, there is no clear pattern of differential allocation. England and Wales was less likely to certify death as due to cancer of the large intestine than the other collaborating centres, whereas the Federal Republic of Germany had a clear excess of deaths assigned to liver cancer. The European centres were more likely to ascribe death to lung cancer than the USA. It is the results for breast cancer which are perhaps the most striking, the USA and England and Wales being much the same, France some 10% higher, the Federal Republic of Germany substantially lower. For prostate cancer, while the United States and the Federal Republic of Germany were much the same, France was higher and England and Wales much lower. France and the Federal Republic of Germany were more likely to choose an ill-defined site than the USA or England and Wales, but the frequency of choice of unspecified sites was much lower in France and somewhat higher in the Federal Republic of Germany than in the other two centres.

Table 3.3. Number of 1246 death certificates with mention of cancer coded to similar ICD-8 categories in the USA, France, England & Wales and the Federal Republic of Germany

ICD-8 Rubric	Site of cancer	USA	France	England & Wales	Germany, FR
140–209	Cancer of any site	1088	1164	1116	1164
140–149	Buccal cavity and pharynx	145	147	133	137
150	Stomach	31	32	29	32
151	Oesophagus	7	7	7	6
153	Large intestine	108	111	91	99
154	Rectum	30	34	30	35
155	Liver	8	12	7	28
162	Lung	77	96	91	90
174	Breast	84	95	87	65
180	Cervix uteri	23	22	21	20
182	Uterus	11	14	11	11
185	Prostate	47	56	39	45
188–189	Urinary organs	55	57	53	55
191–192	Brain and nervous system	55	42	47	47
195	Ill-defined sites	40	49	36	48
199	Unspecified site	50	37	57	62
200–209	Lymphatic and haematopoietic	156	170	100	161
	Disease of circulatory system	90	54	77	59
	Other diseases	68	28	53	23

Source: Percy & Dolman (1978); Percy & Muir (1989)

This exercise could be expected from the beginning to result in differing frequencies. The certificates were laid out in the USA format, albeit in conformity with international recommendations, and used the nomenclature and turns of phrase of that country. Two of the centres listed in Table 3.3 were not of English mother tongue. The two English-speaking countries were more likely to choose an underlying cause of death outside the neoplasms chapter. (This study has now been repeated using the 9th Revision of the ICD (WHO, 1977) and its more extensive indexing; improved comparability was observed (Percy & Muir, 1989)).

The significance of the Percy–Dolman and the Percy–Muir studies is quite clear—the way that coders interpret the rules for the selection of underlying cause of death can lead to substantial differences in the apparent mortality rate for a particular neoplasm. It is impossible to predict the effect that the differences which emerge from these special studies would have on routine death certificate coding in the EEC countries.

While cancers of the buccal cavity and pharynx are exceedingly common in French males and of below or average mortality in England and Wales in males, the converse is largely true in females and it seems difficult to imagine that there would be differential coding of these diagnoses by sex. The same observation holds good for cancer of the oesophagus. It is unlikely that French physicians would systematically under-certify cancer of the stomach and large bowel, while in both studies, the French National Statistics Office tended, using US practice as a reference point, to overestimate these sites (Table 3.3). With regard to lung cancer, the European centres assigned this cause to considerably more death certificates than in the USA, but this would not preclude under-diagnosis by certifying physicians. There was a tendency to over-code breast cancer in France in comparison to the USA and England And Wales. Yet, as will be seen in chapter 5, mortality rates for breast cancer in France are generally below the EEC average, those in the Federal Republic of Germany average, and those in England and Wales above average.

Paradoxically, death certificate coders in France were less likely to code a diagnosis made in the USA to unspecified sites (ICD-8 199) than their colleagues in England and Wales and in the Federal Republic of Germany, although these diagnoses are much more frequent in both sexes in France (see maps 3 and 4).

Coding of cancer death certificates in the EEC

Several EEC working parties have addressed the comparability of diagnosis and of mortality coding for selected groups of disease, although unfortunately not for the full range of malignant neoplasms.

In one such study, some 70 to 80 doctors in eight of the countries featured in this atlas (Luxembourg was not included) were asked to fill in a death certificate for each of 10 case specimen histories as if they were dealing with actual deaths (Kelson & Heller, 1983). The case histories, in the relevant national language, contained the clinical details necessary to reach a diagnosis. Age, occupation and smoking habits, relevant or not, were given for all. The completed death certificates were coded in the usual manner at the appropriate national vital statistics offices. Coded death certificates were then sent to a WHO reference centre. The overall response was 65%. Differences were found not only between countries but also within countries in the cause of death assigned. Further, coding practices were not standard across the EEC. When the nationally assigned codes were compared against a standard coding procedure, more than 10% of cases overall and over 20% of the Belgian and French cases were assigned to different diagnostic categories. The greatest discrepancy in coding lay between the Belgian offices (there are 10 provincial coding offices) and the reference centre.

The study mentioned above was complemented by another (Kelson & Farebrother, 1987) in which 22 case histories were compiled in England, France and Italy and after being tested on physicians in each of the eight countries in the study; 10 of the case histories were selected for use. Among the intended underlying causes of death were one each of the following diagnoses—bladder cancer, stomach cancer, carcinoma of the cervix uteri, malignant melanoma and mesothelioma (Table 3.4). Although this exercise pertains to only five cancers, it is possible to come to some conclusions as to the types of inter-country diffcrence observed. When the 'correct' underlying cause of death was not chosen, it was usual to find that death had been assigned to malignant neoplasms of unspecified site (ICD-8 199) or to respiratory disease, coders having failed to distinguish between immediate cause and underlying cause. For cancer of the cervix uteri, 9% of death certificates were assigned to uterus NOS, the highest proportions being recorded in France, FR Germany and Italy. Malignant melanoma was on the whole accurately coded, with the exception of Belgium where malignant melanoma was confused with multiple myeloma (ICD-8 203).

The fifth example in Table 3.4 is in some ways the most instructive. Although the case history clearly stated that the person in question had a biopsy of the pleura and histological examination showed malignant mesothelioma of the pleura, many of the death certificates did not mention the pleura. For this reason, coders in England and Wales and, to a lesser extent Ireland, followed the ICD, which does not contain a code for mesothelioma of site unspecified, and correctly coded these cases to ICD 199.1. Several countries, notably Denmark, assigned a considerable proportion of these to lung. Since pleural mesothelioma is a somewhat uncommon form of cancer, such errors are likely to exert a large influence on the calculated rates for this cancer associated with exposure to asbestos.

This exercise thus brings out once again the weak points of mortality statistics, namely, the failure of the certifying physician to use all the information available to him when writing the death certificate and the differences in coding practice between national vital statistics offices. The decentralization of coding, as in Belgium and the Federal Republic of Germany, adds a further source of potential inconsistency and error.

Thus, the mutually inverse regional distribution of non-Hodgkin lymphoma and multiple myeloma within the Netherlands may or may not be due to regional differences in interpretation and classification. There is a possibility that the high levels of brain and nervous system cancers seen in Belgium are due neither to high mortality nor to the availability of neurosurgical and neuropathological services but rather to a failure to distinguish between primary and metastatic brain tumours on the death certificate. While these explanations are possible, they require to be substantiated as the areal differences may be true. There is thus a clear need to mount a well-planned study of the type undertaken by Percy and Dolman (1978) and Percy and Muir (1989), and including a wide spectrum of death certificates covering all forms of cancer, to have a better appreciation of current differences in coding practices within the EEC.

Denominator problems

While attention is frequently focused on the reliability of the numerator, that is, the number of deaths assigned to cancer, the denominator—the population among which these deaths occurred—frequently receives less consideration. Each country normally has a population census every 10 years and these, by international agreement, usually take place in the years ending in '0' or '1'. Between censuses quite substantial changes may occur in the population or in the composition of a population dwelling in a given area. The births and deaths are

Table 3.4. Comparison of 'correct' underlying cause of death and assigned underlying cause of death for EEC–9 countries

'Correct' underlying cause of death		Percentage of death certificates coded to 'correct' cause								
		Belgium	Denmark	France	Germany FR	Ireland	Italy	Nether-lands	UK (England and Wales)	All
1.	Bladder	96	92	93	95	78	84	98	88	90
	Neoplasm site unspecified[a]	4	–	6	–	–	3	–	2	2
2.	Stomach	94	96	85	95	85	94	98	86	91
	Neoplasm site unspecified[a]	2	2	6	3	6	–	2	6	4
3.	Cervix uteri	86	90	72	82	94	82	98	100	
	Neoplasm uterus NOS[a]	10	8	21	13	2	18	–	–	9
4.	Melanoma	66*	94	89	95	89	94	96	92	89
5.	Pleura	72	54	79	85	23	54	78	32	57
	Neoplasm lung[a]	–	14	6	3	8	–	–	4	5
	Neoplasm site unspecified[a]	8	–	2	5	32	4	–	50	14

* 30% were coded as multiple myeloma (see text)

[a] The proportion coded to other cancer sites

Source: Kelson & Farebrother (1987): for further details see text

normally readily accounted for, but unless appropriate mechanisms exist, as in several Nordic countries, the estimation of changes due to migration in and out of a region may be imprecise. In the European Community, workers from Community countries are entitled to seek jobs in whichever member states they choose. Freedom to provide services is assured for the professions and already doctors, dentists, nurses and midwives can (in theory at least) practise anywhere in the Community. Migration, however, normally affects younger people coming into or leaving a region to seek work and, as most cancer deaths occur over the age of 50, should have little influence on the age-standardized mortality rates. A more important source of distortion would occur in so-called retirement areas with an influx of elderly persons, as in Florida, resulting in some distortion of mortality. Again, this question is not addressed in this atlas. We believe, however, that imprecisions in the denominator would not distort the overall patterns observed in this atlas. Nonetheless, there are sizeable migrant groups within the EEC such as Maghrebians in France, Turks in the Federal Republic of Germany and Indians, Pakistanis and West Indians in Great Britain. Their mortality has been little studied other than in England and Wales (Marmot *et al.*, 1984).

One important source of bias can occur if the cancer patient dies in hospital or a terminal care home, away from his usual place of residence, and the cancer death is assigned to the place of death rather than the place of usual residence. It is normal practice for the death to be assigned to the place of usual residence but on occasion, as is well illustrated for the district of Stone in the cancer mortality atlas for England and Wales (Gardner *et al.*, 1984), this may not occur.

In conclusion, therefore, one has to ask whether the factors listed above can 'explain' at least part of the differences in mortality observed in the maps in Chapter 5, and if so, are these sufficient to negate comparison and conclusions?

In our estimation, while there are undoubtedly such biases, they are not sufficient to explain the differences seen and the maps thus reflect relatively—if not absolutely—the differences in mortality. It is of the greatest importance for future studies that there be a better quantification of such sources of bias. This implies institution of measures to improve the quality of death certification. A major advance would be to make death certificates nominal and devise and use mechanisms, such as exist in Great Britain, for the follow-up of imprecise death certificates and for the inclusion in the official cause of death of information which becomes available later, such as histological examination of tissue obtained at autopsy. Periodic comparative coding of a sample of death certificates from each country, rather than from one, would be most valuable in pinpointing areas of disagreement and their causes. Percy and Muir (1989) have already started to do this but the exercise involved translation into English from the national languages of the death certificates and this, by itself, may induce distortions.

For the purpose of the present atlas, one further topic needs to be considered in some detail and that is the reality of the low cancer mortality rate observed for most, but not all, cancer sites in southern Italy.

Reality of low rates in southern Italy

Within Italy the mortality rates for many cancer sites are, in general, very much higher in the north than in the south and one must ask whether this gradient reflects real differences in cancer mortality or is an artefact produced by a combination of factors including regional variations in the level of medical care, in the quality of death certification and in the reliability of methods of population estimates. An influx of low-risk southern Italians to the north could be expected to reduce, by dilution, the higher rates in the north and thus give a false impression of the magnitude of the risk differential. However, such migrants may return 'home' to die and by virtue of a long stay in the higher-risk north increase the 'normal' cancer mortality in the south.

The net effect, for all sites of cancer combined, is a two-fold difference between the mortality rates in Lombardia (I-I) and Molise (I-K) in males; the differential is about the same for females when Lombardia is compared with Basilicata (I-B), contiguous to Molise. Granted that the number of deaths is 30 to 50 times greater in Lombardia than in the southern provinces cited, such large differences are not likely to have arisen by chance. Ideally, one would like to search hospital, autopsy and physicians' records for a period of time in the low-risk provinces to see whether cancer was really uncommon. Even this might not suffice if, for some reason, the populations in question did not seek medical care for their cancers, or if, for socio-cultural reasons, cancer was not an acceptable cause of death to write on the death certificate.

(*a*) *Quality of death certificates*

If death certificates are of poorer quality in southern Italy, one would expect the category 'Deaths assigned to symptoms, signs and ill-defined conditions' to be proportionately larger than in the north of the country. This is in fact so, but the differences are comparatively small, with crude rates for these categories of 23.9 in the north/centre and 30.4 in the south. Even if one assumes that the entire difference in mortality rates for these ill-defined categories represents uncertified and/or unrecognized cancers, there would still remain a substantial difference between north and south in overall cancer mortality (see Table 3.5).

(*b*) *Evidence from cancer registration*

There is, however, good evidence, both direct and indirect, that both cancer incidence and mortality are lower in southern Italian people than in the population in the north.

Incidence data for Varese (I12) in Lombardia and Ragusa (I88) in Sicilia are presented, for common cancer sites, in Table 3.6, together with the corresponding mortality figures. It is quite clear that incidence rates are substantially lower in Ragusa than in Varese for most of the cancer sites listed. This differential could be due to inefficient registration in Ragusa. However, rates in males for the relatively inaccessible tumours of brain and nervous system were marginally higher in Ragusa than in Varese (the lower rate in females is based on only six cases), and rates for the more accessible cervix and corpus uteri were approximately equal in both areas. The proportion of cancer of uncertain primary site is somewhat lower in Ragusa than in Varese.

Table 3.5. Mortality rates for broad disease groups in north/centre and south of Italy, 1983

	North + Centre	South	Total
Infections and parasitic diseases	6.3	5.1	5.9
Neoplasms	271.7	148.2	227.5
Mental disorders + diseases of nervous system	17.6	10.5	15.1
Diseases of circulatory system	490.4	402.4	459.0
Diseases of respiratory system	69.2	68.8	69.0
Diseases of digestive system	59.2	48.5	55.3
Other diseases	65.0	70.3	66.9
Symptoms, signs and ill-defined conditions	23.9	30.4	26.2
External causes	55.8	36.6	48.9
Total	1059.2	820.8	974.0

Source: Adapted from *Annuario Statistico Sanitario*, Edizioni 1985, Istituto Centrale di Statistica

Table 3.6. Age-standardized incidence and mortality rates for selected common cancers in Varese, northern Italy and Ragusa, Sicily

ICD Rubric[a]		Varese				Ragusa			
		Incidence[b]		Mortality[c]		Incidence[d]		Mortality[c]	
		M	F	M	F	M	F	M	F
150	Stomach	39.0	17.1	35.7	16.4	18.6	7.6	17.6	8.7
153–154	Large bowel	37.9	25.5	30.7	18.7	19.4	12.1	14.4	9.8
162	Lung	80.5	6.2	64.8	6.5	28.5	2.2	26.6	3.0
174	Breast	–	59.7	–	25.8	–	40.0	–	19.7
180	Cervix uteri	–	10.1	–	0.8	–	9.6	–	1.2
182	Corpus uteri	–	12.5	–	10.0[e]	–	12.1	–	14.3[e]
185	Prostate	20.4	–	15.0	–	14.2	–	10.5	–
188	Bladder	27.3	4.0	9.2	1.1	9.7	0.5	6.2	0.8
191–192	Brain and nervous system	5.5	5.4	4.0	3.3	6.0	1.8	1.9	1.8
201	Hodgkin's disease	4.7	2.5	3.2	1.3	3.7	2.1	1.3	1.3
204–208	Leukaemia	9.9	8.0	9.3	4.9	6.4	5.0	4.7	3.3
	Primary site uncertain	8.4	5.5	12.8	7.4	4.5	4.0	10.4	10.0
	All sites numbers	6152	5163	5296	3850	662	537	1099	994

[a] Incidence data based on the 9th Revision of ICD; mortality data on the 8th Revision
[b] 1978–81
[c] 1975–79
[d] 1981–82
[e] Cervix and corpus combined
Incidence data kindly made available by Dr F. Berrino (Varese) and Professor L. Dardononi (Ragusa).

It could be argued that such differences in incidence and mortality, although consistent, do not, of themselves, resolve the question of underdiagnosis of cancer in southern Italy. However, in a study carried out by Crosignani *et al.* (1986), comparison of the cancer incidence rates for the indigenous population of Varese with those for immigrants to Varese from southern Italy showed differences of the same order of magnitude as those currently existing between the Varese and Ragusa registries. These findings lend support to the existence of a real difference in incidence and, in consequence, in mortality. Vigotti *et al.* (1988) conclude '... the observation that area of birth is often a more important determinant of cancer rates than area of residence provides indirect evidence that cancer death certification in various Italian geographic areas is satisfactorily reliable and consistent.'

(*c*) *Denominator considerations*

A Eurostat publication *Demographic Statistics (in EEC Countries) in 1986* contains the following statement :

> 'Italy: A census of population took place on 25 October 1981 and the results reveal that the estimated figures for the total resident population were too high by a substantial margin, mainly due to the failure by persons leaving the country to notify the registration authorities of their departure.'

In other words, in Italy a *de jure* population definition is used, (and this was the case in previous censuses as well). It is further known that there is in general more migration and mobility within the south than in the north. This means that population estimates in the south are more prone to errors than those in the north.

The median ages of the populations in the north and south of Italy are quite different (Figure 3.1). If there is a deficit of old persons, there will be few people in the 'cancer ages' and the mortality rates, even when age-standardized, will be lower.

(*d*) *Correspondence of numerator and denominator*

Van Poppell (1981) observed :

> 'It has been suggested that the explanation for the favourable position of southern Italy lies partly in the methods of calculating death rates, based on the number of deaths of the *de facto* population in the numerator and the *de jure* population in the denominator. This leads to an overestimation of the expectation of life in the emigrant regions of the south'.

As a corollary, there are probably deaths which occur in the north among (permanent or temporary) migrants from the south. An unknown proportion of these deaths is added to the numerator of the mortality rates in the north, but this group of migrants as a whole is part of the denominator of the mortality rates in the south.

(*e*) *Conclusion*

The above arguments do not entirely resolve this problem. None the less, the editors believe that on the currently available evidence, the differences in risk within Italy are likely to be real, although probably not as large as the maps and tables would suggest.

CHAPTER 4

THE EUROPEAN ECONOMIC COMMUNITY

This chapter provides a brief description of the topography, population size and age-structure (Table 4.1), broad economic activity (Table 4.2) and a few health indicators (Table 4.3) for each member of the European Economic Community represented in this Atlas. The publication *A Journey Through the EC*, from which some of the following information is drawn, outlines the common heritage of the countries forming the EEC (CEC, 1986).

'The economic and social developments that followed in the wake of industrialization have confronted every European government — at different times in different places — with the task of exploiting change for the benefit of the individual and of containing the threat posed by the concentration of economic power. Not all politicians have found it easy to change their way of thinking and some misused technical progress and economic resources to serve their aggressive policies. When in 1925 the French Prime Minister, Edouard Herriot, advocated a united Europe, the other European governments failed to respond. Nor did a similar initiative from his successor, Aristide Briand, in 1929, find any echo after the death of the German Foreign Minister, Gustav Stresemann.'

The Treaty establishing the European Coal and Steel community (ECSC) was signed in 1951, followed in 1957 by the Treaties establishing the European Economic Community (EEC) and the European Atomic Energy Community (Euratom). There were six founder-members: Belgium, France, Germany, Italy, Luxembourg and the Netherlands. Three more countries joined in 1973: Denmark, Ireland and the United Kingdom. In 1981, Greece became the tenth member, and with the accession of Portugal and Spain in 1986, the Community now numbers 12.

The institutions of the three Communities — ECSC, EEC and Euratom — were merged in 1967 and the term 'European Community' is now commonly used to mean all three together.

'Today the Member States of the Community are engaged in a continuous dialogue, trying to accommodate each other's interests and reach agreements in which none feels disadvantaged. This is indispensable because, unlike other international organizations, the European Community can enact legislation that is binding on all its 320 million citizens. Community institutions (Parliament, Commission, Council and Court of Justice) draw up, adopt and enforce Community legislation, and this body of Community law takes precedence over national law.'

The labour market

On the common labour market, workers from Community countries are entitled to seek jobs in whichever Member States they choose. Freedom to provide services is assured for the professions, and the legal and administrative provisions still hindering the right to set up in business are being removed.

Already, doctors, dentists, nurses and midwives can practise anywhere in the Community. Since expensive social provisions can often be put into effect only when they are also applied simultaneously by competitors in neighbouring countries, the Community in 1974 decided upon a social action programme

Table 4.1. Age structure and broad categories of employment in nine EEC countries around 1980

Country	Percentage of total population		Females as % of population	Female % of civilian labour force	Labour force as % of population (1983)	Proportion of labour force employed in		
	under 15	over 65				Agriculture	Industry	Services
Belgium	19	14	50	32	43	3	31	66
Denmark	19	15	51	48	53	9	26	66
Germany, FR	16	15	52	33	45	6	42	52
France	22	13	51	33	43	8	34	58
Ireland	30	11	50	22	37	17	30	53
Italy	21	13	51	27	41	12	36	52
Luxembourg	18	13	51	28	44	5	36	60
The Netherlands	21	12	51	27	41	5	28	67
United Kingdom	20	15	51	37	48	3	34	64

Source: CEE (1986)

which should help to improve the lot of workers generally. There is a European Centre for the Development of Vocational Training in Berlin and a European Foundation for the Improvement of Living and Working Conditions in Dublin.

Although the EEC countries share many common features, none the less, each one, in addition to language, has its own distinctive features, notably the economy.

Table 4.2 shows the gross domestic product per head of population: this varies approximately twofold between member countries. The proportions of agriculture, forestry and fisheries in the gross domestic product also show substantial differences, being greatest in Ireland. Each member country has its own spectrum of industrial activity and the share of industry in the gross domestic product is again variable. Table 4.2 also indicates the major exports, expressed as a percentage of the total value of exports.

Health care in the EEC

Not only do national economies differ but so do several of the health indicators appearing in Table 4.3. There is comparatively little difference in life expectation, the survival of females being greater everywhere. Infant mortality shows a much greater range of values, that in Denmark being less than half the rate in Italy. There is remarkable similarity in the proportion of deaths due to cancer; there is a male excess in all countries except Ireland. The number of physicians per 10 000 population shows considerable variation, ranging from 13 to 29. Cochrane *et al.* (1978) have examined the relation between the number of physicians and mortality, finding this to be inverse. The provision of hospital beds again shows a roughly twofold variation.

Table 4.3 also indicates the total number of cancer patient beds and the number of cancer establishments, but these figures are not really comparable in that, in several countries, cancer patients are treated in general or district hospitals, as well as in special centres. Thus, in France, about 50% of cancer patients are treated outside the anti-cancer centre network (Centres Anticancéreux).

Each of the EEC countries has a health insurance scheme. In several, the diagnosis and treatment of cancer patients are essentially free. If populations are willing to seek medical advice, there is thus no reason why cancer should not be diagnosed. It is possible, however, that there are differences in the likelihood that cancer would be mentioned on a death certificate as there are still residual prejudices (see Chapter 3). Unfortunately, statistics on the proportion of deaths autopsied are not available for several countries (Table 3.1). In general there is a north–south gradient which would result in more previously undiagnosed cancer deaths being detected at autopsy in northern Europe.

The figures appearing in Tables 4.2 and 4.3 pertain to a somewhat later period than the mortality data presented in the maps. However, these are not likely to have changed significantly.

Further information can be obtained from the publication *Health Services in Europe* (WHO, 1981)

Existing community actions against cancer

The need to protect workers and the public against the long-term effects, in particular cancer, of dangerous chemical, biological and physical agents has been the objective of many actions at Community level, in the fields of radiation protection, occupational health and safety, internal market, agriculture and environment. Research programmes and epidemiological and statistical studies have been undertaken in support of these actions.

The Commission has undertaken a series of actions which, in various ways, contribute to the fight against cancer. These include the promulgation and widespread dissemination of the European Code Against Cancer and the publication of a monograph entitled *Reducing the Risk of Cancer* (Heller *et al.*, 1989).

The remainder of this chapter outlines some of the characteristics of each of the nine EEC countries covered by this atlas, with a more detailed analysis of the methods used for the collection of mortality data by the relevant national vital statistics office.

Table 4.2. Gross domestic product per head of population

Country	GDP (ECU)	Share of agriculture forestry & fisheries in GDP (%)	Share of industry in GDP (%)	Major exports	
Belgium	10 000	2	34	Machinery and vehicles	22
				Iron and steel products	13
				Chemicals	12
				Textiles and clothing	7
Denmark	13 595	6	28	Foodstuffs (meat and preserved goods, dairy products, fish and fish preserves, etc.)	29
				Finished goods (furniture, clothing etc.)	25
				Machinery and transport equipment	24
				Chemicals (medicines, pharmaceuticals)	8
Germany, FR	12 750	2	41	Road vehicles	17
				Machinery	15
				Chemicals	14
				Electrical appliances	10
				Iron and steel	4
				Food, beverages and tobacco	5
France	11 381	5	36	Machinery and vehicles	34
				Manufactured goods	27
				Chemicals	13
				Foodstuffs	13
Ireland	6 256	10	37	Machinery and transport equipment (office machines and equipment, electrical appliances, etc.)	26
				Food products (meat, dairy produce, etc.)	25
				Manufactured goods (textiles, etc.)	22
				Chemicals	14

Table 4.2 (contd)

Country	GDP (ECU)	Share of agriculture forestry & fisheries in GDP (%)	Share of industry in GDP (%)	Major exports	
Italy	7 866	6	40	Machinery and vehicles	32
				Textiles and clothing	18
				Chemicals	8
				Food products	7
Luxembourg	11 155	2	30	Steel and other heavy-industry products	up to 90
				Chemicals, agricultural produce	
The Netherlands	10 942	5	34	Minerals	24
				Finished goods: Textiles, etc.	18
				Food, beverages and tobacco:	
				Dairy products, fresh meat, canned and bottled products, fish, cocoa, chocolate, tobacco	18
				Vehicles and electrical appliances	16
				Chemical products	16
United Kingdom	9 577	2	40	Machinery and transport equipment	30
				Manufactured goods	25
				Mineral fuels	22
				Chemicals	11

Source: CEC, 1986

Table 4.3. Health indicators (1979 figures)

Country	Population mid yr '79	Life expectancy at birth (years)		Infant mortality per 1000	% of deaths due to cancer		Total no. of physicians	Physicians per 10 000 population	Total no. of hospital beds	Population per bed	Total no. of cancer patient beds[a]	No. of cancer establish-ments[b]
		Male	Female		Male	Female						
Belgium	9 842 000	69.9	76.6	15.3	26	21	24 536	24.9	60 067	160	412	8
Denmark	5 116 000	71.4	77.6	8.7	24	26	10 572	20.7	41 842	122	460	6
Germany, FR	61 328 000	69.7	76.5	14.7	22	21	139 431	22.7	707 710	87	1 203	22
France	53 383 000	70.6	79.0	11.3	26	19	91 442	17.2	646 188	82	4 766	31
Ireland	3 368 000	69.3	75.1	15.6	18	19	4 340	13.1	33 028	103	258	6
Italy	56 828 000	71.0	77.7	20.8	24	20	164 555	29.0	554 595	103	1 071	28
Luxembourg	362 000	69.0	76.2	na	23	21	505	14.0	4 157	86	na	na
Netherlands	14 013 000	72.5	79.2	9.6	28	25	25 947	18.5	177 265	80	593	10
United Kingdom	55 901 000	68.9	75.1	8.9	21	19	90 533	16.1	na	na	2 550	53

na, not available

[a] In several countries, cancer patients are also treated in general or district hospitals. In France, for example, about 50% of cancer patients are treated outside the network of anti-cancer centres.

[b] For further information see *International Directory of Specialized Cancer Research and Treatment Establishments* (UICC, 1986)

Sources: Data extracted from relevant editions of Encyclopaedia Britannica, United Nations Statistical Yearbook, World Health Statistics Annual

Detailed population figures for the areas mapped in this atlas are presented in the first table of Annex 1 (pp. 130–131)

BELGIUM

Belgium has an area of 30 519 km2 and extends 230 km north to south and 290 km east to west. The Belgian North Sea coast is 66 km long. Inland from the coast are fertile polders, the sandy Flanders plain, the heaths and woods of the Campine (Kempen). Between these northern lowlands and the wooded Ardennes and Belgian Lorraine in the south lie the alluvial, fertile central plateaux. The country's highest point is the Signal de Botrange (694 m) in the Hautes Fagnes (Eifel). The main rivers are the Scheldt and the Meuse. The Scheldt rises in northern France and flows through Ghent, Antwerp and a delta-like estuary in the Netherlands into the North Sea. The Meuse flows out of the French Vosges, through eastern Belgium (Namur and Liège) into the Netherlands. 47% of the land surface is used for agriculture and 20% is wooded. The capital is Brussels (population 990 000).

Belgium has a population of 9.9 million, with an average density of 323 inhabitants per km2 (1983). In the Flemish region (57% of the population), the official language is Dutch; in the Walloon region (33% of the population) it is French; but in the east of the province of Liège (65 000 inhabitants) it is German. The Brussels area (10% of the population) constitutes the fourth language region, where French and Dutch have equal status. The age-structure and broad categories of employment are given in Table 4.1.

Of the 891 000 foreigners living in Belgium, 521 000 come from other Community countries and more than half of those from Italy (1983).

Belgium's nine provinces of Antwerp, Brabant, Oost-Vlaanderen (East Flanders), Hainaut, Limburg, Liège, Luxembourg, Namur and West-Vlaanderen (West Flanders) are each administered by a Provincial Governor.

MORTALITY DATA COLLECTION IN BELGIUM

Anonymous death certificates were introduced in Belgium in 1930, but were not in general use throughout the country until 1954.

The death certificate currently in use was introduced in 1979, and slightly modified in 1983. There are two versions — one for recording stillbirths and deaths of infants up to one year of age and the other for deaths of people older than one year.

The death certificate is divided into four sections (A, B, C and D). Only section A contains the name and address of the deceased. Sections B and D contain the information on age, sex, etc., necessary for compiling general mortality statistics. Section C is used exclusively by the certifying doctor to report cause of death; this section is sealed by the doctor.

Section A is detached from the death certificate and retained by the communal administration. Sections B, C and D are sent to the Provincial Health Inspectorate, where a medical civil servant codes the underlying cause of death according to the International Classification of Diseases (ICD), and enters the code number on section B. (The statistics presented in this atlas were compiled using the 8th Revision of the ICD, although the 9th revision is now in use.) Section C is then detached by the Health Inspector, who sends sections B and D to the National Institute of Statistics.

BELGIAN POPULATION STATISTICS

In Belgium, full national population censuses are taken each decade: thus censuses were held on 31 December 1970 and 1 March 1981. For years between censuses, population figures are estimated by counting new enrolments (births and immigrations) and de-registrations (deaths and emigrations) in the communal population registries. In 1981, because the census was held on 1 March, two population estimates were made, one for the period 1 January to 28 February and the other for the period 1 March to 31 December.

The census measures *de jure* population, that is, persons residing in the country at the time of the census. Population figures are available for all levels of administrative sector (kingdom, region, province, district and commune). Estimates of the populations according to age and sex are made at the district level.

On 1 January 1977 new administrative boundaries were drawn up in Belgium, and some communes, or parts of communes, were transferred to other districts, or even to other provinces. On the whole, the changes in district or province population figures which resulted from this operation were rather limited. Those districts whose populations changed most were Eeklo (minus 8283, or 9.4%), Tielt (plus 7167, or 9.3%) and Huy (minus 7683, or 8.1%). At the provincial level, the greatest changes occurred in Namur (plus 6871, or 1.8%). These changes are not likely to have had a major influence on the cancer rates presented in this atlas.

STATISTICAL PUBLICATIONS

Government publications

Tables of general mortality data (giving information on age, sex, civil status, residence, etc.) are published (in French and Dutch) by the Belgian National Institute of Statistics in a series of monthly brochures entitled *Demographic Statistics*. The brochure on causes of death mainly contains information at the national level. Tables of causes of death classified according to abridged lists of mortality causes (lists A and B of the 8th revision of the ICD, and the basic tabulation list of the 9th revision) are available down to the town or district level.

Publications

André, R., Gossiaux, A.M. & Lemonnier, A. (1981) Causes of Death in Belgium per District and per Region, *Service of the Prime Minister, Scientific Policy Programme, three volumes, 5A, 5B and 5C (in French)*

Annual Brochure on Causes of Death, National Institute of Statistics, Brussels (published in French and in Dutch since 1954)

Data on Cancer Morbidity in Belgium, Public Health and Family Ministry, Centre for Information Processing, Belgian Review for Cancer, Service of Statistics (Brochure covering 1955–1958, followed by an annual brochure) (in French and Dutch)

Directory of Public Health, Public Health Ministry, Brussels (in French and Dutch)

National Registry of Cancer, Belgian League for Cancer, Public Health and Family Ministry (annual brochure since 1985) (in French and Dutch)

Rykeboer, R., Janssens, G. & Thiers, G.L (1983) *Atlas of Cancer Mortality in Belgium (1969–1976)*, Brussels, Public Health Ministry, IHE (in French and Dutch)

Statistical Directory of Belgium, National Institute of Statistics, Brussels (in French and Dutch)

Other publications

Beckers, R., Pleysier, R., Klinkenborg, L. & Schots, A. (1981) *Mortality Due to Cancer in Belgium 1960–1979, First Analysis*. Study group biomedical information system (in French and Dutch)

Grosclaude, A., Lux, B., van Houte-Minet, M. & Wunsch, G. (1978) Regional mortality and differential behaviour. Masculine mortality determinants [in French] *Population et Famille*, **48**, 1–43

van Houte-Minet, M. & Wunsch, G. (1978) Mortality in adult men – a regional analysis essay [in French]. *Population et Famille*, **43**, 37–68

Address: Institut National de Statistique, 44, rue de Louvain, 1000 Brussels

DENMARK

Denmark has an area of 43 080 km2. It consists of the Jutland Peninsula, which has a 67 km-long frontier with north Germany at its base, and 483 islands of which about 100 are inhabited. The seaboard along the North Sea, Skagerrak, Kattegat and the Baltic runs for some 7300 km. Denmark is a flat country, rising to only 173 m at its highest point. The longest river is the Gudena (160 km) which rises in central Jutland and flows into Randers Fjord. 66% of the area is agricultural land, and 11% is wooded. Of growing importance are the oil and natural gas deposits in the Danish waters of the North Sea.

The capital is Copenhagen (population around 1.2 million, including suburbs), the largest city in Scandinavia. It lies on the island of Sjaelland and the nearby island of Amager.

Denmark has a population of 5.1 million, excluding Greenland and the Faeroes, and the average population density is 119 per km2 (1983 figures). The age-structure and broad categories of employment are given in Table 4.3.

Of the 101 726 migrant workers in Denmark, one quarter come from Community countries, predominantly Britain and the Federal Republic of Germany.

Denmark is divided into 14 counties plus the metropolitan region of Copenhagen with Frederiksberg. The Faeroes have had home rule since 1948; they have their own assembly and, unlike Denmark proper, are not in the European Community. Greenland has belonged to Denmark since 1721; it obtained home rule following a referendum in 1979 and withdrew from the Community on 1 February 1985.

MORTALITY DATA COLLECTION IN DENMARK

The international form of death certificate was introduced in Denmark in 1951. Anonymous death certificates were introduced in January 1966 and the current form has been in use since 1977.

The completed and sealed death certificate is given to the next of kin, who passes it to the local vicar who will be responsible for the burial. The vicar checks the name and personal number of the deceased and notifies the local population register of the death. He then sends the death certificate itself to the Medical Officer of Health, who checks the information on it before sending it to the Department of Health Statistics at the National Board of Health (a division within the Ministry of the Interior), where it is again checked and coded manually for later computerization. (Since 1969, cause of death has been coded according to the 8th revision of the International Classification of Diseases (ICD). The 8th revision will continue to be used until the 10th revision is available.) The Department of Health Statistics can ask for supplementary information for coding the death certificates received. In 1984, for example, additional information was requested for 8% of deaths.

After they have been coded, the death certificates are sent to the Central Bureau of Statistics (Danmarks Statistik), which checks the personal number of the deceased with the entry in the Central Population Register. When the coding of death certificates is completed, the information is transferred to magnetic tapes which are available for each quarter year and for the whole year.

For all natural deaths, the death certificate is filled out by the physician of the deceased or, if the person was under treatment at the time of death, by the attending physician. If examination of the body raises doubt about the mode of death, the physician must inform the police, who must also be informed if there is suspicion that death was due to suicide, accident or criminal acts. In such cases, a legal examination must be undertaken. In 1984, legal examination took place following 11% of all deaths. If, after a legal examination, there is still doubt about the cause of death, an autopsy must be carried out. An autopsy was performed for 33% of all deaths occurring in Denmark; this figure includes both legal and hospital autopsies.

In 1984, 56% of all deaths took place in hospitals and autopsies were performed for more than half (55%) of those hospital deaths.

DANISH POPULATION STATISTICS

Data on the size, composition and mobility of the Danish population are compiled from entries in local (council) population registers, which contain, for each individual, information on place of residence, civil status, sex, age and nationality.

Information from all the local registers is collected together in the Central Population Register. The local registers are updated as births, deaths, changes of address, marriages and divorces are notified; all such changes must be reported to the Central Population Register within 40 days. Information from the Central Population Register is transferred to the Central Bureau of Statistics, which is responsible for publishing population statistics.

STATISTICAL PUBLICATIONS

Since 1943, the registers of causes of death have consisted of microfilm copies of individual death certificates. From 1970, the information from the registers, as well as non-medical data from death certificates, has also been stored on magnetic tape. These tapes are used primarily by the Central Bureau of Statistics for generating population statistics and by the Department of Health Statistics for compiling statistics on causes of death, but are also available for use in medical research, by the National Board of Health and by physicians for follow-up studies, etc. In addition, the Danish Institute for Clinical Epidemiology maintains registers of causes of death, based on the data available at the National Board of Health.

Official publications

Changes of the Population, Central Bureau of Statistics (published annually in Danish)

Statistical Yearbook, Central Bureau of Statistics (published annually in Danish)

Johansson, B. (1946) *The Danish Morbidity and Mortality Statistics*, Copenhagen (in Danish)

The Health Status of the Danish Population, Ministry of the Interior and National Board of Health, Copenhagen, 1985 (in Danish)

Causes of Death in Denmark, National Board of Health (published annually in Danish)

Regulations of 10 March 1977, Concerning the Issuing of Death Certificates, National Board of Health, Copenhagen, 1977 (in Danish)

The Danish Cancer Registry uses the information on causes of deaths for improvement of the registration of cases of cancer as well as for cancer research. The following are examples of publications based on the available cancer mortality data:

Andersen, O. (1985) *Mortality and Occupation 1970–80, Statistical Investigations Number 41*, Central Bureau of Statistics

Ewertz, M. & Jensen, O.M. (1981) Cancer mammae in Denmark 1943–1976, Cancer Statistics No 3 [in Danish] *Ugeskr. Læger*, 143, 2758–60

Juel, K. & Jacobsen, P. (1984) *Mortality 1956/80 in Thyborøn-Harboøre and in a Control Area*, DIKE and National Board of Health

Lynge, E. (1979) *Mortality and Occupation 1970–5, Statistical Investigations Number 37*, Central Bureau of Statistics

Mellemgaard, A. & Lynge, E. (1987) Colorectal cancer in Denmark 1943–1982, Cancer Statistics No. 16 [in Danish] *Ugeskr. Læger*, 149, 188–191

Østerlind, A. (1986) Diverging trends in incidence and mortality of testicular cancer in Denmark, 1943–1982. *Br. J. Cancer*, **53**, 501–505

Storm, H.H. (1984) *Validity of Death Certificates for Cancer Patients in Denmark 1977*, Copenhagen, Danish Cancer Society

Storm, H.H. (1986) Percentage of autopsies in cancer patients in Denmark in 1971/1980. *Ugeskr. Læger*, **148**, 1110–1114

Address: Statistical Division, National Board of Health, 1 Store Kongensgade, 1264 Copenhagen K

FRANCE

France has an area of 544 000 km2. The seaboard on the English Channel, the Atlantic and the Mediterranean is some 3120 km long, and the land frontiers extend roughly 2170 km. The Pyrenees in the south-west, the western Alps in the south-east, the Jura and the Rhine in the east are also natural frontiers.

58% of the land surface is used for agriculture. The most important crop is wheat, followed by oats and maize. Fruit and vegetables are grown in all regions, but particularly in the south. Vines cover extensive areas, especially in Languedoc and Burgundy and around Bordeaux. Woodland covers 27% of the country.

France has iron ore deposits in Lorraine, coal in the north-east, natural gas in the south-west, potash in Alsace and bauxite in Provence.

The capital is Paris (population: city 2.04 million; conurbation 10 million).

France has a population of 54.3 million and an average population density of 100 inhabitants per km2 (1983). The age-structure and broad categories of employment are given in Table 4.3. The official language is French, but several other languages or dialects, such as Breton, Alsatian, Basque, Corsican and Catalan, are to be heard in the provinces.

The proportion of foreign residents is around 6.8%. Of the 162 000 or so migrant workers from other Community countries, two thirds come from Italy.

Metropolitan France is divided into 22 regions and 95 departments. The regions are: Nord-Pas-de-Calais, Ile-de-France, Centre, Picardie, Basse Normandie (Lower Normandy), Haute Normandie (Upper Normandy), Bretagne (Brittany), Pays de la Loire (Loire Valley), Poitou-Charentes, Limousin, Aquitaine, Midi-Pyrénées, Champagne-Ardennes, Alsace, Lorraine, Bourgogne (Burgundy), Auvergne, Franche-Comté, Rhône-Alpes, Languedoc-Roussillon, Alpes-Provence-Côte-d'Azur, Corse (Corsica).

The overseas departments and territories are not represented in this Atlas.

MORTALITY DATA COLLECTION IN FRANCE

The death certificate currently used in France is based on the international model proposed by WHO and was introduced in 1958. The physician can indicate one or more diseases leading directly or indirectly to death. Cause of death is coded according to the International Classification of Diseases (ICD); the ninth revision of the ICD (ICD-9) has been used since 1979.

The present system of recording death information has been used since 1968. When someone dies, a physician fills in a two-part death certificate.

- The date and time of death, identification information (name, surname, age, residence) are entered in the first part.
- The place and date of death, and medical causes of death, are entered in the second part. This is sealed by the physician to preserve confidentiality.

Another certificate (Bulletin 7), completed by the town council, contains information on socio-professional status, place of residence and places and dates of birth and death, but no information on identity. The physician certifies the death and fills in the medical certificate. These documents are sent to the town council of the place of death, where the nominal part is removed. The sealed part of the death certificate and the corresponding Bulletin 7 are sent to the Direction Départementale de l'Action Sanitaire et Sociale (DDASS), which uses the anonymous death certificate to follow variations in the number of deaths associated with some diseases.

The anonymous Bulletin 7 and the corresponding medical certificate are sent to the unit of the National Institute of Health and Medical Research (INSERM) responsible for studies of medical causes of death. This unit codes medical causes of death according to ICD-9, notes this code on the Bulletin 7, removes the anonymous part of the death certificate and sends it to the National Institute of Statistics and Economic Studies (INSEE), which thus receives only socio-demographic information and codes of causes of death.

INSERM provides interim statistics from an interim file. The yearly and monthly interim statistics provide only partial information: sex, place of death, medical causes of death.

INSEE performs the computerized data management of death certificates and provides the results (final statistics) to INSERM. It sends also a copy of magnetic tapes containing anonymous socio-professional information and medical causes of death. This information is not completely anonymous, because dates and places of birth and death can be sufficient to identify any individual.

Numbers of deaths are recorded very accurately in France, but the accuracy of data on the causes of death varies widely. The proportion of undefined causes of death decreased from 10.4% in 1971 to 7.6% in 1978 at the national level, but varies according to death place and age. In 1975, for example, it varied from 3.5% in Bas-Rhin to 15.3% in Charentes, excluding Alpes-Maritimes and Corse where the proportions were anomalously high (37.2% and 33.2%, respectively). In the same year, the proportion of undefined causes was 11.7% for persons less than 45 years, 5% between 45 and 65 years, 6.3% between 65 and 84 years and 14.8% for persons older than 85 (Rezvani *et al.*, 1986).

FRENCH POPULATION STATISTICS

Information on the size and composition of the resident population of France is gathered by census, carried out under the supervision of INSEE.

From 1815 to 1945, a national census was performed every five years. However, because of wars, the 1871 census was delayed for one year and the 1916 and 1941 censuses were not carried out at all. Since 1946, censuses have been carried out at intervals of 6–8 years; the most recent was performed in 1990. Data are collected by investigators specially employed by INSEE, who visit about 500 households each, over a period of a month, and explain how to answer the questions. One week later, the investigators return, check and complete the data. If an investigator finds nobody at home, he returns several times; omissions are thus very low. Information on occupation is recorded only for the head of household. Aliens may or may not be included in the results. On the whole, the quality of data is high.

STATISTICAL PUBLICATIONS

Population statistics (census results) are published by INSEE. Preliminary data are published on a 20% random sample of the general population. Updated figures are published every year. Composition by age is given in 18 five-year categories: 0–4, 5–9, ... 75–79, 85+. This composition has been obtained by adding the results of all the *départements*, except Corse, for which a 20% random sample was taken. Data for Corse have been obtained from a complementary survey. Thus, composition by age of the French population is little different from that published by INSEE.

Official publications of mortality and population statistics

Statistics of Medical Causes of Death. Volume I, *Data for the Whole of France, Volume II, Data by Region* (for the years 1968 to 1982) [in French], Paris, INSERM

General Census of the Population of 1975. Results of the Survey of 1/5 by Department [in French]. Paris, INSEE

General Census of the Population of 1982. Results of the Survey of 1/4: Population, Employment. Households, Families, Accommodation [in French]. 'Green' Series, 96 Departmental volumes, Paris, INSEE, 1984–1985

Addresses: Institut National de la Statistique et des Etudes Economiques, 18 boulevard Adolphe Pinard, 75014 Paris.

Institut National de la Santé et de la Recherche Médicale, 101 rue de Tolbiac, 75654 Paris cedex 13.

GERMANY, FEDERAL REPUBLIC

The description that follows refers to the Federal Republic as constituted at the period covered by the data in this atlas, before the unification with the German Democratic Republic in 1990.

The Federal Republic of Germany covers an area of 248 867 km2, made up of mountain areas, uplands and plains. To the north the country is bounded by the North Sea and the Baltic, to the south by the Alps, Lake Constance and the Rhine, which also forms the border in the south-west. The main rivers are the Rhine, the Danube, the Elbe, the Weser and the Moselle. The highest mountain is the Zugspitze (2963 m) in the Alps. Other upland areas rise to 1500 m. 49% of the land is used for agriculture and 29% is wooded.

The Federal Republic's mineral resources include lignite, coal, iron and copper ores and potash.

The capital is Bonn (population 290 000), which has its origins in a Roman fortress.

The Federal Republic of Germany has a population of 61.4 million, with an average density of 247 inhabitants per km2 (1983). The age-structure and broad categories of employment are given in Table 4.3.

The number of foreign residents (1983) stands at 4.5 million (7.4%) — 565 000 from Italy, 292 000 from Greece, 109 000 from the Netherlands, 88 000 from the United Kingdom, 72 000 from France and 18 000 from Belgium.

The Federal Republic is a democratic, parliamentary State with a federal constitution. It is divided into 10 Länder: Schleswig-Holstein, Hamburg, Bremen, Niedersachsen (Lower Saxony), Nordrhein-Westfalen, Rheinland-Pfalz (Rhineland-Palatinate), Saarland (Saar), Hessen, Baden-Württemberg and Bayern (Bavaria). West Berlin has a special status.

MORTALITY DATA COLLECTION IN THE FEDERAL REPUBLIC OF GERMANY

In the Federal Republic of Germany, mortality statistics are collected by each federal state independently. Statistics are compiled from information provided by physicians on death certificates which, in most states, are based on the international model proposed by WHO. Since 1968 cause of death has been coded according to the 8th revision of the International Classification of Diseases (ICD). Mortality statistics are based solely on underlying cause of death.

The death certificate consists of two parts:

- an open part containing identification data (name, sex, date of birth, place of residence, place and time of death, and mode of death (natural, violent or unknown))
- A confidential part, on which the physician indicates all causes contributing to the death. In the case of accidental death (for example, following a road accident), the physician must code the type of accident. In most states, the physician may also make a request for an autopsy on the death certificate. Once filled in, the confidential part is sealed.

The physician who certifies the death sends the death certificate to the registrar's office of the town where the person died. A registration sheet, containing identification data and a registration number, is set up for every death; information on this sheet is used to compile population statistics. The death certificate is then sent to the Local Health Authority (Gesundheitsamt), where the information on the confidential part is checked by a physician (requests for clarification are very rare). Violent deaths and deaths from unknown causes must be reported to the police or public prosecutor's office.

In most states, the Local Health Authority sends the confidential death certificate to the State Board of Statistics (Statistisches Landesamt), where cause of death is coded; in Hamburg, deaths are coded by the Health Authority itself. The ICD code corresponding to the underlying cause of death, indicated by the physician, is marked on the registration sheet; contributing causes are not recorded. The registration sheet is then sent to the registrar's office of the place where the deceased person was last resident. If the last place of residence is in a different state, the registration sheet is sent to the corresponding State Board of Statistics.

Once checked and corrected, data are pooled monthly, quarterly and annually in the state mortality statistics. On an annual basis, each of the 11 federal states transfers pooled data (on state of residence, year of death, sex, nationality, cause of death (four digits), age (in standard age classes) and, in census years, civil status) to the Federal Board of Statistics (Statistisches Bundesamt), which uses these data to compile and publish annual national mortality statistics.

Validity

To guarantee the homogeneity of death coding in the different federal states, and to ensure the correct application of WHO instructions for selecting the underlying cause of death, the Federal Board of Statistics runs annual training courses for coders. In addition, the Federal Ministry of Health is currently financing a research project to investigate whether mortality statistics could be improved by taking into account contributing causes of death, as indicated on death certificates. One problem is deciding which of the previous findings should be considered as contributing to the actual cause of death.

GERMAN POPULATION STATISTICS

Demographic data other than age, sex and civil status are only available through the census. The last two censuses, covering all residents in the Federal Republic of Germany, were held in 1970 and in May 1987. For years between censuses, population size and composition are estimated by counting the births, deaths and migrations reported to the State Boards of Statistics, and relating these figures to the last census data available. As for mortality statistics, population statistics are compiled by each federal state independently. The information from each of the State Boards of Statistics is reported to the Federal Board of Statistics, pooled and then published. As changes of residence are not always reported to the population registry, population data based on this information might be slightly overestimated.

STATISTICAL PUBLICATIONS

Each State Board of Statistics publishes its own mortality and population statistics annually in a series of *Statistical Reports*.

The Federal Board of Statistics publishes national statistics annually. Mortality statistics are published in *Fachserie 12, Gesundheitswesen, Reihe 4, Todesursachen* (Public Health — Causes of Death), and population statistics in *Fachserie 1, Bevölkerung und Erwerbstätigkeit, Reihe 2* (since 1981 *Reihe 1*) *Gebiet und Bevölkerung* (Population and Employment - Territory and Population). (Before 1975, national mortality statistics were published in *Fachserie A Gesundheitswesen, Reihe 7, Bevölkerung und Kultur* (Public Health — Population and Culture), and national population statistics in *Fachserie A, Bevölkerung und Kultur, Reihe 2.*)

The results of the 1987 census are being published separately by the Federal Board of Statistics in *Fachserie 1, Bevölkerung und Erwerbstätigkeit,* Volumes 1 to 13.

In addition, articles on specific topics of mortality statistics are published, irregularly, by the Federal Board of Statistics and the State Boards of Statistics. The following are some important publications, in German, from the Federal Board of Statistics in its series *Wirtschaft und Statistik*:

Cause-Specific Deaths in 1980, Volume 5, 1982
Diseases, Accidents and Deaths among Children, 1978 to 1981, Volume 5, 1983
Relevance of Important Causes of Death to Mortality and Expectation of Life, Volume 3, 1985
Regional Mortality Comparison for Selected Causes of Death, Volume 4, 1987

Other important publications from the Federal Board of Statistics include:

Statistical Yearbook of the Federal Republic of Germany
Population Structure and Economic Resources of the Federal States

Address: Statistisches Bundesamt, Gustav-Stresemann-Ring 11, 6200 Wiesbaden

IRELAND

The total area of the Republic of Ireland is 68 900 km^2. The greatest length from north to south is 486 km and the greatest width from east to west is 275 km.

Ireland comprises a large central lowland of limestone with a relief of hills and a number of coastal mountains, the highest of which is Carantuohill (1040 m). The Shannon is the longest river, 370 km. There are many lakes.

Roughly 81% of the total land is used for agriculture, mostly for grassland pasture. About 5% is wooded. Ireland is a major base-metal producer. Water, peat and natural gas are important indigenous sources of energy.

The country is divided into four provinces (Connaught, Leinster, Munster and Ulster). Dublin, the capital, is in Leinster and is situated on the east coast at the mouth of the river Liffey. The population of the greater Dublin area is approximately 1 million.

The population has been on the increase since 1961, reaching approximately 3.5 million, with an average density of 51 inhabitants per km^2, by 1983. The age-structure and broad categories of employment are given in Table 4.3. Ireland has the youngest population of the EEC-9 countries.

The official languages are Irish and English. Irish (Gaelic) is a Celtic language — one of the oldest written languages in Europe, and it is the first official language. All official documents are published in both languages.

MORTALITY DATA COLLECTION IN IRELAND

General registration of deaths in Ireland began in January 1864, following the Births and Deaths Registration (Ireland) Act 1863. The responsibility for the administration of the registration system, the compilation of death records and the issuing of certificates is vested in the Registrar General, who in turn is responsible to the Minister for Health.

The registration service comprises local registrars in each of 633 districts throughout the country, under the supervision of 30 Superintendent Registrars responsible for all the registrations within larger areas, generally counties and county boroughs. Deaths are registered initially at local offices and the Registrar's books are subsequently forwarded to the Registrar General.

Deaths must be registered within five days of their occurrence. A relative of the deceased, or a person present at the death, delivers to the Registrar's Office the medical certificate, signed by the attending doctor and indicating the cause of death. The person registering the death also completes a special statistical form, which is sent, with any medical certificates, to the Central Statistics Office for coding and analysis. Any queries arising due to unclear indication of cause of death on the certificates are referred back to the certifying doctor for clarification.

In cases where there was no doctor in attendance, a post-mortem may be required and the death may be registered on the basis of a coroner's certificate. About 10% of deaths in Ireland are registered following inquests or post-mortems.

About 60% of deaths in Ireland take place in hospitals, nursing homes and other institutions.

The coding and statistical analysis of deaths is carried out on behalf of the Minister for Health by the Central Statistics Office. The causes of death are currently coded in accordance with the 9th revision of the International Classification of Diseases.

IRISH POPULATION STATISTICS

The census of population is the main source of population statistics for Ireland. Decennial censuses were undertaken from 1821 until 1911 and, following a break in 1921, were resumed in 1926. Quinquennial censuses have been undertaken since 1946 with the exception of 1976, although a census with restricted content was carried out in 1979. For years between censuses, annual population estimates are produced.

The usual range of questions on the census questionnaire cover such topics as age, marital status, sex, place of birth, principal economic status, occupation and industry.

STATISTICAL PUBLICATIONS

Summaries of mortality data are compiled by the Central Statistics Office every quarter, approximately six months after the quarter to which they refer. A detailed report on each year is also prepared and published approximately three years after the year concerned.

Annual Report on Vital Statistics (published annually for the years 1864–1984), Department of Health/Central Statistics Office

Quarterly Report on Vital Statistics (published quarterly for the years 1899–1986), Department of Health/Central Statistics Office

Health Statistics (published annually for the years 1976–1986), Department of Health

Address: Central Statistics Office, Earlsford Terrace, Dublin 2

ITALY

Italy has an area of 301 046 km2. The independent Republic of San Marino and the Vatican City State are surrounded by Italian territory. The southern fringe of the Alps falls steeply down to the plain of the River Po, south of which extends the 1000 km long and 130–250 km wide Apennine peninsula. The sparsely forested Apennines run down almost the entire length of Italy, the highest peak being the Gran Sasso (2914 m). To the west lies Sardinia, and the west coast is dotted with smaller, mostly mountainous, islands such as Elba, Ponza, Capri and Ischia. At the southern tip of the peninsula lies the island of Sicily, with Europe's biggest volcano, Mount Etna (3326 m). Other volcanoes are Vesuvius near Naples and Stromboli on the Lipari Islands. The longest river is the Po (652 km), which rises in the Cottian Alps and flows through a delta-like estuary into the Adriatic Sea. The main rivers rising in the Apennines are the Arno, which passes through Florence, and the Tiber, on whose banks Rome is built.

58% of the land surface is used for agriculture and 20% is wooded. Italy is poor in minerals; the only important ones are sulphur in Sicily, bauxite and lead ore in the south, and the marble quarries at Carrara. The capital is Rome (population 3.1 million).

The population of Italy is 56.7 million, with an average density of 188 inhabitants per km2. The age-structure and broad categories of employment are given in Table 4.3. Many of the considerable number of foreigners in Italy come from other Community countries, predominantly from France, Germany and the United Kingdom. There has recently been some immigration from developing countries.

The national language is Italian, and other languages spoken in the regions include German (Alto Adige), French (Valle d'Aosta), Slovene (Trieste and Gorizia) and Ladin (some areas of the Alto Adige).

For administrative purposes, Italy is divided into 20 regions, with considerable autonomy. Five of them — Valle d'Aosta, Trentino-Alto Adige, Sicilia (Sicily), Sardegna (Sardinia) and Friuli-Venezia Giulia — have special constitutions giving them a wider degree of autonomy than the other 15 — Piemonte (Piedmont), Liguria, Lombardia (Lombardy), Veneto, Emilia Romagna, Toscana (Tuscany), Marche, Umbria, Lazio (Latium), Abruzzio, Molise, Campania, Puglia (Apulia), Basilicata and Calabria.

MORTALITY DATA COLLECTION IN ITALY

Demographic registries were first established in Italy in 1865, during the unification of the country. All deaths, from whatever cause, have been recorded for the whole country since 1887. Each of the 8090 Italian communes has its own registry office where births, marriages and deaths are recorded. The death certificate currently used in Italy is based on the international model proposed by WHO.

Deaths must be reported to the communal registry office within 24 hours. When a death is notified, a two-part data sheet is prepared.

- The first part is completed by a civil servant and contains demographic and social data
- The second part is completed by the medical practitioner who certified the death, and contains comprehensive medical data, including the initial (underlying) cause of death, intermediate causes, final causes and any other relevant health conditions; for each of these items, the date of occurrence is recorded (in years, months or days before the death). However, unless otherwise specified, only the initial

cause is taken into account in compiling mortality statistics.

The data sheets are sent to the provincial registry office, where they are checked, and then to the Central Institute of Statistics (ISTAT), where the data are coded by medical personnel. If necessary, supplementary information may be requested at this stage, but usually this does not lead to any change in the basic information. The coded data sheets are then stored in archives, for conformity tests (the error rate usually amounts to less than 1%). Until 1981 these errors were identified and corrected but this has proved too costly.

Although ISTAT stores the data sheets bearing the names of the deceased, only anonymous data are used to compile tables of causes of death by age, sex and region. These tables are published in directories of health statistics. Other tables are also published in demographic statistics yearbooks, but without any identification of death causes.

In addition to data published by ISTAT, scientists may request direct access to codified data and to anonymous reports.

Various reliability tests are made on the mortality data stored in the ISTAT files by comparing different archives (mortality registries of communal health offices with hospital archives, for example). Such verifications allow optimal compilation of data and lead to a good classification according to cause.

The quality of the information on the death certificate depends to a great extent on whether the death occurs in a hospital or other health institutions or at home.

The tendency for people to die outside their commune of residence seems to be increasing; the rate is currently 30% of all deaths. However, mortality statistics are compiled on the basis of usual residence, not on place of death.

In general, autopsies are rarely carried out in Italy to determine cause of death. In theory, the low incidence of autopsies should not affect the quality of mortality data, but in reality, autopsies can lead to a more precise definition of cause of death. This phenomenon is particularly important in the town of Trieste, which has a great anatomo-pathological tradition: autopsies are performed very frequently here, with the result that the mortality data are of higher quality than elsewhere.

The system of mortality data collection is currently being revised. For example, copies of death certificates must now be sent to the local health authorities who can therefore generate their own data files. The national statistics system has not yet been changed; however, certain modifications have allowed an improvement in the quality of certification.

ITALIAN POPULATION STATISTICS

In Italy, full population censuses are carried out in the autumn of the second year of each decade. A form is delivered to each household, and collected a few days later by an enumerator who checks the correctness of replies and, if necessary, asks the family to provide further information. The occasion is also used to correct errors in legal residence.

In addition, since 1800 each commune has maintained its own population register, which contains records of all vital events (births, marriages, deaths) which occur within the commune, and of all vital events concerning residents of the commune which take place outside the communal territory. Until 1970, freedom to change from the original residence was limited by law for the numerous people who were living in towns, who were obliged to maintain their legal residence in their former commune. For the 1971 census, however, it was established that any individuals who were recorded outside their communes should transfer their legal address, unless their residence elsewhere was only temporary. Certain fiscal features of tax declarations attached to secondary residence did not reflect the actual reality of residence. At the end of the year, each commune calculates its population on the basis of the data in its register.

Communal offices also send information on vital events and on any movements of their registered resident population to ISTAT. Therefore it should be possible to calculate the number of residents in a given commune on a monthly basis. In fact, for administrative reasons, registrations and deregistrations are often recorded at certain times only, and data are therefore only valid if they refer to a wider region or a longer time interval.

STATISTICAL PUBLICATIONS

Population statistics

12th General Census of Population, 25 October 1981, various volumes, ISTAT, Rome, 1984

Inter-census estimates on provincial basis are available on request from the National Institute of Health (Istituto Superiore di Sanita), Rome

Mortality statistics

Cause-of-death data by year are published annually by ISTAT in its *Annuario*; before 1985 they were published in the Year Books on Health Statistics (*Annuari di Statistiche Sanitarie*)

Data from 1969 to 1988 are available, with constraints of confidentiality, on computer media.

Mortality by cause and Local Health Units are published by ISTAT in collaboration with the National Institute of Health

Historical cause-of-death data from 1861 to 1955 are available from ISTAT.

Provisional data by place of death are published in the *Monthly Bulletin of Statistics* (ISTAT)

Address: Istituto Centrale di Statistica, Viale Liegi 13, 00100 Rome

LUXEMBOURG

The Grand Duchy of Luxembourg has an area of 2586 km^2. It is bounded by France, the Federal Republic of Germany and Belgium. Luxembourg is a hilly country, rich in woodland. As the 'Department of Forests', Luxembourg was one of the nine departments formed by France from the territories of the Austrian Netherlands annexed in 1795. The independence and neutrality of the country were confirmed by the treaty of London in 1867.

The main topographical features of the country are the Oesling, a 450 m high plateau, part of the Ardennes, and the Gutland which rises to an average height of 250 m. The main rivers are the Moselle, the Our and the Sûre. 49% of the land area (127 422 ha) is used for agriculture and 32% is wooded; vines are cultivated in the Moselle valley over an area of 1155 ha.

The capital city is Luxembourg (population 80 000).

Luxembourg has a population of 366 000, with an average density of 141 inhabitants per km^2. The age-structure and broad categories of employment are given in Table 4.3. The proportion of foreigners is around 26%, many being employed in the iron industry. 'Letzburgesch' is the national language, spoken by all strata of the population. French and German are used for administrative purposes.

Luxembourg is one of the seats of the European Community, housing a series of Community organizations. The country is one of the most important banking centres in Europe.

The administrative regions used in this atlas are Grevenmacher, Diekirch and Luxembourg with Esch-sur-Alzette.

Grevenmacher, to the east of the country, along the valley of the Moselle, is mainly agricultural (including vineyards) with a few light industries.

Diekirch, in the north of the country, is situated at the border of the hilly and wooded Ardennes. The northern region is largely agricultural with light industries in the areas of the main cities (Diekirch, Ettelbruck, Wiltz).

Luxembourg, to the south of the country, is both industrial (administration, business, light industry) and agricultural (farmlands and woods).

Esch-sur-Alzette, in the extreme south of the country, contains the iron and steel industry and has the highest population density of the country.

MORTALITY DATA COLLECTION IN LUXEMBOURG

Death certificates specifying the cause of death were introduced in 1923. The medical certification of death has been compulsory since 1963. These death certificates are anonymous and are sent to the Public Health Officer (Médecin-inspecteur, Direction de la Santé).

The death certificate now in use was introduced in 1967. There are two types: a specific form for perinatal deaths (stillbirths and neonatal deaths up to 10 days of age) and a general one for all other deaths.

The death certificate is divided into three sections:

section A is a nominative part identifying the deceased,

section B is an anonymous part identifying the deceased,

section C reports the cause of death: it is filled in and sealed by the certifying doctor.

Section A is kept at the registry office of the municipality, which transmits a special form to the National Institute of Statistics (Service Central de la Statistique et des Etudes Economiques). Sections B and C are sent to the Direction de la Santé, where section B is coded by office staff, and section

C is coded by a social nurse for underlying and immediate cause of death, according to the 9th revision of the ICD.

The Direction de la Santé produces annual statistics on causes of deaths and transmits them to the National Institute of Statistics.

LUXEMBOURG POPULATION STATISTICS

In Luxembourg a general population census is carried out every ten years; the last one was held on 31 March 1981. For years between censuses, population figures are estimated each year by adding the natural (births/deaths) and the migration (arrivals/departures) balance.

The census measures two categories of persons:

(1) Those resident in the municipality where they are counted (resident population),

(2) Those who are temporarily present at the moment of the census but do not have their usual residence in that municipality (non-resident population).

Population figures are available for the different levels of administration (county, district, municipality).

The municipalities have to carry out a 'fiscal census' every year on 15 October in order to deliver the 'taxation bulletin' for taxes on salaries. In 1977 and 1979, the *National Institute of Statistics* used these data to produce some population statistics.

STATISTICAL PUBLICATIONS

The Direction de la Santé, Service des Statistiques Sanitaires publishes an annual brochure on the causes of death (all causes by sex and age groups of the deceased). The figures relate to all deaths which occurred in the country ('de facto' deaths), without separation of foreign from Luxembourg citizens.

The National Institute of Statistics publishes in its *Statistical Annual* (*a*) general mortality data (*de jure* deaths) using the information provided by the municipalities (demographic statistics), and (*b*) the causes of death, listed according to the WHO basic tabulation list ('de facto' deaths) provided by the Direction de la Santé.

Much detailed information is available even though it is not published regularly.

Address: Division de la Médecine Préventive et Sociale, Direction de la Santé, 22 rue Goethe, 1637 Luxembourg

THE NETHERLANDS

The Netherlands has an area of 41 473 km^2, and extends roughly 300 km north to south and about 200 km east to west. Behind the North Sea coast lie the 'polders' - land partly reclaimed from the sea. The islands in Zeeland and South Holland provinces are linked by secure dikes to prevent the recurrence of disasters caused by storm tides. About 27% of the country's total area is below sea level, and the land is criss-crossed by a network of lakes, rivers and canals. Land over 100 m above sea level is to be found only in the south-east corner of the country.

71% of the land (excluding water) area is used for agriculture or horticulture and 9% is wooded. Mineral resources include coal, oil and natural gas.

The capital is Amsterdam (population 676 000), but the seat of government and most central government departments is The Hague (population 445 000).

The Netherlands has a population of 14.3 million, with an average density of 346 inhabitants per km^2 (1983), making it nearly the most densely populated country in the world. The age-structure and broad categories of employment are given in Table 4.3. Of the 66 000 migrant workers from Community countries, more than one third come from Belgium. About two thirds of the 108 000 migrant workers from non-community countries come from Turkey and Morocco.

Dutch is the national language. There is a Frisian minority, speaking its own language in the north of the country.

The Netherlands is divided into 12 provinces: Groningen, Friesland, Drenthe, Overijssel, Flevoland (established in 1986), Gelderland, Utrecht, North Holland, South Holland, Zeeland, North Brabant and Limburg. Each province has a Provincial Council and a Provincial Executive (responsible for day-to-day business), both chaired by a Queen's Commissioner appointed by the Government.

MORTALITY DATA COLLECTION IN THE NETHERLANDS

The principles of the present system for notification of death and compilation of cause-of-death statistics date from 1927.

When a natural death occurs, the attending physician prepares two documents: a death certificate (called the A-letter), and a cause-of-death certificate (called the B-letter). In the case of non-natural death or cremation, notification of death is given by the coroner (always a physician). The B-letter is a strictly confidential document on which the name of the deceased does not appear. It is inserted in an envelope which is then sealed. A perforated slip of paper attached to this envelope bears the name of the deceased. Notification of death takes place when both the A- and B-letters are presented at the office of the Local Registrar of the municipality where the death occurred.

In the Local Registrar's Office, the death certificate (A-letter) is numbered and the death entered in the municipal register of births, deaths and marriages. This certificate number and the name of the municipality are written on the envelope containing the B-letter. The slip of paper bearing the name is then removed from the envelope. The personal card of the deceased, which is part of the population register, is removed from the register and the occurrence of the death and death certificate number are recorded on it. Each month the Local Registrars send the closed envelopes with the B-letters, together with the personal cards of deceased persons, to the Netherlands Central Bureau of Statistics (CBS).

If the deceased person has been resident in a municipality other than the one in which he or she died, the personal card must first be sent to the municipality in which the death occurred and from there to the CBS.

At the CBS, the personal cards of the deceased are forwarded to the Department of Population Statistics, while the envelopes with the B-letters are forwarded to the Medical Officer of the Department of Health Statistics. Demographic data from the personal cards (date of death, date of birth, marital status, etc.) are processed by the Department of Population Statistics, while the envelopes of the B-letters are opened by the Medical Officer and the information on the cause of death is coded according to the instructions of the 9th revision of the ICD.

After coding and processing of the demographic information and cause of death have been completed, linking of the two data sets occurs by means of the certificate number (and the number of the municipality where the death occurred). The final and complete data set on cause of death is used to produce statistics on cause of death differentiated by various characteristics.

Information on cause of death is available for the following characteristics: primary and secondary cause of death, municipality where the death occurred; date of death; date of birth; sex; religion (until the end of 1983); nationality; marital status; date of marriage or divorce; municipality of residence; municipality of birth (for infants only); place of death (hospital or at home); and whether a post-mortem examination was performed.

In about 5% of cases, the B-letter contains incomplete or inconsistent information or is missing. Whenever possible, the Medical Officer of the CBS requests the attending physician to provide the missing information or to resolve inconsistencies. As a result of such efforts, 90% of these cases can be coded satisfactorily. The percentage of cases where the cause of death is described as 'unknown or badly described' (ICD rubrics 780–799) was 3.4 in 1983. The percentage of known autopsies in the Netherlands is around 12%; in 71% of the deaths, no post-mortem was held, while for 17% of deaths, no information was available (in 1981 and 1982). Nearly half of the deaths (46%) occurred in hospitals in 1985; 47% occurred elsewhere and for the remaining 7% no information was available.

DUTCH POPULATION STATISTICS

Information on the size and composition of the population of the Netherlands is provided by the system of continuous population enumeration which is based on the population registers. These registers are maintained by the Local Registrars in the different municipalities and comprise all the personal cards of the *de jure* resident population of these municipalities. New personal cards are made out for births and migrants into The Netherlands. All changes in personal situation, such as marriage, divorce, change of residence or death, are entered on this card. When a person moves to another municipality his or her personal card is forwarded to the municipality of the new residence. In the case of emigration or death, the personal card is removed from the register. A number of regulations, measures and checks are in force to make the registers as accurate as possible (van den Brekel, 1977).

With the information from the population registers, the municipalities are able to obtain at regular intervals information on their population size and composition. One of the duties of the Local Registrars is to send monthly figures from their municipalities on vital events (births, deaths, marriages and dissolutions of marriages) and on migration to CBS, where these are processed and analysed. Using the population figures from the 1971 census as the base, changes in population size and composition for The Netherlands as a whole are determined annually by addition and subtraction of figures on vital events and migration which have been received from the different municipalities. As a result, CBS is able to compile statistics (mostly annually, but some monthly) on the size and composition of the population. Information is available on population size by, for example, age, sex, municipality of residence, province, marital status and nationality.

As the last census in the Netherlands was held in 1971, it is possible that population figures obtained with the system of continuous population enumeration have become increasingly inaccurate. This is, however, considered unlikely because of the existence of various control measures built into this system. A study was made in 1983 comparing population figures by several characteristics from the CBS system of continuous population enumeration with corresponding figures obtained from the various municipalities themselves. Discrepancies proved on the whole to be small and adjustments were made in the system of continuous population enumeration to make it similar to the registers maintained in the different municipalities. This study was also used to check the accuracy of the registers of aliens in the Netherlands. Once more, minor discrepancies were observed: there were 1.3% more aliens counted in the municipal registers than there were in the CBS system. These discrepancies are too small to have a measurable impact on the denominators of cause-specific mortality rates.

Over the years, a number of changes have occurred in municipal boundaries. The few small changes in boundaries between 1976 and 1980 do not affect the comparability of the data presented.

STATISTICAL PUBLICATIONS

Provisional monthly figures on deaths by age and sex for the country as a whole, as well as for the large municipalities, are published by the CBS in the *Monthly Bulletin of Population Statistics*. Provisional monthly figures on cause of death by age and sex according to the Adapted Mortality (AM) list are published in the *Monthly Bulletin of Health Statistics*. Articles in these bulletins and in most other CBS publications mentioned below are in Dutch with English summaries. Annual figures on mortality in general are published in the *Monthly Bulletin of Population Statistics* and on causes of death in the *Vademecum of Health Statistics of the Netherlands* (of which the most recent issue was published in 1991) and in the *Monthly Bulletin of Health Statistics*. Detailed annual figures on causes of death (three-digit figures and AM-list) by age, sex, province, large municipalities and a few other variables are published annually in six volumes (Series A1, A2, B1, B2, B3 and C). Detailed figures on mortality in general and by cause of death with emphasis on trends were published in the *Compendium of Health Statistics of The Netherlands* (1986). Two other important CBS publications are *Life Tables for The Netherlands, 1976–1980* and *Life Tables for The Netherlands by Main Causes of Death, 1976–1980.*

Articles on special topics concerning mortality in general and cause of death are published both in the *Monthly Bulletin of Population Statistics* and the *Monthly Bulletin of Health Statistics*. In addition, CBS issues regular publications on special topics relating to mortality. *Cancer: Morbidity and Mortality, 1975/1976*, published by CBS in collaboration with the Medical Records Foundation, contains data on mortality from and incidence of cancer at various sites. Figures on the 'clinical incidence' of cancers at various sites were obtained from the registration scheme in hospitals organized by the Medical Records Foundation. Data are shown on 'clinical incidence' for 1975/1976, together with the corresponding mortality rates as determined by CBS. (Since 1976, such data have been published regularly in the *Monthly Bulletin of Health Statistics*, and since 1982 in the *Monthly Bulletin of Health Statistics*.)

Atlas of Cancer Mortality in the Netherlands, 1969–1978 (in both English and Dutch) consists of maps, supplemented by graphs and tables, showing average standardized mortality ratios for the period

1969–1978 of cancers from a large number of sites by corop area (the country is divided into 40 such areas for statistical purposes; Eurostat, 1981). The graphs and tables also show standardized mortality ratios of cancers of various sites by five periods of two years between 1969 and 1979 in corop areas, provinces and large municipalities.

In addition to these CBS publications, various articles on mortality and on cause of death appear regularly in a number of Dutch medical journals. Two particularly important journals are *Nederlands Tijdschrift voor Geneeskunde* and *Tijdschrift voor Sociale Gezondheidszorg*; the articles in these journals are in Dutch with English summaries.

Address: Department of Health Statistics, Netherlands Central Bureau of Statistics, Prinses Beatrixlaan 428, P.O. Box 959, 2270 AZ Voorburg

UNITED KINGDOM

The United Kingdom of Great Britain and Northern Ireland has an area of 244 111 km2. Nowhere is further than 120 km from the sea. In general, a line from Bristol to the Wash on the east coast divides mainland Britain into a hilly north-western zone and the lowlands of the south-east. The 240 km-long Pennine Chain runs down from the Cheviot Hills on the Scottish border to the Midlands; north-western England is dominated by the Cumbrian Mountains of the Lake District. The highest point here is Scafell Pike (977 m). Wales is dominated by the north–south range of the Cumbrian mountains (Snowdon 1085 m). Scotland is also mountainous (Ben Nevis 1342 m), principally to the north of the central Forth–Clyde lowlands. The north-west highlands, deeply indented by sea lochs, are one of the most scenically impressive areas of Europe.

About 77% of the land surface is used for agriculture. There is little heavily wooded country in Britain (9%), but large areas of heaths, moors and common land abound.

Coal and iron have been mined for centuries, and in the past two decades natural gas and offshore oil deposits have been increasingly exploited.

The capital of the United Kingdom is London (population 7 million). Edinburgh (460 000) is the capital of Scotland, and Cardiff (280 000) the capital of Wales. The province of Northern Ireland is governed from Belfast (360 000).

The population of the United Kingdom is about 56.4 million, with an average density of 231 inhabitants per km2 (1983). The age-structure and broad categories of employment are given in Table 4.3.

Besides the English (80%), the Scots (9%), the Welsh (5%) and the Northern Irish (3%), the UK population includes some 2–3 million Commonwealth immigrants, of whom a third live in London. Of the estimated 313 000 migrant workers from Community countries, two thirds come from Ireland.

The official language is English, but Welsh is spoken in Wales. Gaelic speakers are found in western Scotland and in the Hebrides.

Following the local government reforms of 1974, England is divided into 46 counties; Wales has 8 counties and Scotland 12 regions for local government. There are 26 districts in Northern Ireland.

MORTALITY DATA COLLECTION IN THE UNITED KINGDOM

The present system of registration of deaths in the United Kingdom dates from the Births and Deaths Registration Act 1836 for England and Wales, the Registration of Births, Deaths and Marriages (Scotland) Act 1854, and the Registration of Births and Deaths (Ireland) Act 1863.

Mortality data are derived from the medical certificate of cause of death issued by the attending medical practitioner and from information provided by the informant at the time of registration of the death. In 1980, about 60% of deaths in the United Kingdom occurred in hospitals and institutions for the care of the sick, and 35% at home (the percentage of deaths at home was slightly higher in Northern Ireland).

The doctor completes the registration form (similar to that recommended by WHO), stating cause of death and indicating whether information from an autopsy has been taken into account, or might be available later: in 1980, autopsies were performed for about 28% of deaths in England and Wales (16% in Scotland and 6% in Northern Ireland). The doctor can also indicate whether the death has been reported to the coroner (procurator fiscal in Scotland) or whether other information might be available at a later date. If this latter section is completed, a standard enquiry form is sent at the time of registration of death; such enquiries are made for about 5% of all deaths, and about one third of the replies eventually result in reassignment of cause-of-death codes.

The death certificate is delivered to the Registrar of Births and Deaths in the registration district in which the death occurred. The informant may be a relative of the deceased, a person present at the death, the occupier or an inmate of the institution in which the death occurred, or a person responsible for disposal of the body. The informant is expected to provide information about the deceased, including date and place of birth, occupation and usual address.

A registrar may report a death to the coroner (or in Scotland to the procurator fiscal) if: (i) the deceased person was not attended during his or her last illness by a medical practitioner; (ii) the registrar has been unable to obtain a certificate of cause of death; (iii) information on the certificate of cause of death indicates that the deceased was seen neither after death nor within 14 days before death by the certifying practitioner; (iv) the cause of death is unknown; (v) the registrar has reason to believe that death resulted from an unnatural cause, violence, neglect, abortion or suspicious circumstances; (vi) death appears to have occurred from an operation or before recovery from an anaesthetic; or (vii) from the contents of the certificate, it appears that death was due to industrial disease or poisoning. Depending on the results of preliminary enquiries into whether death was from natural causes, the coroner may issue a notification of the cause of death without holding an inquest, having in some circumstances had an autopsy carried out. In fact, autopsies are performed for the majority of deaths referred to the coroner (about 82% in 1980). However, not all deaths referred to the coroner are certified by him; in 1980, just over 10% of the deaths initially referred to the coroner were finally certified by a doctor.

Death certificates, together with all the particulars obtained at death registration, are forwarded weekly by the registrars to the Office of Population Censuses and Surveys (OPCS) in England and Wales, or the General Registrar Offices (GRO) in Scotland and Northern Ireland. There, the information is coded (for example, area of residence of the deceased is coded to a postcode, and cause of death to the appropriate four-digit ICD code), and entered into a computer. For about 3% of deaths there are difficulties in coding cause of death; in these cases further enquiries may be sent to the certifying practitioner. Finally, by collaboration between the Vital Statistics Section and the Statistics Branch of the Computer Division of OPCS (between the GRO and the Computer Division in Scotland and Northern Ireland), the master file of mortality data is assembled; this is used for routine publications, and is available for *ad hoc* enquiries.

UK POPULATION STATISTICS

National population censuses

A national census has been held every 10 years since 1901, with the exception of 1941; there was an additional 'mid-term' census in 1966 involving a 10% sample of the population.

The vast majority of the population are counted at the census in their (or someone else's) home, usually on a Sunday in April, by specially appointed enumerators. There are also arrangements for enumerating people present in institutions. The number of questions asked of respondents reached a peak of 30 in 1971, and was reduced to 21 in 1981.

A major improvement in the 1966 census was the substitution of date of birth for the previous census question on age; this improved the accuracy of much of the age data.

From the point of providing a denominator for calculating rates, the main demographic items are sex, age and marital status. More extended epidemiological analyses can be performed using the other material.

The initial coverage of the census is checked by attempting to repeat the enumeration for a sample of households, shortly after census day, using a skilled team of field staff. In 1981, it was estimated that 0.62% of people had been missed, but about 0.17% had been counted twice. This indicates that net underenumeration was less than 0.5% (Britton & Birch, 1985).

Annual population estimates

In years between censuses, annual population estimates are produced, which take account of the occurrence of births and deaths and migration into and out of the country or locality since the last census. These estimates have been prepared for the country and large towns since the 19th century, and for local authority areas since 1911; in Northern Ireland they have been produced for both levels since 1926.

In England and Wales the differences between the population estimates carried forward from the 1971 census and the estimates derived from the 1981 census data have been calculated for each local government area (OPCS, 1982). For England and Wales as a whole, the estimates were 0.2% lower than the census, with larger errors for various age groups. At the local level the differences were considerably greater (1–5%), because of inadequate information about people moving between local authority areas. Populations of the larger districts tended to be overestimated and those of the smaller underestimated.

The differences for individual age groups were again much larger than the overall difference.

STATISTICAL PUBLICATIONS

From 1840 to 1974, the Registrar General published an Annual Report containing statistics for England and Wales. After 1954, *The Registrar General's Statistical Review of England and Wales* was published in three parts — medical tables, population tables, and a commentary. Detailed tables were provided, giving particulars of deaths and death rates by cause, sex, age, locality, etc.

In 1974 this publication was replaced by an annual series of volumes containing subsets of the mortality statistics. The intention was that individual components of this series would be published with the least delay; individuals could acquire the subset of material that was of particular interest to them. This series, known as series DH, is produced in five parts:

DH1 — Mortality Statistics

DH2 — Mortality Statistics by Cause

DH3 — Mortality Statistics, Childhood and Maternity

DH4 — Mortality Statistics, Accidents and Violence

DH5 — Mortality Statistics, Area.

The main tables are those in DH2 volume which present, at ICD three- and four-digit levels, the numbers of deaths by age and sex; more detailed analyses, providing rates, appear in the general DH1 volume.

Area and occupational mortality statistics have been published approximately every 10 years since 1851, initially as supplements to the Registrar General's Annual Reports, and later as specific decennial supplements produced by the Registrar General or OPCS. The latest publications are:

OPCS Area Mortality Tables, Decennial Supplement 1969–73. Series DS No. 4, England and Wales (for the years 1969–1973, published in 1981)

The Registrar General's Decennial Supplement, England and Wales, Occupational Mortality. Series DS No. 1 (for 1970–1972, published in 1978)

The Registrar General's Decennial Supplement, Great Britain, Occupational Mortality. Series DS No 6 (for 1979–80, 1982–83, published in 1986)

Until 1974, the Registrar General also published a Weekly Return and a Quarterly Return. In 1974 the Weekly Return was replaced by a monitor, particularly devoted to statistics on infectious diseases, and the Quarterly Return by a quarterly journal, *Population Trends*, which includes articles on specific topics and regular tables, with limited analyses on mortality.

Address: Office of Population Censuses and Surveys, St Catherine's House, 10 Kingsway, London WC2B 6JP

Scotland

The Registrar General for Scotland publishes an Annual Report. Section B summarizes recent Scottish mortality trends, Section C covers deaths by cause and age group, and Sections D and E cover stillbirths and infant deaths. In addition, the Registrar General for Scotland publishes a Vital Statistics Return (VSR) every four weeks. The following are some of the articles appearing in recent issues of this publication.

Measures of Mortality in Scotland. VSR, 1986, weeks 13–16

Manual/Non-Manual Mortality Analysis of Scottish Local Government Districts. VSR, 1986, weeks 45–48

Mortality Rates for Ages 45–74 in Scotland Compared with England and Wales, Northern Ireland and 9 Selected Countries, VSR, 1987, weeks 1–4

Several unpublished reports, available from the Vital Statistics Branch of the General Register Office (Scotland), also contain mortality statistics for Scotland. Examples are *A Comparison of Male Mortality in Selected Countries* and *Data on Occupational Mortality in Scotland 1979–83.*

Address: General Register Office for Scotland, Ladywell House, Ladywell Road, Edinburgh EH12 7IF

Northern Ireland

From 1863 to 1921, Northern Ireland Statistics were included in the Annual Reports of the Registrar General for Ireland. After 1922, the Registrar General published annual statistics for Northern Ireland, with detailed tables giving particulars of deaths and death rates by cause, sex, age, locality, etc. From 1924 to 1969, the Registrar General published weekly and quarterly returns, but from 1970 only quarterly returns have been published.

Address: General Register Office, Department of Health and Social Security, Oxford House, 49–55 Chichester Street, Belfast BT1 4HL

CHAPTER 5

EEC CANCER MORTALITY PATTERNS BY SITE

Introduction

In this chapter the patterns of distribution of mortality throughout the nine EEC countries are examined for the common forms of cancer, following the order of the 8th revision of the International Classification of Diseases (WHO, 1967).

Not all sites of cancer have been mapped, for three reasons. First, the level of detail supplied by national vital statistics offices varies, which means that for some sites data have had to be presented for broad groupings. Thus, ICD-8 rubrics 140–149, which cover such diverse cancers as those of the lip, mouth, tongue, salivary gland, nasopharynx and the various parts of the pharynx, have had to be presented as a group although, in the commentary, information is given about most of these sites separately.

Second, the numbers of deaths from a variety of cancers such as those of the small intestine (ICD-8 152), the mediastinum (ICD-8 164) and the eye (ICD-8 190) were too small to merit mapping. Any differences seen could well have been due to statistical chance.

Third, for some cancers, diagnosis is imprecise. Thus, cancer of the liver (ICD-8 155) presents many problems in that until fairly recently the reliability of diagnosis was poor. Even today, it is not always possible to separate cancers arising in the liver from those which are metastatic. The difficulty of distinguishing between cervix and corpus cancer of the uterus on death certificates is well known, with deaths from the former frequently appearing as cancer of the uterus on death certificates. This inability to distinguish the cervix from the remainder of the uterus in mortality data in several countries is to be regretted, as the risk factors for these cancers are quite different.

Although Hodgkin's disease (ICD-8 201) is mapped separately, the various forms of non-Hodgkin lymphoma (ICD-8 200, 202) have been grouped together as there are national differences in the nomenclature and classification of these forms of malignant disease. All the forms of leukaemia have had to be grouped together (ICD-8 204–208) because death certificates frequently cite leukaemia without further specification, the cell type involved not being mentioned.

Secondary cancers and those of unknown primary site are, however, mapped as these reflect the level of imprecision in certification of cancer deaths.

The atlas is accompanied by two transparent overlays. One gives the code numbers for the regions mapped, the key appearing in Table 1.2. Thus, B10 represents Antwerpen (Antwerp) in Belgium, F69 the *département* of the Rhône in France, S12 the Western Isles of Scotland. On this overlay, the national boundaries are only lightly emphasized in order to permit examination of the pattern of cancer distribution in an uninterrupted manner. A second overlay gives the national and regional boundaries so that the observer can determine whether a given pattern stops at a frontier. This overlay also identifies the regions given in the tables.

Following each cancer site title there appear four figures, these being the average age-standardized mortality rates for males and females for EEC-9, followed by the proportion of the total cancer deaths that the site represents, again for males and females. For example, lung: ICD-8 162 (M53.5, F7.8; M28.8%, F7.1%).

Following a description of spatial patterns, attention is drawn to the regions with the highest and lowest rates for each sex. For this comparison, only rates based on 100 or more deaths are presented. When two or more regions had the same mortality rate, the region with the greatest number of deaths has been chosen. All rates are age-standardized to the 'world' standard population and are expressed as average annual rates per 100 000 population (see Chapter 2 and Boyle & Parkin, 1991).

To place the European mortality rates in a wider context, they are compared with those seen around 1978 in the USA, Japan and Australia, nations with a similar socio-economic level. Japan has been chosen as representing an industrialized country with a standard of living comparable to that of the EEC, but with major differences in life-style and risk. Australia has sizeable communities of migrants from several EEC countries.

In the descriptions which follow, the emphasis is on regional differences and patterns rather than dissection of variation at the EEC level III areas. The reader should bear in mind that a given colour on the maps may, for common cancers, embrace quite a large variation in level of mortality. Thus, for male lung cancer, the yellow areas which represent 40% of all values cover age-adjusted rates which lie between 37.5 and 55.0. Conversely, for infrequent cancers, the range covered by one colour may be quite small — the yellow areas for male malignant melanoma represent the much narrower range of 5.0 to 7.6. Further, the ranges of mortality represented by a given colour may differ quite considerably between the sexes.

In formulating their comments, the editors have tended to ignore isolated 'hot spots', preferring to draw attention to regions where there seem to be groups of areas with high or low mortality rates such as oesophageal and laryngeal cancer in western and north-eastern France. (Some problems in interpretation of these patterns are presented in Alexander & Boyle (1992)). Gastric cancer mortality in virtually all of the north of Italy is high and low in most of the south of France. Similarly, the great excess of breast cancer mortality in the British Isles contrasts with the much lower levels in southern Italy, a contrast all the more interesting in that there is a gradient of mortality in between. In so doing the editors have in a sense dismissed local pockets of risk which may indeed reflect truly elevated risk due to the presence of a regional exposure.

It may be argued that many of the differences seem to stop at national boundaries and this reflects habits of death certification rather than a true difference in risk (see Chapter 3). For example, the high levels of prostate cancer mortality in parts of north-west Germany continue into southern Belgium but cease abruptly at the French border. Oesophageal cancer, so common in west and north-east France, again is much rarer on the other side of the Belgian border. There may also be artefactual variations within countries. However, some of these go in opposite directions — thus the relatively low levels of large bowel cancer in the south of France contrast with the higher levels of cancer of the bladder. It is highly unlikely that these two sites would be confounded. Within Italy the validity of the lower mortality rates for many sites in the south than in the centre or north has already been examined (Chapter 3).

International comparison is further complicated by the fact that mortality is influenced to a certain degree by effectiveness of treatment and hence the death rate for a cancer of equal incidence may be different from one country to another. However, we believe that such differences are not likely to be sufficiently great to materially influence the appearance of the maps.

Following the description of the patterns for each site, comments are presented on the known causes of the respective cancer, and, where possible, on how they may relate to the pattern observed. As many cancers have several component causes, it may not be possible to 'explain' more than a proportion of the tumours seen. These comments are not meant to be exhaustive, with review papers frequently cited rather than original articles. When possible, recent research undertaken in the EEC is described.

At the conclusion of each section, a series of diagrams illustrates (*a*) the range of mortality rates present in each country and (*b*) the age-specific mortality rates for each sex in each of the countries mapped, plus the aggregate of all the countries. The former data are presented as 'box-and-whisker' plots (Tukey, 1977), with the exception of Luxembourg, where asterisks are used to denote the values recorded in the three areas, respectively. The box denotes the inter-quartile range, with a further mark towards the centre of the box indicating the median rate. Observations denoted by an asterisk are deemed to be extreme values, being more than 1.5 times the inter-quartile range outside the box, and observations denoted by a circle are more than 3.0 times the inter-quartile range outside the box.

Ill-defined and secondary sites: *ICD-8 195–199* (Maps 3 and 4)

This pair of maps is, from the point of view of interpretation of data, one of the most important in the atlas, showing clearly that there is a greater degree of imprecision in death certificates mentioning cancer in France than in other countries. The fact that considerable numbers of deaths ascribed to cancer—up to 10% of the total—did not have the site of origin mentioned means that the rates for other specified sites are likely to be underestimated but the degree of underestimation is likely to vary from site to site. On this criterion, the best quality data are to be found in the British Isles, Denmark, the Netherlands and parts of Italy.

The mortality from these cancers ranged from 23.3 in Ile de France to 6.2 in Denmark in males, and from 13.9 again in Ile de France to 5.1 in Wales in females.

Cancer of ill-defined and secondary sites accounted for 6.8% and 7.5% of all cancers in the USA, for 10.4% and 8.8% in Japan and for 4.1% and 4.5% in Australia in males and females respectively.

Ill-defined and secondary sites: ICD-8 195-199

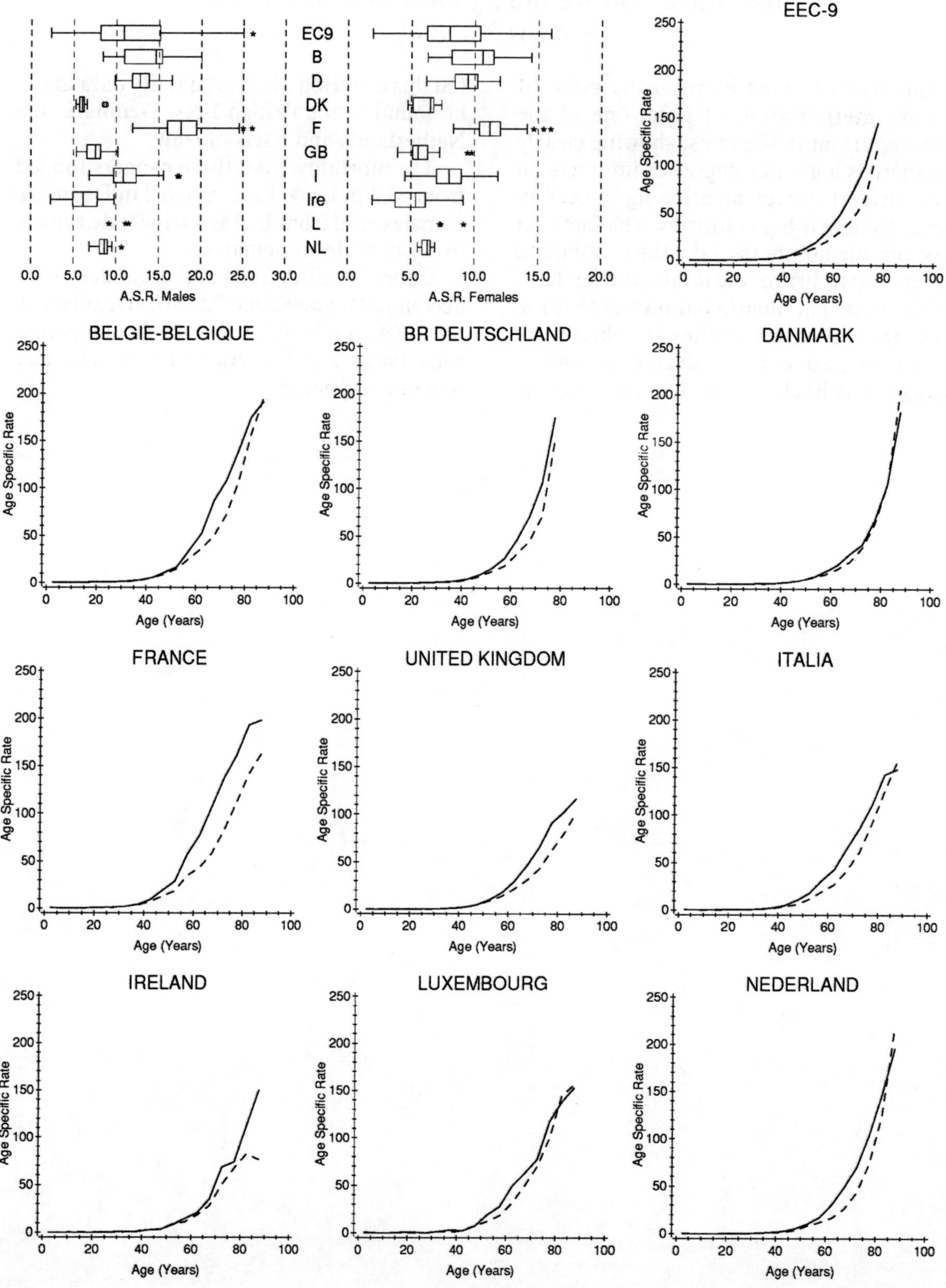

Oral cavity: *ICD-8 140–149* (M6.5, F1.0: M3.5%, F0.9%) (Maps 5 and 6)

The outstanding feature of the map depicting mortality from cancer of these sites in males is the higher levels of mortality in France in general, with concentrations of excess in the north-west and north-east of the country.

The distribution of areas of high cancer risk for sites 140–149 combined, shows that within the north-east of France, there is a differential distribution of buccal cavity and pharyngeal tumours. While the higher mortality rates in France end abruptly at the Belgian and German borders (the risk in the latter countries being around one third of that in France), this phenomenon is not seen in the south, with rates in south-east France and in the north of Italy being at similar levels. This finding suggests that there are likely to be comparable exposures in the south, whereas exposures and/or protective agents may be different in the north. In Ireland, Great Britain, northern Belgium, northern Germany and Denmark, most rates are below average. The gradual fall in mortality from north to central and from central to south Italy is readily discernible.

In females, the highest rates are clearly concentrated in Ireland, with above-average levels in central Scotland, central and south-east England. In looking at the map for females, one must bear in mind that the range of mortality rates is very much narrower than that in males, and hence in contrast to males, a false impression of important differences in level of mortality is obtained.

Within the EEC, the range in mortality is from 21.5 in Bretagne to 1.9 in Munster (an 11-fold range) in males, there being much less of a difference in females, in whom mortality ranges from 2.4 in south-east England to 0.7 in the Netherlands.

In the USA, these cancers represented 2.8% of cancer mortality in males and 1.4% in females; in Japan 1.2% and 0.2% and in Australia 2.4% and 1.4% respectively.

Comment

Broad groupings of intra-oral sites may obscure important differences in etiological factors, but several important risk factors have been clearly established (Boyle *et al.*, 1990).

Lip cancer. Risk of lip cancer has generally been found to be increased by smoking cigarettes and pipes, especially the latter. Risk is also consistently found to be increased among those involved in outdoor occupations and highest in the lower socio-economic status groups. Together with eye (uveal) cancer, this is the only form of cancer whose incidence rate is consistently higher in rural than in urban populations in most cancer registration areas where separate rates are provided (Muir *et al.*, 1987).

Tongue cancer, mouth cancer and pharyngeal cancer have been combined in the majority of analytical studies. These are important forms of cancer with incidence and mortality rates rising among younger persons in many parts of the world (Boyle *et al.*, 1990). Cigarette smoking and alcohol consumption have been found to be independent risk factors for oral cancer; their combined effects seem to be multiplicative. After 5 or 10 years of smoking cessation, risk among non-smokers reduces to a level similar to that in lifelong non-smokers. Use of oral snuff (Winn *et al.*, 1981) and use of a fine homeground tobacco powder (Sankaranarayanan *et al.*, 1989) have been associated with an increased risk of oral cancer. Poor dental hygiene may be an independent contributory factor (Zheng *et al.*, 1990). Cancer risk is reduced by frequent consumption of fruits and vegetables (McLaughlin *et al.*, 1988; Zheng *et al.*, 1991).

Nasopharyngeal cancer has a different epidemiological pattern to the tumours of the mouth which have been discussed above. An association with Epstein-Barr virus infection has been suggested by a large number of ecological observations. Clinical progression of the disease is accompanied by increases in antibody levels and nucleic acid hybridization has shown the presence of EBV DNA in squamous epithelial cells, this latter observation being a strong argument against the virus being a passenger in the process of carcinogenesis. Cigarette smoking is not a major determinant of risk (Boyle *et al.*, 1990). Results from China and Hong Kong indicate increased risks of nasopharyngeal cancer linked to consumption of salted fish, notably in childhood, preserved foods and fermented foods (Yu *et al.*, 1989).

Salivary gland cancer is rare, but the effect of radiation is apparent at all doses ranging from those received from exposure to atmospheric explosions of nuclear devices (Takeichi *et al.*, 1983) to those incurred during diagnostic radiation in the recent past (Preston-Martin *et al.*, 1988).

Oral cavity: ICD-8 140-149

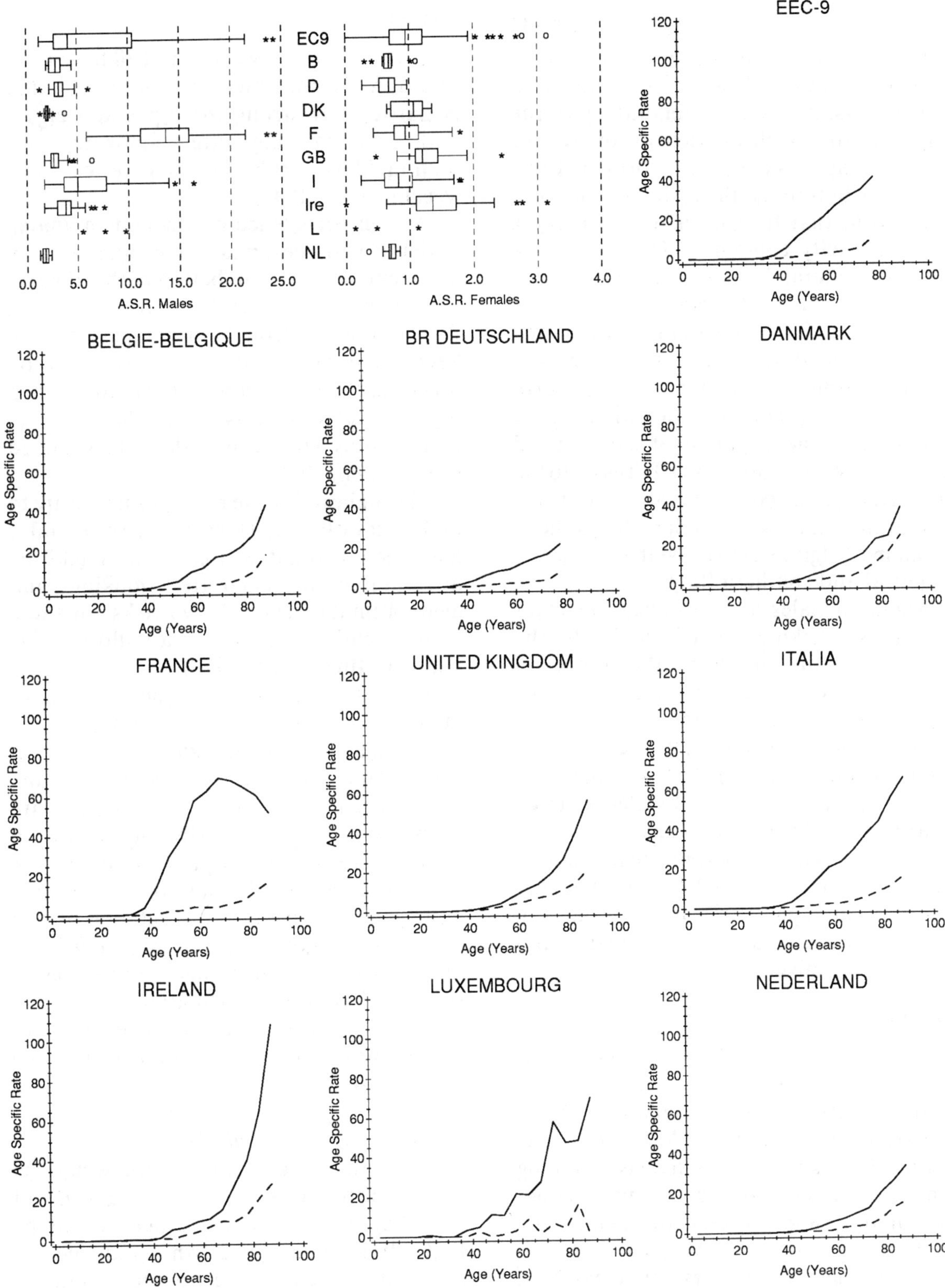

Oesophagus: *ICD-8 150* (M7.1, F1.4 : M3.8%, F1.3%) (Maps 7 and 8)

In males, the salient feature of the map is the concentration of high risk in northern French coastal regions, extending up to the Belgian border, with an extension of areas of above-average risk into the north of Italy. The distribution is thus similar but not identical to that for cancer of the pharynx and oral cavity combined. There is also a band of moderately increased risk passing across the centre of France between the Gironde and Switzerland, extending thereafter northwards along the Franco-German border. Mortality rates in the north and west of Scotland are somewhat higher than those for the remainder of Scotland and England & Wales, rates which fall close to the EEC average. In contrast, rates are below average in Denmark, the Federal Republic of Germany, Belgium and the Netherlands and in central and southern Italy.

Among females, the oesophageal cancer map bears a striking similarity to that for the oral cavity and pharynx, the range of mortality rates for the oesophagus being, however, three times greater.

The highest levels in males were seen in Basse-Normandie (32.3), the lowest in Puglia (1.6), comparable figures in females being 4.5 in Munster and 0.4 in Sardegna.

In the USA, oesophageal cancer accounted for 2.6% and 1.1% of all cancer mortality, in Japan 6.7% and 1.6% and in Australia 2.6% and 1.9% for males and females respectively.

Comment

The most important risk factors for cancer of the oesophagus in developed countries are tobacco smoking (IARC, 1986a) and alcohol intake (IARC, 1988). The risk has been shown to be increased among non-cigarette smokers by consuming alcohol and among non-drinkers of alcohol by smoking cigarettes (La Vecchia & Negri, 1989). In heavy smokers of cigarettes, relative risks of between 5 and 10 have been found. As for the oral cavity, the association is particularly strong for pipes and cigars and, among cigarette smokers, for high-tar/dark tobacco cigarettes (La Vecchia *et al.*, 1991).

A high prevalence of alcoholism among patients with oesophageal cancer and an apparent association between the disease and employment in the production and distribution of alcoholic beverages has long been noted. The role of alcohol consumption was most clearly demonstrated in the French *département* of Ille-et-Vilaine, where the risk rose steadily with dose of alcohol consumed (Tuyns *et al.*, 1977).

The highest disease rates in Europe are to be found in France (Levi *et al.*, 1989) and it has been estimated that 85% could be attributable to cigarette smoking and alcohol intake. The relative risks for these factors tend to combine in a multiplicative manner (Tuyns *et al.*, 1977).

Besides alcohol and tobacco, other factors involved in the etiology of oesophageal cancer include thermal irritation and foodstuffs contamination. Generalized dietary deficiencies are probably a major contributing factor in areas where the diet is poor in vitamins A and C and several other micronutrients and, more generally, fruits and vegetables or rich in maize (Franceschi *et al.*, 1990). A high-maize diet can induce deficiencies of several micronutrients (thiamine, riboflavin and particularly niacin). The risk of oesophageal cancer is also increased among individuals with Barrett's oesophagus (a chronic peptic ulcer of the lower oesophagus) (Levi *et al.*, 1990).

It seems unlikely that there would be major differences in the diagnosis of oesophageal or oral cavity cancer within the EEC. If anything, given the frequency of unspecified site death certificates in France, the mortality rates may be slightly underestimated in that country.

For these cancers the following questions thus need to be answered:

— Is there a sufficient difference in the pattern of alcohol/tobacco consumption between Belgium and the Federal Republic of Germany and France to account for the highly significant and abrupt fall at the French border?

— If not, are there differences in the consumption of protective foods?

— Are the very high rates in the north, west and north-east of France due to the consumption of spirits, the lower risks in the centre and south of France and the north of Italy being linked with wine or do they reflect total ethanol intake?

The completely different pattern in females has already been mentioned. The risk factors for cancers of the upper third of the oesophagus are known to include sideropenic dysphagia. While this lesion may have been common in parts of Scotland (Paterson, 1919) as well as in Sweden (Wynder *et al.*, 1957) some forty to fifty years ago, it is probably now much less prevalent, but the incidence of oesophageal cancer is known to be rapidly increasing in younger people in Scotland (Kemp *et al.*, 1985). The male:female sex ratio here is about two to one, in contrast to the level of twenty-five to one in France. These findings again emphasize the need for multi-centre case–control studies to ascertain how much of the increase in these cancer sites can be attributed to tobacco and alcohol habits, previously uncommon in females, and how much to other factors.

Oesophagus: ICD-8 150

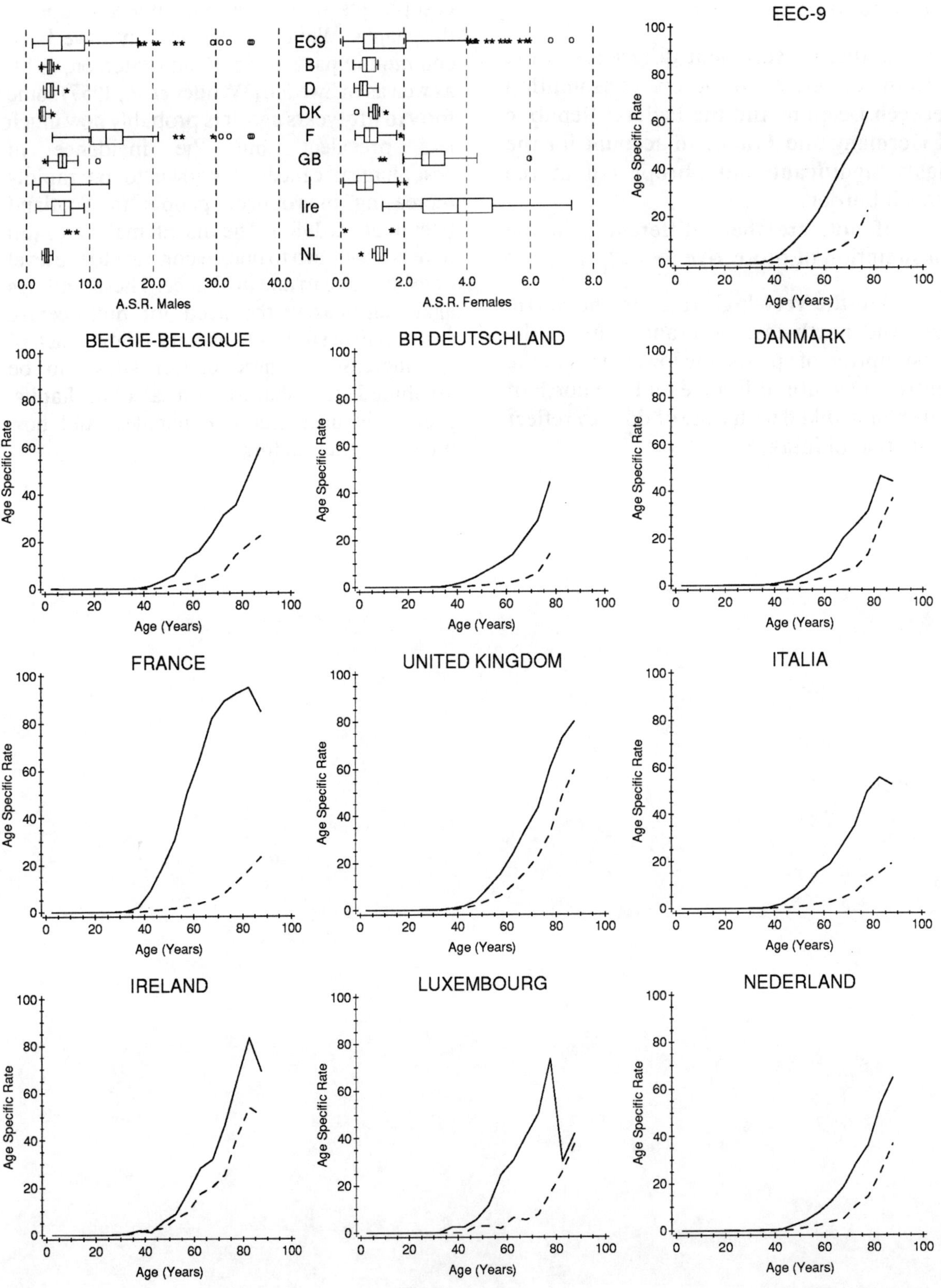

Stomach: *ICD-8 151* (M19.3, F9.3 : M10.4%, F8.4%) (Maps 9 and 10)

Although the mortality rate in males in any given area is normally double that in females, the pattern described below can be observed for both sexes.

There is a band of high and above-average incidence which runs from central Italy, Siena and Grosseto on the west, Macerata on the east which passes up through Emilia-Romagna to the Swiss border. Rates in Piemonte (Piedmont) and in those areas bordering Austria, although lower than elsewhere in the north of Italy, are still above average. This band of high incidence continues through Bayern, notably Oberpfalz and Niederbayern up to virtually the Danish border. In the south of Italy, rates are either average or below average, as in most of France, Great Britain, Ireland and Denmark. Within France the rates are much lower in the southern third of the country, notably from the eastern Pyrénées to the Italian border. The north-west of France shows above-average rates. Within Belgium the rates in the south are similar to those in neighbouring France, whereas rates in northern Belgium, southern Netherlands and Nordrhein-Westfalen and Rheinland-Pfalz and Luxembourg are much the same.

Within the EEC the range in mortality in males is from 36.8 in Lombardia to 10.8 in the Midi-Pyrénées, corresponding figures in females being 18.6 in Emilia Romagna and 5.0 in Midi-Pyrénées.

Gastric cancer was a much less common cause of cancer death in the USA (M3.8%, F 2.8%) than in Europe. In contrast, in Japan 33.7% of fatal cancers in males and 28.2% of those in females arose in the stomach. The proportions in Australia were 7.0% and 5.3% respectively.

Comment

The existence within Europe and within Italy of at least five-fold differences in risk calls for further investigation. Some fifty years ago stomach cancer was the leading cause of death from cancer in males and in the USA. Since then mortality and incidence have fallen virtually everywhere, even in high-risk Japan, but none the less this form of malignant disease remains the second commonest fatal cancer within the EEC countries (Jensen *et al.*, 1990). The reasons for this worldwide decline are not known, although it is suspected that the wider availability of fresh fruit and vegetables and better food preservation (for example, refrigeration rather than salting and pickling) may be responsible. Many studies have shown the risk of stomach cancer to be higher among members of the lower socio-economic classes. While this may be true within a country, the distribution of this disease within the EEC strongly suggests that other factors operate. Alcohol and tobacco seem to have have little influence on this particular cancer (IARC, 1988). The distribution of blood group A, known to carry a 10% greater risk, is not likely to vary sufficiently for this alone to influence mortality substantially.

Attention should thus be turned to investigation of diet, notably consumption of fresh fruit, the so-called green and yellow vegetables and milk. It seems paradoxical that in northern Italy (where fresh fruit and vegetables are likely to be much more readily available than in, say, England and Scotland), the risks should be so much higher. In a study of the role of diet and gastric cancer in this region, La Vecchia *et al.* (1987) found that green vegetables had a protective role, with the risk being three times greater in low consumers than in high consumers. Risk was increased in those consuming polenta (a maize porridge) and cured ham. Buiatti *et al.* (1990) confirmed the association with fruit intake and also demonstrated a possible protective effect for consumption of vegetables such as garlic belonging to the allium family.

Studies of occupational mortality for both Scotland and England & Wales have shown excess risk of stomach cancer in workers exposed to chemicals and metals. The excess risk is not necessarily due to exposure at the workplace, as these individuals may take less fresh fruit and vegetables than others. The risk of stomach cancer has been reported as being elevated among atomic bomb survivors (Shimizu *et al.*, 1987), especially for those individuals exposed at ages of less than twenty years (Preston *et al.*, 1986), and among persons treated for ankylosing spondylitis (Smith & Doll, 1982).

Stomach: ICD-8 151

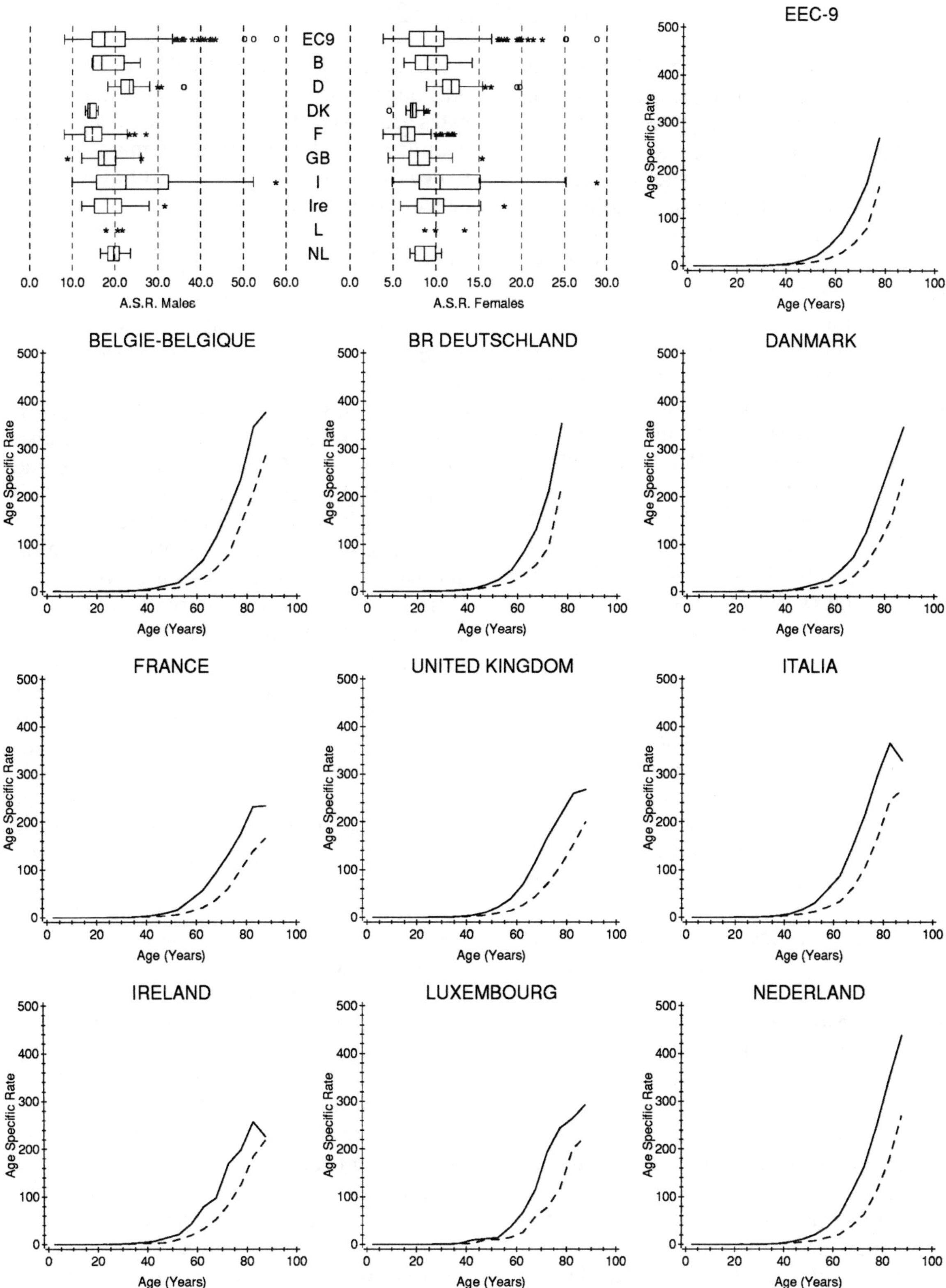

Colon and rectum: *ICD-8 153, 154* (M20.2, F15.2 : M10.9%, F13.8%) (Maps 11 and 12)

As cancer of the large bowel frequently appears on death certificates, a diagnosis allocated by the ICD coding rules to ICD 153, that is the colon, and as there are frequently problems in distinguishing whether a cancer arose in the rectum (ICD 154), sigmoid colon (ICD 153) or recto-sigmoid (ICD 154.1), the editors have decided to combine these two sites. Mortality from colon cancer is normally much the same in males and females, while for cancer of the rectum mortality in males is usually double that for females. It is apparent from the maps that the pattern of geographical distribution in both sexes is substantially the same, with the highest rates being found in the north of Scotland and in a central belt which traverses Ireland from south-west to north-east (particularly noticeable in females). There is a zone of higher than average incidence in both sexes which extends from northern Bavaria through most of the Federal Republic of Germany, where rates tend to be somewhat higher in the west in females, the pattern being much less distinctive in males. Very high rates are also seen in females in eastern Denmark. In southern Belgium in both sexes, the mortality is about the same as in north-east France. However, particularly in females, in northern Belgium, rates are close to those in the southern part of the Netherlands and the contiguous areas of Germany. Within Italy, there are areas of increased mortality in Piemonte and parts of Toscana. The lowest rates for this disease are to be seen in southern Italy and Corse.

Within the EEC, the range in mortality is from 24.2 in Nordrhein-Westfalen to 7.5 in Corse in males, corresponding figures for females being 19.6 (Munster) and 7.1 (Corse).

The proportions of cancer mortality in the USA, Japan and Australia for males and females respectively were 11.6% and 13.4%, 7.8% and 9.7%, and 13.3% and 16.5%. Although the age-standardized mortality rates are lower, these cancers form a greater proportion of the total risk in females than in males due to the burden of alcohol/tobacco cancers in males.

Comment

Colorectal cancer is the third commonest form of cancer worldwide, with high incidence rates in Western Europe and North America. As for stomach cancer, there are up to five-fold differences in mortality between EEC countries, and also substantial differences within some countries (such as Scotland and Italy). Few specific risk factors of a non-dietary nature have been established; inflammatory bowel diseases and familial polyposis syndromes carry a high risk of colorectal cancer in affected individuals but account for only a small proportion of the overall incidence.

It has been fairly consistently found that energy intake is higher in cases of colorectal cancer than in the comparison group (Willett, 1989). Physically active individuals are likely to consume more energy but recent studies suggest that physical activity reduces colorectal cancer risk (Vena *et al.*, 1987; Slattery *et al.*, 1988). The available data, however, suggest a lack of association between obesity and colorectal cancer risk although this is difficult to study since weight loss may be a symptom of this disease. This positive effect of energy does not appear to be merely the result of overeating, therefore, and may reflect differences in metabolic efficiency. Thus individuals who utilize energy more efficiently may be at a lower risk of colorectal cancer.

Intake of dietary fat has been found to be positively related to colorectal cancer risk in ecological studies, animal experiments, case–control and cohort studies, However, many of these studies have failed to demonstrate that the association with fat intake is independent of energy intake.

Inconsistent results have been reported regarding the protective effect of dietary fibre. Most studies in humans have found no protective effect of fibre from cereals but have found a protective effect of fibre from vegetable and, perhaps, fruit sources (see Willett, 1989). This could reflect an association with other components of fruits and vegetables, with 'fibre' intake acting merely as an indicator of their consumption.

Positive associations with alcohol consumption have been reported, but it remains to be proven that the association is with alcohol *per se* and not with the calorie contribution of alcohol. Vitamin E, selenium and vitamin A and/or its precursor beta-carotene may be protective against colon tumours (Zaridze, 1983; Willett, 1989), and lactobacilli, found in some dairy products, may have a favourable effect on the intestine (Goldin & Gorbach, 1984). Eleven studies have indicated negative (protective) associations of coffee consumption with risk of colorectal cancer (IARC, 1991).

In summary, dietary factors are most probably the important determinants of colorectal cancer risk but methodological problems prevent an unequivocal interpretation of the epidemiological data. An effect for saturated fat appears to exist independently of energy intake, and vegetable fibre, directly or indirectly, appears to be protective, as does coffee consumption. Meat intake may also increase risk, but whether this is independent of its fat content or its contribution to calorie intake is unclear; if independent, the risk could be related to mutagenic products formed in the cooking process. Associations with other dietary factors remain open questions.

Colon and rectum: ICD-8 153+154

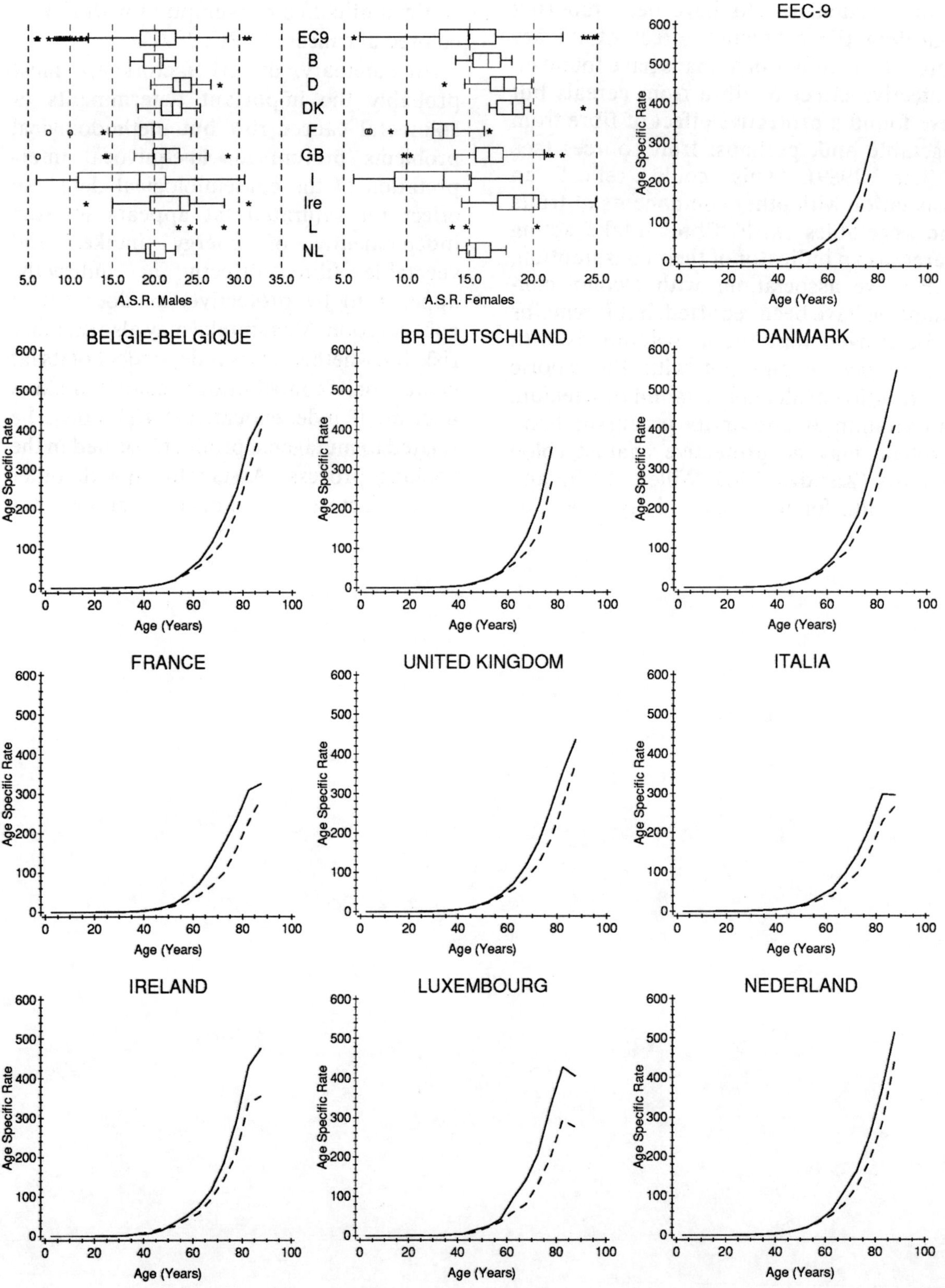

Gallbladder and bile ducts: *ICD-8 156* (M1.5, F2.4 : M0.8%, 2.2%) (Maps 13 and 14)

The distribution of gallbladder and bile duct cancer mortality in EEC-9 is quite unlike that for any other form of malignant disease, with a band of high rates in the centre of the Federal Republic of Germany, extending from south to north. This phenomenon is most clearly seen among females, in whom mortality is greater than among males. Mortality rates in contiguous areas also tend to be above average. The lowest values are found in the British Isles, south and west France and in southern Italy. ICD-8 rubric 156 includes not only the gallbladder cancers but also those arising in the bile ducts outside the liver. Unfortunately, these are not separated in the mortality data available to the editors. In general, the frequency of gallbladder cancer is about the same as that of bile duct cancers in males but double in females (Muir *et al.*, 1987).

In males the highest levels of gallbladder and bile duct cancer mortality were observed in Niedersachsen (3.1), the lowest in Sicilia (0.8): in females the highest levels were recorded in Rheinland-Pfalz (6.3), the lowest in Midi-Pyrénées (1.0).

These cancers accounted for 0.8% and 1.5% of all cancer mortality in the USA; in Japan 2.7% and 4.9% and in Australia 0.9% and 2.2% in males and females respectively.

Comment

The frequencies of gallbladder cancer and of gallstones tend to run in parallel. Thus the high risk of gallbladder cancer seen among American Indians is reflected in a spectrum of gallstone-related disease in this population. The distribution of gallstones shares many of the features of gallbladder cancer, including female predominance. Most epidemiological studies have examined the characteristics of patients with gallstones rather than the much rarer gallbladder cancer. There have been a few reports of an excess of gallbladder and bile duct tumours in workers in a rubber plant (Mancuso & Brennan, 1970; Krain, 1971) consistent with the ability of several chemicals, including those used in rubber processing, to produce such cancers in laboratory animals.

The striking geographical distribution of gallbladder and bile duct cancer within the EEC again offers opportunities for collaborative epidemiological studies.

Gallbladder and bile ducts: ICD-8 156

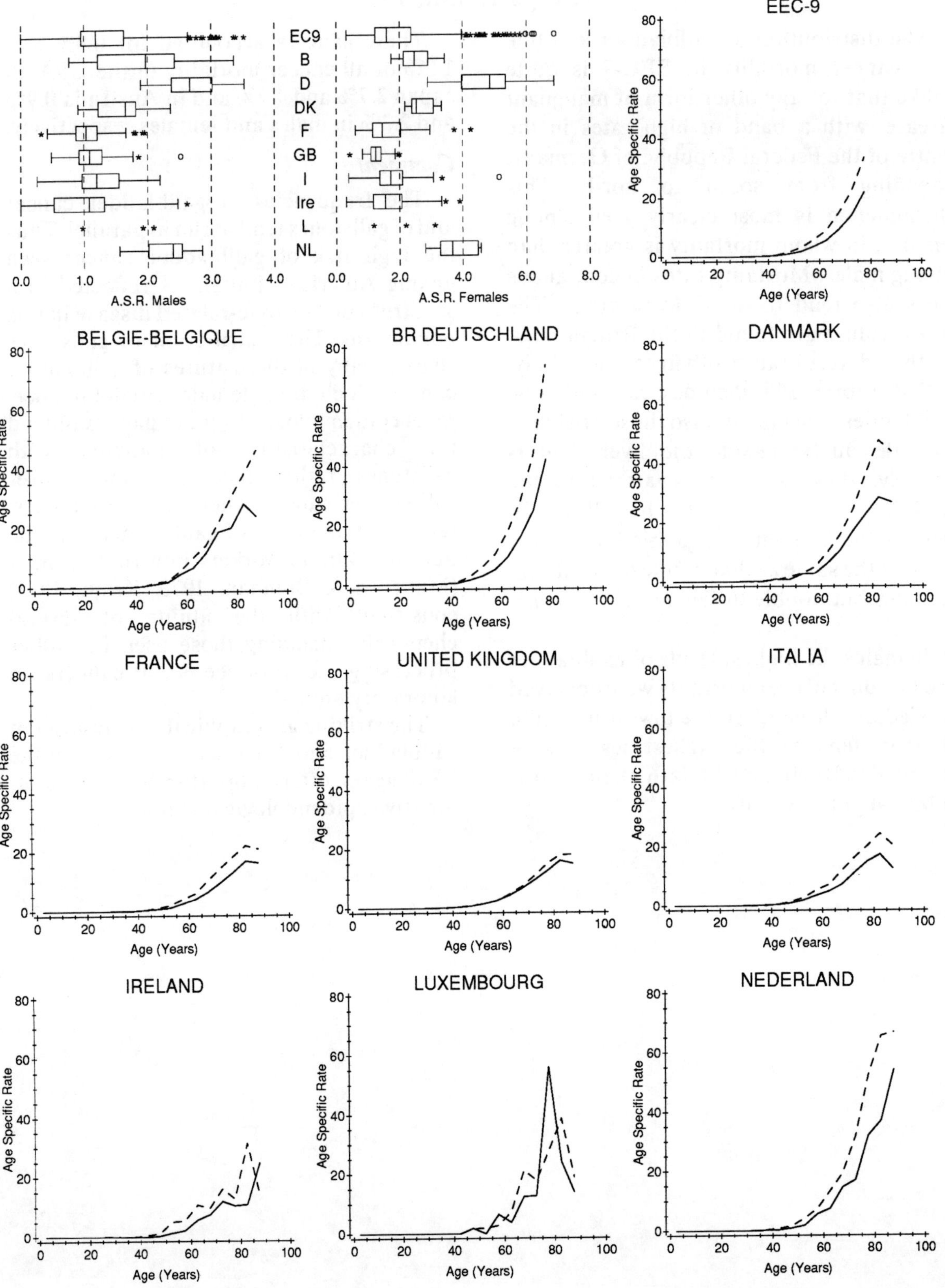

Pancreas: *ICD-8 157* (M7.2, F4.2 : M3.9%, F3.8%) (Maps 15 and 16)

The higher mortality rates for pancreatic cancer in both sexes are to be found in the British Isles and in Ireland. Within the British Isles the mortality tends to be higher, particularly in females, in the north of England and Scotland. This cancer is also fairly common in Denmark, The Netherlands and, in males, the north of Italy. Below average levels are generally observed in most of France and much of Italy.

In both males and females, the highest levels of mortality were observed in Denmark (9.4 and 6.4 respectively); the lowest in Campania (2.7 and 1.7 respectively).

Pancreas cancer mortality accounted for 5.2% and 5.4%, 4.4% and 4.2% and 5.0% and 4.8% of all cancers in males and females respectively in the USA, Japan and Australia.

Comment

The epidemiological study of pancreas cancer suffers seriously from problems of misdiagnosis, particularly underdiagnosis. Pancreas cancer is consistently reported to occur more frequently in men than in women, in blacks than in whites and in urban as compared to rural population groups. In some countries, mortality rates are rising whereas in others declining levels of disease can be seen among members of younger birth cohorts (Boyle *et al.*, 1989).

Analytical studies on patients with pancreas cancer consistently demonstrate that cigarette smoking increases the risk of pancreas cancer (IARC, 1986a) and this at present is the only clearly demonstrated risk factor.

It appears that dietary factors may have a significant role (Howe *et al.*, 1990) and there are now indications that a diet richer in cholesterol and carbohydrate and (perhaps) total energy is associated with elevated risk, while more frequent consumption of green vegetables may be protective. Although an association had been postulated with increased coffee consumption (MacMahon *et al.*, 1981), the overall evidence available does not support this relationship (IARC, 1991). There is minimal evidence linking alcohol consumption to an increased risk (Velema *et al.*, 1986).

Some aspects of medical history, in particular pancreatitis, diabetes and gastrectomy, may be associated with elevated pancreatic cancer risk, while allergies may be linked in some way to reduced risk (Boyle *et al.*, 1989).

Pancreas cancer is possibly related to ionizing radiation. The risk was found to be elevated in a cohort of patients with ankylosing spondylitis who were treated with radiation (Smith & Doll, 1982) and in women treated by radiotherapy for cancer of the cervix (Boice *et al.*, 1985). However, apparent increases reported earlier among atomic bomb survivors (Kato & Schull, 1982) and in workers in the nuclear industry (Gilbert & Marks, 1979) were not confirmed by later observations based on a longer period of follow-up (Tolley *et al.*, 1983; Shimizu *et al.*, 1987).

The associations of pancreas cancer risk with a number of other factors, including occupational exposures, require clarification (Boyle *et al.*, 1989).

Pancreas: ICD-8 157

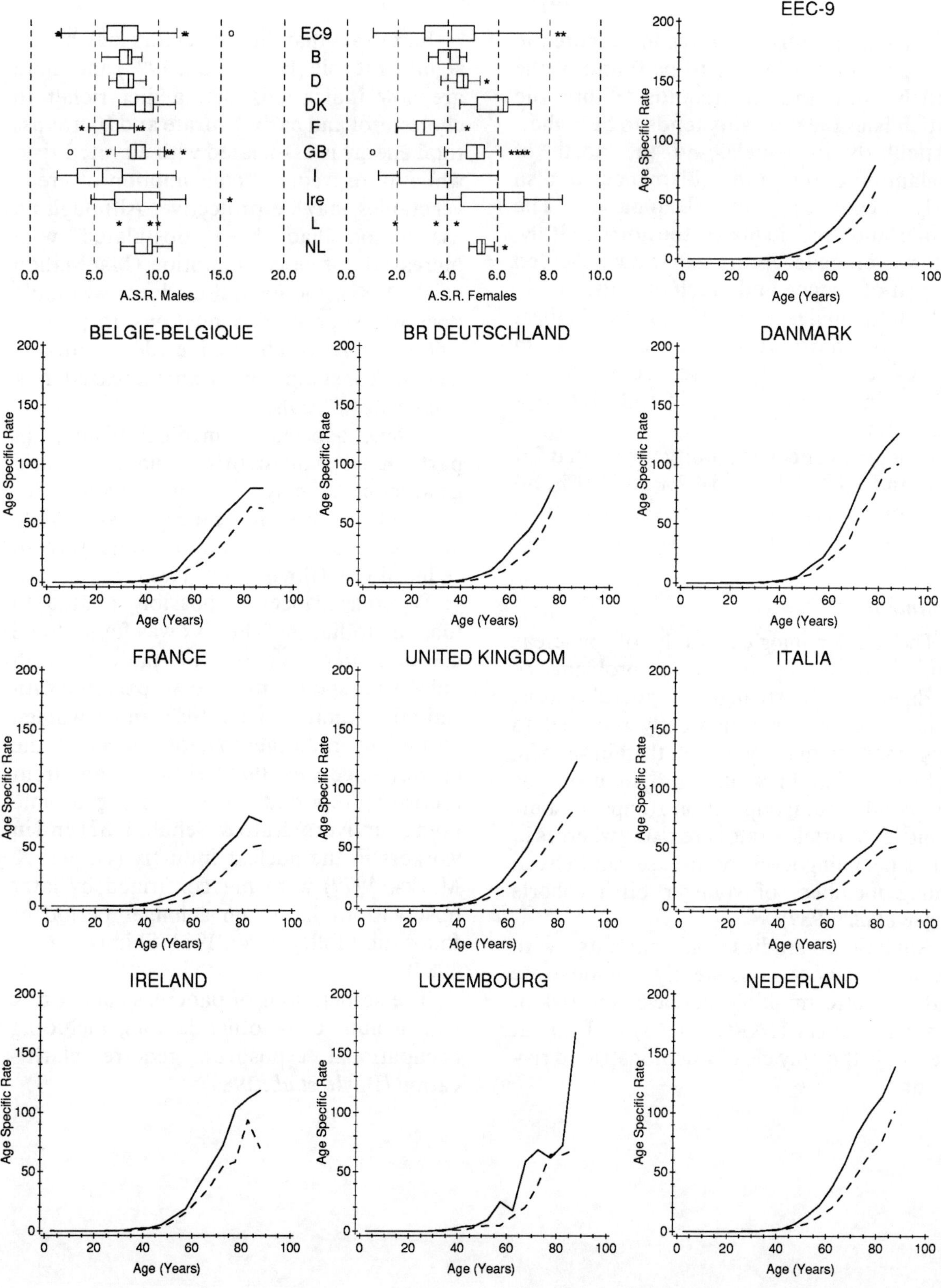

Larynx: *ICD-8 161* (M5.6, F0.3 : M3.0%, F0.3%) (Maps 17 and 18)

The map for laryngeal cancer resembles that for oral cavity cancer, with very high rates in France and parts of the north of Italy, levels being much lower in the British Isles and Denmark. Average or below average values are observed in most of the Federal Republic of Germany and Italy. The picture for females is rather different, with isolated areas of high incidence in northern Denmark, the Federal Republic of Germany, the Netherlands and in central Italy. In the vast majority of areas rates in females are very low.

Within the EEC, the range of mortality in males is between 15.7 in Bretagne and 1.2 in East Anglia, or 13-fold, there being a very much smaller difference in females with mortality ranging from 0.6 in Ile de France to 0.2 in Bayern (some even lower mortality rates were based on very small numbers).

In the USA, Japan and Australia, laryngeal cancers accounted for 1.4% and 0.3%, 0.9% and 0.1%, and 1.5% and 0.3% of cancer mortality in males and females respectively.

Comment

Tobacco smoking (IARC, 1986a) and alcohol consumption (IARC, 1988) are the major established risk factors for laryngeal cancer, as for other upper aerodigestive tract neoplasms. That the relationship between cigarette smoking and laryngeal cancer risk is causal is strongly suggested by the magnitude of the relative risk estimates. There are, however, some quantitative differences in the association with other upper digestive tract cancers, since cancer of the larynx, and particularly the endolarynx, is less strongly associated with alcohol and more strongly with tobacco than that of the oral cavity or oesophagus (Tuyns *et al.*, 1988). This is biologically reasonable since the endolarynx does not come into direct contact with alcohol. The relative risk from smoking was around 10 and black tobacco carried twice the risk of blond tobacco. Alcohol increased risk ten-fold for the hypopharynx and the epilarynx, the increase being smaller (2.5-fold) for the vocal cords. Most investigations have concluded that the combined risk of alcohol and tobacco consumption is multiplicative, or at least greater than additive (Flanders & Rothman, 1982). This further indicates the importance of intervention on at least one factor for subjects exposed to both habits.

Other factors may play an independent role in laryngeal carcinogenesis, such as occupational exposures, possibly including those involving contact with asbestos (Doll & Peto, 1985), and diet. The latter is indirectly suggested by the observation that social class indicators are strongly and inversely related to laryngeal cancer rates, and more directly by a few case–control studies showing that a diet poor in fresh fruit, vegetables and vitamins A and C is associated with higher risk of laryngeal cancer (Graham *et al.*, 1981; De Stefani *et al.*, 1987).

Larynx: ICD-8 161

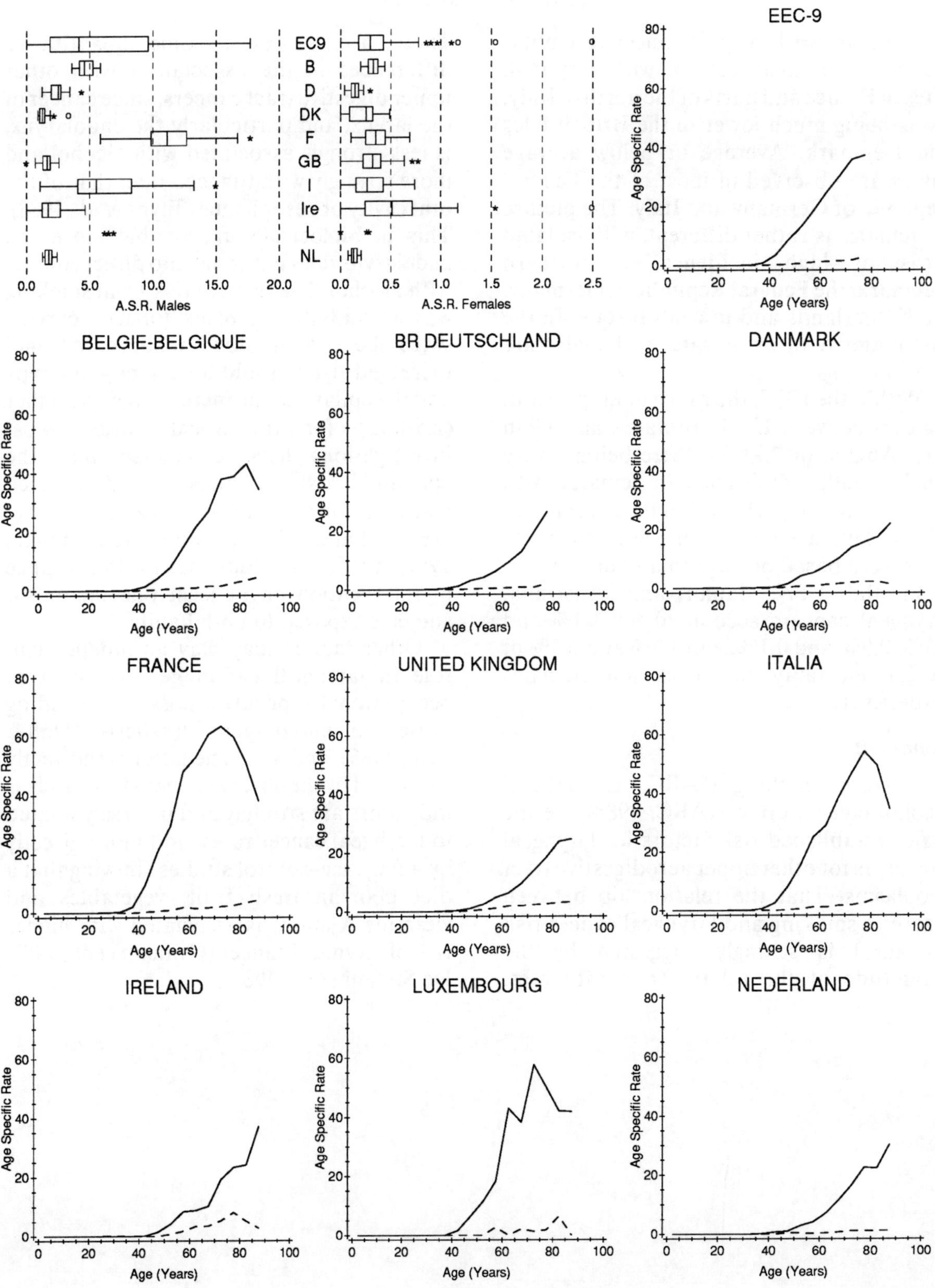

Lung: *ICD-8 162* (M53.5, F7.8 : M28.5%, F7.1%) (Maps 19 and 20)

In males, the highest rates are seen in central and north-east England and central and western Scotland, southern Belgium and western Holland. A group of above-average rates is observed in northern Italy, spreading out from Venice. In the Federal Republic of Germany, France, central and southern Italy, and most of Ireland, rates are either average, below average or low. The map for females is rather different, with all rates in Great Britain being above average, those in southern and central Scotland and around Newcastle, London and Liverpool being very high. In Ire- land rates are again above average, with a concentration of risk in those areas facing the Irish sea. The excess rates seen in males in Belgium and the Netherlands are not observed in women. In Denmark, female rates are above average, being somewhat higher in Copenhagen.

Within the EEC, the mortality from lung cancer ranges from 87.0 in northern England to 20.2 in Basilicata in males and between 20.1 in Scotland and 2.5 in Basilicata in females.

In the USA, Japan and Australia lung cancer represented 33.2% and 14.2%, 15.1% and 7.4% and 29.1% and 9.1% of all cancer mortality in males and females respectively.

Comment

The overwhelming role of tobacco smoking in the causation of lung cancer has been repeatedly demonstrated over the past 50 years (IARC, 1986a). Current lung cancer rates do not necessarily reflect current smoking patterns, since there is an interval of several decades between a change in smoking habits in a population and its consequences on lung cancer rates. Lung cancer rates in self-reported non-smokers from various studies are of the order of 10 to 15 per 100 000. Estimates of the proportions of lung cancer deaths attributable to tobacco smoking in five developed countries (Canada, England and Wales, Japan, Sweden and the USA) ranged between 83% and 92% for males, and 57% and 80% for females (IARC, 1986a).

In males of all European countries, except Portugal, lung cancer is now the leading cause of cancer death. In the USA in both sexes, and in all except a few Scandinavian countries, it is the commonest tumour in terms of incidence as well. The range of geographical variation in lung cancer mortality in Europe is three-fold in both sexes, the highest rates being observed in the United Kingdom, Belgium, the Netherlands and Czechoslovakia, and lowest rates reported in southern Europe but also Norway and Sweden in both sexes (Levi *et al.*, 1989). Because some countries which are now in the lower part of the distribution (such as southern European ones) experienced a later uptake and spread of tobacco use, the elevated rates in younger age groups suggest that these countries will have the highest lung cancer rates in males at the beginning of the next century, in the absence of rapid and adequate intervention. Conversely, lung cancer rates are comparatively low in Scandinavian countries which have adopted, since the early 1970s, integrated policies and programmes against smoking, possibly as a consequence of the limited influence of the tobacco lobby in these countries.

One of the major determinants of tobacco consumption (at least in the short term) is the price of cigarettes. The ratio of price to per capita gross national product shows a difference of more than a factor of seven between the highest (Ireland) and the lowest (France) value, and the countries in the upper part of the distribution (i.e., where cigarettes are relatively expensive) are those now showing lower lung cancer rates in the young.

Among women, rates in most European countries (except Britain and Ireland) are still substantially lower than in the USA, where lung cancer is now the leading cause of cancer death in females. In several countries, including France, Switzerland, Germany and Italy, where smoking is becoming commoner in younger and middle-aged women, upward trends in lung cancer mortality have been registered over the last two decades. The facts that lung cancer is still relatively rare in females and that smoking accounts for a smaller proportion of all lung cancers than in males cannot constitute a reason for delaying interventions against smoking specifically targeted at women.

A proportion of lung cancers that varies across countries and geographical areas may be due to exposures at work, and a small proportion to atmospheric pollution. There are, however, good reasons to believe that the effect of atmospheric pollution in increasing lung cancer risk is chiefly confined to smokers.

Lung cancer risk is elevated in atomic bomb survivors (Shimizu *et al.*, 1987), patients treated for ankylosing spondylitis (Smith & Doll, 1982) and in underground miners whose bronchial mucosa was exposed to radon gas and its decay products (IARC, 1988). A greater risk of lung cancer is generally seen for individuals who are exposed at an older age. Investigations of the interaction with cigarette smoking among atomic bomb survivors suggest that it is additive (Kopecky *et al.*, 1986), but the data from underground miners in Colorado are consistent with a multiplicative effect (Whittemore & McMillan, 1983).

Lung: ICD-8 162

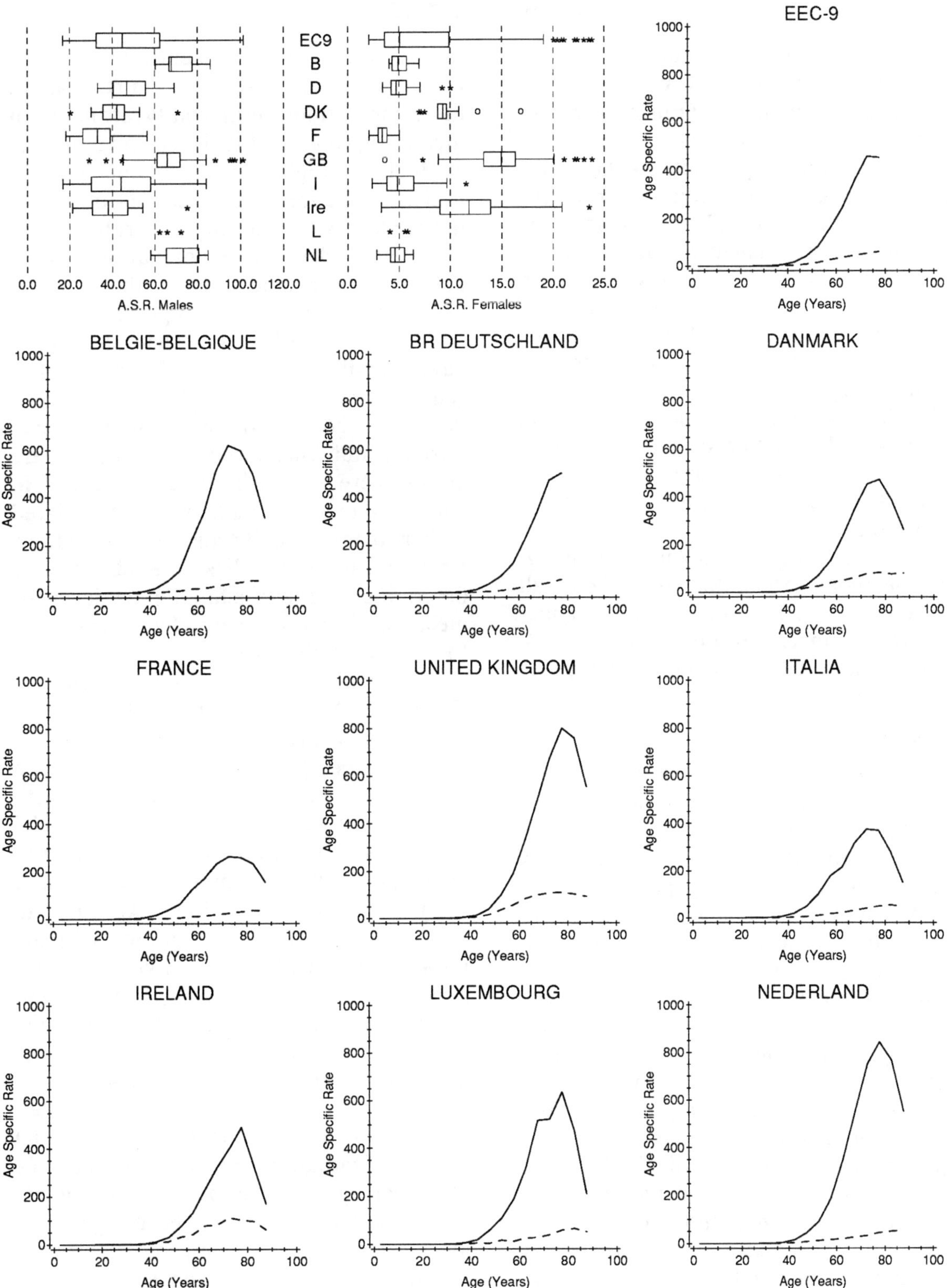

Malignant melanoma of the skin: *ICD-8 172* (M1.0, F0.9: M0.5%, F0.8%) (Maps 21 and 22)

In males there is a quite distinctive pattern of average and below average rates of malignant melanoma in France, southern and central Italy, increasing gradually from northern Italy through southern Germany into Denmark and extending over to the Netherlands. In Scotland, rates tend to be higher in the north than in the south, whereas in Ireland rates are generally higher in coastal areas. In females much the same pattern is noted, although several of the highest rates are to be seen in west Wales and southern England.

The highest levels in males were seen in Denmark (2.1), the lowest in Ile de France (0.6), corresponding figures for females being 1.8 for Denmark and 0.4 for Provence-Alpes-Côte-d'Azur.

In the USA, Japan and Australia malignant melanoma accounted for 2.1% of all male deaths and 1.3% of all female cancer deaths of all cancer mortality, 0.2% and 0.1% and 4.1% and 2.3% in males and females respectively.

Comment

Although cutaneous malignant melanoma is still a relatively rare neoplasm in many populations, incidence rates are increasing around the world. This increase is often of the order of 5% per annum in fair-skinned populations. Because exposure to sunlight is clearly a major cause of the disease in susceptible populations, these trends may be further exacerbated by the postulated depletion of the stratospheric ozone layer. Thus, melanoma is one form of cancer which will become very important in public health terms in coming decades in the absence of effective intervention today. Exposure to strong sunlight in childhood or early adolescence seems to confer a greater risk than exposure in adulthood.

Melanoma is essentially a disease of fair-skinned individuals, among whom the tumour occurs most frequently on the trunk in males and the lower limbs in females. In these populations the mortality rate has been increasing steadily. Incidence and mortality are higher in higher socio-economic groups.

The incidence rate varies 100-fold internationally, with the highest rates being reported in Australian populations, particularly Queensland where the rate is approaching 40 per 100 000 per annum.

Melanoma has been known for decades to have a familial component; blue eyes, fair or red hair and a pale complexion have been demonstrated to increase risk of melanoma. Further, individuals who sunburn easily are at an increased risk. Freckles, either in childhood or as an adult, are also associated with increased risk. Because these traits also tend to run in families it is difficult to determine whether the familial tendency for melanoma is due to genetic characteristics or to the related risk factors.

Investigations in Australia and Denmark (Holman & Armstrong, 1984a,b; Østerlind *et al.*, 1988a,b,c,d) have shown that the presence of palpable naevi on the arms is a good indicator of subsequent risk, those with ten or more such moles having risks 11.3 times greater than those without. A variety of other possibly contributory factors have been suggested, including exposure to fluorescent lighting, consumption of polyunsaturated fats, use of oral contraceptive pills, etc. (Gallagher, 1986). Austin and Reynolds (1986) observed that occupational cohorts engaged in a variety of technologically advanced industries show excesses of malignant melanoma, notably those exposed to unusual chemicals or unusual sources of radiation. However, such persons often belong to the upper socio-economic classes, which are known to be at higher risk and possibly more likely to engage in intermittent leisure sun exposure.

Malignant melanoma of the skin: ICD-8 172

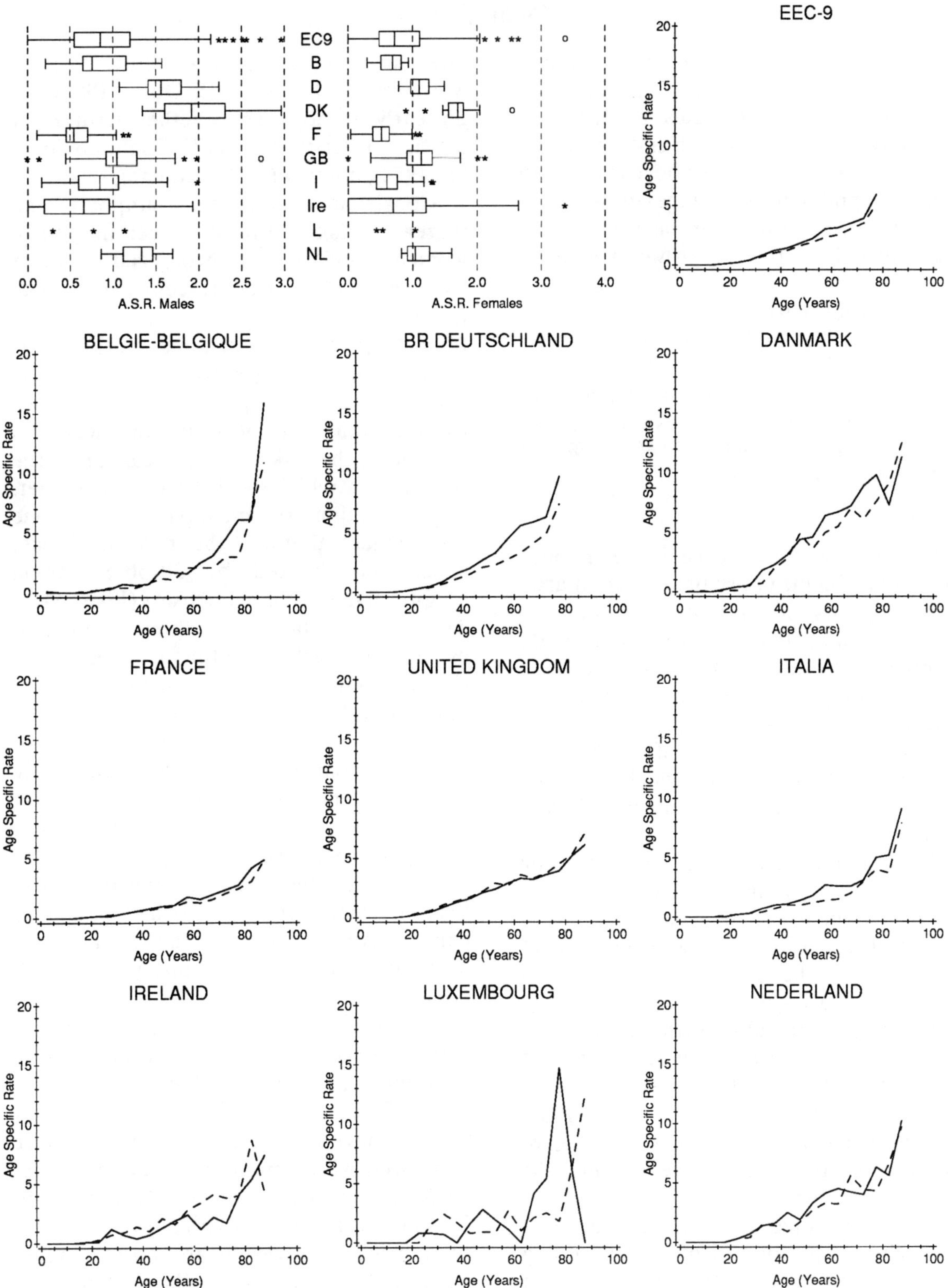

Breast: *ICD-8 174* (M0.3, F21.8: M0.2%, F19.8%) (Map 23)

The distribution of female breast cancer mortality shows a clear north–south gradient. The highest rates are seen in eastern Ireland and southern and south-east England, being somewhat above average in Denmark and below average in southern Italy. In general, except in the British Isles and Italy, risk tends to be fairly even within a given country.

The mortality from male breast cancer is negligible. The highest mortality levels recorded in females were 29.0 in the East Midlands, the lowest 9.6 in Basilicata.

In the USA, Japan and Australia, female breast cancer accounted for 22.5%, 5.1% and 20.5% of fatal cancer.

Comment

Breast cancer incidence is about 30% higher in residents of urban areas compared to rural population groups and similarly elevated among black compared to white members of the same community (Muir *et al.*, 1987). Although a large proportion of breast cancer seems to be related to environmental or life-style factors and, therefore, theoretically avoidable, the factors which influence breast cancer risk are not yet obvious (Boyle, 1988).

The risk of breast cancer is increased by around 50% in nulliparous compared to parous women. Risk increases with increasing age at first birth until a first birth occurring after the age of (approximately) 35 years carries a higher risk than nulliparity, indicating that first childbirth after this age no longer confers protection against breast cancer (MacMahon & Pugh, 1970; Ewertz *et al.*, 1990). Trichopoulos *et al.* (1983) estimated that a 3.5% increase in relative risk is associated with every year of increase in age at first birth.

Proposed protective effects of late age at menarche, of parity and of breast-feeding remain controversial. Risk is increased by a late age at menopause (Bucalossi & Veronesi, 1959; ; Ewertz & Duffy, 1988) and an early menopause, whether natural or artificial (Herity *et al.*, 1975; Trichopoulos *et al.*, 1972), contributes to reducing risk.

Consistent evidence supports an increased risk of breast cancer in 'young' women associated with prolonged use (over five years) of oral contraceptives; 'young' implies less than 35 years and perhaps less than 45 (Prentice & Thomas, 1987). Fortunately, at these ages breast cancer risk is very low and there appears to be no evidence to date that use of oral contraceptives influences the risk of breast cancer at the older ages at which the disease is commoner.

In relation to menopausal hormone replacement therapy, the risk for breast cancer is elevated by 30–50% among long-term (i.e., 5–10 years) users (Pike, 1987). The few data extant on combined estrogen-progestin treatment suggest that the risk may be greater than for estrogens alone (Bergkvist *et al.*, 1989).

Although an anti-estrogenic effect of cigarettes (Baron, 1984) could theoretically lead to some protection against breast cancer, the majority of published studies have given negative results (Ewertz, 1990). Radiation to the breast in high doses has been shown to increase the risk of mammary cancer; exposure around the menarche is associated with a particularly high risk (Boice & Stone, 1978).

The risk of breast cancer appears to rise with increasing body mass index among postmenopausal women (de Waard *et al.*, 1964). Former college athletes have been found to have a reduced risk of breast cancer compared with non-athletes (Frisch *et al.*, 1985), as have ballet dancers (Warren, 1980). This may be associated with physical activity or reduced body weight around menarche, early adolescence or throughout lifetime.

The association with diet, particularly fat intake, is the subject of much research and debate (Willett, 1989). Although an association between risk of breast cancer and saturated fat intake in postmenopausal women is biologically plausible (Boyle & Leake, 1988), the evidence from studies in human subjects with breast cancer is contradictory. Studies in Greece (Katsouyanni *et al.*, 1986) and Italy (La Vecchia *et al.*, 1987) have suggested that green vegetable consumption is an indicator of a low-risk dietary pattern. This may simply reflect low intake of fat or calories, or suggest that some constituent of green vegetables is protective (Minchovicz & Bradlow, 1990). A modest increase in risk of breast cancer with increased alcohol intake has been observed consistently in a large number of studies (Willett *et al.*, 1987; Longnecker *et al.*, 1988).

Of the other factors for breast cancer studied, a positive family history has the effect of increasing the risk of breast cancer (Macklin, 1959), with the maximum effect apparent in premenopausal women who have a first-degree relative with breast cancer at premenopausal ages.

Although probably becoming more homogeneous, diets still vary considerably within the EEC-9 countries, as do national patterns of fertility, age-at-first pregnancy, etc. The existence of a four-fold variation in risk of mortality within the EEC demands investigation. If the age of first full-term pregnancy is truly the major factor in Europe in the determination of risk for this cancer, then incidence of this form of malignancy is bound to increase, unless there are major advances in the success of early diagnosis or treatment.

Breast: ICD-8 174

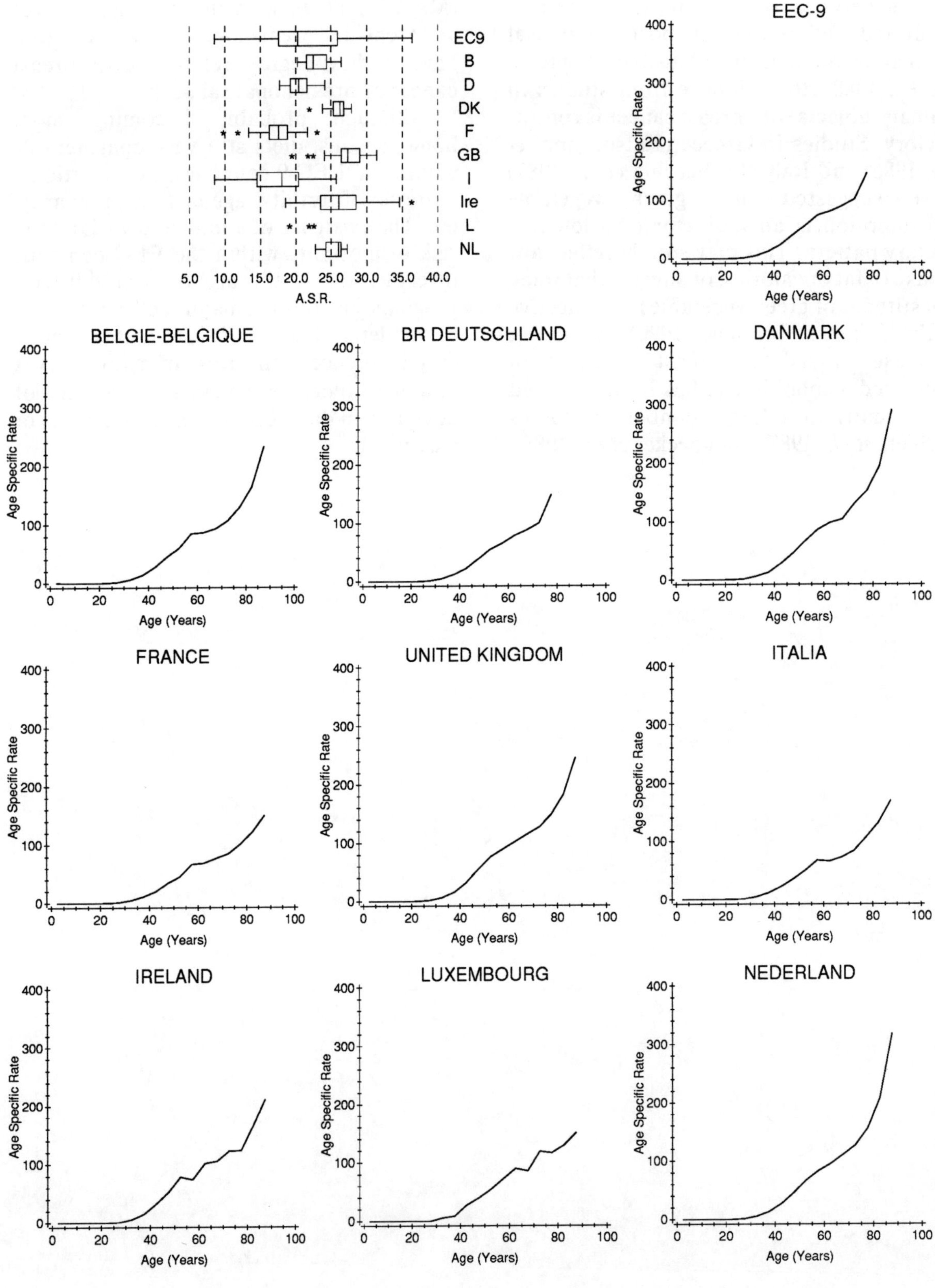

Ovary: *ICD-8 183* (F6.8 : 6.2%) (Map 24)

The distribution for ovary cancer generally resembles that for the breast, with high rates in the United Kingdom and Ireland, and several isolated areas in the highest category. The most notable feature of the map, however, is the strong concentration of high-risk regions in Denmark (where the highest rate in Europe (11.2) is seen), particularly in the eastern part of the country. Germany shows many more areas of above-average rate than on the breast cancer map. A clear north-south gradient is again seen across Europe, with low rates in much of France and Italy, and the lowest rates being recorded in Calabria (1.9).

In the USA, Japan and Australia, ovarian cancer accounted for 6.0%, 2.9% and 6.0% of all cancer deaths in females.

Comment

Epithelial ovarian cancer is the commonest type of ovarian neoplasm and the leading cause of death from gynaecological neoplasms in most western countries. As for other female hormone-related neoplasms, its age–incidence curve tends to flatten off around the age of menopause (Pike, 1987).

These cancers are more frequent in nulliparous than in parous women, with an approximately two-fold elevated risk compared to multiparous women. Increased risks for late age at first birth, early menarche and late menopause have not been found consistently.

Oral contraceptive use is protective, the incidence of invasive epithelial cancer being reduced by approximately 40% in women who have ever used oral contraceptives, and to a greater extent in long-term users (La Vecchia *et al.*, 1991b). Combined oral contraceptives have probably been the major determinant of the decrease in ovarian cancer rates observed in several western countries (Adami *et al.*, 1990).

As for breast and endometrial cancer, nutrition and diet remain major open questions in ovarian cancer epidemiology. Positive correlations with fat, protein and calorie intake are less strong than for endometrial cancer, and again some protection appears to be afforded by green vegetables (La Vecchia *et al.*, 1987). Much further research is required in this area, because diet may be more amenable to intervention than reproductive or menstrual history.

Ovary: ICD-8 183

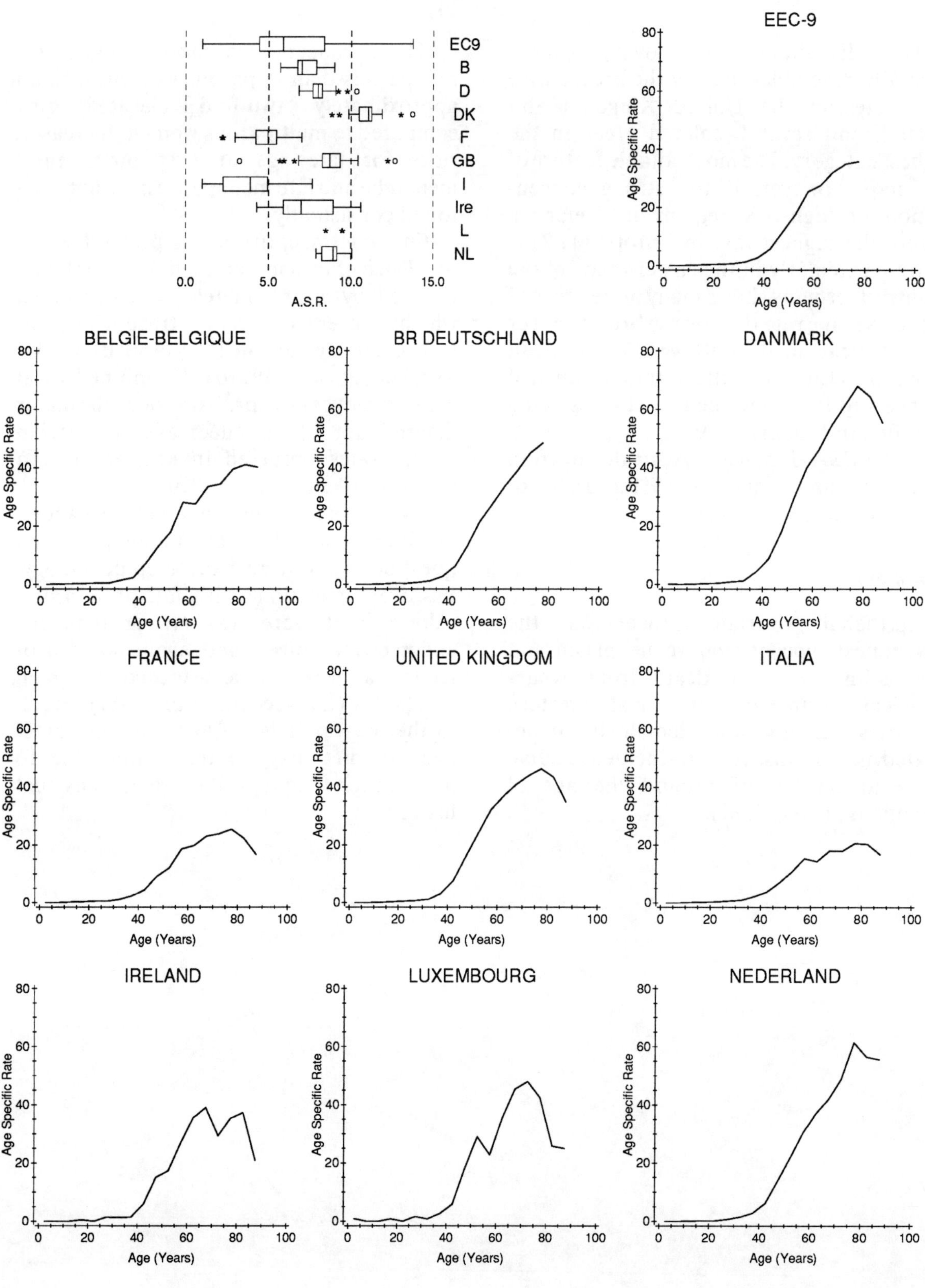

Uterus: *ICD-8 180+182* (F9.1 : F8.3%) (Maps 25 and 26)

Problems in the recording of cervix and corpus cancers on death certificates have been mentioned at the beginning of this chapter. Cervix cancer (ICD-8 180) may be written as 'uterine cancer' on a death certificate and will be coded to 'uterine cancer — not otherwise specified' and counted with cancer of the corpus uteri (ICD-8 182) at a three-digital level (Cuzick & Boyle, 1989; Whittemore & Gong, 1991). The extent of this practice undoubtedly varies between countries, but it is very unlikely that it could, on its own, explain the ten-fold variation seen across Europe. In interpreting the map of cervix cancer, it should therefore be borne in mind that the rates represent the minimal mortality of cervix cancer. The converse would apply for cancer of the corpus, for which the rates are inflated by some misclassified deaths from cervical cancer. Thus, the second map represents the totality of uterine cancer although this undoubtedly could obscure patterns of etiological importance.

It is clear that deaths from cervical cancer are commonest in Denmark, southern Scotland and part of northern England and Wales, with above- average levels being seen in much of the Federal Republic of Germany, the northern portion of Belgium and much of the Netherlands, in contrast to the average rates in France and the below-average levels in virtually all of Italy.

When the map presenting data for the uterus as a whole, i.e. cervix, corpus and uterus unspecified is examined, the picture changes materially. High rates are still found in Denmark, and most of the United Kingdom is average or below average, but Ireland, which in general previously showed average rates, is now well below average, and certain *départements* in France now rank among the top 5%, as does much of Sicilia.

The highest levels of uterine cancer mortality were those in Denmark (12.6), the lowest being recorded in Ulster (6.2).

In the USA, Japan and Australia, uterine cancer accounted for 6.2%, 9.1% and 5.8% of all cancer mortality in females.

Comment

Cancer of the cervix

Cervical cancer resembles in several aspects a sexually transmitted disease. Its incidence is, in fact, inversely related to age at first intercourse, and directly to the number of sexual partners, and apparently independently related to multiparity (Brinton *et al.*, 1987, 1989). Human papilloma virus (HPV) is currently the strongest candidate for the responsible sexually transmitted agent. The fact that the virus cannot grow *in vitro* has made difficult the development of laboratory tests to detect markers of human papilloma virus in human tissues. More than sixty HPV types have been identified, and of these, HPV-16 and to a lesser extent HPV-18 seem to be associated with advanced cervical intraepithelial neoplasia (CIN) or invasive cervical carcinoma.

Cervical cancer risk is elevated in lower social classes, in long-term oral contraceptive users and in cigarette smokers (IARC, 1986a). Pre-vitamin A (carotenoids) or other aspects of a vegetable-rich diet may be protective, or may simply represent indicators of a better diet and hence more health-concerned lifestyles. In terms of prevention and public health, rational use of cytological screening is undoubtedly the key factor for reducing rates of invasive cervical cancer. It has been estimated that screening at three-year intervals for women aged 35 to 64 can reduce the incidence of invasive cervical cancer by over 90% if a nationwide programme is instituted (IARC, 1986b).

Cancer of the uterine corpus

Cancer of the uterine corpus (mainly endometrial cancer) is, in terms of hormonal correlates, the best understood gynaecological malignancy. It is strongly related to elevated levels or availability of exogenous or endogenous estrogens, and comparably low levels of progestogens. It is thus related to anovularity, obesity (which increases endogenous estrogen levels) and estrogen replacement treatment at the menopause. The relative risks for long-term estrogen use and severe obesity are around 5 to 10. Menopausal hormone replacement therapy was the major determinant of the epidemic of endometrial cancer in the USA during the 1970s (Ziel & Finkle, 1975), but in Europe obesity is the main established risk factor (Parrazini *et al.*, 1989).

Use of combined oral contraceptives, and the consequent relative progestin excess, considerably decreases the risk of the disease, giving approximately 50% protection in women who have ever used them, and the risk appears inversely related to duration of use (La Vecchia *et al.*, 1991b).

Other determinants of endometrial cancer include nulliparity, late menopause and perhaps early menarche, diabetes and hypertension (Wynder *et al.*, 1966), but these risk factors may be partly mediated through a mutual association with overweight.

All these established and potential risk factors, however, explain only about 50% of the endometrial cancer in Europe, and cannot account for the 30-fold worldwide variation in incidence; both nutritional status and diet composition appear to be related. Positive correlations with consumption of meat, eggs, milk, proteins, fats and oils and total calorie intake have been found, while green vegetables may be protective, as for so many other cancers (La Vecchia *et al.*, 1987).

Cervix: ICD-8 180

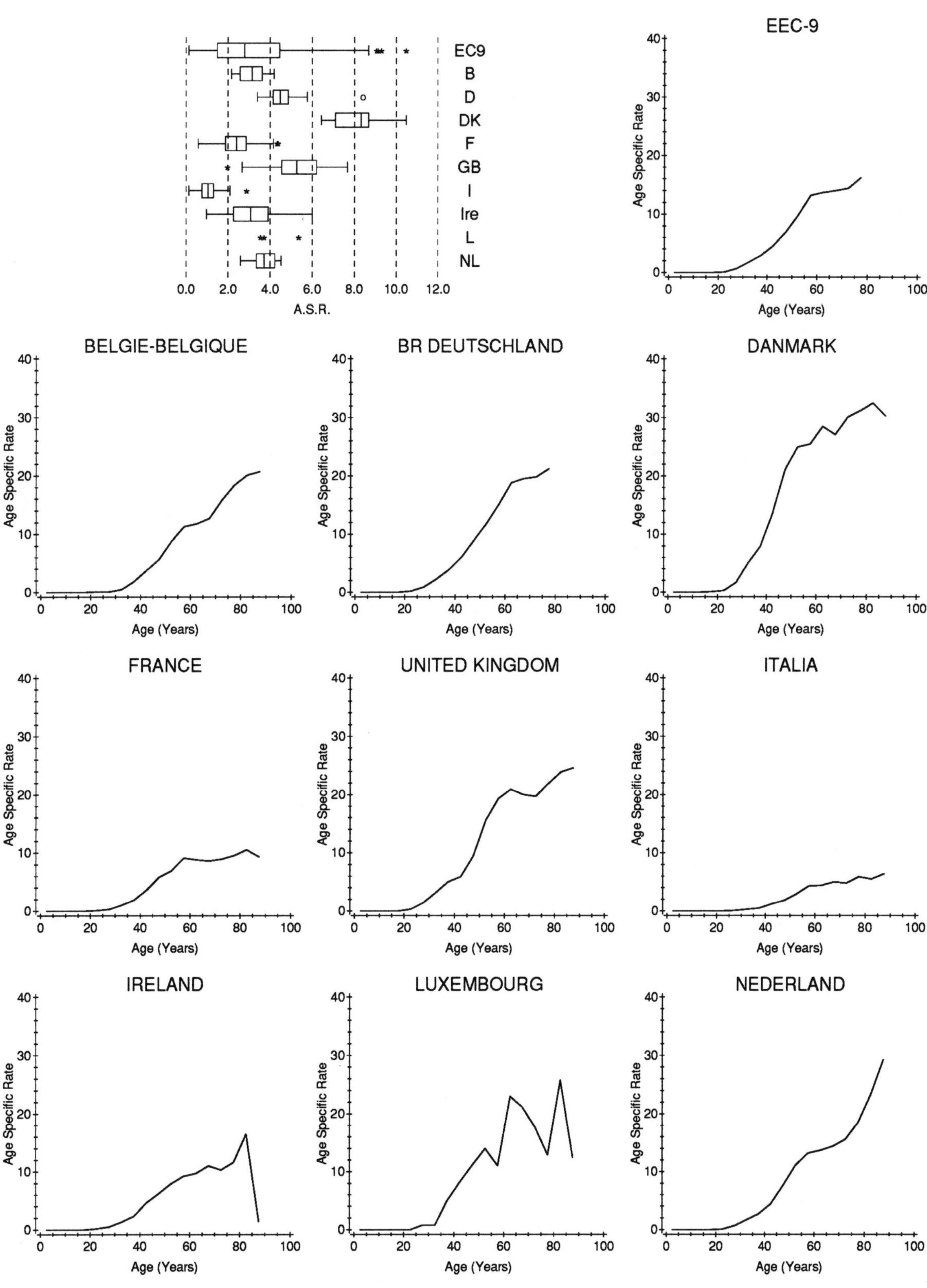

Uterus: ICD-8 180+182

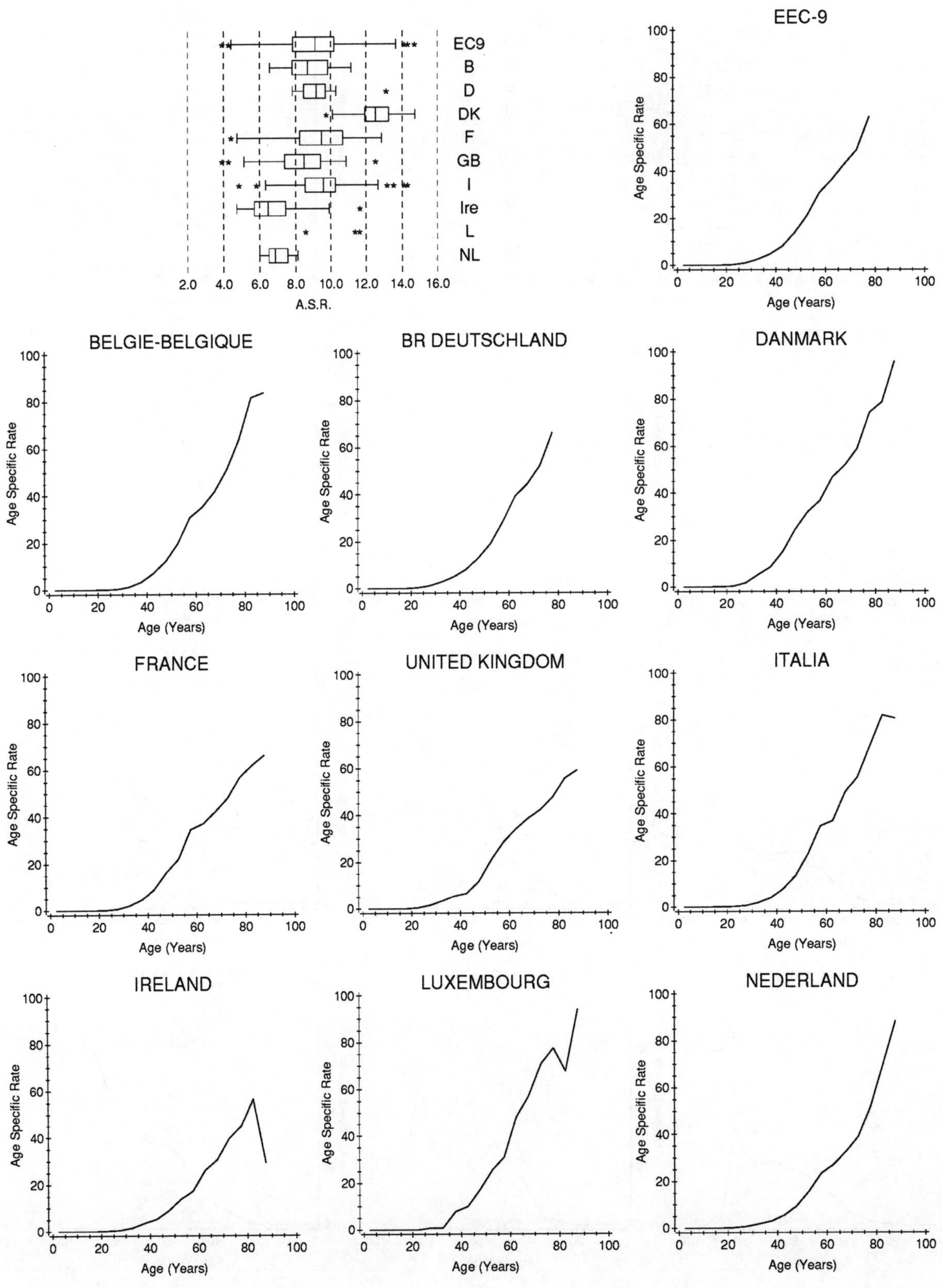

Prostate: *ICD-8 185* (M13.3 : 7.2%) (Map 27)

Testis: *ICD-8 186* (M0.9 : 0.5%) (Map 28)

The distribution of prostate cancer mortality is in many respects quite unlike any other. High rates are seen in part of the west of Ireland, those for Great Britain being either average or below average. In most of Italy mortality is low, the zones of high mortality being found in southern Belgium and parts of the Federal Republic of Germany, as in the west and centre of France.

The contrast with the distribution of testis cancer depicted on the opposite page is outstanding, for which the highest rates are found in largely rural Denmark as well as in Copenhagen and in the north of Germany. The lowest rates are observed in the Flemish-speaking portion of Belgium.

Prostatic cancer mortality ranged between 18.3 in Nordrhein-Westfalen and 6.5 in Corse.

In the USA, Japan and Australia, prostatic cancer accounted for 9.1%, 1.7% and 9.5% of all fatal cancer.

Mortality from testicular cancer in the EEC ranged from 1.7 in Denmark to 0.6 in the Rhône-Alpes region of France.

In the USA, Japan and Australia, testis cancer comprised 0.2%, 0.2% and 0.4% of fatal cancer.

Comment

Cancer of the prostate

Very rare before the age of 50 years, cancer of the prostate is one of the commonest forms of malignant disease but relatively little is known about its etiology. Incidence and mortality rates of cancer of the prostate demonstrate wide international variations according to the most recent statistics (Muir *et al.*, 1987). The lowest rates are observed in countries of south-east Asia and the highest among USA blacks. The incidence of prostate cancer is increasing in many European countries (Zaridze & Boyle, 1987; Hakulinen *et al.*, 1986), but birth cohort studies in US blacks, Australia and England show that the disease is less common in men born after 1900.

The descriptive epidemiology of prostate cancer provides compelling evidence that prostate cancer may be preventable. While the data on blacks in Africa and the USA provide some evidence of a genetic component to prostate cancer risk, the geographic and temporal variations and the results of migrant studies indicate that life-style comprises a large fraction of the causes of prostate cancer.

Sex hormones have been implicated in the etiology of this cancer, primarily on the basis that the growth and development of this organ requires the presence of sex hormones. However, the hormonal hypothesis has received only equivocal support from epidemiological studies and clinical observations. Sexual activity, which is largely an indicator or indirect measure of hormonal status, has been related to the cancer. Prostatic cancer patients seem to have a greater sexual drive than controls, but are less sexually active. They also experience both puberty and first intercourse at a later age than controls.

Prostatic cancer mortality rates are associated with marital status, increasing in the following order: single, married, widowed, divorced. It has also been suggested that among married men the risk of prostatic cancer is higher in those with children than among those without children.

The hypothesis relating prostatic cancer to a high-fat diet, through possible influence on hormone metabolism, has arisen from observation of the international distribution of prostatic cancer occurrence and *per capita* fat intake (Zaridze & Boyle, 1987). Recent interest has focused on three aspects of diet: animal fat intake, beta-carotene intake and milk consumption. Although it is clear that there are dietary determinants of prostate cancer risk, their precise nature remains to be identified. The suggestion that increased intake of beta-carotene, vitamin A and vegetables increases the risk of prostate cancer deserves to be taken seriously in view of the possible protective role of these agents, and their use in chemoprevention, against many common forms of cancer, but evidence is still inconclusive.

Cancer of the testis

The age–incidence curve of testicular cancer has two peaks, one in the twenties and one later in life, possibly reflecting the relative frequency of different histological types (teratomas have an earlier peak incidence than the more frequent seminomas) or reflecting the roles of different risk factors. There is evidence that the incidence is now increasing, predominantly in young men and specifically for teratomas (Boyle *et al.*, 1988) but effective chemotherapy, particularly with cis-platinum, has substantially reduced mortality from the disease over the last decade. Cryptorchidism is the only established risk factor for the disease, with relative risks of the order of 2 to 4 and a population attributable risk of approximately 10% in North America, not restricted to the retrieved testis (Schottenfeld *et al.*, 1980). Correlation studies have suggested an association with high dietary fat intake (Armstrong & Doll, 1975).

Prostate: ICD-8 185

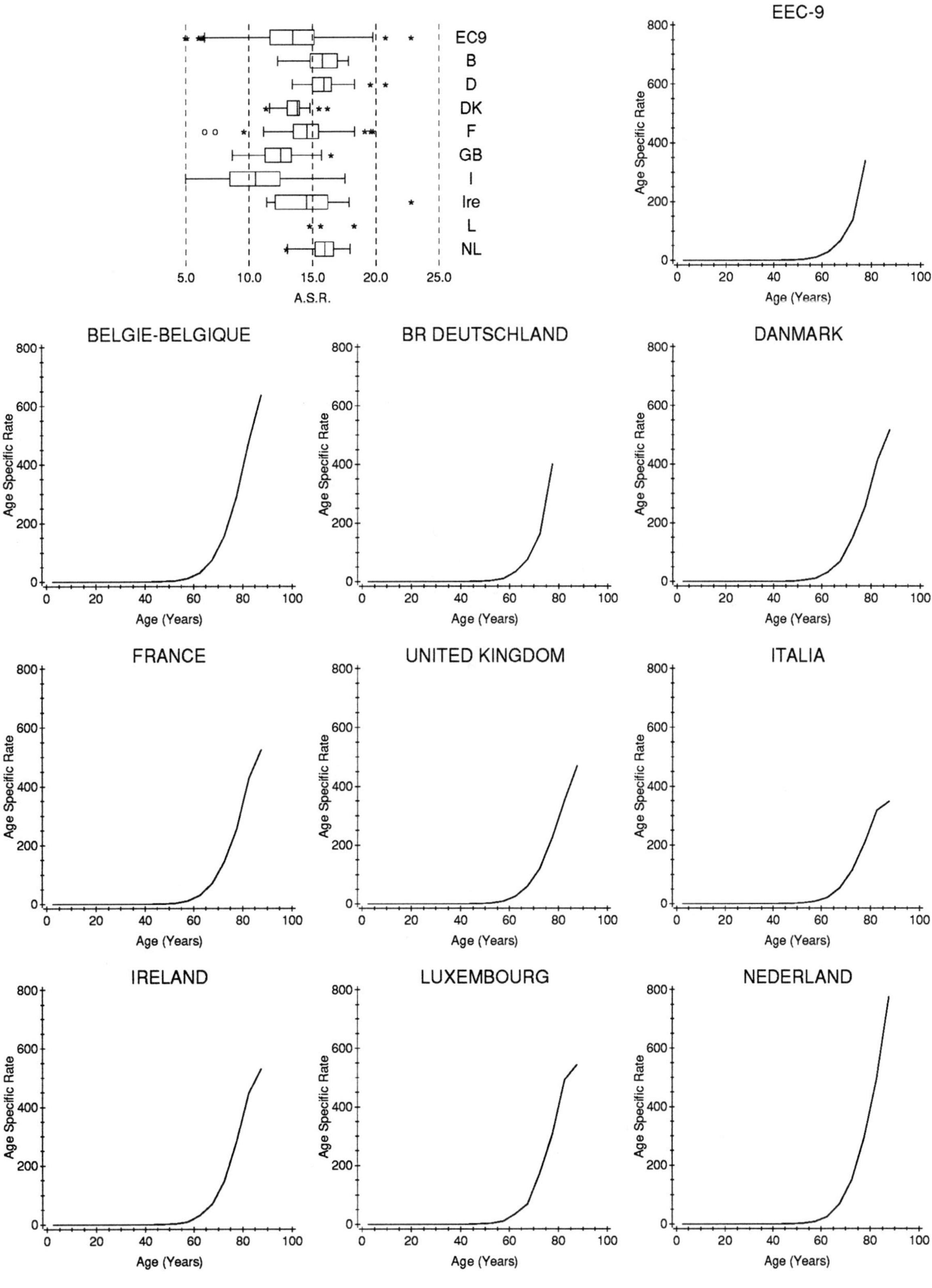

Testis: ICD-8 186

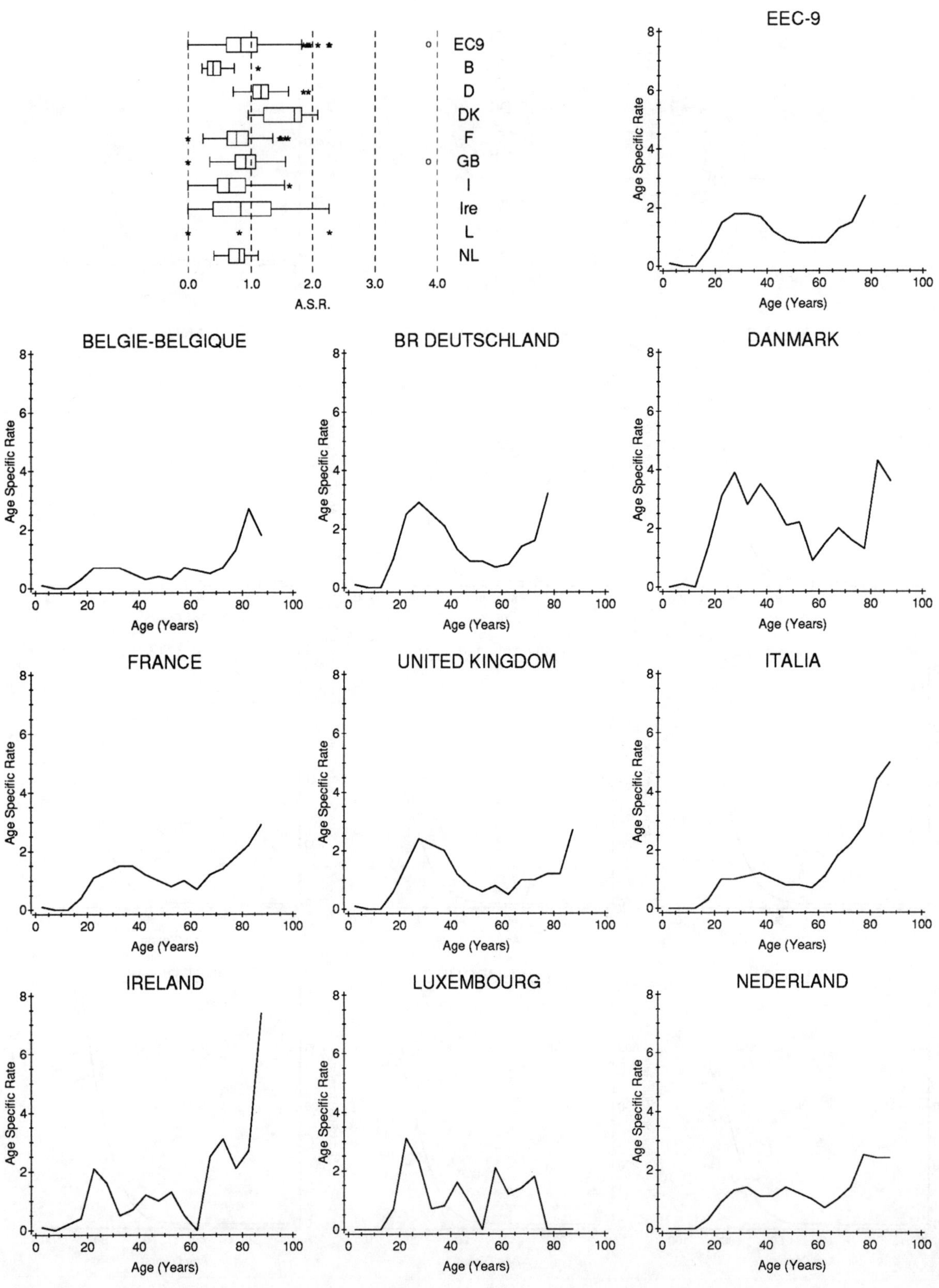

Bladder: *ICD-8 188* (M7.1, F1.7 : M3.8%, F1.5%) (Maps 29 and 30)

The greatest concentration of bladder cancer risk is to be found in Liverpool, around Newcastle in England, in parts of Nordrhein-Westfalen, around Turin, Milan and Genoa in Italy and in the regions of Rome and Naples. There is a moderate increase in risk in much of France. Those *départements* bordering the Mediterranean Sea, with one exception, have higher than average rates. There seems to be an excess of this tumour in some, but not all, heavily industrialized areas. Risk in females in continental Europe tends to follow that in males. However, many of the areas that appear in dark red on the male map are somewhat less intense on the female map due to the much greater concentration of areas of high risk in central and southern Scotland and northern England. Mortality is also high in eastern Denmark.

In males, the mortality from bladder cancer ranged between 9.5 in Liguria to 3.7 in the Pays de la Loire, and between 2.7 (Scotland) and 1.0 (Bretagne) in females.

In the USA, Japan and Australia, bladder cancer comprised 3.2% and 1.7%, 1.7% and 1.0% and 2.8% and 1.7% of all cancer deaths, for males and females respectively.

Comment

The evidence for an association of bladder cancer with cigarette smoking is overwhelming with estimates of relative risk among smokers compared to non-smokers being between 1.2 and 7.3 (La Vecchia *et al.*, 1991a). Furthermore, smokers of black tobacco appear to have a higher risk than smokers of blond cigarettes (Vineis *et al.*, 1984; La Vecchia *et al.*, 1991a). The dominant role of cigarette smoking is reflected in the geographical distribution of the disease, with high rates in predominantly urban areas of Europe and North America, although areas with high concentrations of chemical industries also tend to have high rates.

Several other factors have been related to cancer of the urinary bladder, including occupational exposure to aromatic amines and to coal tar, infection with *Schistosoma haematobium* and some other agents, and use of some drugs such as chlornaphazine and cyclophosphamide (IARC, 1987). A number of studies have reported increased risks of bladder cancer associated with coffee consumption and an IARC Working Group considered that there was some evidence that coffee may be carcinogenic for the human bladder (IARC, 1991). There is some evidence that a diet rich in fresh fruit and vegetables and, possibly, vitamin A is protective. The observation that a number of heterogeneous factors have been related to bladder cancer is not surprising, since most substances or metabolites are excreted through the urinary tract and are consequently in direct contact with the mucosa of the bladder.

Bladder: ICD-8 188

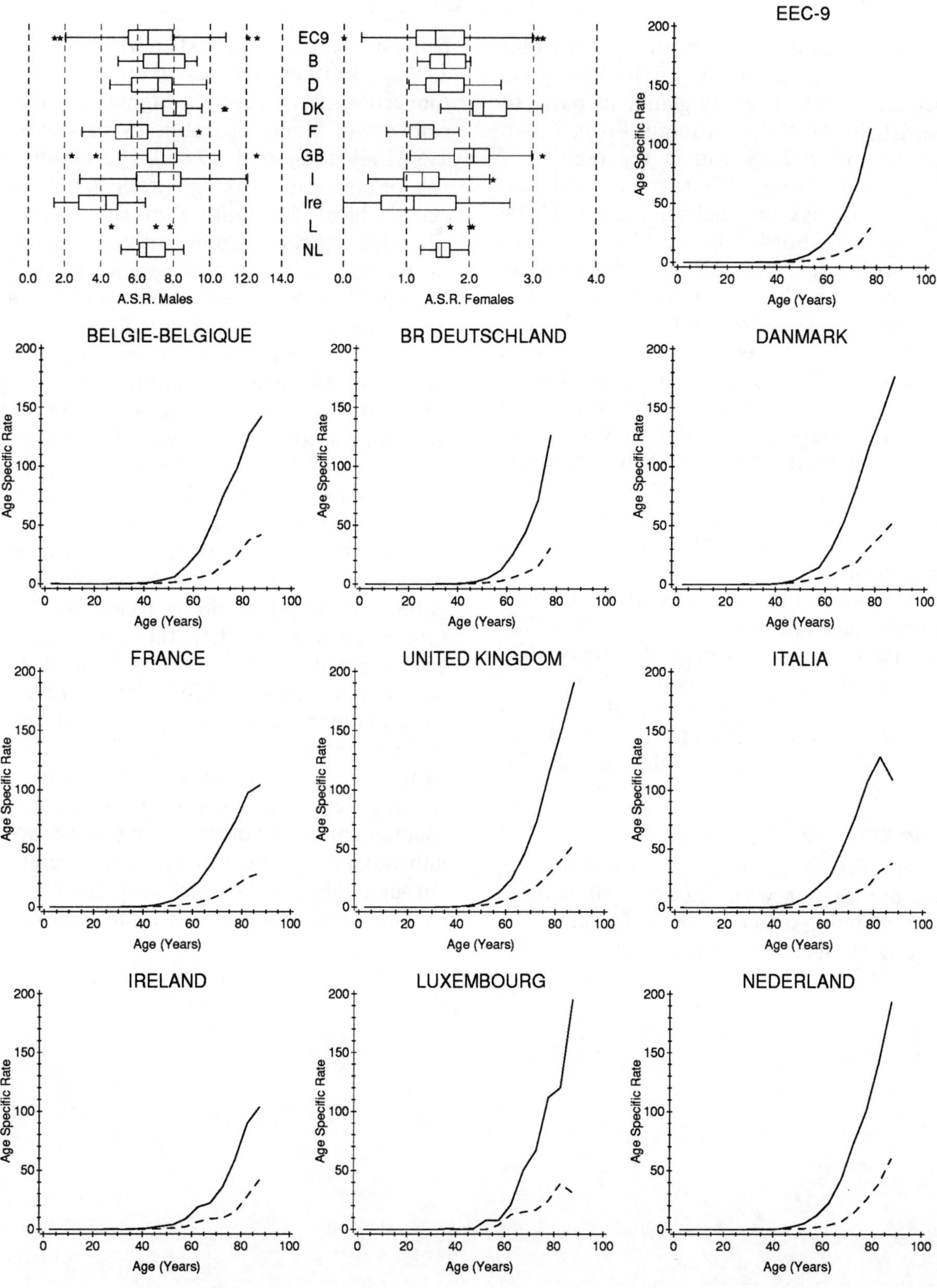

Urinary tract: *ICD-8 188–189* (M10.8, F3.5 : M5.8%, F3.2%) (Maps 31 and 32)

The map showing mortality from cancers of the kidney and bladder combined naturally reflects the influence of the more common bladder tumours. The excess risk in eastern Denmark and the Federal Republic of Germany, in the regions of Milan, Naples, Trieste and Newcastle is even more noticeable for females. The addition of kidney cancers to those for the bladder emphasizes the fact that mortality from urinary tract cancers in Denmark is very high and reinforces the impression of high risk in the Federal Republic of Germany. Indeed in females these cancers appear to be commoner in the Federal Republic of Germany and Denmark than elsewhere in Europe.

The mortality from cancer of the urinary organs, bladder and kidney combined, ranged from 15.1 in males (West Berlin) to 6.6 (Basilicata) and in females from 6.2 in Denmark to 1.6 in Calabria.

In the USA, urinary tract malignancy accounted for 5.4% and 3.3% of all cancer deaths in males and females respectively. Corresponding figures for Japan were 2.6% and 1.6% and for Australia 4.8% and 3.8% respectively.

Comment

In addition to the bladder, the other urinary tract cancers are those arising in the kidney, the pelvis of the kidney and the urethra. From a functional point of view, the tumours of the renal pelvis and bladder form part of the same collecting and storage system and it has been shown that the incidence of renal pelvis and bladder cancers usually parallel each other. Cancer of the kidney is a relatively common cancer in many western countries, and occurs more frequently among males than females, at a ratio of around 2:1. Renal cell adenocarcinoma accounts for about 85% of all kidney cancers. Other histological types include Wilms' tumour in childhood, whose etiology is unknown, but which has been shown to be linked to deletion of specific loci on chromosome 11. Transitional cell cancer of the renal pelvis is related to smoking (McCredie *et al.*, 1983) and probably other factors associated with bladder neoplasms. Further, the abuse of phenacetin and other analgesics has been specifically related to cancers of the renal pelvis (McCredie *et al.*, 1983). The relative risk of cigarette smoking is about two in current versus never smokers, lower than for bladder and most other tobacco-related neoplasms (IARC, 1986a).

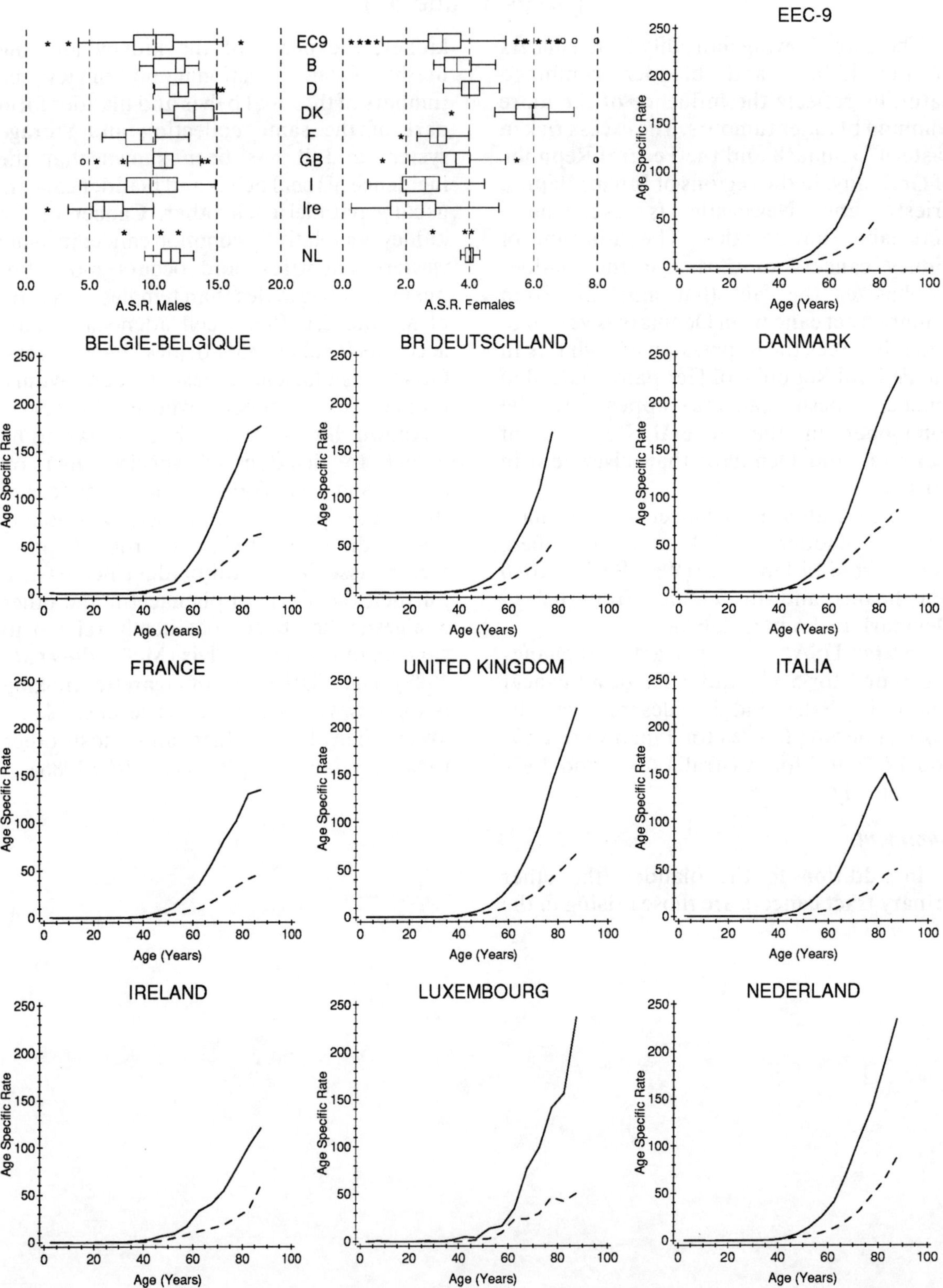

Urinary tract: ICD-8 188+189
EC9
B
D
DK
F
GB
I
Ire
L
NL
0.0
5.0
10.0
15.0
20.0
A.S.R. Males
0.0
2.0
4.0
6.0
8.0
A.S.R. Females
EEC-9
BELGIE-BELGIQUE
BR DEUTSCHLAND
DANMARK
FRANCE
UNITED KINGDOM
ITALIA
IRELAND
LUXEMBOURG
NEDERLAND
Age Specific Rate
Age (Years)

Brain and nervous system: *ICD-8 191–192* (M3.7, F2.5 : M2.0%, F2.3%) (Maps 33 and 34)

The highest levels of mortality in both sexes are to be seen in the British Isles, Ireland, Denmark and Belgium. Given the comparative rarity of these tumours, it is perhaps not surprising that there are inconsistencies between the sexes. Thus in the north of Scotland, the Outer Isles are in the top 5% in males but in the lowest 5% in females, whereas in the northern portions of the Scottish mainland virtually the converse is observed.

Within the EEC, the mortality from cancers of the brain and nervous system ranged from 5.8 in Vlaanderen to 1.9 in Basse-Normandie in males, and from 4.8 again in Vlaanderen to 1.5 in Provence-Alpes-Côte-d'Azur.

In the USA, Japan and Australia, brain and nervous system cancers accounted for 2.3% and 2.1%, 0.5% and 0.5%, and 2.9% and 2.9% of all cancer deaths in males and females respectively.

Comment

As these cancers are often difficult to diagnose, the mortality level must be influenced by the availability of specialized neurosurgical centres. At present only a small proportion of brain tumours can be attributed to a defined cause; there is more suspicion than proof for several postulated risk factors.

Gliomas, meningiomas and other intracranial neoplasms have generally been grouped together in epidemiological studies, despite the fact that gliomas and meningiomas are derived from different tissues and the various histological types have different prognosis and biological behaviour (Helseth & Mork, 1989). Adult brain tumours have been noted to occur more frequently in a number of different occupational groups including a number of professional and managerial occupations (Milham, 1983) and some occupations with potential carcinogenic exposures in the workplace such as rubber industry workers (McMichael *et al.*, 1974), farming (Howe & Lindsay, 1983; Reif *et al.*, 1989) and individuals employed in thc electrical industries (Thomas *et al.*, 1987). When cancer incidence rates are examined subdivided by histology, it has been found that the risk of astrocytoma was elevated among automobile repair workers, workers in justice, public order and safety, police and fire protection officers, and machinists; farmers had an increased risk for non-astrocytoma cell types (Brownson *et al.*, 1990). The risk of brain tumours has been shown to be increased by cigarette smoking (Burch *et al.*, 1987) but this has not been a consistent finding (Choi *et al.*, 1970; Preston-Martin, 1978; Brownson *et al.*, 1990).

Primary tumours of the brain and nervous system are the second commonest cancer in children (Parkin *et al.*, 1988a). Exposure to ionizing radiation appears to be a risk factor, the increased risk being found among children exposed *in utero* when mothers had pelvimetry late in pregnancy (Stewart *et al.*, 1958; MacMahon, 1962) and among cohorts of children who received X-ray treatment for ringworm of the scalp (Shore *et al.*, 1976). Head trauma during birth (Choi *et al.*, 1970) or early life (Preston-Martin *et al.*, 1982) also appears to increase the risk of childhood brain tumours. Trauma at birth may also explain the finding of more tumours among first-born (Gold *et al.*, 1978).

Brain and nervous system: ICD-8 191+192

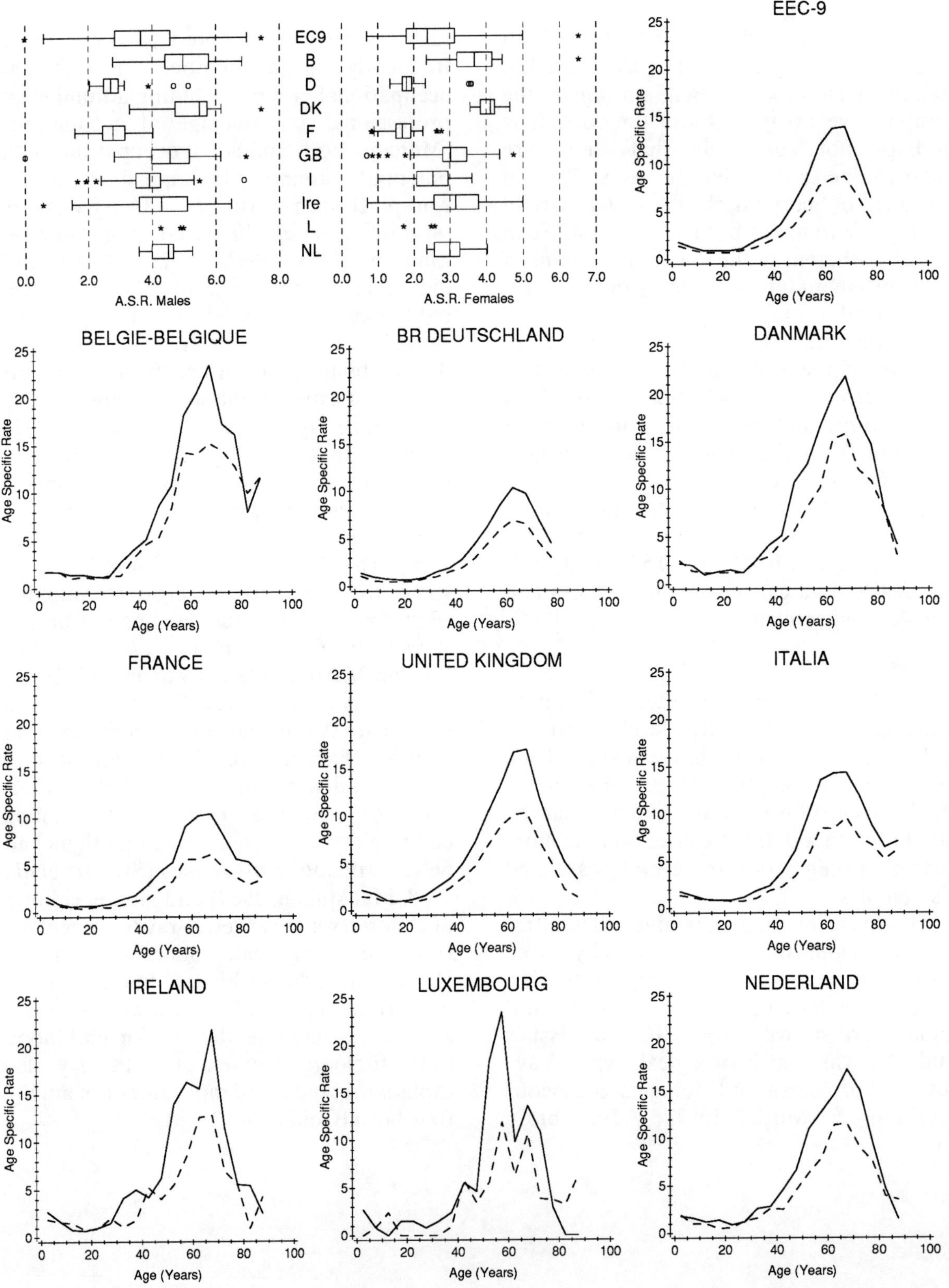

Thyroid: *ICD-8 193* (M0.5, F0.7 : M0.3%, F0.6%) (Maps 35 and 36)

In both sexes mortality from thyroid cancer seems to cluster round the mountainous areas surrounding Switzerland and Austria. It is probable that maps of the distribution of this cancer in these countries would show a similar pattern. In Ireland both sexes show an excess in some counties but these not infrequently border counties with very low mortality, suggesting random fluctuation.

Mortality from thyroid cancer ranged from 0.9 in Bayern to 0.3 in south-east England in males, and from 1.3 in Baden-Wurttemberg to 0.5, again in south-east England, in females.

In the USA, Japan and Australia these cancers constituted 0.2% and 0.4%, 0.2% and 0.8% and 0.1% and 0.5% of all fatal cancers in males and females respectively.

Comment

Thyroid cancer is a rare form of cancer, which is characterized by the wide variation in the degree of malignancy exhibited by the various histological types (Franceschi *et al.*, 1991). In many developed countries, mortality has been decreasing while inci- dence has been increasing (Kerr *et al.*, 1985), but many factors complicate the interpretation of thyroid cancer trends (Saxén, 1982); in particular, changing diagnostic practices have led to an inflation of thyroid cancer rates.

Ionizing radiation is the best defined risk factor for thyroid cancer. The thyroid tissue is particularly susceptible to radiation at younger ages, and considerable excess rates have been observed in Hiroshima and Nagasaki (Prentice *et al.*, 1982) and in subjects irradiated for thyroid hypertrophy during childhood (Hempelmann *et al.*, 1975). Prior thyroid diseases, benign nodules and goitre are also associated with substantially elevated risk (Silverberg & Vidone, 1966).

Little is conclusively known about other etiological factors. Iodine deficiency has been suspected to increase risk and if this is so, the incidence should have fallen in mountainous areas following the introduction of iodized salt. The scanty available data suggest that a poorer diet, particularly if containing natural goitrogens, is associated with elevated risk. Positive associations have been reported also with nulliparity, late age at first birth and the use of oral contraceptives or menopausal replacement treatment, but remain to be confirmed (Franceschi *et al.*, 1991).

Thyroid: ICD-8 193

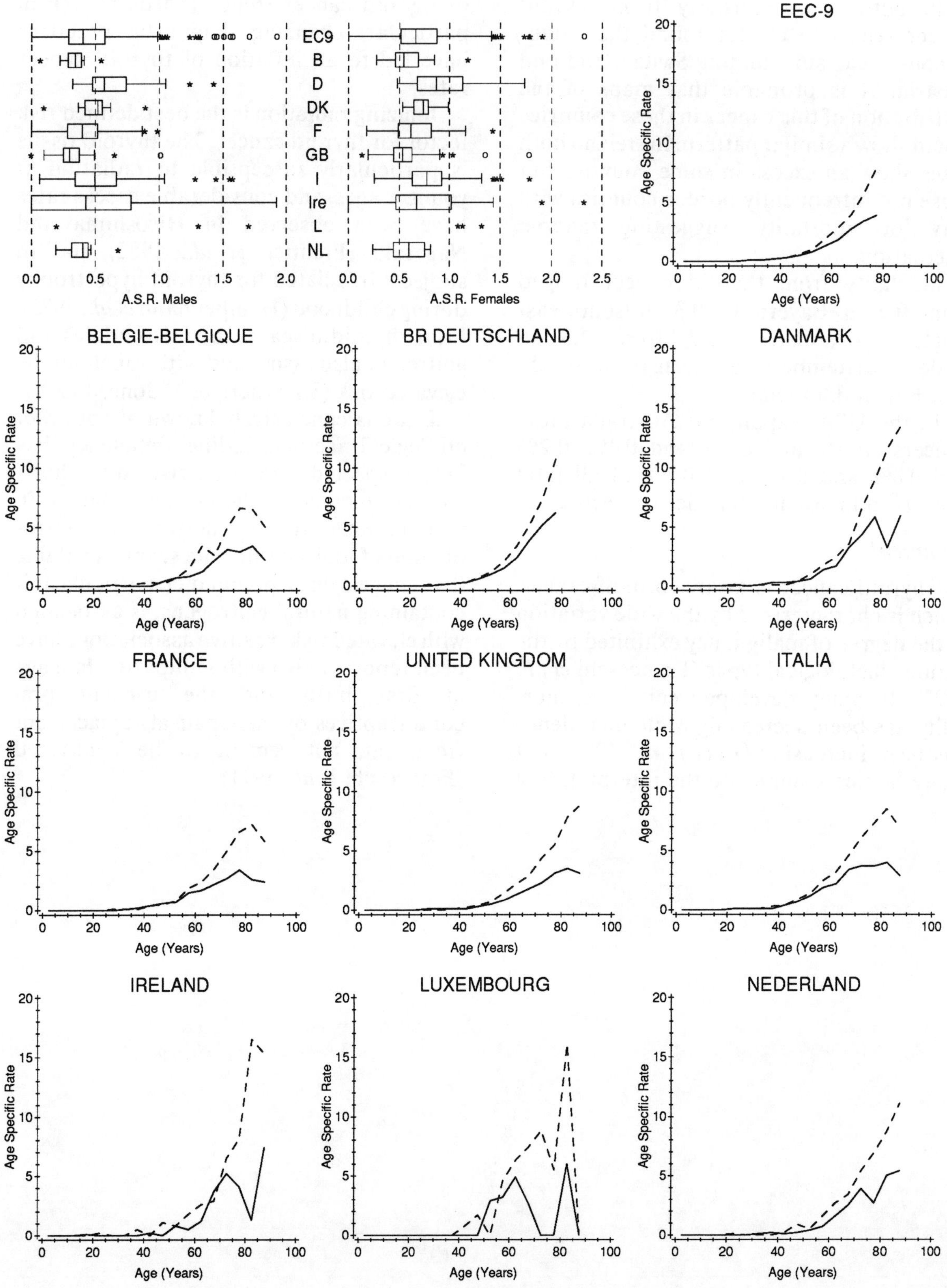

Hodgkin's disease: *ICD-8 201* (M1.5, F0.8 : M0.8%, F0.7%) (Maps 37 and 38)

Both sexes show a grouping of areas with high mortality rates from Hodgkin's disease in northern and central parts of Italy. Indeed rates in most parts of that country are above average. There is a similar grouping in Ireland both in the north and the Irish Republic. However, these maps have to be read in conjunction with those for non-Hodgkin lymphoma where the picture is rather different, rates in Italy being on the whole average (although a few provinces have somewhat higher rates). Those for France and the Federal Republic of Germany are again on the whole average whereas in Denmark, most of the Netherlands and most of Great Britain the rates for non-Hodgkin lymphoma are well above average. It is possible that these differences reflect varying national practice in certifying deaths due to these two groups of diseases. However, when the maps for multiple myeloma, a form of malignancy not readily confused with the other variants of malignant lymphoma, are examined, a picture substantially similar to that for non-Hodgkin lymphoma emerges.

The mortality from Hodgkin's disease ranged from 2.4 in Lombardia to 1.0 in south-west England in males, and from 1.4, again in Lombardia, to 1.3 in south-east England.

In the USA, Japan and Australia, Hodgkin's disease accounted for 0.6% and 0.5%, 0.3% and 0.2% and 0.6% and 0.6% of fatal cancer in males and females respectively.

Comment

Hodgkin's disease has been one of the few neoplasms which has experienced considerable advances in survival over the past twenty years through the impact of effective treatment (Boyle *et al.*, 1988). The age–incidence curve is bimodal: incidence rates rise early in life, peak in the late 20's and then decline to around age 45. Thereafter the incidence increases with age. The suggestion that this is due to two distinct etiological processes (MacMahon, 1957) is supported by the observation that among younger adults (15 to 39 years of age) Hodgkin's disease of the nodular sclerosing type predominates but at older ages the predominant type changes to the mixed cellularity form (Newell *et al.*, 1970). Geographical variation of Hodgkin's disease rates is greatest among younger adults.

The similarity of the age distribution of Hodgkin's disease with that of paralytic poliomyelitis and Epstein–Barr Virus (EBV) infections led to the formulation of the 'late-host-response' model (Gutensohn & Cole, 1980). This excludes the effect of direct contagion but proposes that early exposure to some relatively common agent is benign and confers subsequent immunity but later exposure can (although not commonly) lead to Hodgkin's disease.

Although the 'late-host-response' model for Hodgkin's disease does not require evidence for social contact between cases, numerous studies have addressed this issue, presumably motivated initially by anecdotal reports.

Hodgkin's disease: ICD-8 201

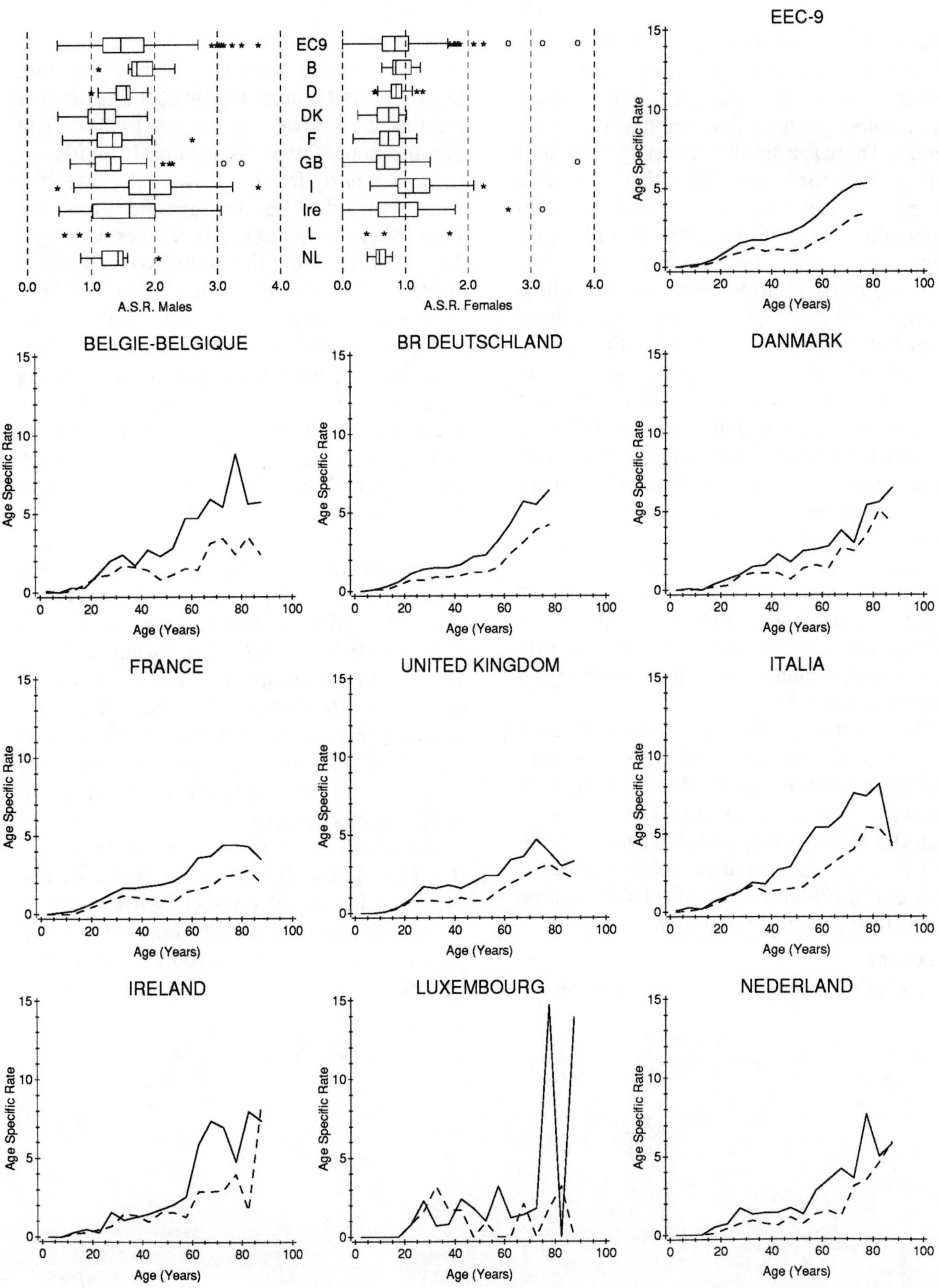

Non-Hodgkin lymphoma: *ICD-8 200 + 202* (M2.6, F1,5 : M1.4%, F1.4%) (Maps 39 and 40)

The geographical distributions of non-Hodgkin lymphoma are broadly similar in males and in females. Rates in both males and females are generally high in the United Kingdom with the highest rate in males being seen in Scotland (3.6), although the areas with the highest rates are not geographically contiguous. Rates in Denmark are also high in both sexes. A striking feature is the aggregation of areas of high mortality rate in the Netherlands in both males and females. Little consistent pattern is evident in France, Belgium and Germany but Italy again shows decreasing rates towards the south. In males, for example, the lowest rate was found in Campania (1.7). In females, the highest and lowest rates were in the Netherlands (2.4) and 1.1 in Baden- Wurttemburg, respectively.

In the USA, Japan and Australia, non-Hodgkin lymphomas represented 3.4% and 3.7%, 2.1% and 1.7% and 1.8% and 2.9% of all fatal cancer in males and females respectively.

Comment

This disease grouping includes a wide spectrum of cyto- (and almost certainly etio-) pathological entities (Non-Hodgkin's Lymphomas Classification Project, 1982) whose incidence and mortality have generally been rising in most developed countries during the past decades, possibly in association with improvements in diagnosis and certification.

For some histological types there is a recognised viral etiology as, for example, in Burkitt's lymphoma. This disease is a well defined pathoclinical entity comprising an undifferentiated, monoclonal lymphoma composed of malignant B-cells. It is common in children in many parts of sub-Saharan Africa, where the incidence rate is up to 8 per 100 000 compared to the usual 0.1 to 0.3 per 100 000 in European children (Parkin *et al.*, 1988b).

Markers of Epstein–Barr virus (DNA or antigens) are found in 96% of cases living in endemic areas of Africa but in only 15% of the sporadic tumours (Lenoir & Bornkamm, 1987): the corollary is that EBV is unlikely to be involved in the etiology of Burkitt's lymphoma in 85% of the cases outside Africa. The causal role of EBV in the etiology of Burkitt's lymphoma is supported by an association between high antibody titres to EBV and the risk of developing Burkitt's lymphoma (de-Thé *et al.*, 1978) but the molecular basis of EBV-induced B-cell proliferation is not yet understood.

B-cell lymphomas occur more frequently than expected in subjects with depressed immune systems and most of these lymphoproliferations are (at least at the beginning of the disease) polyclonal B-cell malignancies, in contrast to the monoclonal Burkitt's lymphoma. These malignancies are com- moner in organ transplant recipients, treated with immunodepressants to reduce the risk of organ rejection, and among patients with virus-induced immuno-deficiencies such as acquired immuno-deficiency syndrome (AIDS) or genetic immunodeficiencies. Etiological links with aspects of disturbed or aberrant immunity were first suggested by a British case–control study which showed significant associations with past history of several diseases including skin conditions, malignancies, pneumonia, scarlet fever and diabetes (Cartwright *et al.*, 1988).

Higher risk of non-Hodgkin lymphoma has been associated with agricultural activity which may be linked to a possible viral etiology (La Vecchia *et al.*, 1989), although exposure to phenoxyacid herbicides, chlorophenols, organic solvents and insecticides has also been postulated as being involved (Hardell *et al.*, 1981). Increased risks have also been suspected among workers exposed to wood, meat and other food processing and certain chemical agents.

Non-Hodgkin lymphoma: ICD-8 200+202

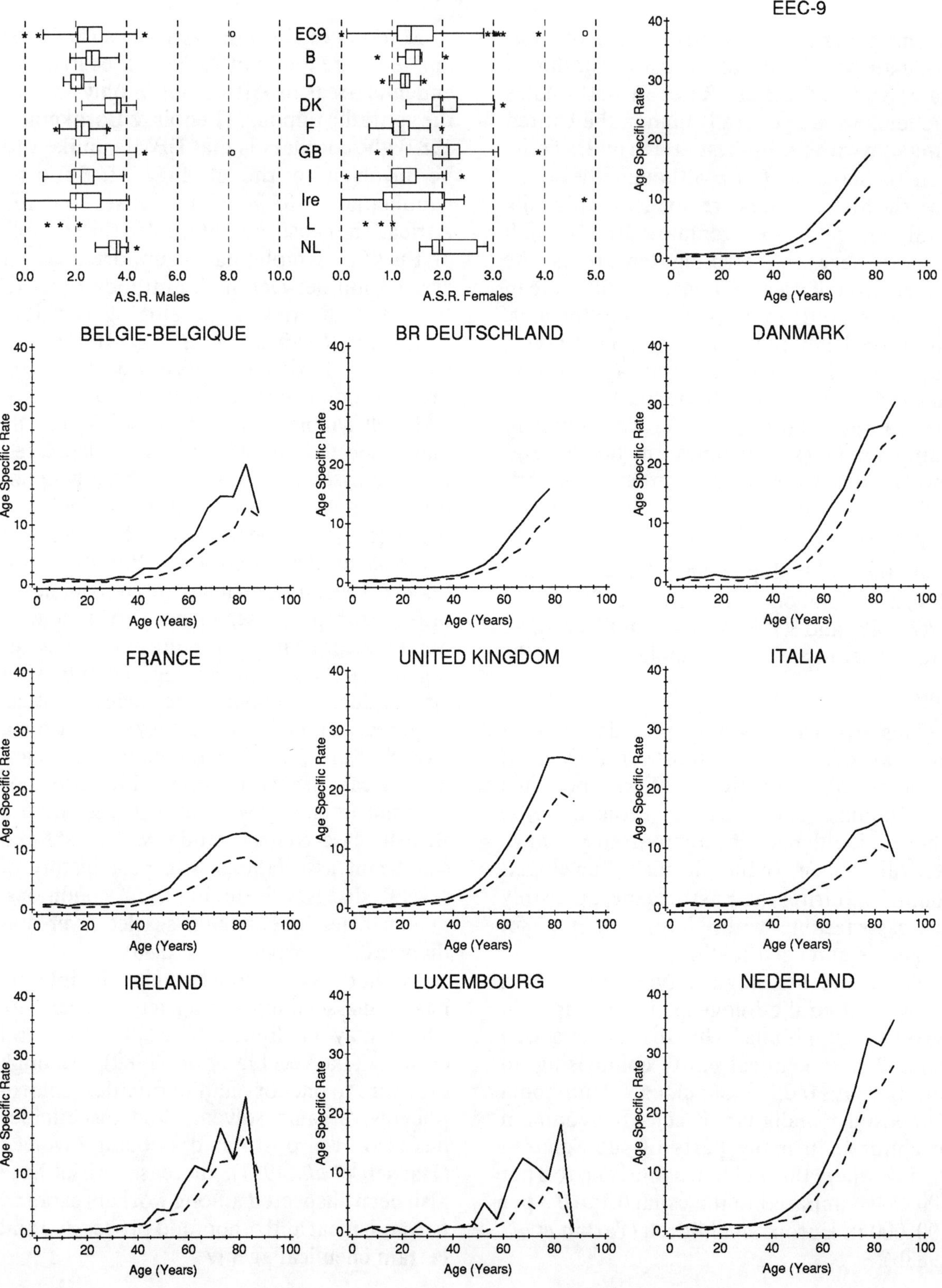

Multiple myeloma: *ICD-8 203* (M1.7, F1.2 : M0.9%, F1.1%) (Maps 41 and 42)

There are similarities in the maps for males and females regarding the geographical distribution of multiple myeloma, and they also somewhat resemble those for non-Hodgkin lymphoma. The highest rate in males is found in Leinster (2.9) and rates are generally high in Ireland and the United Kingdom. Rates are also high in both sexes in Denmark and the Netherlands, where the highest rate in females (1.8) is recorded. Italy has higher rates in the north than in the south, with the lowest rates in both males (1.0) and females (0.8) being recorded in Sicilia.

In the USA, Japan and Australia, multiple myeloma comprised 1.5% and 1.6%, 0.7% and 0.7% and 1.1% and 1.3% of all fatal cancer in males and females respectively.

Comment

Ionizing radiation is the sole established risk factor for multiple myeloma (Cuzick, 1981) but it seems unlikely that this is responsible for the geographical variations seen on the maps. Like many kinds of leukaemia, multiple myeloma can be produced by irradiation to the bone marrow. A small increased risk of multiple myeloma observed in atomic bomb survivors (Shimizu *et al.*, 1987) and among cervical cancer patients treated by radiotherapy (Boice *et al.*, 1985) became evident after a longer latent period than that for leukaemia. Among personnel employed in the nuclear industry, no consistent increase in multiple myeloma has been detected (Smith & Douglas, 1986; Gilbert *et al.*, 1989).

This association is interesting since, although radiation is linked to myeloid leukaemia, there is little evidence of association with chronic lymphatic leukaemia which, like myeloma, is a tumour of B lymphocytes. The elevated risk of myeloma becomes evident ten years after exposure, and persists for up to 30 years.

Multiple myeloma: ICD-8 203

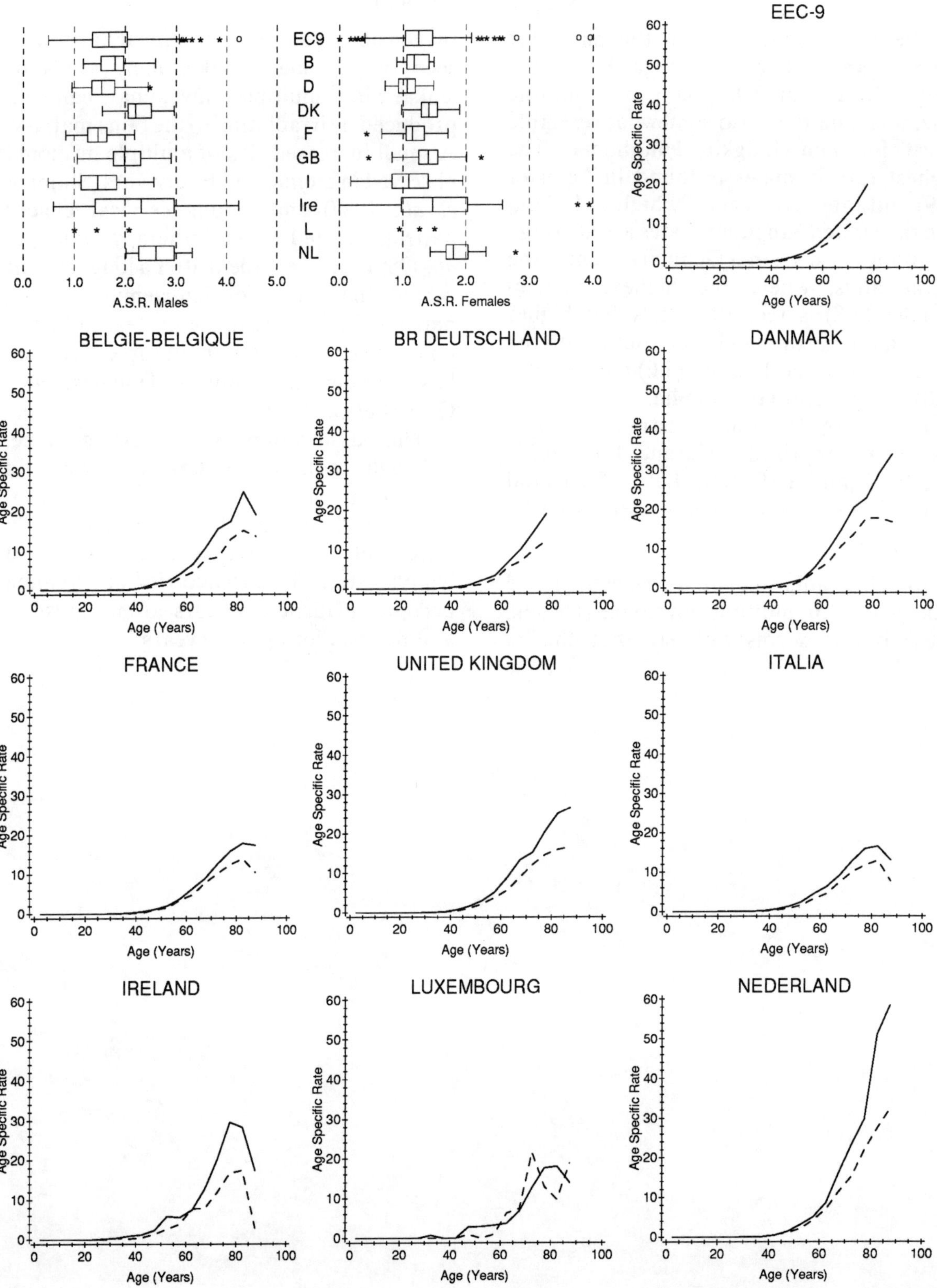

Leukaemia: *ICD-8 204–207* (M6.4, F4.2 : M3.4%, F3.8%) (Maps 43 and 44)

There is some consistency in the patterns of leukaemia observed in males and females, although somewhat less than that observed for non-Hodgkin lymphoma and multiple myeloma.

Death rates from leukaemia seem to be higher in northern Italy and central France. In both males (7.9) and females (5.2) the highest rates were reported from Lombardia. The north/south gradient within Italy is less conspicuous than that observed for many other forms of cancer. Rates are generally low in the United Kingdom and Ireland, with the lowest rates observed in Europe being found in the north of England in males (5.1) and Leinster in females (3.0).

In the USA, Japan and Australia, leukaemia constituted 4.1% and 3.8%, 3.0% and 3.0%, and 3.9% and 3.8% of fatal cancer among males and females respectively.

Comment

There have been reports of increases in leukaemia around atomic power stations and nuclear reprocessing plants in the United Kingdom (Gardner *et al.*, 1990) but neither in France (Hill & Laplanche, 1990) nor in the USA (Jablon *et al.*, 1990), and following therapeutic radiation. In certain areas of south-west Japan and China, an unusual form of leukaemia has been shown to be due to a virus. However, the causes of most leukaemias are still not known.

Ionizing radiation is an undoubted cause (Finch, 1984) and the observations originally made from the Hiroshima and Nagasaki cohorts have never seriously been contradicted. Age at exposure influences both the type of the resultant leukaemia and the latent interval: exposure at a young age is likely to cause acute lymphoblastic leukaemia with a short latency, while at older ages at first exposure it is more likely that acute myeloid leukaemia will result with a much longer latency. Chronic myeloid leukaemia appears at any age and apparently at a rate that is unaffected by age.

The issue of leukaemia risk due to exposure to low doses of ionizing radiation remains controversial. A modest increased risk of childhood leukaemia associated with X-ray exposure *in utero* (Bithell & Stiller, 1988; Monson & MacMahon, 1984) has now largely disappeared as a result of a combination of changes in clinical practice and in the X-ray equipment, which have resulted in lower doses (Mole, 1990). No excess leukaemia risk has been shown to result from the similarly small doses given for investigatory reasons to children or adults. Similarly, radiologists themselves have little or no apparent increase in risk nowadays (Smith & Doll, 1981).

Studies of workers in the nuclear industry whose occupational gamma doses are known have not shown statistically significant excesses of leukaemia to date, although some have demonstrated non-significant excesses. Despite a 1000-fold decline in gamma dose resulting from atomic weapon atmospheric tests since 1960, there has been no parallel decline in the rates of childhood (Darby & Doll, 1987) or adult leukaemias. The situation with household gamma radiation, which has the potential for individual doses greater than terrestrial doses, has yet to be investigated by direct measures. There are no data available on beta-emitters in the environment. The radiobiology of alpha emitters is such that the tissue dose is very difficult to measure. Thorium dioxide exposure (through Thorotrast use, an obsolete medical procedure) produced large numbers of leukaemia and liver angiosarcoma cases (Faber, 1978), but exposure to plutonium (various isotopes) or radium 224 has not been shown to produce excess leukaemia risk (Voelz *et al.*, 1985; Spiers *et al.*, 1983). Experimental work on alpha sources in animals has shown that very low doses do have biological effects, and fractionated doses produce greater biological response than the equivalent single dose (Adams, 1989). Overall, several lines of evidence indicate that alpha radiation may prove to be an important etiological factor for leukaemia. The marrow doses in houses with high levels of radon gas, a source of alpha particle activity, are quite considerable and may have a direct biological effect: geographical correlation studies support an association with the induction of leukaemia (Alexander *et al.*, 1990; Henshaw *et al.*, 1990).

A suggestion that genetic damage caused in fathers by ionizing radiation increases the risk of childhood leukaemia (Gardner *et al.*, 1990) was based on very small numbers of cases. However, the implication that certain parental exposures may cause mutations conferring substantial risk of childhood leukaemia deserves attention.

Other known risk factors for leukaemia are exposures to chemotherapeutic agents used in the treatment of prior malignant diseases, producing mainly adult acute myeloid leukaemia (Lilleyman, 1987; IARC, 1987) and chronic benzene exposure (Cronkite *et al.*, 1985; IARC, 1987). The risk of childhood leukaemia, both acute lymphocytic leukaemia and acute myeloid leukaemia, is greatly increased by the use of chloramphenicol (Shu *et al.*, 1987), a drug with restricted use systemically due to its ability to induce aplastic anaemia among users. Employment in 'electrically' related occupations is associated with an increased risk of adult leukaemia (Coleman & Beral, 1988). The occupational groups investigated include linemen, power station workers, telecommunication workers, electrical engineers, nuclear shipyard electricians, radio and television repairers and assembly line workers, and it has not yet been convincingly demonstrated that these workers have a greater exposure to electromagnetic fields than the general population.

It has long been suspected that infectious agents play an etiological role in leukaemia, and certain viruses are known to be leukaemogenic in animals (Onions & Jarret, 1987). The evidence is, however, highly inconclusive, and no specific organism has been definitely implicated other than the human T-cell leukaemia virus in Western Japan.

Families of cases of haematopoietic malignancy, especially Hodgkin's disease and other lymphomas, have an increased risk of leukaemias (Linet, 1985). A family history of other conditions including immunopathologic disease (Till *et al.*, 1979), multiple sclerosis and infectious mononucleosis (McKinney *et al.*, 1991) also appears to increase the risk of leukaemia. However, the current evidence does not suggest that childhood leukaemia is a genetic disease (Narod, 1990).

Leukaemia: ICD-8 204-207

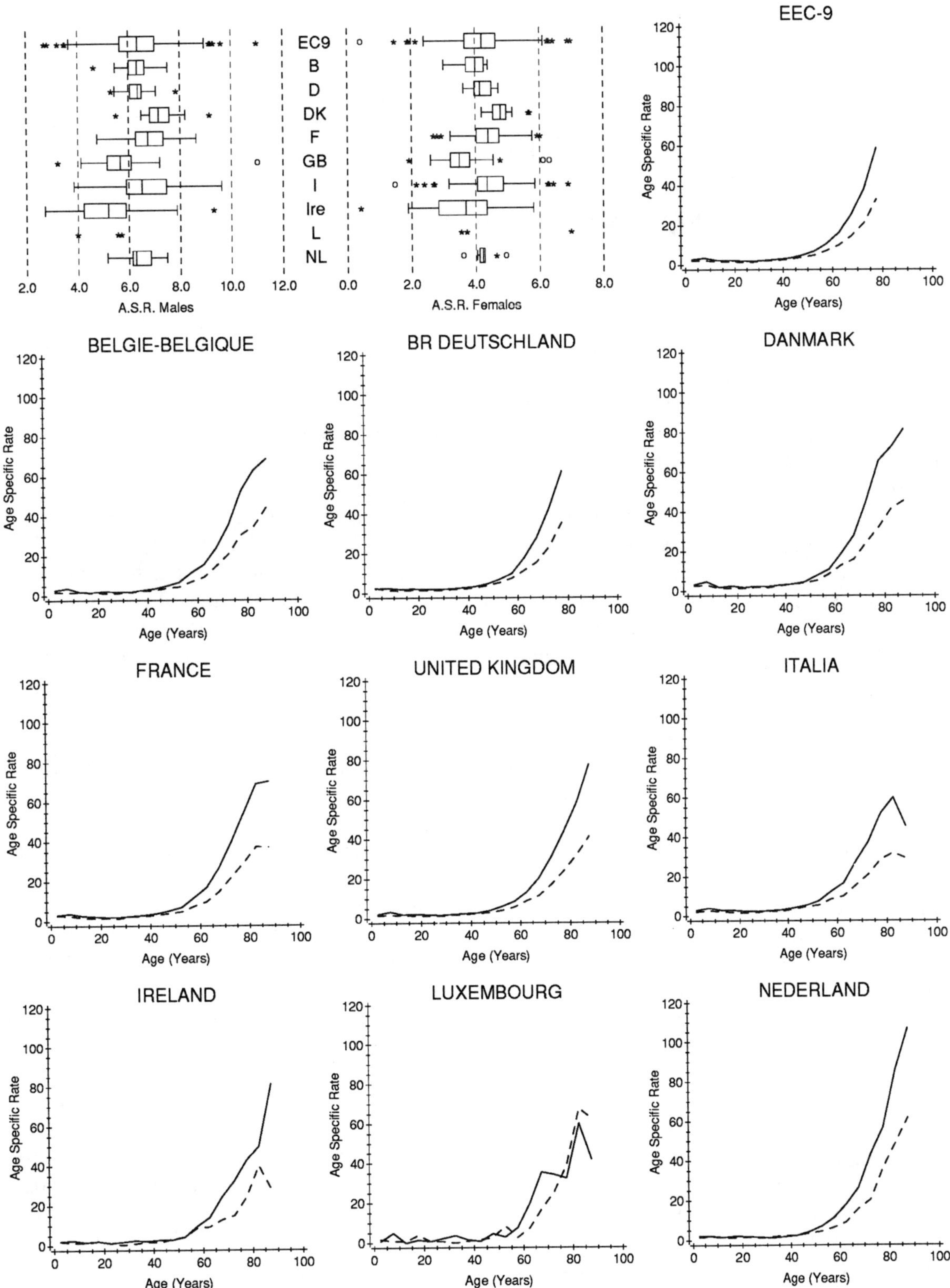

CHAPTER 6

POTENTIAL FOR PREVENTION

While an atlas of cancer mortality is of interest *per se* in that patterns of distribution are uncovered, its main value lies in the hypotheses as to the causes of cancer that may emerge from examination of the patterns of distribution, in demonstrating where studies to test such hypotheses would best be undertaken, and in pointing to priority areas for prevention. In Tables 6.1 and 6.2, the seven leading sites of cancer mortality are presented for each of the countries represented in this atlas: the implications for prevention for several of these, and for some other forms of cancer, are examined below.

In *males*, lung and stomach cancer rank first and second respectively in all nine countries, prostate being in third place except in Ireland and Italy. Colon is in fourth place, except in Italy and Ireland where these cancers occupy third rank and in France where they are fifth. France is the only country to have oesophagus in fourth place; other than Ireland, it is the only country in which this site appears in the top seven.

In *females*, breast cancer is in first place everywhere. The second ranking site is either colon or, less commonly, stomach. Only in the United Kingdom is lung cancer in second place; elsewhere it occupies fifth or sixth rank. (Currently lung cancer has displaced breast cancer from first rank in the United Kingdom.) Ovarian cancer is usually found in sixth or fifth place but in the Netherlands, it ranks second.

In Table 6.3 the range of age-standardized mortality rates for the major cancers in EEC-9 are presented (rates based on less than 10 deaths have been excluded). For many sites, the ratios of the highest to the lowest rates are very high. *It is the lowest rates that should be the target levels to be achieved by preventive measures.*

Lung

In several EEC countries, notably the United Kingdom, lung cancer mortality has begun to fall in males as a consequence of a diminution in the number of men smoking, rather than as a result of improvements in treatment. Unfortunately, at present, the mortality rates continue to rise steadily for females and in the United Kingdom, for example, there are now more deaths each year in women from lung cancer than there are from breast cancer. While voluntary bodies must continue to emphasize the dangers of tobacco, coordinated government intervention, notably in ensuring that taxation of tobacco rises at a rate above that of inflation, is of paramount importance.

The steadily accumulating epidemiological evidence of the dangers of inhaling other people's tobacco smoke (so-called passive or involuntary smoking), evidence supported by the demonstration that side-stream smoke contains higher concentrations of known cancer-causing chemicals than main-stream smoke, recently led the US Surgeon-General to estimate that passive smoking may cause over 2000 additional lung cancer deaths in the US each year. These findings reinforce the need for continuous governmental and public

Table 6.1. The seven commonest cancers in the EEC and the constituent member states in rank order of the age-standardized mortality rates (ASMR) in males

	Belgium		Denmark		Germany (FR)		France		Ireland	
Rank	Site	ASMR	Site	ASMR	Site	ASMR	Site	ASMR	Site	ASMR
1.	Lung	69.8	Lung	48.6	Lung	50.2	Lung	35.9	Lung	46.3
2.	Stomach	19.4	Stomach	14.4	Stomach	23.3	Stomach	15.0	Stomach	18.3
3.	Prostate	15.7	Prostate	14.2	Prostate	15.5	Prostate	14.2	Colon	15.3
4.	Colon	12.6	Colon	12.4	Colon	13.6	Oesophagus	14.0	Prostate	14.6
5.	Unknown	9.8	Rectum	10.4	Rectum	9.3	Colon	12.5	Pancreas	8.7
6.	Rectum	7.8	Pancreas	9.4	Unknown	7.7	Larynx	11.6	Rectum	7.9
7.	Bladder	7.8	Bladder	8.6	Pancreas	7.5	Secondary	7.9	Oesophagus	6.1

	Italy		Luxembourg		Netherlands		United Kingdom		EEC	
Rank	Site	ASMR	Site	ASMR	Site	ASMR	Site	ASMR	Site	ASMR
1.	Lung	48.6	Lung	66.3	Lung	76.8	Lung	72.9	Lung	53.5
2.	Stomach	24.5	Stomach	18.9	Stomach	19.1	Stomach	18.2	Stomach	19.3
3.	Colon	11.1	Prostate	15.9	Prostate	15.8	Prostate	12.2	Prostate	13.3
4.	Prostate	10.8	Colon	14.0	Colon	13.0	Colon	12.2	Colon	12.4
5.	Bladder	7.8	Rectum	9.6	Pancreas	9.3	Rectum	9.0	Rectum	7.8
6.	Larynx	6.7	Pancreas	7.7	Bladder	7.3	Pancreas	8.3	Pancreas	7.2
7.	Rectum	6.2	Bladder	7.2	Rectum	6.6	Bladder	7.8	Bladder	7.1

Table 6.2. The seven commonest cancers in the EEC and the constituent member states in rank order of age–standardized mortality rates (ASMR) in females

	Belgium		Denmark		Germany (FR)		France		Ireland	
Rank	Site	ASMR	Site	ASMR	Site	ASMR	Site	ASMR	Site	ASMR
1.	Breast	23.7	Breast	26.2	Breast	20.8	Breast	18.3	Breast	26.0
2.	Colon	11.7	Colon	12.1	Stomach	12.0	Colon	9.5	Colon	14.5
3.	Stomach	9.8	Lung	11.7	Colon	11.9	Uterus	6.9	Lung	14.4
4.	Uterus	7.2	Ovary	11.2	Ovary	8.1	Stomach	6.9	Stomach	9.8
5.	Unknown	7.1	Cervix uteri	8.7	Lung	5.5	Unknown	5.7	Ovary	7.3
6.	Uterus	5.6	Stomach	7.5	Rectum	5.5	Ovary	4.9	Pancreas	6.0
7.	Lung	5.5	Pancreas	6.4	Unknown	5.3	Secondary	4.2	Rectum	4.2

	Italy		Luxembourg		Netherlands		United Kingdom		EEC	
Rank	Site	ASMR	Site	ASMR	Site	ASMR	Site	ASMR	Site	ASMR
1.	Breast	18.9	Breast	21.6	Breast	26.1	Breast	27.8	Breast	21.8
2.	Stomach	12.0	Colon	10.5	Colon	11.9	Lung	16.4	Colon	10.6
3.	Colon	9.1	Stomach	9.6	Ovary	8.8	Colon	11.2	Stomach	9.3
4.	Uterus	8.7	Ovary	8.7	Stomach	8.3	Ovary	8.7	Lung	7.8
5.	Lung	5.7	Uterus	6.4	Pancreas	5.5	Stomach	8.3	Ovary	6.8
6.	Secondary	4.1	Lung	5.5	Lung	5.4	Cervix uteri	5.4	Uterus	5.5
7.	Ovary	4.0	Cervix uteri	5.0	Cervix uteri	3.9	Pancreas	5.1	Rectum	4.5

Table 6.3. Range of age-standardized cancer mortality rates for selected sites within EEC–9, between 1973 and 1980 with ratio of highest to lowest rates recorded

ICD–8	Site	Sex	Highest rate[a]			Lowest rate[a]			Ratio
140–149	Buccal cavity	M	F56	Morbihan	24.3	DBO	Berlin (West)	1.3	20.5
	and pharynx	F	JW	N. Ireland (Western)	2.4	B40	Vlaanderen (Oost)	0.3	3.8
150	Oesophagus	M	F61	Orne	35.7	I71	Foggia	1.1	32.5
		F	R17	Meath	7.3	D97	Schwaben	0.4	18.3
151	Stomach	M	I19	Cremona	57.7	F06	Alpes Maritimes	8.1	7.1
		F	I40	Forli	28.8	F06	Alpes Maritimes	3.8	7.6
153–154	Colon–rectum	M	R15	Lough	31.1	I86	Enna	6.0	5.2
		F	R20	Roscommon	24.9	I84	Agrigento	5.8	4.3
157	Pancreas	M	R01	Carlow	15.8	I83	Messina	2.1	7.5
		F	R13	Limerick	8.5	I65	Salerno	1.3	6.5
161	Larynx	M	F29	Finistere	17.7	G55	Suffolk	0.9	19.7
		F	R04	Cork	0.9	D81	Stuttgart	0.1	8.0
162	Lung	M	G14	Tyne & Wear	101.3	I86	Enna	16.7	6.1
		F	G12	Merseyside	23.8	F32	Gers	2.1	11.3
188–189	Urinary organs	M	K15	Copenhagen	16.9	R08	Kerry	4.1	4.1
		F	S12	Western Isles	8.0	I62	Benevento	0.8	6.2
201	Hodgkin's disease	M	I20	Mantova	3.6	F06	Alpes Maritimes	0.5	7.2
		F	I05	Asti	2.3	F06	Alpes Maritimes	0.3	7.7
204–207	Leukaemias	M	S12	Western Isles	11.0	S09	Dumfries + Galloway	3.2	5.7
		F	LE	Grevenmacher	7.0	I85	Caltanisetta	2.2	2.7
172	Malignant melanoma	M	K25	Roskilde	3.0	B50	Hainault	0.2	1.5
		F	K25	Roskilde	2.5	B50	Hainault	0.3	8.3
174	Breast	F	R15	Louth	36.4	I77	Matera	8.5	4.3
182	Uterus	F	K30	Vestsjaelland	14.7	JS	N. Ireland (South)	4.3	3.4
185	Prostate	M	R14	Langford	22.8	I95	Oristano	5.0	4.6
140–209	All sites	M	I19	Cremona	267.9	I86	Enna	94.2	2.8
		F	R15	Louth	143.3	F06	Alpes Maritimes	61.3	2.3

[a]Areas with rates based on less than 10 deaths have been excluded. When two or more areas had the same age–standardized mortality rate, the area with the larger number of cases has been presented.

pressure to ensure that the non-smoker is protected.

There is abundant evidence to show that persons following unskilled occupations are more likely to smoke and hence die from lung cancer than the more favoured socio-economic groups. It is here that educational efforts need to be concentrated in males. In females, in contrast, smoking is much more widely distributed among all social and occupational groups; educational campaigns need to be designed accordingly.

Oesophagus and oropharynx

As Tuyns has elegantly shown for cancers of the oesophagus, reduction in either the amount of tobacco smoked or the quantity of alcohol consumed reduces risks very substantially, as the effects of these two habits are not additive but multiplicative. The social problems related to excessive of use of alcohol are outside the scope of this atlas; none the less, control of this major public health problem would result in considerable falls in cancer incidence and mortality.

It would be instructive to consider what the mortality rates would be if alcohol-tobacco related cancers were to disappear. Assuming that these sites are the buccal cavity and pharynx, oesophagus, larynx and lung only and ignoring the contribution of smoking to other cancers such as those of the pancreas and urinary tract, removal of these tumours would reduce the total EEC cancer mortality in males by no less than 39% (Table 6.4).

Stomach

Although cancer of the stomach is in second place in males in all the countries represented in this atlas and, on average, in third place in females and is thus still a very important cause of death, the incidence and mortality for this form of malignant disease are decreasing on a worldwide basis. It would seem not unreasonable to expect that mortality rates will eventually fall from the current levels of 15-25 to those currently obtaining in the USA (around 8). The possible reasons for this fall have been mentioned earlier. These include improved food preservation through refrigeration with concomitant reduction in pickling, smoking and salting, and an increased availability of fresh fruit and vegetables throughout the year. Case-control studies have shown that consumption of fresh fruit and vegetables seems to be protective. Although two microscopic types of gastric cancer have been recognized, the intestinal and the diffuse, the former disappearing more rapidly, fresh fruit and vegetables seem to be protective against both. Cancer of the stomach is frequently preceded by a change in the gastric mucosa denoted intestinal metaplasia, as the cells of the mucosa lose their characteristic appearance and come to resemble those lining the small intestine. It has been suggested that there are three types of such metaplasia, that associated with high levels of sulfomucins being most likely to become malignant. The implications of these findings, if confirmed, for prevention are, however, not clear.

Table 6.4. Estimated proportions of cancer deaths in males in the EEC countries due to consumption of alcohol and/or tobacco

Country	%	Country	%
Belgium	40 %	Italy	37 %
FR Germany	33 %	Ireland	36 %
Denmark	33 %	Luxembourg	42 %
France	40 %	Netherlands	42 %
UK	44 %	EEC	39 %

It would thus seem highly desirable to promote the consumption of fresh fruit and vegetables as these protect against not only stomach cancer but possibly cancers at other sites as well (see below). While these items of diet are apparently abundant in northern Italy, levels of stomach cancer are high, an inconsistency requiring further study. La Vecchia *et al.* (1987), in a case–control study of gastric cancer in Milan, confirmed the protective role of green vegetables, noting that consumption of polenta (maize porridge) and ham increased risk (relative risks 2.3 and 1.6 respectively).

Breast

The risk factors for two other major causes of death from cancer within the EEC, breast and large bowel, are currently much less well understood. It is unlikely that the age of first full-term pregnancy will continue to fall within Europe and preventive measures will thus have to rely on other actions. As noted elsewhere, it is by no means certain that high levels of dietary fat are a major risk factor for this disease. A study in Athens by Katsouyanni *et al.* (1986) has indicated that breast cancer cases reported significantly less frequent consumption of vegetables, and specifically of cucumber, lettuce and raw carrot, which would imply that rational prevention was possible. These authors noted that comparing the highest quintile of vegetable consumers with the lowest quintile gave a relative risk of 0.09. In other words, the lowest quintile of vegetable consumers had about ten times the breast cancer risk of the highest. The availability of good quality fruit and vegetables could thus be of major public health importance; Kemp *et al.* (1985) have already drawn attention to the probable inequalities in their distribution in Scotland.

Large bowel

While, as for cancer of the breast, a high intake of fat has been suggested as being an important cause of large bowel cancer, the evidence is frequently conflicting. The underlying hypothesis was that a high intake of fat resulted in a high level of production of bile acids which were either carcinogens or carcinogen precursors. The effect of the presence of these bile acids could be mitigated by consumption of dietary fibre, the result of which was to dilute the concentration of these chemicals in the faeces by increasing faecal bulk. As a considerable amount of dietary fibre comes from fresh fruits and vegetables, it is rather difficult to separate the action of fibre itself from that of other components of fresh fruit and vegetables. Current belief is that there are other substances in fresh fruit and vegetables, particularly vegetables of the brassica family, which reduce large bowel cancer risk.

Dietary studies are notoriously difficult to undertake, as dietary items are frequently interrelated and few people can describe their usual diet quantitatively with any precision. None the less, if rational preventive measures are to be implemented, this is clearly a priority area for research.

Malignant melanoma of skin

The incidence of malignant melanoma of the skin and mortality from this disease is rising sharply in all fair-skinned populations. As this rate of increase is such that incidence doubles every ten to fifteen years, preventive measures need to be applied urgently. The major known risk factor for malignant melanoma is exposure to sunlight. Such exposures are frequently short but intense during vacations, and result in burning of the skin. Studies of migrants to Australia suggest that for at least one form of malignant melanoma (superficial spreading melanoma), exposure in childhood is important. The results of studies in Denmark (Østerlind *et al.*, 1988a,b,c,d) and Australia (Holman & Armstrong, 1984b), which have shown that the number of palpable pigmented naevi on the skin is a good indicator of risk, have yet to be incorporated into public information campaigns.

While it is believed that the use of protective sun screens may reduce the risk, this has yet to be scientifically proven. Preventive measures must thus run counter to the current, strongly promoted, desire to be heavily sun-tanned, reverting to the concept that a pale skin is interesting and laying emphasis on the fact that sun exposure leads to premature skin damage and wrinkling.

Cervix uteri

The evidence that cancer of the cervix uteri is in essence a venereal disease has become increasingly convincing with the demonstration of a link between this form of cancer and infection with certain human papilloma virus types. While a vaccine against this virus will probably be difficult to prepare, introduce and evaluate, systematic and nationwide implementation of cervical cytology screening programmes will continue to do much to reduce the morbidity and mortality from this form of cancer. It has been convincingly shown that only nationwide screening programmes are effective (Hakama *et al.*, 1986). While the incidence of and mortality from cancer of the cervix uteri have been falling in the EEC countries, as elsewhere, since at least 1955, there is a suggestion of an increase in women in their twenties and preventive strategies may need to be revised to take this into account.

Prostate

Although the most rational interpretation of current evidence lies in a link between diet, possibly fat, and cancer of the prostate, such an association is by no means proven and hence precise advice on preventive measures for this increasingly frequent cancer cannot yet be given.

Industrial pollution

While there is now general agreement that exposure to carcinogens in the work-place accounts for no more than 3–4% of all cancers in males and a much smaller proportion in females, most of these cancers are none the less preventable. There can be no place for complacency, as this comparatively low figure includes small industrial groups which have a much higher level of risk. For bladder cancer, for example, it has been estimated that perhaps as many as one third of all cases in males are in some way linked to an exposure at work.

Care must be taken to distinguish between an excess risk observed in a particular occupational group due to exposures at work and that due to the way of life of persons in that group. As noted above, high levels of lung cancer are more likely to reflect smoking habits than any occupational exposure, but the possibility that there may be an occupational component must always be borne in mind. The well known multiplicative effect of asbestos exposure and cigarette smoking resulted in risks some 60 to 80 times greater than in the non-smoker who was not industrially exposed to asbestos.

Potential for prevention in the Community

While within the EEC–9, there is comparatively little difference in the overall mortality from all forms of cancer combined (the highest values, 207 in males and 133 in females, are 20% and 30% higher than the lowest values respectively), there is a much wider range of mortality for several cancers (Table 6.3). Community actions should aim to reduce cancer occurrence everywhere to the lowest levels observed anywhere.

The Community has undertaken a series of actions which, in various ways, contribute to the fight against cancer.

The need to protect workers and the public against the long-term effects, in particular cancer, of dangerous chemical, biological and physical agents, has been the objective of many actions at Community level. These have been contained in a number of different sectorial activities, namely radiation protection, occupational health and safety, internal market regulations covering human and veterinary medicinals and food additives, agriculture and the environment. Research programmes in epidemiology and statistical studies have been undertaken in support of these actions (EEC, 1988), and 1989 was the 'European Cancer Year'.

In 1988, the Community published a series of posters containing the following advice:

1. **Do not smoke:** Smokers, stop as quickly as possible and do not smoke in the presence of others.

2. **Moderate your consumption of alcoholic drinks**, beers, wines or spirits.

3. **Avoid excessive exposure to sun.**

4. **Follow health and safety instructions**, especially in the working environment concerning production, handling or use of any substance which may cause cancer.

5. **Eat frequently fresh fruits and vegetables and cereals with a high fibre content.**

6. **Avoid becoming overweight**, and limit your intake of fatty foods.

More cancers will be cured if detected early:

7. **See a doctor if you notice a lump or observe a change in a mole or abnormal bleeding.**

8. **See a doctor if you have persistent problems**, such as a persistent cough, a persistent hoarseness, a change in bowel habits or an unexplained weight loss.

9. **Have a cervical smear regularly**.

10. **Check your breasts regularly,** and, if possible, undergo mammography at regular intervals above the age of 50.

Conclusion

While most cultures have a proverb to the effect that prevention is better than cure, for cancer the public and their elected governments frequently act as if they preferred to wait for the still elusive 'cure'. Such an attitude is understandable when the causes for particular cancers are unknown or debatable—it is incomprehensible when the causes are known.

REFERENCES

Adami, H.O., Bergstrom, R., Persson, I. & Sparen, P. (1990) The incidence of ovarian cancer in Sweden, 1960–1984. *Am. J. Epidemiol.*, **132**, 446–452

Adams, G.E.D. (1989) *Reverse Dose Rate Effects and Similar Phenomena*, Harwell, United Kingdom, Atomic Energy Authority

Alexander, F.E. & Boyle, P., eds (1993) *Statistical Methods for Investigating Localized Clusters of Disease* (IARC Scientific Publications), Lyon, International Agency for Research on Cancer (in press)

Alexander, F.E., McKinney, P.A. & Cartwright, R.A. (1990) Radon and leukaemia. *Lancet*, **335**, 1336–1337

Annuario Statistico Sanitario (1985) Rome, Istituto Centrale di Statistica

Armstrong, B. & Doll, R. (1975) Environmental factors and cancer incidence and mortality in different countries, with special reference to dietary practices. *Int. J. Cancer*, **15**, 617–631

Austin, D.F. & Reynolds, P. (1986) Occupation and malignant melanoma of the skin. In: Gallagher, R.P., ed., *Epidemiology of Malignant Melanoma* (Recent Results in Cancer Research, Vol. 102), Berlin, Heidelberg, New York, Springer-Verlag, pp. 98–108

Baron, J.A. (1984) Smoking and estrogen-related disease. *Am. J. Epidemiol.*, **119**, 9–22

Bergkvist, L., Adami, H.O., Persson, I., Hoover, R. & Schairer, C. (1989) The risk of breast cancer after estrogen and estrogen-progestin replacement. *New Engl. J. Med.*, **321**, 293–297

Bithell, J.F. & Stiller, C.A. (1988) A new calculation of the carcinogenic risk of obstetric X-raying. *Stat. Med.*, **7**, 587–602

Boice, J.D. & Stone, B.J. (1978) Interaction between radiation and other breast cancer risk factors. In: *Late Biological Effects of Ionizing Radiation*. Vol. I, Vienna, International Atomic Energy Agency, pp. 231–249

Boice, J.D. and 35 other authors (1985) Cancer risk following radiation treatment for cervical cancer. An international collaboration among cancer registries. *J. Natl Cancer Inst.*, **74**, 955–975

Boyle, P. (1988) Epidemiology of breast cancer. *Bailliere's Clin. Oncol.*, **2**, 1–59

Boyle, P. (1989) Relative value of incidence and mortality data in cancer research. In: Boyle, P., Muir, C. & Grundmann, E., eds, *Cancer Mapping* (Recent Results in Cancer Research, Vol. 114), Berlin, Heidelberg, New York, Springer-Verlag, pp. 41–63

Boyle, P. & Leake, R. (1988) Progress in understanding breast cancer: epidemiological interactions. *Breast Cancer Res. Treat.*, **11**, 91–112

Boyle, P. & Parkin, D.M. (1991) Statistical methods for registries. In: Jensen, O.M., Parkin, D.M., MacLennan, R., Muir, C.S. & Skeet, R.G., eds, *Cancer Registration: Principles and Methods* (IARC Scientific Publications No. 95), Lyon, International Agency for Research on Cancer, pp. 126–158

Boyle, P., Zaridze, D. & Smans, M. (1985) Descriptive epidemiology of colorectal cancer, *Int. J. Cancer*, **36**, 9–18

Boyle, P., Kaye, S.B. & Robertson, A.G. (1987) Changes in testicular cancer in Scotland. *Eur. J. Cancer Clin. Oncol.*, **23**, 827–830

Boyle, P., Soukop, M., Scully, C., Robertson, A.G., Burns, H.J.G., Gillis, C.R. & Kaye, S.B. (1988) Improving prognosis of Hodgkin's disease in Scotland. *Eur. J. Cancer Clin. Oncol.*, **24**, 229–234

Boyle, P., Hsieh, C.-C., Maisonneuve, P., La Vecchia, C., Macfarlane, G.J., Trichopoulos, D. & Walker, A.M. (1989) Epidemiology of pancreas cancer. *Int. J. Pancreatol.*, **5**, 327–346

Boyle, P., Macfarlane, G.J., McGinn, R., Zheng, T., La Vecchia, C., Maisonneuve, P. & Scully, C. (1990) International epidemiology of head and neck cancer. In: DeVries, N. & Gluckman, J. (eds) *Multiple Primary Tumours in the Head and Neck*, Stuttgart, Georg Thieme Verlag

Brinton, L.A., Reeves, W.C., Brenes, M.M., Herrero, R., Gaitan, E., Tenorio, F., de Britton, R.L., Garcia, M. & Rawls, W.E. (1989) The male factor in the etiology of cervical cancer among sexually monogamous women. *Int. J. Cancer*, **44**, 199–203

Brinton, L.A., Reeves, W.C., Brenes, M.M., Herrero, R., Gaitan, E., Tenorio, F., de Britton, R.L., Garcia, M. & Rawls, W.E. (1989) The male factor in the etiology of cervical cancer among sexually monogamous women. *Int. J. Cancer*, **44**, 199–203

Brinton, L.A., Tashima, K.T, Lehman, H.F., Levine, R.S., Mallin, K., Savitz, D.A., Stolley, P.D. & Fraumeni, J.F., Jr (1987) Epidemiology of cervical cancer by cell type. *Cancer Res.*, **47**, 1706–1711

Britton, M. & Birch, F. (1985) *1981 Cancer Post-Enumeration Survey,* London, Her Majesty's Stationery Office

Brownson, R.C., Reif, J.S., Chang, J.C. & Davis, J.R. (1990) An analysis of occupational risks for brain cancer. *Am. J. Public Health*, **80**, 169–172

Bucalossi, P. & Veronesi, U. (1959) Researches on the etiological factors in human breast cancer. *Acta Un. Int. Cancr.*, **15**, 1056–1060

Buiatti, E., Palli, D., DeCarli, A., Amadovi, D., Avellini, C., Bianchi, S., Bonaguri, C., Cipriani, F., Cocco, P., Giacosa, A., Marubini, E., Minacci, C., Puntoni, R., Russo, A., Vindigni, C., Fraumeni, J.F., Jr & Blot, W.J. (1990) A case-control study of gastric cancer and diet in Italy: II. Association with nutrients. *Int. J. Cancer*, **45**, 896–901

Burbank, F. (1971) *Patterns in Cancer Mortality in the United States 1950–1967* (National Cancer Institute Monograph 33), Washington DC, US Government Printing Office

Burch, J.D., Craib, K.J.P., Choi, B.C.K., Miller, A.B., Risch, H. & Howe, G.R. (1987) An exploratory case-control study of brain tumours in adults. *J. Natl Cancer Inst.*, **78**, 601–609

Cairns, J. (1977) *Cancer, Science and Society*, San Francisco, Freeman

Cameron, H.M. & McGoogan, E. (1981) A prospective study of 1,152 hospital autopsies. I. Inaccuracies in death certification. *J. Pathol.*, **133**, 273–283

Cartwright, R.A., McKinney, P.A., O'Brien, C., Richards, I.D.G., Roberts, B., Lauder, I., Darwin, C.M., Bernard, S.M. & Bird, C.C. (1988) Non-Hodgkin's lymphoma: case control epidemiological study in Yorkshire. *Leukaemia Res.*, **12**, 81–92

CEC (Commission of the European Communities) (1986) *A Journey through the EC*, Luxembourg, Office for Official Publications of the European Communities

Choi, N.W., Schuman, L.M. & Gullen, W.H. (1970) Epidemiology of primary central nervous system neoplasms. II. Case-control study. *Am. J. Epidemiol.*, **91**, 467–485

Cochrane, A.L., St Leger, A.S. & Moore, F. (1978) Health service 'input' and mortality 'output' in developed countries. *J. Epidemiol Commun. Health*, **32**, 200–205

Coleman, M. & Beral, V. (1988) A review of epidemiological studies on the health effects of living near or working with electricity generation and transmission equipment. *Int. J. Epidemiol.*, **17**, 1–13

Cronkite, E.P., Drew, R.T., Inove, T. & Bullis, J.E. (1985) Benzene hepatoxicity and leukaemogenesis. *Am. J. Ind. Med.*, **7**, 447–456

Crosignani, P., Macaluso, M., Berrino, F. & Vigano, C. (1983) Migrations internes et cancer dans la province de Varese. *Groupe pour l'épidemiologie et l'enregistrement du cancer dans les pays de langue latine. Communications présentées à la VIII réunion. Raguse 12–13 Mai 1983*

Cuzick, J. (1981) Radiation-induced myelomatosis. *N. Engl. J. Med.*, **304**, 204–210

Cuzick, J. & Boyle, P. (1989) Trends in cervix cancer mortality. *Cancer Surv.*, **7**, 417–439

Darby, S. & Doll, R. (1987) Fallout, radiation doses near Dounreay and childhood leukaemia. *Br. Med. J.*, **294**, 603–697

De Stefani, E., Correa, P., Oreggia, F., Leiva, J., Rivero, S., Fernandez, G., Deneo-Pellegrini, H., Zavala, D. & Fontham, E. (1987) Risk factors for laryngeal cancer. *Cancer*, **60**, 3087–3091

de-Thé, G., Geser, A., Day, N.E., Tukei, P.M., Williams, E.H., Beri, D.P., Smith, P.G., Dean, A.G., Bornkamm, G.W., Feorino, P. & Henle, W. (1978) Epidemiological evidence for causal relationship between Epstein-Barr virus and Burkitt's lymphoma from Uganda prospective study. *Nature*, **274**, 756–761

de Waard, F., Baanders-van Halewijn, E.A. & Huizinga, J. (1964) The bimodal age distribution of patients with mammary carcinoma. *Cancer*, **17**, 141–151

Doll, R. & Peto, J. (1985) *Effects on Health of Exposure to Asbestos*, London, Her Majesty's Stationery Office

Doll, R., Payne, P. & Waterhouse, J.A.H. (1966) *Cancer Incidence in Five Continents*, Vol. I, Berlin, Heidelberg, New York, Springer-Verlag

Eurostat (1981) *Nomenclature of Territorial Units for Statistics, at 1/1/1981*, Luxembourg, Statistical Office of the European Community

Ewertz, M. & Duffy, S.W. (1988) Risk of breast cancer in relation to reproductive factors in Denmark. *Br. J. Cancer*, **58**, 99-104

Ewertz, M., Duffy, S.W., Adami, H.O., Kvåle, G., Lund, E., Meirik, O., Mellengaard, A., Soini, I. & Tulinius, H. (1990) Age at first birth, parity and risk of breast cancer: a meta-analysis. *Int. J. Cancer*, **46**, 597-603

Faber, M. (1978) Malignancies in Danish thorotrast patients. *Health Phys.*, **35**, 153-157

Finch, S.C. (1984) Leukaemia and lymphoma in atomic bomb survivors. In: Boice, J.D. & Fraumeni, J.F., eds, *Radiation Carcinogenesis: Epidemiology and Biological Significance*, New York, Raven Press

Flanders, W.D. & Rothman, K.J. (1982) Interaction of alcohol and tobacco in laryngeal cancer. *Am. J. Epidemiol.*, **115**, 371-379

Franceschi, S., Boyle, P., Maisonneuve, P., La Vecchia, C., Burt, A.D., Kerr, D.J., MacFarlane, G.J. & Alexander, W.D. (1991) The epidemiology of thyroid cancer. *Epidemiol. Rev.* (in press)

Franceschi, S., Bidoli, E., Baron, A.E. & La Vecchia, C. (1990) Maize and risk of cancers of the oral cavity, pharynx and esophagus in northeastern Italy. *J. Natl Cancer Inst.*, **82**, 1407-1411

Frentzel-Beyme, R., Leutner, R., Wagner, G. & Wiebelt, H. (1979) *Krebsatlas der Bundesrepublik Deutschland*, Berlin, Heidelberg, New York, Springer-Verlag

Frisch, R.E., Wyshak, G., Albright, N.L., Albright, T.E., Schiff, I., Jones, K.P., Witschi, J., Shiang, E., Kuff, E. & Marguglio, M. (1985) Lower prevalence of breast cancer and cancers of the reproductive system among former college athletes compared to non-athletes. *Br. J. Cancer*, **52**, 885-891

Gallagher, R.P., ed. (1986) *Epidemiology of Malignant Melanoma*, Berlin, Heidelberg, New York, Springer-Verlag

Gardner, M.J., Snee, M.P., Hall, H.A., Powell, C.A., Downes, S. & Terrell, J.D. (1990) Results of a case-control study of leukaemia and lymphoma among young people near Sellafield nuclear plant in West Cumbria. *Br. Med. J.*, **300**, 423-434

Gardner, M.J., Winter, P.D., Taylor, C.P. & Acheson, E.D. (1984) *Atlas of Cancer Mortality in England and Wales, 1968-1978*, Chichester, John Wiley

Gilbert, E.S. & Marks, S. (1979) An analysis of the mortality of workers in a nuclear facility. *Radiat. Res.*, **79**, 122-148

Gilbert, E.S., Petersen, G.R. & Buchanan, J.A. (1989) Mortality of workers at the Hanford site: 1945-81. *Health Phys.*, **56**, 11-25

Gold, E., Gordis, L., Tonascia, J. & Szklo, M. (1978) Increased risk of brain tumours in children exposed to barbiturates. *J. Natl Cancer Inst.*, **61**, 1031-1034

Goldin, B.R. & Gorbach, S.L. (1984) The effect of milk and lactobacillus feeding on human intestinal bacterial enzyme activity. *Am. J. Clin. Nutr.*, **39**, 756-761

Graham, S., Mettlin, C., Marshall, J.R., Priore, R., Rzepka, T. & Shedd, D. (1981) Dietary factors in the epidemiology of cancer of the larynx. *Am. J. Epidemiol.*, **113**, 675-680

Gutensohn, N. & Cole, P. (1980) Epidemiology of Hodgkin's disease. *Seminars in Oncology*, **7**, 92-102

Hakama, M., Miller, A.B. & Day, N.E., eds (1986) *Screening for Cancer of the Uterine Cervix* (IARC Scientific Publications No. 76), Lyon, International Agency for Research on Cancer

Hakulinen, T., Andersen, A.A., Malker, B., Pukkala, E., Schou, G. & Tulinius, H. (1986) Trends in cancer incidence in the Nordic countries. *Acta Pathol. Microbiol. Immunol. Scand.*, **228** (Suppl.), 1-151

Hardell, L., Eriksson, M., Lenner, P. & Lundgren, E. (1981) Malignant lymphoma and exposure to chemicals, especially organic solvents, chlorophenols and phenoxy acids: a case-control study. *Br. J. Cancer*, **43**, 169-176

Haviland, A. (1875) *The Geographical Distribution of Diseases in Great Britain* (1st Ed.), London, Smith Elder

Heasman, M.A. & Lipworth, L. (1968) *Accuracy of Certification of Cause of Death*, London, Her Majesty's Stationery Office

Heller, T., Pavey, B. & Bailey, L., eds (1989) *Reducing the Risk of Cancer*, London, Hodder & Stoughton

Helseth, A. & Mork, S.J. (1989) Neoplasms of the central nervous system in Norway. III. Epidemiological characteristics of intracranial gliomas according to histology. *Acta Pathol. Microbiol. Immunol. Scand.*, **97**, 547–555

Hempelmann, L.H., Hall, W.J., Phillips, M., Cooper, R.A. & Ames, W.R. (1975) Neoplasms in persons treated with X-rays in infancy: fourth survey in 20 years. *J. Natl Cancer Inst.*, **55**, 519–530

Henshaw, D.L., Eatough, J.P. & Richardson, R.B. (1990) Radon: a causative factor in the induction of myeloid leukaemia and other cancers in adults and children. *Lancet*, **335**, 1008–1012

Herity, B.A., O'Halloran, M.J., Bourke, G.J. & Wilson-Davies, K. (1975) A study of breast cancer in Irish women. *Br. J. Prev. Soc. Med.*, **29**, 178–181

Hill, C. & Laplanche, A. (1990) Overall mortality and cancer mortality at French nuclear sites. *Nature*, **347**, 755–757

Holman, C.D.J. & Armstrong, B.K. (1984a) Pigmentary traits, ethnic origin, benign nevi, and family history as risk factors for cutaneous malignant melanoma. *J. Natl Cancer Inst.*, **72**, 257–266

Holman, C.D.J. & Armstrong, B.K. (1984b) Cutaneous malignant melanoma and indicators of total accumulated exposure to the sun: an analysis separating histogenetic types. *J. Natl Cancer Inst.*, **73**, 75–82

Howe, G.M. (1963) *National Atlas of Disease Mortality in the United Kingdom*, London, Nelson

Howe, G.M. (1970) *National Atlas of Disease Mortality in the United Kingdom*, revised edition, London, Nelson

Howe, G.R. & Lindsay, J.P. (1983) A follow-up study of a ten percent sample of the Canadian labor force. I. Cancer mortality in males, 1965-1973. *J. Natl Cancer Inst.*, **70**, 37–44

Howe, G.R., Jain, M. & Miller, A.B. (1990) Dietary factors and risk of pancreatic cancer: results of a Canadian population-based case-control study. *Int. J. Cancer*, **45**, 604–608

IARC (1986a) *IARC Monographs on the Evaluation of the Carcinogenic Risk of Chemicals to Humans*, Vol. 38, *Tobacco Smoking*, Lyon, International Agency for Research on Cancer

IARC (1986b) IARC Working Group on Evaluation of Cervical Screening Programmes. Screening for squamous cervical cancer: duration of low risk after negative results of cervical cytology and its implication for screening policies. *Br. Med. J.*, **293**, 659–664

IARC (1987) *IARC Monographs on the Evaluation of Carcinogenic Risks to Humans*, Supplement 7, *Overall Evaluations of Carcinogenicity: Volumes 1–42*, Lyon, International Agency for Research on Cancer

IARC (1988) *IARC Monographs on the Evaluation of Carcinogenic Risks to Humans*, Vol. 44, *Alcohol Drinking*, Lyon, International Agency for Research on Cancer

IARC (1991) *IARC Monographs on the Evaluation of Carcinogenic Risks to Humans*, Vol. 51, *Coffee, Tea, Mate, Methylxanthines and Methylglyoxal*, Lyon, International Agency for Research on Cancer

Jablon, S., Hrubec, Z., Boice, J.D. & Stone, B.J. (1990) *Cancer in Populations Living Near Nuclear Facilities* (NIH Publication No. 98–874), Washington, DC, US Government Printing Office

Jensen, O.M., Estève, J., Møller, H. & Renard, H. (1990) Cancer in the European Community and its member states. *Eur. J. Cancer*, **26**, 1167–1256

Kato, H. & Schull, W.J. (1982) Studies of A-bomb survivors. 7. Mortality, 1950–1978. Part I. Cancer mortality. *Radiat. Res.*, **90**, 395–432

Katsouyanni, K., Trichopoulos, D., Boyle, P., Xirouchaki, E., Trichopoulou, A., Lisseos, B., Vasilaros, S. & MacMahon, B. (1986) Diet and breast cancer: a case-control study in Greece. *Int. J. Cancer*, **38**, 815–820

Kelson, M. & Farebrother, M. (1987) The effect of inaccuracies in death certification and coding practices in the European Economic Community (EEC) on international cancer mortality statistics. *Int. J. Epidemiol.*, **16**, 411–414

Kelson, M.C. & Heller, R.F. (1983) The effect of death certification and coding practices on observed differences in respiratory disease mortality in 8 EEC countries. *Rev. Epidemiol. Santé Publique*, **31**, 423–432

Kemp, I., Boyle, P., Smans, M. & Muir, C., eds (1985) *Atlas of Cancer in Scotland 1975–1980: Incidence and Epidemiological Perspective* (IARC Scientific Publications No. 72), Lyon, International Agency for Research on Cancer

Kerr, D.J., Burt, A.D., Brewin, T.B. & Boyle, P. (1985) Divergence between mortality and incidence rates of thyroid cancer in Scotland. *Lancet*, **2**, 149–150

Kopecky, K.J., Yamamoto, T., Fujikura, T., Tokuoka, S., Monzen, T., Nishimori, I., Nakashima, E. & Kato, H. (1987) *Lung Cancer, Radiation Exposure and Smoking among A-bomb Survivors, Hiroshima and Nagasaki, 1950–1980* (Radiation Effects Research Foundation Technical Report 13-86), Hiroshima, Radiation Effects Research Foundation

Krain, L.S. (1971) The rising incidence of cancer of the pancreas — further epidemiological studies. *J. Chron. Dis.*, **23**, 685–690

La Vecchia, C. & Negri, E. (1989) The role of alcohol in oesophageal cancer in non-smokers and of tobacco in non-drinkers. *Int. J. Cancer*, **43**, 784–785

La Vecchia, C., Decarli, A., Fasoli, M. & Gentile, A. (1986) Nutrition and diet in the etiology of endometrial cancer. *Cancer*, **57**, 1248–1253

La Vecchia, C., Decarli, A., Negri, E., Parazzini, F., Gentile, A., Cecchetti, G., Fasoli, M. & Franceschi, S. (1987a) Dietary factors and the risk of epithelial ovarian cancer. *J. Natl Cancer Inst.*, **79**, 663–669

La Vecchia, C., Negri, E., Decarli, A., D'Avanzo, B. & Francheschi, S. (1987b) A case-control study of diet and gastric cancer in northern Italy. *Int. J. Cancer*, **40**, 484–489

La Vecchia, C., Negri, E., D'Avanzo, B. & Franceschi, S. (1989) Occupation and lymphoid neoplasms. *Br. J. Cancer*, **60**, 385–388

La Vecchia, C., Bidoli, E., Barra, S., D'Avanzo, B., Negri, E., Talamini, R. & Franceschi, S. (1990) Type of cigarettes and cancers of the upper digestive and respiratory tract. *Cancer Causes and Control*, **1**, 69–74

La Vecchia, C., Boyle, P., Franceschi, S., Maisonneuve, P., Negri, E., Lucchini, F. & Smans, M. (1991a) Smoking and cancer with emphasis on Europe. *Eur. J. Cancer*, 27, 94–104

La Vecchia, C., Levi, F., Franceschi, S. & Boyle, P. (1991b) An assessment of screening for cancer. *Int. J. Tech. Assess. and Hlth Care*, 7, 275–285

Lenoir, G.M. & Bornkamm, G.W. (1987) Burkitt's lymphoma, a human cancer model for the study of the multistep development of cancer: proposal for a new scenario. *Adv. Viral Oncol.*, **7**, 173–206

Levi, F., Maisonneuve, P., Filiberti, R., La Vecchia, C. & Boyle, P. (1989) Cancer incidence and mortality in Europe. *Sozial- und Präventivmedizin*, **34** (Suppl. 2), 1–84

Levi, F., Ollyo, J.B., La Vecchia, C., Boyle, P., Monnier, P. & Savary, M. (1990) The consumption of tobacco, alcohol, and the risk of adenocarcinoma in Barrett's oesophagus. *Int. J. Cancer*, **45**, 852–854

Lilleyman, J.S. (1987) Secondary leukaemia. In: Whittaker, J.A. & Delamare, I.W., eds, *Leukaemia*, Oxford, Blackwell Scientific Publications

Linet, M.S. (1985) *The Leukaemias: Epidemiologic Aspects*, Oxford, Oxford University Press

Longnecker, M.P., Berlin, J.A., Orza, M.J. & Chalmers, T.C. (1988) A meta-analysis of alcohol consumption in relation to risk of breast cancer. *J. Am. Med. Assoc.*, **260**, 252–256

Macklin, M.T. (1959) Comparison of the number of breast-cancer deaths observed in relatives of breast-cancer patients, and the number expected on the basis of mortality rates. *J. Natl Cancer Inst.*, **22**, 927–951

MacMahon, B. (1957) Epidemiological evidence on the nature of Hodgkin's disease. *Cancer*, **10**, 1045–1050

MacMahon, B. (1962) Prenatal x-ray exposure and childhood cancer. *J. Natl Cancer Inst.*, **28**, 1173–1191

MacMahon, B. & Pugh, T.F. (1970) *Epidemiology: Principles and Methods*, Boston, Little Brown

MacMahon, B., Yen, S., Trichopoulos, D., Warren, K. & Nardi, G. (1981) Coffee and cancer of the pancreas. *New Engl. J. Med.*, **304**, 630–633

Mancuso, T.F. & Brennan, M.S. (1970) Epidemiological considerations of cancer of the gallbladder, bile ducts and salivary glands in the rubber industry. *J. Occup. Med.*, **12**, 333–341

Marmot, M.G., Adelstein, A.M. & Bulusu, L. (1984) *Immigrant Mortality in England and Wales 1970–1978* (Studies on Medical and Population Subjects No. 47), London, Office of Population Censuses and Surveys

Mason, T.J., McKay, F.W., Hoover, R., Blot, W.T. & Fraumeni, J.F., Jr (1975) *Atlas of Cancer Mortality for US Counties: 1950–1969* (DHEW Publication No. 75-780), Washington, US Government Printing Office

Mason, T.J., McKay, F.W., Hoover, R., Blot, W.J. & Fraumeni, J.F. (1976) *Atlas of Cancer Mortality among US Non-whites: 1950–69*, Bethesda, US Department of Health, Education and Welfare

McCredie, M., Stewart, J.H. & Ford, J.M. (1983) Analgesics and tobacco as risk factors for cancer of the ureter and renal pelvis. *J. Urol.*, **130**, 28–30

McKinney, P.A., Alexander, F.E., Cartwright, R.A., Parker, L., Craft, A.W., Bailey, C. & Lewis, I. (1991) Childhood leukaemia in Cumbria, North Humberside and Gateshead and maternal and paternal occupations. *Br. Med. J.*, **302**, 681–687

McLaughlin, J.K., Gridley, G. & Block, G. (1988) Dietary factors in oral and pharyngeal cancer. *J. Natl Cancer Inst.*, **15**, 1237–1243

McMichael, A.J., Spirtas, R. & Kupper, L.L. (1974) An epidemiologic study of mortality within a cohort of rubber workers, 1964–1972. *J. Occup. Med.*, **16**, 457–464

Milham S. (1983) *Occupational Mortality in Washington State, 1950–1979* (DHHS Publ. No. 83-116), Washington, DC, US Government Printing Office

Minchovicz, J.J. & Bradlow, H.L. (1990) Induction of estradiol metabolism by dietary indole-3-carbinol in humans. *J. Natl Cancer Inst.*, **82**, 947–949

Mole, R.H. (1990) Childhood cancer after prenatal exposure to diagnostic X-ray examinations in Britain. *Br. J. Cancer*, **62**, 152–168

Monson, R.R. & MacMahon, B. (1984) Prenatal X-ray exposure and cancer in children. In: Boice, J.D. & Fraumeni, J.F., eds, *Radiation Carcinogenesis: Epidemiology and Biologic Significance*, New York, Raven Press

Muir, C., Waterhouse, J., Mack, T., Powell, J. & Whelan, S., eds (1987) *Cancer Incidence in Five Continents*, Vol. V (IARC Scientific Publications No. 88), Lyon, International Agency for Research on Cancer

Narod, S. (1990) Radiation, genetics and childhood leukaemia. *Eur. J. Cancer*, **26**, 661–665

Netherlands Central Bureau of Statistics (1980) *Atlas of Cancer Mortality in the Netherlands, 1969–1978*, The Hague, Staatsuitgeverij

Newell, G., Cole, P., Mietinen, O. & MacMahon, B. (1970) Age differences in the histology of Hodgkin's disease. *J. Natl Cancer Inst.*, **45**, 311–317

Non-Hodgkin's Lymphoma Classification Project (1982) National Cancer Institute sponsored study of classifications of non-Hodgkin's lymphomas. Summary and description of a working formulation for clinic usage. *Cancer*, **49**, 2112-2135

Onions, D. & Jarrett, O. (1987) Viral oncogenesis: lessons from naturally occurring cancer viruses. *Cancer Surveys*, **6**, 161–180

OPCS, Population Statistics Division (1982) *A Comparison of the Registrar General's Annual Population Estimates for England and Wales with the Results of 1981 Census*. Occasional Paper 29, London, Office of Population Censuses and Surveys

Østerlind, A., Tucker, M.A., Hou-Jensen, K., Stone, B.J., Engholm, G. & Jensen, O.M. (1988a) The Danish case-control study of cutaneous malignant melanoma. I. Importance of host factors. *Int. J. Cancer*, **42**, 200–206

Østerlind, A., Tucker, M.A., Stone, B.J. & Jensen, O.M. (1988b) The Danish case-control study of cutaneous malignant melanoma. II. Importance of UV-exposure. *Int. J. Cancer*, **42**, 319–324

Østerlind, A., Tucker, M.A., Stone, B.J. & Jensen, O.M. (1988c) The Danish case-control study of cutaneous malignant melanoma. III. Hormonal and reproductive factors in women. *Int. J. Cancer*, **42**, 821–824

Østerlind, A., Tucker, M.A., Stone, B.J. & Jensen, O.M. (1988d) The Danish case-control study of cutaneous malignant melanoma. IV. No association with nutritional factors, alcohol, smoking or hair dyes. *Int. J. Cancer*, **42**, 825–828

Parazzini, F., La Vecchia, C., Negri, E. & Gentile, A. (1989) Menstrual factors and the risk of epithelial ovarian cancer. *J. Clin. Epidemiol.*, **42**, 443–448

Parkin, D.M., Stiller, C.A., Bieber, C.A., Draper, G.J., Terracini, B. & Young, J.L., eds (1988a) *International Incidence of Childhood Cancer* (IARC Scientific Publications No. 87), Lyon, International Agency for Research on Cancer

Parkin, D.M., Läärä, E. & Muir, C.S. (1988b) Estimates of the worldwide frequency of sixteen major cancers in 1980. *Int. J. Cancer*, **41**, 184–197

Paterson, D.R. (1919) A clinical type of dysphagia. *J. Laryngol. Otol.*, **34**, 289–291

Percy, C. & Dolman, A. (1978) Comparison of the coding of death certificates related to cancer in seven countries. *Publ. Health Rep.*, **93**, 335–350

Percy, C. & Muir, C.S. (1989) The international comparability of cancer mortality data. Results of an international death certificate study. *Am. J. Epidemiol.*, **129**, 934–946

Percy, C., Stanek, E. & Gloeckler, L. (1981) Accuracy of cancer death certificates and its effect on cancer mortality statistics. *Am. J. Publ. Health*, **71**, 242–250

Pike, M.C. (1987) Age-related factors in cancers of the breast, ovary, and endometrium. *J. Chron. Dis.*, **40**, Suppl. 2, 595–695

Pike, M.C., Chilvers, C.E.D., Bobrow, L.G. (1987) Classification of testicular cancer in incidence and mortality statistics. Short communication. *Br. J. Cancer*, **56**, 83–85

Prentice, R.L. & Thomas, D.B. (1987) On the epidemiology of oral contraceptives and disease. *Adv. Cancer Res.*, **49**, 285–401

Prentice, R.L., Kato, H., Yoshimoto, K. & Mason, M. (1982) Radiation exposure and thyroid cancer incidence among Hiroshima and Nagasaki residents. *Natl Cancer Inst. Monogr.*, **62**, 207–212

Preston, D.L., Kato, H., Kopecky, K.J. & Fujita, S. (1986) *Life Span Study Report 10, Part 1: Cancer Mortality among A-Bomb Survivors in Hiroshima and Nagasaki, 1950-1982* (Radiation Effects Research Foundation Technical Report 1-86), Hiroshima, Radiation Effects Research Foundation

Preston-Martin, S., (1978) Abstract: A case-control study of intracranial meningiomas in women. *Am. J. Epidemiol.*, **108**, 233–234

Preston-Martin, S., Thomas, D.C, White, S.C. & Cohen, D. (1988) Prior exposure to medical and dental X-rays related to tumors of the parotid gland. *J. Natl Cancer Inst.*, **80**, 943–949

Preston-Martin, S., Yu, M.C., Benton, B. & Henderson, B.E. (1982) N-Nitroso compounds and childhood brain tumours: a case-control study. *Cancer Res.*, **42**, 5240–5245

Puffer, R.R. & Wynn-Griffith, G. (1967) *Patterns of Urban Mortality* (Scientific Publication No. 151) Washington DC, Pan American Health Organization

Reif, J.S, Pearce, N. & Fraser, J. (1989) Occupational risks for brain cancer: a New Zealand cancer registry-based study. *J. Occup. Med.*, **31**, 863–867

Rezvani A., Doyon, F. & Flamant, R. (1986) *Atlas de la Mortalité par Cancer en France*, Paris, INSERM

Sankaranarayanan, R., Duffy, S.W., Padmakuimary, G., Day, N.E. & Padmanabuam, T.K. (1989) Tobacco chewing, alcohol and nasal snuff in cancer of the gingivae in Kenuli, India. *Br. J. Cancer*, **60**, 638–643

Saxén, E.A. (1982) Trends: facts or fallacy. In: Magnus, K., ed., *Trends in Cancer Incidence. Causes and Practical Implications*, Washington, DC, Hemisphere, pp. 5–16

Schottenfeld, D., Warshauer, M.E., Sherlock, S., Zauber, L.A., Leder, M. & Payne, R. (1980) The epidemiology of testicular cancer in young adults. *Am. J. Epidemiol.*, **112**, 232–246

Segi, M. (1960) *Cancer Mortality for Selected Sites in 24 Countries (1950-57)*. Department of Public Health, Tohoku University School of Medicine, Sendai, Japan

Shimizu, Y., Kato, H., Schull, W.J., Preston, D.L., Fujita, S. & Pierce, D.A. (1987) *Life Span Study Report 11, Part 1: Comparison of risk Coefficients for Site Specific Cancer Mortality Based on the DS86 and T65DR Shielded Kerma and Organ Doses* (Radiation Effects Research Foundation Technical Report 12-87) Hiroshima, Radiation Effects Research Foundation

Shore, R.E., Albert, R.E. & Pasternack, B.S. (1976) Follow-up study of patients treated by x-ray epilation for tinea capitis. *Arch. Environ. Health*, **31**, 17–24

Shu, X.O., Linet, M.S., Gao, R.N., Gao, Y.T., Brinton, L.A., Jin, F. & Fraumeni, J.F. (1987) Chloramphenicol use and childhood leukaemia in Shanghai. *Lancet*, **2**, 934–937

Silverberg, S.G. & Vidone, R.A (1966) Adenomas and carcinoma of the thyroid. *Cancer*, **19**, 1053–1062

Slattery, M.L., Schumacher, M.L., Smith, K.R. & West, D.W. (1988) Physical activity, diet and risk of colon cancer in Utah. *Am. J. Epidemiol.*, **128**, 989–999

Smith, P.G. & Doll, R. (1981) Mortality from cancer of all causes among British radiologists. *Br. J. Radiol.*, **54**, 187–192

Smith, P.G. & Doll, R. (1982) Mortality among patients with ankylosing spondylitis after a single treatment course with x-rays. *Br. Med. J.*, **284**, 449–454

Smith, P.G. & Douglas, A.J. (1986) Mortality of workers at the Sellafield plant of British Nuclear Fuels. *Br. Med. J.*, **293**, 845–854

Smithers, D.W. (1960) *Monograph on Neoplastic Disease. Introductory Volume. A Clinical Prospect of the Cancer Problem*, Edinburgh, Livingstone, p. 140

Spiers, F.W., Lucas, H.F., Purdo, J. & Anast, G.A. (1983) Leukaemia incidence in United States dial workers. *Health Phys.*, **44**, 5–20

Stocks, P. (1936) *Distribution in England and Wales of Cancer of Various Organs.* 13th Annual Report of British Empire Cancer Campaign, London, pp. 239–280

Stocks, P. (1937) *Distribution in England and Wales of Cancer of Various Organs.* 14th Annual Report of British Empire Cancer Campaign, London, pp. 198–223

Stocks, P. (1939) *Distribution in England and Wales of Cancer of Various Organs.* 16th Annual Report of British Empire Cancer Campaign, London, pp. 308–343

Takeichi, N., Hirose, F., Yamamoto, H., Ezaki, H. & Fujikura, T. (1983) Salivary gland tumours in the atomic bomb survivors, Hiroshima, Japan. II. Pathologic study and supplementary epidemiologic observations. *Cancer*, **52**, 377–385

Thomas, T.L., Stolley, P.D., Stemhagen, A., Fontham, E.T.H., Bleecker, M.L., Stewart, P.A. & Hoover, R.N. (1987) Brain tumor mortality risk among men with electrical and electronics jobs: a case-control study. *J. Natl Cancer Inst.*, **79**, 233–238

Till, M., Rapson, N. & Smith, P.G. (1979) Family studies in acute leukaemia in childhood: a possible association with autoimmune disease. *Br. J. Cancer*, **40**, 62–71

Tolley, H.D., Marks, S., Buchanan, J.A. & Gilbert, E.S. (1983) A further update of the analysis of mortality of workers in a nuclear facility. *Radiat. Res.*, **95**, 211–213

Trichopoulos, D., MacMahon, B. & Cole, P. (1972) Menopause and breast cancer risk. *J. Natl Cancer Inst.*, **48**, 605–613

Trichopoulos, D., Hsieh, C., MacMahon, B., Lin, T., Lowe, C.R., Mirra, A.P., Ravnihar, B., Salber, E.J., Valaoras, V.G. & Yuasa, S. (1983) Age at any birth and breast cancer risk. *Int. J. Cancer*, **31**, 701–704

Tukey, J.W. (1977) *Exploratory Data Analysis* Reading, MA, London, Addison-Wesley

Tuyns, A.J., Péquignot, G. & Jensen, O.M. (1977) Le cancer de l'oesophage en Ille-et-Vilaine en fonction des niveaux de consommation d'alcool et de tabac. Des risques qui se multiplient. *Bull. Cancer*, **64**, 45–60

Tuyns, A.J., Estève, J., Raymond, L., Berrino, F., Benhamou, E., Blanchet, F., Boffetta, P., Crosignani, P., del Moral, A., Lehmann, W., Merletti, F., Péquignot, G., Riboli, E., Sancho-Garnier, H., Terracini, B., Zubiri, A. & Zubiri, L. (1988) Cancer of the larynx/hypopharynx, tobacco and alcohol. *Int. J. Cancer*, **41**, 481–483

Van den Brekel, J.C. (1977) *The Population Register: The Example of the Netherlands System* (Scientific Reports Series No. 31), Chapel Hill, NC, University of North Carolina, International Program of Laboratories for Population Statistics

Van Poppel, F.W. (1981) Regional mortality differences in western Europeans: a review of the situation in the seventies. *Soc. Sci. Med.*, **D15**, 341–352

Velema, J.P., Walker, A.M. & Gold, E.B. (1986) Alcohol and pancreatic cancer: insufficient epidemiologic evidence for a causal relationship. *Epidemiol. Rev.*, **8**, 28–41

Vena, J.E., Graham, S., Zielezny, M., Brasure, J. & Swanson, M.K. (1987) Occupational exercise and risk of cancer. *Am. J. Clin. Nutr.*, **45**, 318–327

Vigotti, M.A., Cislaghi, C., Balzi, D., Giorgi, D., La Vecchia, C., Marchi, M., Decarli, A. & Zanetti, R. (1988) Cancer mortality in migrant populations within Italy. *Tumori*, **74**, 107–128

Vineis, P., Estève, J. & Terracini, B. (1984) Bladder cancer and smoking in males: types of cigarettes, age at start, effect of stopping and interaction with occupation. *Int. J. Cancer*, **34**, 165–170

Voelz, G.L., Grier, R.S. & Hempelmann, R. (1985) A 37-year medical follow-up of Manhattan Project PO workers. *Health Phys.*, **48**, 249–254

Warren, M.P (1980) The effects of exercise on pubertal progression and reproduction function in girls. *J. Clin. Endocrinol. Metab.*, **51**, 1150–1157

Whittemore, A.S. & Gong, G. (1991) Poisson regression with misclassified counts: application to cervical cancer mortality rates. *Appl. Stat.*, **40**, 81–93

Whittemore, A.S. & McMillan, A. (1983) Lung cancer mortality among US uranium miners: a reappraisal. *J. Natl Cancer Inst.*, **71**, 489–499

WHO (World Health Organization) (1967) *Manual of the International Classification of Diseases, Injuries and Causes of Death* (Based on the Recommendations of the Eighth Revision Conference, 1965), Geneva

WHO (World Health Organization) (1977) *Manual of the International Statistical Classification of Diseases, Injuries, and Causes of Death* (Based on the recommendations of the Ninth Revision Conference, 1975), Geneva

WHO (World Health Organization) (1981) *Health Services in Europe*, Copenhagen, World Health Organization, Regional Office for Europe

WHO (World Health Organization) (1989) *World Health Statistics Annual*, Geneva, pp. xvii–xxvi

Willett, W.C. (1989) The search for the causes of breast and colon cancer. *Nature*, **338**, 389–394

Willett, W.C., Stampfer, M.J., Colditz, G.A., Rosner, B.A., Hennekens, C.H. & Speizer, F.E. (1987) Moderate alcohol consumption and the risk of breast cancer. *New Engl. J. Med.*, **316**, 1174–1180

Winn, D.M., Blot, W.J., Shy, C.M., Pickle, L.W., Toledo, A. & Fraumeni, J.F. (1981) Snuff dipping and oral cancer among women in the southern United States. *New Engl. J. Med.*, **305**, 745–749

Wynder, E.L., Hultberg, S., Jacobsson, F. & Bross, I.J. (1957) Environmental factors in cancer of the upper alimentary tract. A Swedish study with special reference to Plummer-Vinson (Paterson-Kelly) syndrome. *Cancer*, **10**, 470–487

Wynder, E.L., Escher, G.C. & Mantel, N. (1966) An epidemiological investigation of cancer of the endometrium. *Cancer*, **19**, 489–520

Yu, M.C., Huang, T.B. & Henderson, B.E. (1989) Diet and nasopharyngeal carcinoma: a case-control study in Guangzhou, China. *Int. J. Cancer*, **43**, 1077–1082

Zaridze, D.G. (1983) Environmental etiology of large-bowel cancer. *J. Natl Cancer Inst.*, **70**, 389–400

Zaridze, D.G. & Boyle, P. (1987) Cancer of the prostate: epidemiology and aetiology. *Br. J. Urol.*, **59**, 493–503

Zheng, T., Boyle, P., Hu, H., Duan, J., Jiang, P., Ma, D., Shui, L., Niu, S., Scully, C. & McMahon, B. (1990) Dentition, oral hygiene and risk of oral cancer: a case-control study in Beijing, People's Republic of China. *Cancer Causes and Control*, **1**, 235–241

Zheng, T., Boyle, P., Willett, W.C., Hu, H.F., Duan, J., Evstifeeva, T., Niu, S. & MacMahon, B. (1991) A case-control study of oral cancer in Beijing, People's Republic of China: I. The associations with nutrient intakes. *Int. J. Cancer* (in press)

Ziel, H.K. & Finkle, W.D. (1975) Increased risk of endometrial carcinoma among users of conjugated estrogens. *New Engl. J. Med.*, **293**, 1167–1170

ANNEX 1

TABLES

BELGIE-BELGIQUE (1971-78)

BRUSSEL-BRUXELLES					
B21	1275	32.3	20.0++	0.58	17
VLAANDEREN					
B10	746	12.1	8.4--	0.32	252
B29	751	20.9	14.6++	0.55	102
B30	1138	26.8	18.6++	0.57	31
B40	904	17.3	11.4--	0.40	160
B70	253	9.1	9.3--	0.59	222
B-V	3792	17.2	12.3	0.21	
WALLONIE					
B25	217	21.1	14.7+	1.02	99
B50	1223	23.8	16.0++	0.47	78
B60	872	22.1	14.7++	0.51	99
B80	140	16.2	11.2	0.98	169
B90	225	14.8	10.6--	0.72	186
B-W	2677	21.5	14.5++	0.29	
B.0	7744	20.1	13.9++	0.16	

BR DEUTSCHLAND (1976-80)

BADEN-WURTTEMBERG					
D81	1122	13.5	9.9--	0.31	207
D82	931	16.4	11.9	0.41	152
D83	724	16.4	12.0	0.47	151
D84	468	13.0	10.0--	0.49	206
D-A	3245	14.7	10.8--	0.20	
BAYERN					
D91	1788	20.5	14.1++	0.35	110
D92	562	24.0	16.5++	0.73	68
D93	513	22.2	16.3++	0.75	70
D94	487	19.7	12.9	0.62	133
D95	746	20.8	13.8+	0.53	115
D96	525	18.4	12.9	0.59	133
D97	773	21.4	14.0++	0.53	112
D-B	5394	20.8	14.2++	0.20	
BERLIN(WEST)					
DB0	1006	23.5	13.7+	0.47	120
BREMEN					
D40	390	23.7	14.6+	0.78	102
HAMBURG					
D20	948	24.5	13.8+	0.49	115
HESSEN					
D64	1907	18.1	12.2	0.30	143
D66	535	18.9	11.4-	0.53	160
D-F	2442	18.3	12.0-	0.26	
NIEDERSACHSEN					
D31	747	19.1	12.2	0.47	143
D32	946	19.5	12.2	0.42	143
D33	632	18.1	12.2	0.52	143
D34	866	17.1	12.7	0.45	137
D-G	3191	18.4	12.3	0.23	
NORDRHEIN-WESTFALEN					
D51	2212	17.9	13.5++	0.30	125
D53	1437	15.3	12.7	0.35	137
D55	969	16.7	14.5++	0.49	105
D57	766	17.9	13.1	0.49	129
D59	1747	19.8	15.0++	0.38	92
D-H	7131	17.5	13.7++	0.17	
RHEINLAND-PFALZ					
D71	561	17.2	11.3--	0.50	167
D72	165	14.7	10.5-	0.86	192
D73	682	15.8	11.0--	0.45	175
D-I	1408	16.2	11.0--	0.31	
SAARLAND					
DA0	424	16.5	11.4-	0.58	160
SCHLESWIG-HOLSTEIN					
D10	1268	20.3	13.0	0.39	131
D.0	26847	18.3	12.7	0.08	

DANMARK (1971-80)

K15	613	10.1	6.4--	0.26	316
K20	88	5.8	5.3--	0.57	344
K25	84	9.0	8.6--	0.95	249
K30	140	10.3	6.0--	0.54	329
K35	160	12.4	6.5--	0.55	312
K40	35	14.7	8.8-	1.60	241
K42	231	10.4	6.1--	0.42	326
K50	101	8.3	5.6--	0.57	340
K55	89	8.6	6.1--	0.67	326
K60	154	9.8	6.2--	0.52	323
K65	105	8.2	5.6--	0.57	340
K70	230	8.3	6.0--	0.41	329
K76	109	9.5	5.7--	0.58	339
K80	223	9.4	6.0--	0.42	329
K.0	2362	9.4	6.2--	0.13	

FRANCE (1971-78)

ALSACE					
F67	998	28.9	23.4++	0.77	6
F68	671	26.8	22.5++	0.91	8
F-A	1669	28.0	23.0++	0.59	
AQUITAINE					
F24	420	28.8	15.1++	0.80	88
F33	1265	31.0	21.1++	0.62	10
F40	367	32.8	19.4++	1.08	26
F47	296	26.0	14.9+	0.92	94
F64	605	29.3	18.3++	0.78	35
F-B	2953	29.9	18.6++	0.36	
AUVERGNE					
F03	495	33.4	18.6++	0.90	31
F15	177	26.7	15.1+	1.19	88
F43	212	26.4	15.1+	1.11	88
F63	553	24.3	17.5++	0.77	51
F-C	1437	27.5	17.2++	0.48	
BASSE-NORMANDIE					
F14	511	23.4	20.3++	0.92	15
F50	476	27.3	20.5++	0.97	13
F61	248	21.7	15.9++	1.05	79
F-D	1235	24.4	19.3++	0.56	
BOURGOGNE					
F21	398	22.2	16.6++	0.86	66
F58	283	28.9	15.1+	0.99	88
F71	568	25.3	16.3++	0.73	70
F89	413	34.8	19.8++	1.07	21
F-E	1662	26.8	16.9++	0.44	
BRETAGNE					
F22	597	29.3	20.0++	0.86	17
F29	894	28.7	19.6++	0.68	23
F35	678	25.1	20.3++	0.80	15
F56	507	23.0	17.5++	0.80	51
F-F	2676	26.6	19.4++	0.39	
CENTRE					
F18	360	28.7	17.6++	0.99	48
F28	305	22.7	15.6++	0.94	81
F36	298	30.5	16.3++	1.05	70
F37	474	25.5	18.0++	0.87	42
F41	294	26.5	16.2++	1.02	75
F45	503	25.9	18.1++	0.85	40
F-G	2234	26.3	17.1++	0.38	
CHAMPAGNE-ARDENNE					
F08	308	24.8	19.9++	1.18	19
F10	322	28.7	19.5++	1.16	25
F51	419	19.9	16.7++	0.84	63
F52	176	20.7	15.2+	1.19	87
F-H	1225	23.0	17.8++	0.53	
CORSE					
F20	280	29.2	19.4++	1.21	26
FRANCHE-COMTE					
F25	275	14.6	13.8	0.85	115
F39	177	18.6	11.9	0.94	152
F70	185	21.2	14.7	1.15	99
F90	117	22.9	20.5++	1.93	13
F-J	754	17.9	14.2++	0.54	
HAUTE-NORMANDIE					
F27	353	21.1	16.3++	0.90	70
F76	1014	22.0	18.3++	0.59	35
F-K	1367	21.8	17.8++	0.49	
ILE-DE-FRANCE					
F75	3418	40.2	25.0++	0.45	2
F77	681	22.6	18.9++	0.75	29
F78	864	20.0	21.0++	0.73	11
F91	676	18.4	19.9++	0.78	19
F92	1685	30.0	24.1++	0.60	4
F93	1281	24.2	23.1++	0.66	7
F94	1314	27.7	24.5++	0.69	3
F95	788	23.6	23.7++	0.86	5
F-L	10707	27.8	23.2++	0.23	
LANGUEDOC-ROUSSILLON					
F11	400	38.4	19.6++	1.08	23
F30	525	27.3	17.2++	0.79	58
F34	726	29.1	17.6++	0.70	48
F48	101	33.6	18.4++	1.95	34
F66	365	31.5	16.4++	0.92	69
F-M	2117	30.6	17.6++	0.41	
LIMOUSIN					
F19	324	34.4	18.0++	1.09	42
F23	228	39.8	19.1++	1.41	28
F87	416	30.4	17.4++	0.92	53
F-N	968	33.6	18.0++	0.63	
LORRAINE					
F54	549	19.2	16.1++	0.71	76
F55	197	24.5	18.0++	1.35	42
F57	688	17.0	16.3++	0.64	70
F88	318	20.4	15.7++	0.92	80
F-O	1752	18.9	16.3++	0.40	
MIDI-PYRENEES					
F09	166	30.3	13.6	1.16	124
F12	305	28.2	15.0++	0.92	92
F31	725	24.1	16.7++	0.64	63
F32	225	32.2	16.8++	1.21	61
F46	153	26.0	14.8	1.39	96
F65	226	25.5	15.5++	1.07	84
F81	314	23.7	13.4	0.82	126
F82	215	30.0	17.4++	1.28	53
F-P	2329	26.3	15.5++	0.34	
NORD-PAS-DE-CALAIS					
F59	2089	21.2	18.2++	0.41	37
F62	1119	20.4	16.7++	0.51	63
F-Q	3208	20.9	17.6++	0.32	
PAYS DE LA LOIRE					
F44	894	24.8	20.7++	0.71	12
F49	537	21.8	16.6++	0.75	66
F53	230	22.7	17.0++	1.16	60
F72	415	21.6	15.3++	0.78	86
F85	434	24.9	17.2++	0.87	58
F-R	2510	23.4	17.8++	0.37	
PICARDIE					
F02	518	24.4	18.0++	0.84	42
F60	526	21.6	18.6++	0.84	31
F80	540	25.6	18.0++	0.82	42
F-S	1584	23.7	18.2++	0.48	
POITOU-CHARENTES					
F16	315	23.9	14.8+	0.89	96
F17	425	21.9	13.4	0.69	126
F79	277	20.8	13.1	0.84	129
F86	384	27.4	17.3++	0.93	56
F-T	1401	23.4	14.5++	0.41	
PROVENCE-ALPES-COTE D'AZUR					
F04	128	28.5	15.6+	1.48	81
F05	112	28.9	18.7++	1.84	30
F06	1041	33.8	18.2++	0.62	37
F13	2284	35.7	26.1++	0.56	1
F83	872	35.4	22.0++	0.78	9
F84	403	26.0	17.6++	0.92	48
F-U	4840	33.8	21.8++	0.33	
RHONE-ALPES					
F01	301	19.9	14.5+	0.87	105
F07	304	30.3	18.2++	1.11	37
F26	298	21.1	14.6+	0.89	102
F38	743	21.8	18.1++	0.68	40
F42	718	24.5	17.9++	0.69	47
F69	1284	22.9	19.7++	0.56	22
F73	256	21.0	16.1++	1.04	76
F74	338	18.8	16.8++	0.94	61
F-V	4242	22.5	17.6++	0.28	
F.0	53150	25.8	18.8++	0.08	

UNITED KINGDOM (1976-80)

EAST ANGLIA					
G25	192	11.2	8.6--	0.64	249
G46	310	15.6	8.9--	0.52	236
G55	218	12.3	8.0--	0.56	269
G-A	720	13.1	8.5--	0.33	
EAST MIDLANDS					
G30	318	12.1	7.8--	0.45	274
G44	242	9.8	6.9--	0.46	303
G45	172	10.9	7.0--	0.55	300
G47	175	11.5	7.7--	0.60	278
G50	263	9.2	6.4--	0.40	316
G-B	1170	10.6	7.1--	0.21	
NORTHERN					
G14	506	14.9	10.2--	0.47	199
G27	134	8.0	6.3--	0.55	320
G29	184	13.4	8.3--	0.62	254
G33	253	14.2	9.6--	0.62	214
G48	94	11.0	6.8--	0.73	306
G-C	1171	12.9	8.8--	0.26	
NORTH-WEST					
G11	1030	13.3	9.4--	0.30	218
G12	612	13.7	9.6--	0.40	214
G26	279	10.4	7.6--	0.46	283
G43	399	10.1	6.2--	0.32	323
G-D	2320	12.3	8.5--	0.18	

SOUTH-EAST					
G01	2460	12.3	7.6--	0.16	283
G22	141	9.5	7.6--	0.65	283
G23	232	11.5	9.0--	0.60	233
G24	145	9.2	7.4--	0.62	291
G34	334	18.7	8.2--	0.49	259
G35	471	11.2	7.7--	0.36	278
G37	469	10.7	7.9--	0.37	272
G39	281	10.1	7.6--	0.47	283
G41	43	13.3	7.1--	1.17	298
G42	470	11.1	7.1--	0.34	298
G51	191	11.4	9.9--	0.76	207
G56	284	9.8	6.6--	0.40	311
G58	288	16.2	8.1--	0.51	266
G-E	5809	11.8	7.7--	0.10	
SOUTH-WEST					
G21	327	12.3	7.8--	0.44	274
G28	172	14.4	8.2--	0.65	259
G31	395	14.3	7.6--	0.41	283
G32	252	15.2	7.4--	0.50	291
G36	172	11.9	7.7--	0.61	278
G53	156	12.9	7.9--	0.66	272
G59	125	8.1	6.2--	0.57	323
G-F	1599	12.8	7.5--	0.20	
WEST MIDLANDS					
G15	836	10.4	7.3--	0.26	294
G38	227	12.7	8.4--	0.58	252
G52	117	10.9	7.5--	0.71	290
G54	244	8.3	6.3--	0.41	320
G57	115	8.3	6.4--	0.62	316
G-G	1539	10.1	7.2--	0.19	
YORKSHIRE AND HUMBERSIDE					
G13	400	10.4	6.8--	0.35	306
G16	732	12.2	8.2--	0.31	259
G40	247	10.0	6.8--	0.44	306
G49	218	11.2	7.0--	0.49	300
G-H	1597	11.2	7.4--	0.19	
WALES					
G61	117	10.6	6.5--	0.62	312
G62	97	10.3	6.0--	0.63	329
G63	118	9.2	5.9--	0.55	335
G64	65	9.9	5.8--	0.75	337
G65	170	10.8	7.7--	0.60	278
G66	34	10.7	5.9--	1.06	335
G67	130	11.6	8.0--	0.72	269
G68	131	12.4	8.0--	0.72	269
G-I	862	10.7	6.9--	0.24	
SCOTLAND(1975-80)					
S01	76	13.6	9.2--	1.08	227
S02	179	13.4	9.3--	0.72	222
S03	129	11.2	7.4--	0.68	291
S04	84	8.4	6.1--	0.68	326
S05	280	13.0	9.3--	0.57	222
S06	27	9.4	5.3--	1.09	344
S07	63	7.9	5.5--	0.72	343
S08	769	10.9	8.2--	0.30	259
S09	42	10.0	6.5--	1.05	312
S10	6	11.3	7.2	3.10	297
S11	9	14.4	8.8	3.01	241
S12	15	17.1	7.8-	2.15	274
G-J	1679	11.2	8.0--	0.20	
NORTHERN IRELAND					
JE	145	8.8	7.6--	0.66	283
JN	67	7.4	6.4--	0.80	316
JS	44	6.6	6.0--	0.94	329
JW	58	9.6	8.8--	1.20	241
G-K	314	8.2	7.2--	0.42	
G.0	18780	11.6	7.7--	0.06	

ITALIA (1975-79)

ABRUZZI					
I66	124	16.9	10.6-	0.99	186
I67	83	12.5	8.2--	0.92	259
I68	94	13.5	9.9--	1.05	207
I69	118	13.2	8.9--	0.84	236
I-A	419	14.0	9.4--	0.47	
BASILICATA					
I76	103	10.0	7.3--	0.75	294
I77	61	12.1	10.1	1.31	203
I-B	164	10.7	8.1--	0.65	
CALABRIA					
I78	187	10.5	8.8--	0.65	241
I79	176	9.6	8.2--	0.63	259
I80	204	14.0	10.2--	0.74	199
I-C	567	11.2	9.0--	0.39	
CAMPANIA					
I61	214	12.0	11.0-	0.76	175
I62	111	15.4	10.3-	1.02	198
I63	914	13.1	13.8++	0.46	115
I64	133	12.3	8.9--	0.79	236
I65	271	11.0	9.3--	0.57	222
I-D	1643	12.6	11.7--	0.29	
EMILIA-ROMAGNA					
I33	128	18.4	10.6-	1.00	186
I34	198	20.4	11.4	0.83	160
I35	177	17.8	11.1	0.87	173
I36	196	13.8	10.1--	0.75	203
I37	294	13.0	8.3--	0.50	254
I38	140	14.9	9.3--	0.80	222
I39	115	13.1	8.2--	0.79	259
I40	221	15.3	10.7--	0.73	182
I-E	1469	15.3	9.7--	0.26	
FRIULI-VENEZIA GIULIA					
I30	227	17.7	11.4	0.77	160
I31	51	14.5	9.4-	1.33	218
I32	117	16.8	9.0--	0.89	233
I93	96	14.7	10.5	1.11	192
I-F	491	16.4	10.4--	0.48	
LAZIO					
I56	110	16.8	10.5-	1.03	192
I57	78	21.9	12.4	1.48	140
I58	1282	14.4	12.9	0.37	133
I59	124	11.9	10.9	0.99	177
I60	174	15.6	11.2	0.88	169
I-G	1768	14.7	12.3	0.30	
LIGURIA					
I08	125	22.5	12.4	1.16	140
I09	152	20.6	11.7	0.98	156
I10	536	20.8	12.1	0.54	149
I11	138	23.3	13.7	1.20	120
I-H	951	21.3	12.3	0.41	
LOMBARDIA					
I12	265	14.1	12.8	0.84	136
I13	330	18.0	14.8++	0.84	96
I14	76	17.7	14.2	1.65	109
I15	1723	17.7	15.5++	0.38	84
I16	386	18.0	17.4++	0.91	53
I17	473	19.3	17.3++	0.80	56
I18	281	22.1	12.6	0.78	139
I19	168	20.7	13.7	1.09	120
I20	193	20.8	13.2	0.98	128
I-I	3895	18.1	15.0++	0.25	
MARCHE					
I41	106	13.1	8.7--	0.87	245
I42	144	14.0	9.1--	0.78	230
I43	110	15.5	9.7--	0.97	212
I44	124	14.5	10.2--	0.93	199
I-J	484	14.2	9.4--	0.44	
MOLISE					
I70	80	13.9	9.5--	1.09	217
I94	42	18.1	10.9	1.75	177
I-K	122	15.1	9.8--	0.92	
PIEMONTE					
I01	976	16.8	13.8++	0.46	115
I02	239	24.7	14.5	1.00	105
I03	227	18.5	12.2	0.84	143
I04	182	13.4	7.7--	0.60	278
I05	110	20.5	10.2-	1.06	199
I06	255	22.0	10.4--	0.69	195
I-L	1989	18.0	12.1	0.28	
PUGLIA					
I71	200	11.9	9.7--	0.71	212
I72	372	10.6	9.1--	0.48	230
I73	155	11.3	10.8-	0.87	181
I74	136	14.3	12.2	1.06	143
I75	248	13.7	11.4	0.73	160
I-M	1111	11.9	10.2--	0.31	
SARDEGNA					
I90	160	15.3	10.9	0.89	177
I91	134	19.7	13.9	1.30	113
I92	281	16.0	14.9+	0.90	94
I95	74	19.1	11.4	1.45	160
I-N	649	16.7	13.1	0.53	
SICILIA					
I81	143	13.9	8.9--	0.78	236
I82	571	19.9	15.6++	0.67	81
I83	256	15.6	10.7--	0.69	182
I84	178	14.9	10.4--	0.81	195
I85	109	15.1	11.9	1.18	152
I86	74	14.7	10.6	1.29	186
I87	306	12.6	9.8--	0.57	210
I88	95	14.4	10.4-	1.10	195
I89	158	16.3	13.0	1.05	131
I-O	1890	15.7	11.7--	0.28	
TOSCANA					
I45	71	14.3	8.9--	1.09	236
I46	177	19.0	11.6	0.91	158
I47	124	19.4	12.1	1.12	149
I48	518	18.0	11.2--	0.51	169
I49	184	21.9	13.7	1.03	120
I50	174	18.6	10.9-	0.86	177
I51	130	16.9	10.1--	0.90	203
I52	92	14.5	7.3--	0.81	294
I53	107	19.4	11.1	1.10	173
I-P	1577	18.2	10.9--	0.28	
TRENTINO-ALTO ADIGE					
I21	171	16.2	14.1	1.11	110
I22	209	19.5	13.9	0.99	113
I-Q	380	17.9	14.0	0.74	
UMBRIA					
I54	206	14.7	9.2--	0.66	227
I55	64	11.4	6.9--	0.88	303
I-R	270	13.7	8.5--	0.53	
VALLE D'AOSTA					
I07	40	14.0	10.6	1.72	186
VENETO					
I23	349	18.7	14.3+	0.78	108
I24	240	13.8	11.7	0.76	156
I25	86	15.9	10.6	1.18	186
I26	250	14.6	11.9	0.77	152
I27	265	13.0	10.7--	0.67	182
I28	266	13.6	11.3	0.70	167
I29	113	18.2	12.4	1.19	140
I-T	1569	15.0	11.9-	0.31	
I.0	21448	15.6	11.7--	0.08	

IRELAND (1976-80)

CONNAUGHT					
R07	32	7.4	4.6--	0.86	350
R12	5	6.7	2.3--	1.06	355
R16	26	8.9	3.9--	0.78	352
R20	19	13.3	6.8--	1.62	306
R21	13	9.4	5.8--	1.72	337
R-A	95	8.8	4.7--	0.51	
LEINSTER					
R01	10	10.1	8.3	2.67	254
R06	180	7.6	8.3--	0.63	254
R09	20	7.9	9.8	2.24	210
R10	11	6.2	4.6--	1.43	350
R11	8	6.1	5.2--	1.88	347
R14	7	8.7	5.6--	2.16	340
R15	12	5.6	5.0--	1.47	348
R17	17	7.3	6.3--	1.56	320
R19	6	4.0	2.6--	1.10	354
R24	12	7.9	5.3--	1.60	344
R25	23	9.4	6.8--	1.45	306
R26	22	10.5	9.4	2.05	218
R-B	328	7.6	7.3--	0.41	
MUNSTER					
R03	22	10.0	7.0--	1.53	300
R04	99	9.9	8.3--	0.86	254
R08	41	13.2	8.7--	1.43	245
R13	35	8.8	7.8--	1.36	274
R22	29	8.4	6.0--	1.17	329
R23	25	11.4	9.4	1.93	218
R-C	251	10.1	7.9--	0.51	
ULSTER					
R02	11	7.8	4.9--	1.54	349
R05	21	6.7	3.9--	0.89	352
R18	12	9.1	6.5--	1.94	312
R-D	44	7.5	4.7--	0.74	
R.0	718	8.5	6.8--	0.26	

LUXEMBOURG (1971-80)

LE	28	15.4	9.2	1.80	227
LN	46	17.4	11.2	1.73	169
LS	195	15.3	11.6	0.85	158
L.0	269	15.6	11.2-	0.70	

NEDERLAND (1976-80)

N01	191	14.0	9.6--	0.72	214
N02	160	11.2	7.6--	0.64	283
N03	105	10.1	6.9--	0.69	303
N04	284	11.3	9.0--	0.55	233
N05	429	10.3	8.1--	0.40	266
N06	276	12.7	10.7--	0.66	182
N07	676	11.7	8.7--	0.34	245
N08	935	12.4	9.1--	0.30	230
N09	125	14.7	8.7--	0.82	245
N10	452	8.9	8.6--	0.41	249
N11	236	8.9	8.1--	0.53	266
N.0	3869	11.2	8.7--	0.14	

EEC-9

EEC	135187	17.8	12.6	0.04	

BELGIE-BELGIQUE (1971-78)

BRUSSEL-BRUXELLES					
B21	1390	31.2	12.4++	0.38	21
VLAANDEREN					
B10	750	11.9	6.3--	0.25	258
B29	726	19.8	11.2++	0.45	58
B30	1102	25.4	14.5++	0.47	4
B40	994	18.5	9.8++	0.34	111
B70	207	7.7	6.4--	0.45	250
B-V	3779	16.9	9.6++	0.17	
WALLONIE					
B25	252	23.5	11.6++	0.81	44
B50	1243	22.8	10.6++	0.34	80
B60	1000	23.7	11.4++	0.40	51
B80	141	15.8	7.7	0.71	189
B90	276	17.2	8.7	0.58	156
B-W	2912	22.0	10.5++	0.22	
B.0	8081	20.2	10.3++	0.13	

BR DEUTSCHLAND (1976-80)

BADEN-WURTTEMBERG					
D81	1455	16.3	7.9--	0.23	183
D82	1135	18.3	8.4	0.28	167
D83	872	18.0	8.4	0.32	167
D84	606	15.7	7.9--	0.35	183
D-A	4068	17.1	8.1--	0.14	
BAYERN					
D91	2200	23.5	10.4++	0.25	89
D92	653	24.9	11.5++	0.49	47
D93	605	23.9	10.9++	0.48	68
D94	616	22.0	8.8	0.40	150
D95	918	23.0	9.6+	0.35	122
D96	622	20.1	9.1	0.40	140
D97	1042	26.2	11.3++	0.39	54
D-B	6656	23.5	10.3++	0.14	
BERLIN(WEST)					
DB0	1035	19.5	6.2--	0.24	267
BREMEN					
D40	521	28.1	12.0++	0.61	26
HAMBURG					
D20	1153	25.8	9.0	0.33	145
HESSEN					
D64	2860	25.2	10.9++	0.23	68
D66	817	26.3	10.2++	0.40	95
D-F	3677	25.4	10.8++	0.20	
NIEDERSACHSEN					
D31	927	21.6	8.8	0.34	150
D32	1219	22.4	8.9	0.30	147
D33	816	22.1	9.7+	0.38	116
D34	1076	19.8	10.1++	0.34	100
D-G	4038	21.4	9.3++	0.17	
NORDRHEIN-WESTFALEN					
D51	2782	20.2	9.8++	0.20	111
D53	1932	19.2	10.1++	0.25	100
D55	1243	19.9	11.3++	0.34	54
D57	1039	21.9	10.1++	0.34	100
D59	2296	23.8	11.8++	0.27	37
D-H	9292	20.9	10.5++	0.12	
RHEINLAND-PFALZ					
D71	602	16.9	7.4--	0.34	196
D72	173	13.9	6.8--	0.58	231
D73	724	15.3	7.2--	0.30	208
D-I	1499	15.8	7.2--	0.21	
SAARLAND					
DA0	539	18.9	8.8	0.42	150
SCHLESWIG-HOLSTEIN					
D10	1534	22.8	9.4+	0.27	130
D.0	34012	21.2	9.3++	0.06	

DANMARK (1971-80)

K15	758	11.4	4.8--	0.19	330
K20	105	7.0	4.7--	0.49	333
K25	92	10.1	7.4	0.80	196
K30	136	10.2	4.9--	0.45	328
K35	185	14.5	6.3--	0.51	258
K40	38	16.2	7.0	1.25	218
K42	264	11.8	5.5--	0.37	301
K50	164	13.4	6.7--	0.56	235
K55	124	12.2	7.4	0.70	196
K60	218	13.7	7.2--	0.52	208
K65	135	10.8	6.8--	0.61	231
K70	270	9.6	5.1--	0.33	321
K76	153	13.7	6.8--	0.59	231
K80	261	11.1	5.7--	0.38	288
K.0	2903	11.4	5.6--	0.11	

FRANCE (1971-78)

ALSACE					
F67	840	23.2	12.7++	0.49	19
F68	661	25.5	13.7++	0.61	9
F-A	1501	24.2	13.1++	0.38	
AQUITAINE					
F24	422	27.6	11.7++	0.68	41
F33	1143	25.9	12.2++	0.42	24
F40	311	26.5	11.1++	0.75	61
F47	307	25.7	11.6++	0.79	44
F64	641	29.0	13.8++	0.63	8
F-B	2824	26.8	12.3++	0.27	
AUVERGNE					
F03	474	30.3	12.3++	0.68	23
F15	139	20.6	9.8	0.98	111
F43	212	25.2	10.6+	0.90	80
F63	537	22.7	11.9++	0.59	32
F-C	1362	25.0	11.6++	0.37	
BASSE-NORMANDIE					
F14	456	19.8	11.5++	0.60	47
F50	420	22.5	11.8++	0.66	37
F61	228	18.8	9.5	0.73	127
F-D	1104	20.5	11.1++	0.38	
BOURGOGNE					
F21	336	18.2	10.0	0.61	103
F58	313	31.0	12.8++	0.88	16
F71	522	22.5	10.4++	0.55	89
F89	334	27.4	10.9++	0.73	68
F-E	1505	23.5	10.8++	0.33	
BRETAGNE					
F22	528	24.5	11.4++	0.57	51
F29	703	21.2	10.2++	0.44	95
F35	628	21.5	11.5++	0.51	47
F56	438	19.0	9.7	0.52	116
F-F	2297	21.5	10.6++	0.25	
CENTRE					
F18	321	24.9	10.9++	0.74	68
F28	284	21.2	11.4++	0.80	51
F36	300	30.1	14.1++	1.01	5
F37	521	26.5	14.7++	0.74	3
F41	269	23.4	10.4+	0.77	89
F45	444	22.4	11.0++	0.59	65
F-G	2139	24.5	12.1++	0.31	
CHAMPAGNE-ARDENNE					
F08	236	19.0	11.1++	0.81	61
F10	279	24.2	12.0++	0.83	26
F51	383	18.0	10.5++	0.60	87
F52	176	20.6	10.7+	0.92	77
F-H	1074	20.0	11.0++	0.38	
CORSE					
F20	223	25.9	12.0++	0.92	26
FRANCHE-COMTE					
F25	264	13.9	9.3	0.62	133
F39	173	17.8	8.5	0.75	165
F70	208	23.3	11.3++	0.92	54
F90	103	20.1	11.1	1.24	61
F-J	748	17.5	9.7+	0.40	
HAUTE-NORMANDIE					
F27	332	19.4	11.6++	0.71	44
F76	848	17.7	10.6++	0.40	80
F-K	1180	18.1	10.8++	0.35	
ILE-DE-FRANCE					
F75	3581	36.3	15.5++	0.30	2
F77	612	20.1	12.4++	0.57	21
F78	727	16.8	11.7++	0.48	41
F91	624	16.8	13.1++	0.58	13
F92	1496	25.3	14.1++	0.40	5
F93	1057	20.0	13.6++	0.45	10
F94	1122	22.6	13.6++	0.45	10
F95	637	18.8	13.5++	0.58	12
F-L	9856	24.3	13.9++	0.16	
LANGUEDOC-ROUSSILLON					
F11	366	32.7	12.8++	0.83	16
F30	458	22.6	10.9++	0.59	68
F34	691	25.7	12.0++	0.53	26
F48	72	23.9	9.7	1.41	116
F66	303	24.2	10.2+	0.71	95
F-M	1890	25.6	11.4++	0.31	
LIMOUSIN					
F19	245	24.8	9.9	0.76	106
F23	214	35.3	12.2++	1.11	24
F87	424	29.1	11.7++	0.68	41
F-N	883	29.0	11.1++	0.46	
LORRAINE					
F54	492	16.9	10.4++	0.51	89
F55	163	19.8	9.7	0.90	116
F57	631	15.8	10.9++	0.46	68
F88	314	19.3	9.7	0.63	116
F-O	1600	17.1	10.3++	0.28	
MIDI-PYRENEES					
F09	161	28.7	11.0+	1.06	65
F12	265	23.2	9.9	0.72	106
F31	650	20.4	11.2++	0.50	58
F32	176	25.1	10.3	0.92	93
F46	155	25.4	9.9	0.94	106
F65	226	24.2	11.8++	0.92	37
F81	294	21.2	9.6	0.67	122
F82	152	20.2	9.6	0.92	122
F-P	2079	22.4	10.5++	0.27	
NORD-PAS-DE-CALAIS					
F59	2221	21.7	12.9++	0.31	14
F62	1128	19.6	11.1++	0.36	61
F-Q	3349	21.0	12.2++	0.24	
PAYS DE LA LOIRE					
F44	727	18.9	10.6++	0.44	80
F49	552	21.1	11.8++	0.58	37
F53	250	23.2	11.9++	0.86	32
F72	405	20.1	10.9++	0.62	68
F85	424	23.0	11.5++	0.64	47
F-R	2358	20.7	11.2++	0.26	
PICARDIE					
F02	474	22.1	11.9++	0.63	32
F60	530	21.9	12.9++	0.63	14
F80	577	26.2	14.0++	0.67	7
F-S	1581	23.3	12.9++	0.37	
POITOU-CHARENTES					
F16	320	23.1	10.7++	0.70	77
F17	411	20.2	9.3	0.54	133
F79	268	19.7	9.9	0.72	106
F86	357	24.6	11.9++	0.75	32
F-T	1356	21.8	10.3++	0.33	
PROVENCE-ALPES-COTE D'AZUR					
F04	117	26.3	12.7++	1.34	19
F05	82	21.0	10.6	1.38	80
F06	1026	29.7	12.8++	0.49	16
F13	1969	29.5	16.0++	0.40	1
F83	680	26.7	12.0++	0.52	26
F84	340	21.4	10.9++	0.66	68
F-U	4214	27.9	13.6++	0.24	
RHONE-ALPES					
F01	299	19.8	10.2+	0.68	95
F07	308	29.4	11.2++	0.76	58
F26	276	18.8	9.6	0.66	122
F38	582	16.8	9.9+	0.45	106
F42	689	22.4	11.0++	0.48	65
F69	1224	20.9	12.0++	0.38	26
F73	247	20.0	10.7+	0.77	77
F74	245	13.6	8.3	0.58	171
F-V	3870	19.9	10.7++	0.19	
F.0	48993	22.8	11.9++	0.06	

UNITED KINGDOM (1976-80)

EAST ANGLIA					
G25	179	10.6	5.4--	0.44	311
G46	340	16.4	6.9--	0.42	224
G55	234	13.2	6.0--	0.43	274
G-A	753	13.6	6.2--	0.25	
EAST MIDLANDS					
G30	300	10.9	5.5--	0.35	301
G44	256	10.1	5.3--	0.37	316
G45	191	11.9	6.0--	0.48	274
G47	162	10.3	5.5--	0.47	301
G50	298	10.0	5.1--	0.32	321
G-B	1207	10.5	5.4--	0.17	
NORTHERN					
G14	540	14.9	7.1--	0.34	213
G27	149	8.6	5.1--	0.45	321
G29	223	15.3	7.0--	0.53	218
G33	240	12.9	6.7--	0.46	235
G48	102	11.5	5.2--	0.56	318
G-C	1254	13.1	6.5--	0.20	
NORTH-WEST					
G11	1059	12.8	6.3--	0.22	258
G12	667	13.8	6.7--	0.28	235
G26	286	10.2	5.6--	0.35	294
G43	455	10.6	4.6--	0.25	336
G-D	2467	12.2	5.9--	0.13	

SOUTH-EAST					
G01	2751	12.6	5.7--	0.12	288
G22	107	7.3	4.5--	0.46	340
G23	228	11.3	6.3--	0.45	258
G24	137	8.8	4.6--	0.42	336
G34	429	20.0	6.2--	0.38	267
G35	492	11.2	5.5--	0.28	301
G37	478	11.1	5.5--	0.27	301
G39	352	12.1	6.4--	0.36	250
G41	48	13.3	5.0--	0.87	326
G42	575	12.8	5.7--	0.27	288
G51	211	13.5	7.0--	0.53	218
G56	312	10.2	4.6--	0.28	336
G58	314	15.6	5.1--	0.35	321
G-E	6434	12.4	5.6--	0.08	

SOUTH-WEST					
G21	343	12.0	5.4--	0.33	311
G28	198	15.3	6.1--	0.48	272
G31	461	15.8	6.2--	0.34	267
G32	290	15.7	5.6--	0.39	294
G36	186	12.2	5.8--	0.48	281
G53	188	14.9	5.6--	0.45	294
G59	166	10.8	5.5--	0.46	301
G-F	1832	13.8	5.7--	0.15	

WEST MIDLANDS					
G15	900	10.9	5.8--	0.21	281
G38	237	12.8	6.7--	0.47	235
G52	120	10.8	5.6--	0.56	294
G54	266	8.8	5.0--	0.33	326
G57	148	10.4	5.5--	0.49	301
G-G	1671	10.7	5.7--	0.15	

YORKSHIRE AND HUMBERSIDE					
G13	416	10.4	5.3--	0.28	316
G16	806	12.6	5.9--	0.23	280
G40	316	12.1	5.7--	0.35	288
G49	266	13.3	5.8--	0.40	281
G-H	1804	12.0	5.7--	0.15	

WALES					
G61	134	11.3	4.8--	0.48	330
G62	109	10.8	4.5--	0.48	340
G63	121	9.0	4.5--	0.44	340
G64	65	9.2	3.9--	0.58	348
G65	195	11.8	6.4--	0.50	250
G66	32	10.1	4.3--	0.85	345
G67	139	11.5	5.5--	0.54	301
G68	119	10.4	5.4--	0.53	311
G-I	914	10.7	5.1--	0.19	

SCOTLAND(1975-80)					
S01	76	13.3	6.4--	0.82	250
S02	210	14.7	7.2--	0.56	208
S03	160	12.8	5.7--	0.50	288
S04	118	11.3	5.7--	0.58	288
S05	330	14.0	6.7--	0.40	235
S06	30	9.6	4.4--	0.91	344
S07	71	8.6	4.7--	0.61	333
S08	780	10.2	5.4--	0.21	311
S09	64	14.5	7.3	0.99	203
S10	5	9.2	4.0-	1.97	346
S11	14	22.9	9.5	2.89	127
S12	16	17.7	6.9	2.00	224
G-J	1874	11.6	5.9--	0.15	

NORTHERN IRELAND					
JE	195	11.6	7.2--	0.55	208
JN	69	7.5	4.8--	0.62	330
JS	58	8.5	5.4--	0.76	311
JW	98	16.0	9.8	1.06	111
G-K	420	10.8	6.7--	0.35	
G.0	20630	12.0	5.8--	0.04	

ITALIA (1975-79)

ABRUZZI					
I66	111	14.4	7.1-	0.75	213
I67	86	12.8	7.3	0.85	203
I68	102	14.1	8.7	0.92	156
I69	98	10.6	5.6--	0.61	294
I-A	397	12.9	7.0--	0.38	

BASILICATA					
I76	130	12.5	8.0	0.75	177
I77	60	11.9	8.5	1.14	165
I-B	190	12.3	8.1	0.62	

CALABRIA					
I78	216	12.0	7.9	0.57	183
I79	227	12.3	8.2	0.58	174
I80	226	15.1	8.8	0.64	150
I-C	669	13.0	8.3	0.34	

CAMPANIA					
I61	253	13.8	10.5+	0.68	87
I62	132	17.9	10.3	0.97	93
I63	1034	14.2	11.3++	0.36	54
I64	169	15.4	8.8	0.73	150
I65	303	12.0	8.0	0.48	177
I-D	1891	14.0	10.3++	0.25	

EMILIA-ROMAGNA					
I33	73	10.1	4.5--	0.58	340
I34	186	18.2	7.7	0.64	189
I35	153	14.9	7.0--	0.60	218
I36	204	13.8	7.3--	0.54	203
I37	309	12.7	6.0--	0.37	274
I38	139	14.0	6.9--	0.62	224
I39	96	10.4	4.6--	0.50	336
I40	164	11.0	6.3--	0.53	258
I-E	1324	13.1	6.3--	0.19	

FRIULI-VENEZIA GIULIA					
I30	254	18.7	8.7	0.60	156
I31	57	14.9	7.1	1.03	213
I32	121	15.1	5.6--	0.57	294
I93	90	13.1	6.5--	0.76	244
I-F	522	16.2	7.2--	0.35	

LAZIO					
I56	115	17.3	9.3	0.90	133
I57	71	19.7	9.6	1.28	122
I58	1262	13.4	9.3	0.27	133
I59	111	10.7	8.3	0.80	171
I60	165	14.5	8.0	0.68	177
I-G	1724	13.6	9.0	0.23	

LIGURIA					
I08	117	19.5	7.5	0.77	194
I09	134	17.0	7.7	0.72	189
I10	581	20.5	9.2	0.43	137
I11	121	19.0	7.7	0.76	189
I-H	953	19.6	8.5	0.31	

LOMBARDIA					
I12	248	12.4	7.4--	0.50	196
I13	255	13.0	8.0	0.54	177
I14	60	13.7	7.4	1.01	196
I15	1542	14.8	9.7++	0.26	116
I16	350	15.8	10.6++	0.59	80
I17	430	16.9	10.6++	0.54	80
I18	271	20.0	8.4	0.57	167
I19	155	18.0	8.4	0.73	167
I20	194	19.8	8.9	0.69	147
I-I	3505	15.4	9.3++	0.17	

MARCHE					
I41	107	12.9	6.3--	0.68	258
I42	140	12.7	6.4--	0.59	250
I43	116	15.7	7.5	0.74	194
I44	114	12.8	6.5--	0.65	244
I-J	477	13.4	6.7--	0.33	

MOLISE					
I70	89	14.8	7.6	0.87	193
I94	33	13.7	7.0	1.31	218
I-K	122	14.5	7.4	0.72	

PIEMONTE					
I01	879	14.4	8.7	0.31	156
I02	220	20.8	8.6	0.66	162
I03	205	15.6	7.4-	0.58	196
I04	232	16.9	7.8	0.56	187
I05	114	20.3	8.8	0.95	150
I06	282	22.8	8.9	0.61	147
I-L	1932	16.6	8.4-	0.21	

PUGLIA					
I71	210	12.3	8.3	0.60	171
I72	417	11.5	8.0	0.42	177
I73	151	10.8	8.2	0.69	174
I74	125	12.6	9.1	0.84	140
I75	225	11.7	8.1	0.56	176
I-M	1128	11.7	8.2-	0.26	

SARDEGNA					
I90	162	15.2	9.8	0.83	111
I91	93	13.4	8.0	0.90	177
I92	237	13.3	10.2+	0.69	95
I95	66	17.0	10.0	1.36	103
I-N	558	14.2	9.6	0.43	

SICILIA					
I81	182	17.0	9.1	0.72	140
I82	542	18.1	11.9++	0.54	32
I83	291	16.8	9.4	0.59	130
I84	165	13.8	9.0	0.74	145
I85	104	14.1	9.5	0.97	127
I86	53	10.3	6.4-	0.93	250
I87	333	13.3	9.1	0.52	140
I88	113	16.6	10.0	0.99	103
I89	150	15.5	10.9+	0.92	68
I-O	1933	15.6	9.9++	0.24	

TOSCANA					
I45	80	15.1	6.9-	0.83	224
I46	197	19.6	8.6	0.69	162
I47	103	15.2	7.2-	0.78	208
I48	518	16.8	7.9-	0.38	183
I49	154	17.4	8.7	0.76	156
I50	160	16.3	6.9--	0.60	224
I51	103	13.1	6.4--	0.67	250
I52	89	13.6	5.8--	0.68	281
I53	63	11.2	5.8--	0.82	281
I-P	1467	16.0	7.4--	0.21	

TRENTINO-ALTO ADIGE					
I21	153	14.1	9.4	0.79	130
I22	190	16.9	9.1	0.73	140
I-Q	343	15.5	9.3	0.53	

UMBRIA					
I54	206	14.3	7.1--	0.53	213
I55	71	12.3	6.5--	0.82	244
I-R	277	13.7	6.9--	0.44	

VALLE D'AOSTA					
I07	34	12.0	6.8	1.23	231

VENETO					
I23	297	15.2	8.7	0.54	156
I24	214	11.8	7.3--	0.53	203
I25	84	14.4	6.9-	0.82	224
I26	214	12.0	6.6--	0.49	242
I27	243	11.3	7.1--	0.48	213
I28	222	10.9	6.5--	0.46	244
I29	105	16.2	8.6	0.89	162
I-T	1379	12.6	7.3--	0.21	
I.0	20825	14.5	8.4--	0.06	

IRELAND (1976-80)

CONNAUGHT					
R07	35	8.6	5.2--	0.94	318
R12	8	12.3	6.7	2.82	235
R16	31	11.2	6.0-	1.20	274
R20	15	11.7	5.2-	1.44	318
R21	15	11.2	6.3	1.81	258
R-A	104	10.3	5.7--	0.61	

LEINSTER					
R01	3	3.2	1.9--	1.14	354
R06	199	7.8	6.0--	0.45	274
R09	8	3.4	2.8--	1.03	352
R10	15	9.0	6.2	1.70	267
R11	4	3.4	2.4--	1.20	353
R14	8	10.9	6.5	2.45	244
R15	8	3.7	2.9--	1.12	351
R17	16	7.3	5.5-	1.48	301
R19	12	8.7	6.3	1.89	258
R24	3	2.0	1.9--	1.12	354
R25	24	10.1	7.0	1.51	218
R26	26	12.4	9.2	1.94	137
R-B	326	7.4	5.6--	0.33	

MUNSTER					
R03	18	8.8	5.1--	1.29	321
R04	95	9.6	6.1--	0.67	272
R08	23	7.9	4.0--	0.89	346
R13	32	8.2	5.6--	1.05	294
R22	24	7.4	4.7--	1.03	333
R23	27	12.5	7.8	1.60	187
R-C	219	9.1	5.6--	0.41	

ULSTER					
R02	8	6.3	3.5--	1.31	350
R05	28	9.4	4.9--	1.03	328
R18	8	6.6	3.8--	1.44	349
R-D	44	8.1	4.3--	0.71	
R.0	693	8.3	5.5--	0.22	

LUXEMBOURG (1971-80)

LE	33	17.2	7.3	1.37	203
LN	43	16.3	7.4	1.22	196
LS	228	17.0	9.2	0.64	137
L.0	304	16.9	8.7	0.53	

NEDERLAND (1976-80)

N01	179	13.0	6.4--	0.52	250
N02	164	11.4	5.8--	0.50	281
N03	118	11.5	6.9--	0.68	224
N04	274	11.0	6.6--	0.42	242
N05	470	11.2	6.7--	0.33	235
N06	251	11.2	6.3--	0.43	258
N07	659	11.1	5.5--	0.24	301
N08	943	12.1	6.2--	0.22	267
N09	103	12.1	5.8--	0.63	281
N10	418	8.4	6.0--	0.31	274
N11	259	9.8	6.5--	0.43	244
N.0	3838	11.0	6.2--	0.11	

EEC-9

EEC	140279	17.5	8.8	0.03

BELGIE-BELGIQUE (1971-78)

BRUSSEL-BRUXELLES

B21	263	6.7	4.5--	0.29	162

VLAANDEREN

B10	173	2.8	2.0--	0.16	321
B29	168	4.7	3.4--	0.27	211
B30	198	4.7	3.4--	0.25	211
B40	159	3.0	2.1--	0.17	317
B70	52	1.9	1.9--	0.27	332
B-V	750	3.4	2.5--	0.09	

WALLONIE

B25	34	3.3	2.5--	0.43	284
B50	243	4.7	3.3--	0.22	221
B60	153	3.9	2.6--	0.22	274
B80	36	4.2	2.9--	0.50	247
B90	74	4.9	3.5--	0.42	206
B-W	540	4.3	3.0--	0.13	
B.0	1553	4.0	2.9--	0.08	

BR DEUTSCHLAND (1976-80)

BADEN-WURTTEMBERG

D81	405	4.9	4.0--	0.20	185
D82	344	6.1	4.8--	0.27	157
D83	245	5.6	4.6--	0.30	161
D84	188	5.2	4.4--	0.33	165
D-A	1182	5.4	4.4--	0.13	

BAYERN

D91	339	3.9	3.0--	0.17	241
D92	93	4.0	3.3--	0.35	221
D93	86	3.7	2.9--	0.32	247
D94	133	5.4	4.0--	0.36	185
D95	157	4.4	3.3--	0.27	221
D96	131	4.6	3.6--	0.33	202
D97	151	4.2	3.2--	0.27	231
D-B	1090	4.2	3.2--	0.10	

BERLIN(WEST)

DB0	82	1.9	1.3--	0.16	354

BREMEN

D40	71	4.3	2.9--	0.36	247

HAMBURG

D20	200	5.2	3.2--	0.24	231

HESSEN

D64	401	3.8	2.8--	0.15	257
D66	93	3.3	2.2--	0.25	308
D-F	494	3.7	2.7--	0.13	

NIEDERSACHSEN

D31	139	3.6	2.5--	0.22	284
D32	187	3.8	2.8--	0.21	257
D33	106	3.0	2.2--	0.23	308
D34	152	3.0	2.4--	0.20	296
D-G	584	3.4	2.5--	0.11	

NORDRHEIN-WESTFALEN

D51	500	4.0	3.2--	0.15	231
D53	313	3.3	2.7--	0.16	266
D55	204	3.5	3.0--	0.22	241
D57	159	3.7	2.9--	0.24	247
D59	382	4.3	3.4--	0.18	211
D-H	1558	3.8	3.1--	0.08	

RHEINLAND-PFALZ

D71	163	5.0	3.6--	0.30	202
D72	88	7.9	6.1	0.67	133
D73	247	5.7	4.4--	0.29	165
D-I	498	5.7	4.3--	0.20	

SAARLAND

DA0	146	5.7	4.1--	0.34	178

SCHLESWIG-HOLSTEIN

D10	215	3.4	2.5--	0.18	284
D.0	6120	4.2	3.2--	0.04	

DANMARK (1971-80)

K15	344	5.7	3.8--	0.21	194
K20	45	3.0	2.7--	0.40	266
K25	22	2.4	2.3--	0.50	305
K30	46	3.4	2.2--	0.34	308
K35	40	3.1	1.7--	0.29	343
K40	7	2.9	2.0--	0.82	321
K42	72	3.3	2.2--	0.26	308
K50	36	2.9	2.0--	0.35	321
K55	29	2.8	2.0--	0.39	321
K60	33	2.1	1.4--	0.25	352
K65	37	2.9	2.1--	0.36	317
K70	73	2.6	1.9--	0.23	332
K76	34	3.0	1.7--	0.31	343
K80	69	2.9	1.9--	0.24	332
K.0	887	3.5	2.4--	0.08	

FRANCE (1971-78)

ALSACE

F67	609	17.6	16.0++	0.66	24
F68	467	18.7	16.9++	0.81	16
F-A	1076	18.1	16.3++	0.51	

AQUITAINE

F24	330	22.7	13.3++	0.77	55
F33	679	16.6	12.1++	0.48	72
F40	223	19.9	12.8++	0.90	62
F47	206	18.1	11.2++	0.83	82
F64	287	13.9	9.3++	0.57	106
F-B	1725	17.5	11.7++	0.29	

AUVERGNE

F03	326	22.0	14.0++	0.82	47
F15	107	16.2	10.1++	1.03	95
F43	150	18.7	12.9++	1.11	60
F63	437	19.2	14.7++	0.72	39
F-C	1020	19.5	13.6++	0.44	

BASSE-NORMANDIE

F14	512	23.4	21.5++	0.96	3
F50	339	19.5	15.0++	0.83	35
F61	213	18.6	14.6++	1.03	42
F-D	1064	21.0	17.5++	0.55	

BOURGOGNE

F21	393	21.9	18.0++	0.94	11
F58	235	24.0	16.0++	1.11	24
F71	446	19.9	14.1++	0.70	46
F89	245	20.7	13.3++	0.93	55
F-E	1319	21.3	15.3++	0.44	

BRETAGNE

F22	591	29.0	21.3++	0.90	4
F29	955	30.6	23.6++	0.78	2
F35	541	20.0	17.0++	0.74	15
F56	663	30.1	24.3++	0.96	1
F-F	2750	27.3	21.5++	0.42	

CENTRE

F18	264	21.1	15.1++	0.98	34
F28	206	15.3	12.2++	0.88	71
F36	240	24.6	15.7++	1.09	29
F37	281	15.1	11.8++	0.73	76
F41	234	21.1	14.9++	1.04	37
F45	313	16.1	12.8++	0.75	62
F-G	1538	18.1	13.5++	0.36	

CHAMPAGNE-ARDENNE

F08	300	24.1	21.2++	1.26	5
F10	233	20.8	16.0++	1.10	24
F51	435	20.7	19.0++	0.93	7
F52	168	19.8	16.4++	1.31	20
F-H	1136	21.4	18.4++	0.56	

CORSE

F20	78	8.1	5.9	0.69	136

FRANCHE-COMTE

F25	247	13.1	13.0++	0.84	58
F39	212	22.3	15.9++	1.14	27
F70	170	19.5	14.4++	1.17	44
F90	77	15.1	14.0++	1.62	47
F-J	706	16.8	14.1++	0.54	

HAUTE-NORMANDIE

F27	274	16.4	14.4++	0.89	44
F76	860	18.7	16.6++	0.58	18
F-K	1134	18.1	16.0++	0.48	

ILE-DE-FRANCE

F75	1800	21.2	15.0++	0.36	35
F77	534	17.7	15.9++	0.71	27
F78	621	14.4	14.9++	0.61	37
F91	517	14.1	15.5++	0.70	31
F92	1110	19.7	16.3++	0.49	23
F93	1099	20.8	19.7++	0.60	6
F94	918	19.3	17.6++	0.59	13
F95	602	18.0	18.4++	0.76	10
F-L	7201	18.7	16.4++	0.20	

LANGUEDOC-ROUSSILLON

F11	170	16.3	8.7++	0.73	108
F30	303	15.7	10.6++	0.63	86
F34	342	13.7	9.5++	0.54	104
F48	52	17.3	10.4+	1.52	88
F66	193	16.7	9.7++	0.74	100
F-M	1060	15.3	9.7++	0.31	

LIMOUSIN

F19	185	19.7	11.9++	0.93	74
F23	146	25.5	13.2++	1.21	57
F87	228	16.7	10.0++	0.71	97
F-N	559	19.4	11.3++	0.51	

LORRAINE

F54	568	19.9	17.6++	0.76	13
F55	191	23.7	18.7++	1.40	8
F57	566	14.0	13.5++	0.58	54
F88	296	19.0	15.2++	0.91	32
F-O	1621	17.5	15.6++	0.39	

MIDI-PYRENEES

F09	70	12.8	6.5	0.86	126
F12	146	13.5	7.8+	0.69	116
F31	318	10.6	7.9++	0.45	114
F32	155	22.2	12.5++	1.08	67
F46	82	13.9	8.1	0.97	111
F65	149	16.8	10.4++	0.89	88
F81	193	14.6	9.0++	0.68	107
F82	128	17.9	11.0++	1.03	84
F-P	1241	14.0	8.9++	0.26	

NORD-PAS-DE-CALAIS

F59	1894	19.2	17.8++	0.42	12
F62	1047	19.1	16.5++	0.52	19
F-Q	2941	19.2	17.3++	0.33	

PAYS DE LA LOIRE

F44	763	21.2	18.6++	0.68	9
F49	343	13.9	11.9++	0.66	74
F53	143	14.1	11.3++	0.96	80
F72	274	14.2	11.3++	0.70	80
F85	266	15.2	11.7++	0.75	77
F-R	1789	16.6	13.9++	0.34	

PICARDIE

F02	419	19.7	16.7++	0.85	17
F60	397	16.3	15.2++	0.78	32
F80	333	15.8	12.5++	0.71	67
F-S	1149	17.2	14.8++	0.45	

POITOU-CHARENTES

F16	241	18.3	13.0++	0.87	58
F17	417	21.5	14.7++	0.76	39
F79	191	14.3	10.5++	0.80	87
F86	208	14.8	10.4++	0.76	88
F-T	1057	17.6	12.4++	0.40	

PROVENCE-ALPES-COTE D'AZUR

F04	47	10.5	6.3	0.98	128
F05	75	19.3	13.6++	1.63	52
F06	363	11.8	7.0	0.39	122
F13	838	13.1	10.1++	0.36	95
F83	430	17.5	12.0++	0.60	73
F84	203	13.1	9.8++	0.71	99
F-U	1956	13.7	9.6++	0.22	

RHONE-ALPES

F01	226	14.9	11.4++	0.78	79
F07	190	18.9	12.8++	0.98	62
F26	207	14.7	10.4++	0.76	88
F38	540	15.8	13.8++	0.60	50
F42	548	18.7	14.7++	0.64	39
F69	866	15.4	13.7++	0.47	51
F73	234	19.2	15.6++	1.04	30
F74	326	18.1	16.4++	0.93	20
F-V	3137	16.6	13.7++	0.25	
F.0	37257	18.1	14.4++	0.08	

UNITED KINGDOM (1976-80)

EAST ANGLIA

G25	39	2.3	1.7--	0.29	343
G46	66	3.3	1.9--	0.25	332
G55	47	2.6	1.8--	0.27	339
G-A	152	2.8	1.8--	0.15	

EAST MIDLANDS

G30	100	3.8	2.6--	0.27	274
G44	81	3.3	2.5--	0.28	284
G45	65	4.1	2.7--	0.34	266
G47	47	3.1	2.4--	0.36	296
G50	106	3.7	2.7--	0.27	266
G-B	399	3.6	2.6--	0.13	

NORTHERN

G14	204	6.0	4.3--	0.31	173
G27	99	5.9	4.7--	0.48	158
G29	46	3.3	2.3--	0.35	305
G33	90	5.1	3.5--	0.38	206
G48	37	4.3	2.6--	0.45	274
G-C	476	5.2	3.7--	0.17	

NORTH-WEST

G11	360	4.6	3.4--	0.19	211
G12	228	5.1	3.8--	0.26	194
G26	101	3.8	2.7--	0.27	266
G43	203	5.2	3.3--	0.24	221
G-D	892	4.7	3.4--	0.12	

SOUTH-EAST					
G01	795	4.0	2.6--	0.09	274
G22	36	2.4	2.0--	0.34	321
G23	43	2.1	1.7--	0.27	343
G24	64	4.1	3.3--	0.42	221
G34	92	5.2	2.7--	0.31	266
G35	124	3.0	2.2--	0.20	308
G37	152	3.5	2.7--	0.22	266
G39	71	2.6	2.0--	0.24	321
G41	18	5.6	3.1--	0.78	235
G42	121	2.9	1.9--	0.18	332
G51	59	3.5	3.3--	0.47	221
G56	80	2.8	1.9--	0.21	332
G58	85	4.8	2.5--	0.28	284
G-E	1740	3.5	2.4--	0.06	
SOUTH-WEST					
G21	96	3.6	2.4--	0.26	296
G28	53	4.4	2.5--	0.37	284
G31	130	4.7	2.5--	0.23	284
G32	64	3.9	2.0--	0.27	321
G36	51	3.5	2.5--	0.36	284
G53	53	4.4	2.5--	0.36	284
G59	49	3.2	2.6--	0.38	274
G-F	496	4.0	2.4--	0.11	
WEST MIDLANDS					
G15	292	3.6	2.6--	0.15	274
G38	75	4.2	2.9--	0.35	247
G52	28	2.6	1.9--	0.38	332
G54	118	4.0	3.1--	0.30	235
G57	45	3.2	2.5--	0.38	284
G-G	558	3.7	2.7--	0.12	
YORKSHIRE AND HUMBERSIDE					
G13	182	4.7	3.2--	0.24	231
G16	289	4.8	3.3--	0.20	221
G40	98	4.0	2.8--	0.29	257
G49	90	4.6	3.1--	0.34	235
G-H	659	4.6	3.1--	0.13	
WALES					
G61	56	5.1	3.3--	0.46	221
G62	46	4.9	2.9--	0.44	247
G63	44	3.4	2.4--	0.37	296
G64	31	4.7	2.9--	0.54	247
G65	59	3.7	2.8--	0.37	257
G66	24	7.6	4.7	1.01	158
G67	45	4.0	2.8--	0.43	257
G68	46	4.4	3.0--	0.46	241
G-I	351	4.4	2.9--	0.16	
SCOTLAND(1975-80)					
S01	21	3.8	2.8--	0.63	257
S02	40	3.0	2.0--	0.33	321
S03	43	3.7	2.4--	0.38	296
S04	40	4.0	3.0--	0.49	241
S05	96	4.5	3.4--	0.36	211
S06	16	5.6	3.1--	0.82	235
S07	37	4.6	3.4--	0.58	211
S08	313	4.4	3.4--	0.20	211
S09	11	2.6	1.8--	0.56	339
S10	5	9.4	6.4	3.01	127
S11	2	3.2	2.9	2.06	247
S12	6	6.8	3.4-	1.51	211
G-J	630	4.2	3.1--	0.13	
NORTHERN IRELAND					
JE	48	2.9	2.5--	0.37	284
JN	23	2.5	2.2--	0.48	308
JS	18	2.7	2.4--	0.59	296
JW	27	4.5	4.1--	0.82	178
G-K	116	3.0	2.6--	0.26	
G.0	6469	4.0	2.8--	0.04	
ITALIA (1975-79)					
ABRUZZI					
I66	52	7.1	5.0-	0.71	152
I67	47	7.1	5.1	0.76	149
I68	37	5.3	4.0--	0.66	185
I69	48	5.4	3.7--	0.55	198
I-A	184	6.2	4.4--	0.33	
BASILICATA					
I76	48	4.7	3.7--	0.54	198
I77	14	2.8	2.4--	0.65	296
I-B	62	4.1	3.2--	0.42	
CALABRIA					
I78	83	4.7	3.9--	0.43	191
I79	73	4.0	3.5--	0.42	206
I80	48	3.3	2.8--	0.42	257
I-C	204	4.0	3.4--	0.24	
CAMPANIA					
I61	54	3.0	2.8--	0.39	257
I62	23	3.2	2.0--	0.42	321
I63	167	2.4	2.5--	0.20	284
I64	27	2.5	1.7--	0.34	343
I65	78	3.2	2.6--	0.30	274
I-D	349	2.7	2.5--	0.13	
EMILIA-ROMAGNA					
I33	75	10.8	6.3	0.76	128
I34	75	7.7	4.5--	0.53	162
I35	92	9.3	6.3	0.69	128
I36	101	7.1	4.9--	0.50	155
I37	144	6.4	4.2--	0.36	175
I38	85	9.1	5.8	0.63	137
I39	58	6.6	4.0--	0.54	185
I40	99	6.8	5.2-	0.53	148
I-E	729	7.6	5.0--	0.19	
FRIULI-VENEZIA GIULIA					
I30	256	19.9	13.6++	0.86	52
I31	52	14.8	10.2+	1.44	93
I32	106	15.2	8.7+	0.88	108
I93	121	18.5	14.0++	1.30	47
I-F	535	17.9	11.9++	0.53	
LAZIO					
I56	43	6.6	4.4--	0.69	165
I57	25	7.0	4.1--	0.84	178
I58	435	4.9	4.4--	0.21	165
I59	49	4.7	4.4--	0.64	165
I60	63	5.6	4.2--	0.55	175
I-G	615	5.1	4.3--	0.18	
LIGURIA					
I08	55	9.9	5.7	0.80	139
I09	62	8.4	5.0-	0.66	152
I10	268	10.4	6.1	0.38	133
I11	51	8.6	5.1	0.75	149
I-H	436	9.8	5.7-	0.28	
LOMBARDIA					
I12	211	11.3	9.6++	0.68	102
I13	207	11.3	9.6++	0.69	102
I14	57	13.3	11.1++	1.49	83
I15	910	9.3	8.0++	0.27	113
I16	240	11.2	10.7++	0.70	85
I17	346	14.2	12.6++	0.68	65
I18	205	16.1	9.9++	0.72	98
I19	146	18.0	12.5++	1.06	67
I20	105	11.3	7.1	0.72	120
I-I	2427	11.3	9.3++	0.19	
MARCHE					
I41	51	6.3	4.4--	0.64	165
I42	70	6.8	4.4--	0.54	165
I43	32	4.5	2.7--	0.51	266
I44	49	5.7	4.1--	0.60	178
I-J	202	5.9	3.9--	0.29	
MOLISE					
I70	32	5.5	3.6--	0.66	202
I94	8	3.5	2.2--	0.80	308
I-K	40	4.9	3.2--	0.52	
PIEMONTE					
I01	553	9.5	7.9++	0.34	114
I02	169	17.4	10.4++	0.83	88
I03	181	14.8	10.2++	0.78	93
I04	153	11.3	7.1	0.60	120
I05	52	9.7	5.5	0.81	144
I06	142	12.2	6.3	0.56	128
I-L	1250	11.3	7.9++	0.23	
PUGLIA					
I71	54	3.2	2.6--	0.36	274
I72	116	3.3	2.8--	0.27	257
I73	57	4.2	4.0--	0.53	185
I74	45	4.7	4.2--	0.64	175
I75	115	6.3	5.3-	0.50	146
I-M	387	4.2	3.6--	0.18	
SARDEGNA					
I90	74	7.1	4.9--	0.59	155
I91	62	9.1	5.7	0.78	139
I92	112	6.4	5.7	0.55	139
I95	40	10.3	6.0	1.03	135
I-N	288	7.4	5.5--	0.34	
SICILIA					
I81	41	4.0	2.9--	0.48	247
I82	91	3.2	2.6--	0.28	274
I83	75	4.6	3.5--	0.42	206
I84	50	4.2	3.1--	0.46	235
I85	24	3.3	2.6--	0.55	274
I86	14	2.8	2.3--	0.63	305
I87	102	4.2	3.4--	0.35	211
I88	19	2.9	2.0--	0.48	321
I89	42	4.3	3.7--	0.58	198
I-O	458	3.8	3.0--	0.14	
TOSCANA					
I45	44	8.9	5.3	0.81	146
I46	104	11.2	6.9	0.70	123
I47	44	6.9	3.8--	0.59	194
I48	171	5.9	3.7--	0.29	198
I49	83	9.9	6.6	0.75	125
I50	81	8.6	5.0-	0.57	152
I51	44	5.7	3.3--	0.51	221
I52	50	7.9	4.1--	0.60	178
I53	48	8.7	5.1	0.76	149
I-P	669	7.7	4.6--	0.18	
TRENTINO-ALTO ADIGE					
I21	95	9.0	8.1	0.84	111
I22	180	16.8	12.9++	0.98	60
I-Q	275	12.9	10.7++	0.66	
UMBRIA					
I54	130	9.3	5.8	0.52	137
I55	51	9.1	5.4	0.77	145
I-R	181	9.2	5.7	0.43	
VALLE D'AOSTA					
I07	50	17.5	12.6++	1.80	65
VENETO					
I23	205	11.0	8.5++	0.60	110
I24	247	14.2	12.4++	0.80	70
I25	112	20.7	14.6++	1.41	42
I26	347	20.2	16.4++	0.90	20
I27	279	13.6	11.5++	0.70	78
I28	225	11.5	9.5++	0.64	104
I29	68	11.0	7.7	0.95	117
I-T	1483	14.2	11.5++	0.30	
I.0	10824	7.9	6.0--	0.06	
IRELAND (1976-80)					
CONNAUGHT					
R07	30	6.9	4.1--	0.81	178
R12	11	14.8	7.7	2.54	117
R16	10	3.4	1.7--	0.56	343
R20	11	7.7	3.5--	1.09	206
R21	6	4.3	2.4--	1.02	296
R-A	68	6.3	3.4--	0.44	
LEINSTER					
R01	7	7.1	6.7	2.61	124
R06	81	3.4	3.8--	0.43	194
R09	13	5.1	6.3	1.81	128
R10	9	5.0	4.7	1.66	158
R11	4	3.1	2.2--	1.19	308
R14	5	6.2	4.1	1.93	178
R15	4	1.9	2.0--	1.01	321
R17	10	4.3	4.0	1.28	185
R19	6	4.0	2.9--	1.21	247
R24	7	4.6	4.4	1.76	165
R25	10	4.1	3.0--	0.98	241
R26	7	3.3	3.9	1.47	191
R-B	163	3.8	3.9--	0.31	
MUNSTER					
R03	10	4.6	3.4--	1.11	211
R04	53	5.3	4.3--	0.62	173
R08	16	5.1	3.0--	0.77	241
R13	25	6.3	5.7	1.18	139
R22	20	5.8	4.5	1.04	162
R23	11	5.0	3.9-	1.21	191
R-C	135	5.4	4.2--	0.37	
ULSTER					
R02	7	4.9	3.1--	1.27	235
R05	17	5.4	3.6--	0.96	202
R18	4	3.0	3.3	1.68	221
R-D	28	4.8	3.5--	0.72	
R.0	394	4.7	3.9--	0.20	
LUXEMBOURG (1971-80)					
LE	22	12.1	7.7	1.72	117
LN	38	14.4	9.7+	1.65	100
LS	92	7.2	5.6	0.59	143
L.0	152	8.8	6.4	0.53	
NEDERLAND (1976-80)					
N01	29	2.1	1.5--	0.30	350
N02	43	3.0	2.4--	0.39	296
N03	22	2.1	1.5--	0.33	350
N04	55	2.2	1.8--	0.25	339
N05	73	1.8	1.4--	0.17	352
N06	44	2.0	1.6--	0.25	349
N07	159	2.7	2.1--	0.17	317
N08	214	2.8	2.2--	0.15	308
N09	18	2.1	1.3--	0.32	354
N10	107	2.1	2.1--	0.20	317
N11	52	2.0	1.8--	0.25	339
N.0	816	2.4	1.9--	0.07	
EEC-9					
EEC	64472	8.5	6.5	0.03	

BELGIE-BELGIQUE (1971-78)

BRUSSEL-BRUXELLES					
B21	112	2.5	1.0	0.11	147
VLAANDEREN					
B10	67	1.1	0.6--	0.09	285
B29	36	1.0	0.6--	0.11	285
B30	56	1.3	0.7-	0.10	247
B40	37	0.7	0.3--	0.05	347
B70	14	0.5	0.4--	0.12	336
B-V	210	0.9	0.5--	0.04	
WALLONIE					
B25	12	1.1	0.7	0.21	247
B50	76	1.4	0.7--	0.09	247
B60	61	1.4	0.7-	0.10	247
B80	17	1.9	1.1	0.29	111
B90	20	1.2	0.7	0.16	247
B-W	186	1.4	0.7--	0.06	
B.0	508	1.3	0.7--	0.03	

BR DEUTSCHLAND (1976-80)

BADEN-WURTTEMBERG					
D81	128	1.4	0.8	0.08	207
D82	97	1.6	0.8	0.09	207
D83	49	1.0	0.5--	0.08	319
D84	64	1.7	1.0	0.13	147
D-A	338	1.4	0.8--	0.05	
BAYERN					
D91	134	1.4	0.7--	0.07	247
D92	28	1.1	0.6--	0.13	285
D93	36	1.4	0.7-	0.12	247
D94	29	1.0	0.5--	0.10	319
D95	71	1.8	0.8	0.10	207
D96	23	0.7	0.4--	0.09	336
D97	44	1.1	0.5--	0.09	319
D-B	365	1.3	0.6--	0.04	
BERLIN (WEST)					
DB0	30	0.6	0.3--	0.06	347
BREMEN					
D40	24	1.3	0.5--	0.12	319
HAMBURG					
D20	88	2.0	0.8	0.10	207
HESSEN					
D64	168	1.5	0.8-	0.07	207
D66	37	1.2	0.5--	0.10	319
D-F	205	1.4	0.7--	0.06	
NIEDERSACHSEN					
D31	65	1.5	0.7--	0.09	247
D32	80	1.5	0.7-	0.10	247
D33	46	1.2	0.6--	0.10	285
D34	51	0.9	0.6--	0.09	285
D-G	242	1.3	0.7--	0.05	
NORDRHEIN-WESTFALEN					
D51	195	1.4	0.8--	0.06	207
D53	141	1.4	0.8-	0.07	207
D55	72	1.2	0.7--	0.09	247
D57	46	1.0	0.5--	0.08	319
D59	111	1.1	0.6--	0.06	285
D-H	565	1.3	0.7--	0.03	
RHEINLAND-PFALZ					
D71	47	1.3	0.6--	0.10	285
D72	19	1.5	0.9	0.21	178
D73	60	1.3	0.7--	0.10	247
D-I	126	1.3	0.7--	0.07	
SAARLAND					
DA0	37	1.3	0.8	0.14	207
SCHLESWIG-HOLSTEIN					
D10	102	1.5	0.7--	0.08	247
D.0	2122	1.3	0.7--	0.02	

DANMARK (1971-80)

K15	180	2.7	1.2++	0.10	83
K20	23	1.5	1.2	0.26	83
K25	9	1.0	0.7	0.24	247
K30	34	2.5	1.3	0.24	57
K35	27	2.1	1.1	0.24	111
K40	5	2.1	0.6	0.30	285
K42	50	2.2	1.1	0.17	111
K50	13	1.1	0.7	0.21	247
K55	19	1.9	1.2	0.29	83
K60	37	2.3	1.4	0.24	42
K65	14	1.1	0.7	0.20	247
K70	40	1.4	0.8	0.14	207
K76	19	1.7	0.8	0.21	207
K80	43	1.8	1.0	0.17	147
K.0	513	2.0	1.1+	0.05	

FRANCE (1971-78)

ALSACE					
F67	55	1.5	0.9	0.14	178
F68	55	2.1	1.3	0.19	57
F-A	110	1.8	1.1	0.11	
AQUITAINE					
F24	35	2.3	1.0	0.19	147
F33	69	1.6	0.8	0.11	207
F40	27	2.3	1.0	0.24	147
F47	23	1.9	0.9	0.22	178
F64	41	1.9	0.9	0.16	178
F-B	195	1.9	0.9	0.07	
AUVERGNE					
F03	37	2.4	1.0	0.22	147
F15	19	2.8	1.4	0.39	42
F43	16	1.9	0.7	0.21	247
F63	43	1.8	1.0	0.17	147
F-C	115	2.1	1.0	0.11	
BASSE-NORMANDIE					
F14	47	2.0	1.3	0.22	57
F50	32	1.7	0.9	0.19	178
F61	19	1.6	0.7	0.20	247
F-D	98	1.8	1.1	0.12	
BOURGOGNE					
F21	34	1.8	1.1	0.22	111
F58	35	3.5	1.5	0.31	28
F71	45	1.9	0.9	0.16	178
F89	28	2.3	1.2	0.28	83
F-E	142	2.2	1.1	0.11	
BRETAGNE					
F22	60	2.8	1.1	0.16	111
F29	74	2.2	1.1	0.16	111
F35	52	1.8	0.9	0.15	178
F56	51	2.2	1.1	0.17	111
F-F	237	2.2	1.1	0.08	
CENTRE					
F18	27	2.1	0.9	0.21	178
F28	29	2.2	1.1	0.24	111
F36	22	2.2	0.9	0.24	178
F37	30	1.5	0.8	0.16	207
F41	29	2.5	1.0	0.24	147
F45	27	1.4	0.8	0.18	207
F-G	164	1.9	0.9	0.08	
CHAMPAGNE-ARDENNE					
F08	31	2.5	1.6	0.32	20
F10	19	1.6	0.9	0.24	178
F51	24	1.1	0.6--	0.14	285
F52	14	1.6	1.1	0.31	111
F-H	88	1.6	1.0	0.12	
CORSE					
F20	11	1.3	0.7	0.24	247
FRANCHE-COMTE					
F25	31	1.6	1.1	0.21	111
F39	19	1.9	1.0	0.26	147
F70	12	1.3	0.8	0.27	207
F90	3	0.6	0.5	0.27	319
F-J	65	1.5	0.9	0.12	
HAUTE-NORMANDIE					
F27	40	2.3	1.3	0.24	57
F76	91	1.9	1.3+	0.15	57
F-K	131	2.0	1.3++	0.13	
ILE-DE-FRANCE					
F75	330	3.3	1.7++	0.10	15
F77	60	2.0	1.3	0.19	57
F78	71	1.6	1.4+	0.17	42
F91	50	1.3	1.2	0.18	83
F92	154	2.6	1.6++	0.14	20
F93	108	2.0	1.6++	0.16	20
F94	103	2.1	1.3+	0.14	57
F95	64	1.9	1.4+	0.19	42
F-L	940	2.3	1.5++	0.05	
LANGUEDOC-ROUSSILLON					
F11	20	1.8	0.6	0.17	285
F30	33	1.6	0.8	0.15	207
F34	41	1.5	0.6--	0.12	285
F48	9	3.0	1.8	0.72	10
F66	29	2.3	0.8	0.17	207
F-M	132	1.8	0.7--	0.08	
LIMOUSIN					
F19	16	1.6	0.6-	0.17	285
F23	19	3.1	1.1	0.31	111
F87	25	1.7	0.6-	0.16	285
F-N	60	2.0	0.7-	0.11	
LORRAINE					
F54	54	1.9	1.2	0.18	83
F55	11	1.3	0.6	0.21	285
F57	71	1.8	1.4+	0.17	42
F88	26	1.6	1.0	0.22	147
F-O	162	1.7	1.2+	0.10	
MIDI-PYRENEES					
F09	11	2.0	0.7	0.27	247
F12	18	1.6	0.6-	0.16	285
F31	50	1.6	0.9	0.15	178
F32	10	1.4	0.4--	0.15	336
F46	8	1.3	0.5-	0.19	319
F65	19	2.0	0.7	0.18	247
F81	24	1.7	0.9	0.21	178
F82	13	1.7	0.5--	0.15	319
F-P	153	1.7	0.7--	0.07	
NORD-PAS-DE-CALAIS					
F59	191	1.9	1.3++	0.10	57
F62	105	1.8	1.1	0.12	111
F-Q	296	1.9	1.2++	0.08	
PAYS DE LA LOIRE					
F44	42	1.1	0.6--	0.11	285
F49	40	1.5	0.8	0.14	207
F53	28	2.6	1.4	0.29	42
F72	50	2.5	1.1	0.18	111
F85	33	1.8	0.7	0.15	247
F-R	193	1.7	0.8	0.07	
PICARDIE					
F02	46	2.1	1.1	0.18	111
F60	45	1.9	1.1	0.20	111
F80	48	2.2	1.2	0.20	83
F-S	139	2.1	1.1	0.11	
POITOU-CHARENTES					
F16	26	1.9	0.8	0.19	207
F17	42	2.1	0.9	0.16	178
F79	27	2.0	0.8	0.19	207
F86	22	1.5	0.6-	0.16	285
F-T	117	1.9	0.8	0.09	
PROVENCE-ALPES-COTE D'AZUR					
F04	9	2.0	0.9	0.34	178
F05	9	2.3	0.9	0.36	178
F06	52	1.5	0.6--	0.10	285
F13	151	2.3	1.3++	0.12	57
F83	63	2.5	1.3	0.18	57
F84	21	1.3	0.8	0.19	207
F-U	305	2.0	1.1	0.07	
RHONE-ALPES					
F01	23	1.5	0.8	0.20	207
F07	25	2.4	1.1	0.26	111
F26	26	1.8	0.7	0.16	247
F38	52	1.5	1.0	0.15	147
F42	49	1.6	0.8	0.14	207
F69	80	1.4	0.8	0.10	207
F73	18	1.5	0.9	0.23	178
F74	19	1.1	0.8	0.19	207
F-V	292	1.5	0.9	0.06	
F.0	4145	1.9	1.1++	0.02	

UNITED KINGDOM (1976-80)

EAST ANGLIA					
G25	21	1.2	0.8	0.19	207
G46	66	3.2	1.3	0.18	57
G55	54	3.1	1.5+	0.23	28
G-A	141	2.5	1.2+	0.12	
EAST MIDLANDS					
G30	69	2.5	1.4+	0.19	42
G44	53	2.1	1.2	0.18	83
G45	44	2.7	1.4	0.23	42
G47	37	2.4	1.5	0.26	28
G50	70	2.3	1.2	0.15	83
G-B	273	2.4	1.3++	0.09	
NORTHERN					
G14	103	2.8	1.5++	0.16	28
G27	36	2.1	1.3	0.23	57
G29	39	2.7	1.2	0.21	83
G33	52	2.8	1.5+	0.23	28
G48	21	2.4	1.2	0.28	83
G-C	251	2.6	1.4++	0.10	
NORTH-WEST					
G11	213	2.6	1.3++	0.10	57
G12	140	2.9	1.6++	0.15	20
G26	72	2.6	1.5++	0.19	28
G43	116	2.7	1.1	0.12	111
G-D	541	2.7	1.4++	0.06	

SOUTH-EAST					
G01	534	2.5	1.2++	0.06	83
G22	24	1.6	1.2	0.25	83
G23	39	1.9	1.1	0.20	111
G24	30	1.9	1.2	0.23	83
G34	74	3.5	1.3	0.19	57
G35	88	2.0	1.1	0.13	111
G37	112	2.6	1.4++	0.14	42
G39	65	2.2	1.3	0.16	57
G41	17	4.7	1.9	0.56	8
G42	103	2.3	1.2	0.13	83
G51	36	2.3	1.2	0.22	83
G56	73	2.4	1.1	0.14	111
G58	61	3.0	1.2	0.19	83
G-E	1256	2.4	1.2++	0.04	
SOUTH-WEST					
G21	72	2.5	1.2	0.16	83
G28	28	2.2	0.9	0.20	178
G31	84	2.9	1.2	0.15	83
G32	52	2.8	1.0	0.17	147
G36	40	2.6	1.4	0.24	42
G53	27	2.1	1.0	0.21	147
G59	24	1.6	0.9	0.20	178
G-F	327	2.5	1.1+	0.07	
WEST MIDLANDS					
G15	167	2.0	1.1	0.09	111
G38	36	1.9	1.0	0.18	147
G52	26	2.3	1.4	0.32	42
G54	86	2.8	1.8++	0.20	10
G57	28	2.0	1.1	0.22	111
G-G	343	2.2	1.2++	0.07	
YORKSHIRE AND HUMBERSIDE					
G13	83	2.1	1.2	0.14	83
G16	170	2.7	1.3++	0.11	57
G40	78	3.0	1.6++	0.19	20
G49	47	2.3	1.1	0.18	111
G-H	378	2.5	1.3++	0.07	
WALES					
G61	33	2.8	1.5	0.29	28
G62	37	3.7	1.5	0.28	28
G63	37	2.8	1.5	0.27	28
G64	14	2.0	1.0	0.33	147
G65	45	2.7	1.3	0.22	57
G66	11	3.5	1.7	0.56	15
G67	43	3.6	1.8++	0.30	10
G68	35	3.1	1.6+	0.29	20
G-I	255	3.0	1.5++	0.10	
SCOTLAND(1975-80)					
S01	15	2.6	1.3	0.38	57
S02	37	2.6	1.3	0.24	57
S03	40	3.2	1.5+	0.28	28
S04	17	1.6	0.9	0.24	178
S05	56	2.4	1.1	0.17	111
S06	4	1.3	0.5	0.25	319
S07	16	1.9	1.4	0.35	42
S08	211	2.7	1.5++	0.11	28
S09	9	2.0	1.0	0.35	147
S10	2	3.7	1.0	0.69	147
S11	1	1.6	0.9	0.92	178
S12	1	1.1	1.0	0.99	147
G-J	409	2.5	1.3++	0.07	
NORTHERN IRELAND					
JE	35	2.1	1.1	0.20	111
JN	17	1.8	1.0	0.26	147
JS	12	1.8	1.2	0.36	83
JW	22	3.6	2.4++	0.55	4
G-K	86	2.2	1.3+	0.15	
G.0	4260	2.5	1.3++	0.02	
ITALIA (1975-79)					
ABRUZZI					
I66	10	1.3	0.5--	0.17	319
I67	3	0.4	0.2--	0.14	351
I68	9	1.2	0.7	0.25	247
I69	18	1.9	1.0	0.25	147
I-A	40	1.3	0.7--	0.11	
BASILICATA					
I76	13	1.2	0.7	0.22	247
I77	3	0.6	0.4-	0.23	336
I-B	16	1.0	0.6-	0.16	
CALABRIA					
I78	22	1.2	0.9	0.21	178
I79	17	0.9	0.6-	0.16	285
I80	14	0.9	0.6-	0.16	285
I-C	53	1.0	0.7-	0.10	

CAMPANIA					
I61	11	0.6	0.5--	0.14	319
I62	8	1.1	0.6	0.24	285
I63	61	0.8	0.6--	0.09	285
I64	6	0.5	0.2--	0.10	351
I65	22	0.9	0.6--	0.13	285
I-D	108	0.8	0.6--	0.06	
EMILIA-ROMAGNA					
I33	10	1.4	0.9	0.32	178
I34	16	1.6	0.6-	0.16	285
I35	26	2.5	1.2	0.25	83
I36	36	2.4	1.3	0.23	57
I37	49	2.0	1.0	0.15	147
I38	24	2.4	1.2	0.28	83
I39	16	1.7	1.0	0.28	147
I40	12	0.8	0.5--	0.16	319
I-E	189	1.9	1.0	0.08	
FRIULI-VENEZIA GIULIA					
I30	40	2.9	1.6+	0.28	20
I31	12	3.1	1.8	0.56	10
I32	30	3.8	1.7+	0.34	15
I93	21	3.1	1.8	0.42	10
I-F	103	3.2	1.7++	0.18	
LAZIO					
I56	4	0.6	0.4--	0.19	336
I57	4	1.1	0.6	0.32	285
I58	142	1.5	1.1	0.09	111
I59	14	1.4	1.1	0.31	111
I60	15	1.3	0.8	0.22	207
I-G	179	1.4	1.0	0.08	
LIGURIA					
I08	15	2.5	1.0	0.29	147
I09	12	1.5	0.8	0.24	207
I10	66	2.3	1.1	0.14	111
I11	15	2.4	1.0	0.28	147
I-H	108	2.2	1.0	0.10	
LOMBARDIA					
I12	29	1.5	1.0	0.20	147
I13	16	0.8	0.6-	0.15	285
I14	7	1.6	0.9	0.37	178
I15	139	1.3	0.9	0.08	178
I16	29	1.3	0.8	0.16	207
I17	43	1.7	1.1	0.17	111
I18	31	2.3	1.0	0.20	147
I19	22	2.6	1.4	0.32	42
I20	14	1.4	0.5--	0.15	319
I-I	330	1.4	0.9	0.05	
MARCHE					
I41	7	0.8	0.5--	0.18	319
I42	20	1.8	0.9	0.23	178
I43	6	0.8	0.3--	0.15	347
I44	8	0.9	0.5-	0.20	319
I-J	41	1.2	0.6--	0.10	
MOLISE					
I70	8	1.3	0.7	0.26	247
I94	6	2.5	1.0	0.42	147
I-K	14	1.7	0.8	0.22	
PIEMONTE					
I01	112	1.8	1.2	0.11	83
I02	26	2.5	1.1	0.24	111
I03	31	2.4	1.1	0.23	111
I04	24	1.7	0.9	0.21	178
I05	12	2.1	1.1	0.37	111
I06	27	2.2	0.9	0.20	178
I-L	232	2.0	1.1	0.08	
PUGLIA					
I71	15	0.9	0.7	0.18	247
I72	38	1.0	0.6--	0.11	285
I73	15	1.1	0.8	0.22	207
I74	6	0.6	0.4--	0.18	336
I75	23	1.2	0.8	0.17	207
I-M	97	1.0	0.7--	0.07	
SARDEGNA					
I90	10	0.9	0.4--	0.15	336
I91	9	1.3	0.8	0.30	207
I92	17	1.0	0.7	0.18	247
I95	5	1.3	0.7	0.30	247
I-N	41	1.0	0.6--	0.11	
SICILIA					
I81	7	0.7	0.4--	0.15	336
I82	26	0.9	0.6--	0.13	285
I83	21	1.2	0.7	0.17	247
I84	14	1.2	0.7	0.20	247
I85	8	1.1	0.7	0.27	247
I86	6	1.2	0.9	0.38	178
I87	32	1.3	1.0	0.18	147
I88	4	0.6	0.3--	0.15	347
I89	6	0.6	0.4--	0.17	336
I-O	124	1.0	0.7--	0.06	

TOSCANA					
I45	6	1.1	0.7	0.30	247
I46	17	1.7	0.8	0.23	207
I47	6	0.9	0.6	0.26	285
I48	57	1.8	1.0	0.14	147
I49	18	2.0	1.2	0.31	83
I50	17	1.7	0.8	0.20	207
I51	12	1.5	0.6	0.20	285
I52	12	1.8	0.9	0.30	178
I53	7	1.2	0.7	0.28	247
I-P	152	1.7	0.9	0.08	
TRENTINO-ALTO ADIGE					
I21	8	0.7	0.6	0.21	285
I22	26	2.3	1.2	0.26	83
I-Q	34	1.5	0.9	0.17	
UMBRIA					
I54	13	0.9	0.4--	0.13	336
I55	11	1.9	1.0	0.32	147
I-R	24	1.2	0.6--	0.13	
VALLE D'AOSTA					
I07	5	1.8	1.2	0.56	83
VENETO					
I23	42	2.2	1.3	0.21	57
I24	32	1.8	1.2	0.23	83
I25	10	1.7	0.8	0.27	207
I26	31	1.7	1.1	0.22	111
I27	41	1.9	1.3	0.21	57
I28	44	2.2	1.5+	0.24	28
I29	8	1.2	0.8	0.29	207
I-T	208	1.9	1.2++	0.09	
I.0	2098	1.5	0.9--	0.02	
IRELAND (1976-80)					
CONNAUGHT					
R07	13	3.2	1.6	0.46	20
R12	0	0.0	0.0--	0.00	354
R16	12	4.3	1.7	0.49	15
R20	2	1.6	1.1	0.83	111
R21	3	2.2	1.3	0.75	57
R-A	30	3.0	1.4	0.26	
LEINSTER					
R01	3	3.2	2.7	1.56	3
R06	44	1.7	1.4	0.22	42
R09	2	0.9	0.8	0.60	207
R10	1	0.6	0.6	0.63	285
R11	1	0.8	0.8	0.80	207
R14	0	0.0	0.0--	0.00	354
R15	4	1.9	1.5	0.79	28
R17	3	1.4	1.0	0.65	147
R19	3	2.2	1.3	0.82	57
R24	4	2.7	1.9	1.00	8
R25	9	3.8	3.1+	1.08	1
R26	3	1.4	1.3	0.76	57
R-B	77	1.7	1.4++	0.17	
MUNSTER					
R03	4	2.0	1.7	0.93	15
R04	31	3.1	2.2++	0.43	6
R08	9	3.1	1.5	0.53	28
R13	7	1.8	1.3	0.53	57
R22	10	3.1	2.3	0.77	5
R23	4	1.8	1.4	0.72	42
R-C	65	2.7	1.9++	0.25	
ULSTER					
R02	4	3.1	2.0	1.10	7
R05	7	2.4	1.1	0.45	111
R18	4	3.3	2.8	1.53	2
R-D	15	2.8	1.7	0.48	
R.0	187	2.2	1.6++	0.12	
LUXEMBOURG (1971-80)					
LE	1	0.5	0.1--	0.14	353
LN	2	0.8	0.5	0.40	319
LS	25	1.9	1.1	0.24	111
L.0	28	1.6	0.9	0.18	
NEDERLAND (1976-80)					
N01	17	1.2	0.6	0.18	285
N02	20	1.4	0.8	0.21	207
N03	14	1.4	0.8	0.24	207
N04	28	1.1	0.7	0.14	247
N05	38	0.9	0.6--	0.10	285
N06	25	1.1	0.7	0.15	247
N07	77	1.3	0.7--	0.09	247
N08	108	1.4	0.8	0.09	207
N09	11	1.3	0.7	0.24	247
N10	48	1.0	0.7-	0.11	247
N11	12	0.5	0.4--	0.10	336
N.0	398	1.1	0.7--	0.04	
EEC-9					
EEC	14259	1.8	1.0	0.01	

BELGIE-BELGIQUE (1971-78)

BRUSSEL-BRUXELLES					
B21	278	7.0	4.4--	0.27	228
VLAANDEREN					
B10	286	4.6	3.3--	0.20	278
B29	195	5.4	3.9--	0.29	249
B30	249	5.9	4.1--	0.27	239
B40	408	7.8	5.1--	0.26	198
B70	65	2.3	2.4--	0.31	320
B-V	1203	5.5	3.9--	0.12	
WALLONIE					
B25	36	3.5	2.5--	0.42	314
B50	307	6.0	4.0--	0.24	244
B60	219	5.6	3.7--	0.26	257
B80	47	5.4	3.5--	0.54	268
B90	79	5.2	3.5--	0.41	268
B-W	688	5.5	3.7--	0.15	
B.0	2169	5.6	3.9--	0.09	

BR DEUTSCHLAND (1976-80)

BADEN-WURTTEMBERG					
D81	384	4.6	3.5--	0.19	268
D82	356	6.3	4.7--	0.26	213
D83	258	5.8	4.3--	0.28	232
D84	164	4.6	3.7--	0.30	257
D-A	1162	5.3	4.0--	0.12	
BAYERN					
D91	344	4.0	2.8--	0.15	304
D92	94	4.0	2.9--	0.31	296
D93	126	5.4	4.0--	0.37	244
D94	158	6.4	4.5--	0.37	226
D95	183	5.1	3.4--	0.26	274
D96	161	5.6	4.0--	0.33	244
D97	171	4.7	3.2--	0.26	284
D-B	1237	4.8	3.3--	0.10	
BERLIN(WEST)					
DB0	339	7.9	4.6--	0.27	220
BREMEN					
D40	96	5.8	3.5--	0.38	268
HAMBURG					
D20	233	6.0	3.7--	0.26	257
HESSEN					
D64	463	4.4	3.1--	0.15	288
D66	137	4.8	3.0--	0.27	293
D-F	600	4.5	3.1--	0.13	
NIEDERSACHSEN					
D31	173	4.4	2.8--	0.23	304
D32	246	5.1	3.3--	0.22	278
D33	208	5.9	3.9--	0.29	249
D34	279	5.5	4.1--	0.26	239
D-G	906	5.2	3.5--	0.12	
NORDRHEIN-WESTFALEN					
D51	772	6.2	4.7--	0.17	213
D53	477	5.1	4.2--	0.20	234
D55	305	5.3	4.6--	0.27	220
D57	222	5.2	3.9--	0.27	249
D59	544	6.2	4.8--	0.21	210
D-H	2320	5.7	4.5--	0.10	
RHEINLAND-PFALZ					
D71	185	5.7	3.7--	0.29	257
D72	96	8.6	6.5	0.69	147
D73	243	5.6	3.9--	0.27	249
D-I	524	6.0	4.2--	0.19	
SAARLAND					
DA0	179	7.0	5.1--	0.40	198
SCHLESWIG-HOLSTEIN					
D10	273	4.4	2.9--	0.19	296
D.0	7869	5.4	3.8--	0.04	

DANMARK (1971-80)

K15	407	6.7	4.3--	0.22	232
K20	55	3.6	3.4--	0.46	274
K25	23	2.5	2.4--	0.51	320
K30	87	6.4	4.0--	0.44	244
K35	83	6.4	3.6--	0.41	264
K40	13	5.5	3.1--	0.87	288
K42	97	4.4	2.5--	0.27	314
K50	41	3.4	2.2--	0.35	328
K55	46	4.4	3.1--	0.47	288
K60	57	3.6	2.2--	0.30	328
K65	36	2.8	2.1--	0.35	331
K70	92	3.3	2.4--	0.26	320
K76	56	4.9	2.7--	0.38	309
K80	90	3.8	2.3--	0.25	325
K.0	1183	4.7	3.1--	0.09	

FRANCE (1971-78)

ALSACE					
F67	608	17.6	15.3++	0.64	24
F68	497	19.9	17.3++	0.81	15
F-A	1105	18.6	16.1++	0.50	
AQUITAINE					
F24	338	23.2	12.4++	0.71	50
F33	667	16.3	11.3++	0.45	70
F40	244	21.8	13.1++	0.89	42
F47	191	16.8	9.2++	0.71	90
F64	319	15.4	9.8++	0.58	81
F-B	1759	17.8	11.2++	0.28	
AUVERGNE					
F03	346	23.4	13.5++	0.77	38
F15	134	20.2	12.2++	1.10	54
F43	191	23.8	13.4++	1.04	40
F63	450	19.8	14.6++	0.71	28
F-C	1121	21.5	13.8++	0.43	
BASSE-NORMANDIE					
F14	753	34.5	30.7++	1.14	5
F50	743	42.7	32.0++	1.20	3
F61	524	45.8	35.7++	1.61	1
F-D	2020	39.8	32.3++	0.73	
BOURGOGNE					
F21	265	14.8	11.4++	0.72	66
F58	217	22.2	12.7++	0.93	49
F71	478	21.3	14.5++	0.70	29
F89	230	19.4	11.7++	0.84	61
F-E	1190	19.2	12.8++	0.39	
BRETAGNE					
F22	891	43.7	29.5++	1.02	6
F29	1074	34.4	24.7++	0.78	7
F35	787	29.1	23.7++	0.86	8
F56	882	40.1	30.8++	1.06	4
F-F	3634	36.1	26.7++	0.46	
CENTRE					
F18	231	18.4	11.6++	0.81	62
F28	223	16.6	11.9++	0.83	59
F36	202	20.7	11.4++	0.87	66
F37	276	14.9	10.6++	0.67	76
F41	212	19.1	12.0++	0.89	56
F45	273	14.0	9.8++	0.62	81
F-G	1417	16.7	11.1++	0.31	
CHAMPAGNE-ARDENNE					
F08	238	19.2	15.8++	1.06	22
F10	172	15.3	11.5++	0.93	64
F51	337	16.0	14.2++	0.79	31
F52	134	15.8	12.3++	1.11	52
F-H	881	16.6	13.6++	0.47	
CORSE					
F20	60	6.3	4.2--	0.56	234
FRANCHE-COMTE					
F25	263	14.0	13.6++	0.86	36
F39	188	19.8	12.9++	0.99	45
F70	165	18.9	13.8++	1.13	35
F90	70	13.7	11.4++	1.40	66
F-J	686	16.3	13.2++	0.52	
HAUTE-NORMANDIE					
F27	373	22.3	18.0++	0.96	12
F76	949	20.6	17.7++	0.58	14
F-K	1322	21.0	17.8++	0.50	
ILE-DE-FRANCE					
F75	1471	17.3	11.6++	0.31	62
F77	425	14.1	12.3++	0.62	52
F78	490	11.4	12.0++	0.55	56
F91	425	11.6	12.8++	0.63	47
F92	903	16.1	13.1++	0.44	42
F93	909	17.2	16.3++	0.55	20
F94	760	16.0	14.3++	0.53	30
F95	497	14.9	15.2++	0.69	25
F-L	5880	15.3	13.1++	0.17	
LANGUEDOC-ROUSSILLON					
F11	146	14.0	7.3	0.65	125
F30	273	14.2	8.8++	0.55	98
F34	315	12.6	7.7	0.46	116
F48	76	25.3	15.2++	1.84	25
F66	166	14.3	7.6	0.63	119
F-M	976	14.1	8.2++	0.28	
LIMOUSIN					
F19	184	19.6	10.8++	0.85	75
F23	158	27.6	12.8++	1.16	47
F87	297	21.7	12.4++	0.76	50
F-N	639	22.2	11.9++	0.51	
LORRAINE					
F54	447	15.7	13.6++	0.66	36
F55	208	25.9	18.7++	1.36	11
F57	573	14.2	13.5++	0.57	38
F88	324	20.8	16.3++	0.93	20
F-O	1552	16.8	14.6++	0.38	
MIDI-PYRENEES					
F09	70	12.8	6.5	0.85	147
F12	187	17.3	9.5++	0.75	86
F31	316	10.5	7.3	0.42	125
F32	110	15.8	7.6	0.77	119
F46	99	16.8	9.0	0.98	95
F65	136	15.3	8.8+	0.79	98
F81	196	14.8	8.3	0.63	103
F82	118	16.5	9.4+	0.91	87
F-P	1232	13.9	8.1++	0.24	
NORD-PAS-DE-CALAIS					
F59	2238	22.7	20.3++	0.44	10
F62	1354	24.7	20.9++	0.58	9
F-Q	3592	23.4	20.5++	0.35	
PAYS DE LA LOIRE					
F44	731	20.3	17.3++	0.65	15
F49	474	19.3	15.4++	0.73	23
F53	469	46.3	35.4++	1.67	2
F72	464	24.1	17.9++	0.86	13
F85	331	19.0	13.9++	0.80	32
F-R	2469	23.0	18.2++	0.38	
PICARDIE					
F02	451	21.2	16.8++	0.83	18
F60	384	15.8	13.9++	0.73	32
F80	380	18.0	13.4++	0.72	40
F-S	1215	18.2	14.7++	0.44	
POITOU-CHARENTES					
F16	269	20.4	12.9++	0.82	45
F17	310	16.0	10.2++	0.61	78
F79	171	12.8	8.6+	0.69	101
F86	208	14.8	9.8++	0.72	81
F-T	958	16.0	10.4++	0.35	
PROVENCE-ALPES-COTE D'AZUR					
F04	63	14.0	8.2	1.09	105
F05	59	15.2	10.3+	1.39	77
F06	271	8.8	4.7--	0.31	213
F13	600	9.4	6.9	0.29	135
F83	360	14.6	9.2++	0.50	90
F84	175	11.3	7.9	0.62	110
F-U	1528	10.7	7.0	0.19	
RHONE-ALPES					
F01	245	16.2	12.0++	0.79	56
F07	266	26.5	16.5++	1.07	19
F26	228	16.2	11.1++	0.77	72
F38	445	13.0	11.1++	0.54	72
F42	587	20.0	14.8++	0.63	27
F69	795	14.2	12.2++	0.44	54
F73	262	21.5	16.9++	1.07	17
F74	291	16.2	13.9++	0.83	32
F-V	3119	16.5	13.1++	0.24	
F.0	38355	18.6	14.0++	0.07	

UNITED KINGDOM (1976-80)

EAST ANGLIA					
G25	107	6.2	4.7--	0.46	213
G46	175	8.8	5.1--	0.40	198
G55	157	8.8	5.7--	0.47	173
G-A	439	8.0	5.2--	0.26	
EAST MIDLANDS					
G30	236	9.0	5.7--	0.38	173
G44	183	7.4	5.3--	0.40	192
G45	138	8.8	5.7--	0.50	173
G47	97	6.3	4.6--	0.48	220
G50	192	6.7	4.6--	0.34	220
G-B	846	7.6	5.2--	0.18	
NORTHERN					
G14	300	8.9	6.1--	0.36	160
G27	144	8.6	6.8	0.57	138
G29	128	9.3	6.0-	0.55	166
G33	115	6.5	4.4--	0.42	228
G48	77	9.0	5.5-	0.64	185
G-C	764	8.4	5.8--	0.21	
NORTH-WEST					
G11	684	8.8	6.3--	0.25	157
G12	488	10.9	7.7	0.36	116
G26	256	9.5	6.9	0.44	135
G43	414	10.5	6.6	0.34	146
G-D	1842	9.8	6.8-	0.16	

SOUTH-EAST					
G01	1564	7.8	4.9--	0.13	207
G22	95	6.4	5.1--	0.54	198
G23	142	7.1	5.6--	0.48	180
G24	113	7.2	5.6--	0.53	180
G34	221	12.4	5.7--	0.41	173
G35	300	7.2	4.9--	0.29	207
G37	338	7.7	5.7--	0.31	173
G39	220	7.9	5.9--	0.41	169
G41	33	10.2	4.5--	0.81	226
G42	333	7.9	5.1--	0.29	198
G51	105	6.3	5.0--	0.51	203
G56	225	7.7	5.2--	0.35	195
G58	214	12.1	6.4	0.47	152
G-E	3903	8.0	5.2--	0.09	
SOUTH-WEST					
G21	194	7.3	4.7--	0.35	213
G28	144	12.1	6.4	0.55	152
G31	301	10.9	6.1--	0.37	160
G32	171	10.3	5.5--	0.45	185
G36	103	7.1	4.6--	0.47	220
G53	98	8.1	4.9--	0.52	207
G59	126	8.1	6.1	0.56	160
G-F	1137	9.1	5.4--	0.17	
WEST MIDLANDS					
G15	666	8.3	5.9--	0.23	169
G38	177	9.9	6.7	0.52	143
G52	95	8.9	6.3	0.67	157
G54	218	7.4	5.5--	0.38	185
G57	116	8.4	6.4	0.61	152
G-G	1272	8.3	6.0--	0.17	
YORKSHIRE AND HUMBERSIDE					
G13	279	7.3	4.8--	0.30	210
G16	476	7.9	5.3--	0.25	192
G40	220	8.9	6.1-	0.42	160
G49	198	10.2	6.3	0.46	157
G-H	1173	8.2	5.5--	0.16	
WALES					
G61	115	10.4	6.4	0.62	152
G62	86	9.2	5.4--	0.61	190
G63	87	6.8	4.6--	0.50	220
G64	63	9.6	5.8	0.75	172
G65	126	8.0	5.7--	0.52	173
G66	31	9.8	6.1	1.14	160
G67	88	7.9	5.5--	0.60	185
G68	119	11.3	7.4	0.69	123
G-I	715	8.9	5.8--	0.22	
SCOTLAND(1975-80)					
S01	64	11.5	8.2	1.05	105
S02	153	11.4	8.0	0.67	107
S03	129	11.2	7.3	0.66	125
S04	89	8.9	6.5	0.71	147
S05	204	9.5	7.0	0.50	132
S06	27	9.4	5.6	1.14	180
S07	75	9.4	6.8	0.80	138
S08	696	9.8	7.5	0.29	122
S09	46	11.0	7.7	1.17	116
S10	3	5.6	3.0-	1.78	293
S11	10	16.0	11.4	3.76	66
S12	11	12.5	6.7	2.28	143
G-J	1507	10.1	7.3	0.19	
NORTHERN IRELAND					
JE	106	6.5	5.5--	0.55	185
JN	38	4.2	3.6--	0.59	264
JS	25	3.8	3.4--	0.72	274
JW	35	5.8	5.2-	0.92	195
G-K	204	5.4	4.6--	0.34	
G.0	13802	8.5	5.7--	0.05	
ITALIA (1975-79)					
ABRUZZI					
I66	40	5.5	3.3--	0.54	278
I67	23	3.5	2.5--	0.53	314
I68	16	2.3	1.6--	0.41	344
I69	24	2.7	1.9--	0.39	337
I-A	103	3.5	2.3--	0.23	
BASILICATA					
I76	30	2.9	2.1--	0.40	331
I77	9	1.8	1.4--	0.49	349
I-B	39	2.5	1.9--	0.31	
CALABRIA					
I78	29	1.6	1.5--	0.28	348
I79	43	2.4	2.0--	0.32	335
I80	39	2.7	1.8--	0.30	339
I-C	111	2.2	1.8--	0.17	

CAMPANIA					
I61	32	1.8	1.7--	0.30	341
I62	13	1.8	1.2--	0.33	353
I63	131	1.9	2.0--	0.17	335
I64	20	1.8	1.3--	0.30	351
I65	49	2.0	1.6--	0.24	344
I-D	245	1.9	1.7--	0.11	
EMILIA-ROMAGNA					
I33	61	8.8	5.0--	0.66	203
I34	65	6.7	3.7--	0.47	257
I35	47	4.7	2.9--	0.44	296
I36	66	4.7	3.2--	0.41	284
I37	121	5.4	3.3--	0.31	278
I38	71	7.6	4.7--	0.56	213
I39	57	6.5	3.9--	0.53	249
I40	81	5.6	3.9--	0.44	249
I-E	569	5.9	3.7--	0.16	
FRIULI-VENEZIA GIULIA					
I30	203	15.8	10.2++	0.73	78
I31	38	10.8	7.2	1.20	129
I32	96	13.8	7.2	0.76	129
I93	121	18.5	13.1++	1.22	42
I-F	458	15.3	9.6++	0.46	
LAZIO					
I56	35	5.3	3.3--	0.57	278
I57	23	6.5	3.7--	0.79	257
I58	293	3.3	2.9--	0.17	296
I59	34	3.3	2.9--	0.51	296
I60	37	3.3	2.3--	0.39	325
I-G	422	3.5	2.9--	0.14	
LIGURIA					
I08	61	11.0	5.6-	0.75	180
I09	47	6.4	3.3--	0.49	278
I10	235	9.1	5.3--	0.35	192
I11	50	8.4	4.7--	0.67	213
I-H	393	8.8	4.9--	0.25	
LOMBARDIA					
I12	182	9.7	8.3	0.64	103
I13	192	10.5	8.7+	0.64	100
I14	42	9.8	7.9	1.24	110
I15	901	9.2	8.0++	0.28	107
I16	218	10.2	9.6++	0.66	85
I17	248	10.1	9.0++	0.58	95
I18	159	12.5	6.9	0.57	135
I19	145	17.9	11.9++	1.02	59
I20	106	11.4	6.8	0.68	138
I-I	2193	10.2	8.3++	0.18	
MARCHE					
I41	33	4.1	2.5--	0.45	314
I42	59	5.7	3.7--	0.49	257
I43	30	4.2	2.4--	0.45	320
I44	36	4.2	2.9--	0.48	296
I-J	158	4.6	2.9--	0.24	
MOLISE					
I70	19	3.3	1.9--	0.45	337
I94	11	4.8	3.1--	0.97	288
I-K	30	3.7	2.3--	0.43	
PIEMONTE					
I01	460	7.9	6.5	0.31	147
I02	111	11.5	7.1	0.69	131
I03	128	10.4	7.0	0.64	132
I04	103	7.6	4.4--	0.46	228
I05	58	10.8	5.2-	0.74	195
I06	135	11.6	5.6--	0.52	180
I-L	995	9.0	6.1--	0.20	
PUGLIA					
I71	26	1.5	1.1--	0.22	354
I72	52	1.5	1.3--	0.19	351
I73	27	2.0	1.8--	0.35	339
I74	11	1.2	1.1--	0.32	354
I75	59	3.3	2.7--	0.35	309
I-M	175	1.9	1.6--	0.12	
SARDEGNA					
I90	34	3.2	2.6--	0.47	312
I91	28	4.1	2.9--	0.59	296
I92	54	3.1	2.8--	0.39	304
I95	15	3.9	2.3--	0.63	325
I-N	131	3.4	2.7--	0.25	
SICILIA					
I81	23	2.2	1.4--	0.31	349
I82	80	2.8	2.1--	0.24	331
I83	43	2.6	1.7--	0.27	341
I84	39	3.3	2.1--	0.35	331
I85	25	3.5	2.5--	0.51	314
I86	19	3.8	2.6--	0.62	312
I87	51	2.1	1.7--	0.24	341
I88	16	2.4	1.6--	0.41	344
I89	32	3.3	2.5--	0.45	314
I-O	328	2.7	2.0--	0.11	

TOSCANA					
I45	59	11.9	7.4	0.99	123
I46	119	12.8	7.9	0.75	110
I47	64	10.0	5.9	0.75	169
I48	258	9.0	5.4--	0.35	190
I49	64	7.6	5.0--	0.64	203
I50	61	6.5	3.6--	0.47	264
I51	59	7.7	4.4--	0.59	228
I52	53	8.4	4.2--	0.59	234
I53	48	8.7	5.0--	0.74	203
I-P	785	9.0	5.3--	0.20	
TRENTINO-ALTO ADIGE					
I21	136	12.9	11.5++	1.01	64
I22	164	15.3	10.9++	0.87	74
I-Q	300	14.1	11.1++	0.66	
UMBRIA					
I54	95	6.8	4.2--	0.43	234
I55	20	3.6	2.2--	0.51	328
I-R	115	5.9	3.6--	0.34	
VALLE D'AOSTA					
I07	31	10.9	7.8	1.42	114
VENETO					
I23	224	12.0	9.1++	0.62	93
I24	193	11.1	9.3++	0.68	89
I25	83	15.4	10.2++	1.15	78
I26	204	11.9	9.7++	0.69	84
I27	236	11.5	9.4++	0.62	87
I28	268	13.7	11.3++	0.70	70
I29	76	12.2	8.4	0.99	102
I-T	1284	12.3	9.7++	0.27	
I.0	8865	6.5	4.8--	0.05	
IRELAND (1976-80)					
CONNAUGHT					
R07	25	5.8	4.1--	0.87	239
R12	8	10.8	6.0	2.28	166
R16	28	9.6	5.7	1.16	173
R20	10	7.0	4.0-	1.34	244
R21	10	7.2	4.1-	1.34	239
R-A	81	7.5	4.7--	0.55	
LEINSTER					
R01	11	11.1	8.9	2.71	97
R06	142	6.0	6.7	0.58	143
R09	15	5.9	7.3	1.94	125
R10	19	10.6	7.9	1.86	110
R11	11	8.4	6.8	2.14	138
R14	3	3.7	3.2-	1.88	284
R15	20	9.3	9.1	2.09	93
R17	21	9.0	7.8	1.73	114
R19	6	4.0	2.8--	1.18	304
R24	16	10.5	7.6	1.93	119
R25	14	5.7	4.8	1.35	210
R26	14	6.7	6.1	1.68	160
R-B	292	6.8	6.6	0.40	
MUNSTER					
R03	11	5.0	3.1--	0.97	288
R04	108	10.8	9.2+	0.91	90
R08	20	6.4	3.9--	0.92	249
R13	32	8.1	7.0	1.27	132
R22	33	9.6	6.5	1.16	147
R23	17	7.7	6.0	1.49	166
R-C	221	8.9	6.8	0.47	
ULSTER					
R02	3	2.1	1.6--	1.02	344
R05	19	6.1	3.9--	0.95	249
R18	9	6.9	4.2-	1.43	234
R-D	31	5.3	3.3--	0.63	
R.0	625	7.4	6.1--	0.25	
LUXEMBOURG (1971-80)					
LE	22	12.1	6.8	1.51	138
LN	32	12.1	8.0	1.47	107
LS	109	8.5	6.4	0.62	152
L.0	163	9.5	6.7	0.54	
NEDERLAND (1976-80)					
N01	73	5.4	3.5--	0.43	268
N02	62	4.3	2.9--	0.39	296
N03	39	3.8	2.4--	0.41	320
N04	106	4.2	3.4--	0.34	274
N05	158	3.8	3.0--	0.25	293
N06	74	3.4	2.8--	0.33	304
N07	279	4.8	3.6--	0.22	264
N08	357	4.7	3.5--	0.19	268
N09	55	6.5	4.1--	0.58	239
N10	168	3.3	3.2--	0.25	284
N11	78	2.9	2.7--	0.31	309
N.0	1449	4.2	3.3--	0.09	
EEC-9					
EEC	74480	9.8	7.1	0.03	

BELGIE-BELGIQUE (1971-78)

BRUSSEL-BRUXELLES					
B21	123	2.8	1.1-	0.12	156
VLAANDEREN					
B10	108	1.7	0.9--	0.09	205
B29	48	1.3	0.7--	0.11	263
B30	103	2.4	1.1-	0.12	156
B40	130	2.4	1.2	0.11	138
B70	21	0.8	0.6--	0.14	291
B-V	410	1.8	1.0--	0.05	
WALLONIE					
B25	9	0.8	0.4--	0.14	333
B50	152	2.8	1.1--	0.10	156
B60	81	1.9	0.8--	0.10	227
B80	17	1.9	0.8--	0.21	227
B90	29	1.8	0.7--	0.14	263
B-W	288	2.2	0.9--	0.06	
B.0	821	2.0	1.0--	0.04	

BR DEUTSCHLAND (1976-80)

BADEN-WURTTEMBERG					
D81	106	1.2	0.5--	0.05	317
D82	92	1.5	0.6--	0.07	291
D83	76	1.6	0.6--	0.08	291
D84	58	1.5	0.7--	0.10	263
D-A	332	1.4	0.6--	0.04	
BAYERN					
D91	113	1.2	0.5--	0.05	317
D92	53	2.0	0.8--	0.13	227
D93	45	1.8	0.7--	0.12	263
D94	45	1.6	0.6--	0.09	291
D95	48	1.2	0.5--	0.07	317
D96	46	1.5	0.6--	0.10	291
D97	46	1.2	0.4--	0.07	333
D-B	396	1.4	0.6--	0.03	
BERLIN(WEST)					
DB0	180	3.4	1.1-	0.11	156
BREMEN					
D40	42	2.3	1.0-	0.17	179
HAMBURG					
D20	93	2.1	0.7--	0.09	263
HESSEN					
D64	157	1.4	0.6--	0.05	291
D66	54	1.7	0.7--	0.10	263
D-F	211	1.5	0.6--	0.05	
NIEDERSACHSEN					
D31	61	1.4	0.5--	0.08	317
D32	101	1.9	0.7--	0.08	263
D33	71	1.9	0.8--	0.10	227
D34	139	2.6	1.2	0.11	138
D-G	372	2.0	0.8--	0.05	
NORDRHEIN-WESTFALEN					
D51	275	2.0	0.9--	0.06	205
D53	166	1.6	0.8--	0.07	227
D55	127	2.0	1.1--	0.10	156
D57	87	1.8	0.8--	0.09	227
D59	210	2.2	1.1--	0.08	156
D-H	865	1.9	0.9--	0.03	
RHEINLAND-PFALZ					
D71	55	1.5	0.7--	0.10	263
D72	15	1.2	0.5--	0.14	317
D73	83	1.8	0.7--	0.08	263
D-I	153	1.6	0.7--	0.06	
SAARLAND					
DA0	53	1.9	0.8--	0.12	227
SCHLESWIG-HOLSTEIN					
D10	148	2.2	0.9--	0.08	205
D.0	2845	1.8	0.7--	0.02	

DANMARK (1971-80)

K15	196	2.9	1.2-	0.09	138
K20	30	2.0	1.4	0.27	113
K25	15	1.6	1.2	0.31	138
K30	34	2.5	1.2	0.22	138
K35	33	2.6	1.2	0.22	138
K40	2	0.9	0.5-	0.37	317
K42	51	2.3	1.1-	0.16	156
K50	24	2.0	1.0	0.23	179
K55	21	2.1	1.0	0.24	179
K60	34	2.1	1.1	0.21	156
K65	19	1.5	0.9-	0.22	205
K70	59	2.1	1.1	0.15	156
K76	23	2.1	1.0	0.22	179
K80	60	2.6	1.2	0.17	138
K.0	601	2.4	1.1--	0.05	

FRANCE (1971-78)

ALSACE					
F67	55	1.5	0.7--	0.11	263
F68	60	2.3	1.2	0.18	138
F-A	115	1.9	0.9--	0.10	
AQUITAINE					
F24	43	2.8	0.9--	0.17	205
F33	107	2.4	1.1--	0.12	156
F40	33	2.8	1.2	0.24	138
F47	23	1.9	0.7--	0.16	263
F64	50	2.3	0.9--	0.15	205
F-B	256	2.4	1.0--	0.07	
AUVERGNE					
F03	37	2.4	0.8--	0.16	227
F15	12	1.8	0.5--	0.20	317
F43	29	3.4	1.1	0.26	156
F63	50	2.1	0.9--	0.15	205
F-C	128	2.4	0.9--	0.09	
BASSE-NORMANDIE					
F14	68	3.0	1.5	0.20	106
F50	54	2.9	1.2	0.18	138
F61	49	4.0	1.9	0.31	94
F-D	171	3.2	1.5	0.12	
BOURGOGNE					
F21	31	1.7	0.8--	0.16	227
F58	25	2.5	0.7--	0.16	263
F71	37	1.6	0.6--	0.11	291
F89	28	2.3	0.9-	0.21	205
F-E	121	1.9	0.7--	0.08	
BRETAGNE					
F22	73	3.4	1.3	0.17	121
F29	101	3.0	1.3	0.14	121
F35	83	2.8	1.3	0.15	121
F56	71	3.1	1.5	0.20	106
F-F	328	3.1	1.3	0.08	
CENTRE					
F18	30	2.3	0.8--	0.17	227
F28	28	2.1	1.0	0.22	179
F36	24	2.4	0.9	0.24	205
F37	46	2.3	0.8--	0.13	227
F41	20	1.7	0.6--	0.17	291
F45	36	1.8	0.8--	0.16	227
F-G	184	2.1	0.8--	0.07	
CHAMPAGNE-ARDENNE					
F08	24	1.9	0.9--	0.20	205
F10	23	2.0	0.9-	0.22	205
F51	33	1.5	0.9--	0.17	205
F52	10	1.2	0.6--	0.24	291
F-H	90	1.7	0.8--	0.10	
CORSE					
F20	16	1.9	0.7--	0.20	263
FRANCHE-COMTE					
F25	25	1.3	0.8--	0.17	227
F39	20	2.1	1.0	0.26	179
F70	21	2.4	1.1	0.30	156
F90	7	1.4	0.7-	0.30	263
F-J	73	1.7	0.9--	0.12	
HAUTE-NORMANDIE					
F27	39	2.3	1.3	0.23	121
F76	110	2.3	1.2	0.13	138
F-K	149	2.3	1.2	0.11	
ILE-DE-FRANCE					
F75	357	3.6	1.5	0.09	106
F77	43	1.4	0.9--	0.15	205
F78	69	1.6	1.1-	0.14	156
F91	51	1.4	1.0--	0.15	179
F92	157	2.7	1.5	0.13	106
F93	135	2.6	1.7+	0.16	99
F94	108	2.2	1.3	0.14	121
F95	62	1.8	1.2	0.17	138
F-L	982	2.4	1.4	0.05	
LANGUEDOC-ROUSSILLON					
F11	33	3.0	1.0-	0.21	179
F30	51	2.5	0.9--	0.14	205
F34	67	2.5	1.0-	0.15	179
F48	12	4.0	1.1	0.44	156
F66	24	1.9	0.6--	0.13	291
F-M	187	2.5	0.9--	0.08	
LIMOUSIN					
F19	36	3.6	1.1	0.23	156
F23	13	2.1	0.5--	0.15	317
F87	41	2.8	0.8--	0.16	227
F-N	90	3.0	0.9--	0.11	
LORRAINE					
F54	78	2.7	1.4	0.18	113
F55	14	1.7	0.7--	0.21	263
F57	54	1.4	1.0--	0.14	179
F88	36	2.2	1.0-	0.19	179
F-O	182	1.9	1.1--	0.09	
MIDI-PYRENEES					
F09	15	2.7	0.5--	0.13	317
F12	31	2.7	1.0-	0.20	179
F31	47	1.5	0.7--	0.12	263
F32	16	2.3	0.7--	0.19	263
F46	15	2.5	0.6--	0.16	291
F65	21	2.2	1.0	0.24	179
F81	23	1.7	0.6--	0.14	291
F82	12	1.6	0.5--	0.14	317
F-P	180	1.9	0.7--	0.06	
NORD-PAS-DE-CALAIS					
F59	339	3.3	1.8++	0.11	96
F62	214	3.7	1.9++	0.14	94
F-Q	553	3.5	1.8++	0.09	
PAYS DE LA LOIRE					
F44	79	2.1	1.0--	0.13	179
F49	45	1.7	0.7--	0.12	263
F53	41	3.8	1.7	0.30	99
F72	40	2.0	0.8--	0.15	227
F85	39	2.1	0.9--	0.18	205
F-R	244	2.1	0.9--	0.07	
PICARDIE					
F02	57	2.7	1.2	0.17	138
F60	58	2.4	1.1	0.17	156
F80	65	3.0	1.3	0.18	121
F-S	180	2.7	1.2	0.10	
POITOU-CHARENTES					
F16	26	1.9	0.7--	0.16	263
F17	42	2.1	0.8--	0.15	227
F79	29	2.1	0.9--	0.19	205
F86	23	1.6	0.6--	0.14	291
F-T	120	1.9	0.7--	0.08	
PROVENCE-ALPES-COTE D'AZUR					
F04	9	2.0	0.9	0.38	205
F05	9	2.3	1.0	0.35	179
F06	55	1.6	0.6--	0.09	291
F13	126	1.9	1.0--	0.10	179
F83	71	2.8	1.2	0.16	138
F84	22	1.4	0.6--	0.15	291
F-U	292	1.9	0.9--	0.06	
RHONE-ALPES					
F01	33	2.2	0.9-	0.19	205
F07	34	3.2	1.3	0.26	121
F26	25	1.7	0.8--	0.17	227
F38	43	1.2	0.6--	0.10	291
F42	62	2.0	0.9--	0.13	205
F69	84	1.4	0.8--	0.09	227
F73	18	1.5	0.8--	0.21	227
F74	26	1.4	0.8--	0.17	227
F-V	325	1.7	0.8--	0.05	
F.0	4966	2.3	1.1--	0.02	

UNITED KINGDOM (1976-80)

EAST ANGLIA					
G25	86	5.1	2.5++	0.30	74
G46	124	6.0	2.6++	0.25	64
G55	105	5.9	2.6++	0.28	64
G-A	315	5.7	2.6++	0.16	
EAST MIDLANDS					
G30	141	5.1	2.6++	0.24	64
G44	154	6.1	3.3++	0.29	36
G45	92	5.7	2.7++	0.30	58
G47	84	5.4	2.5++	0.30	74
G50	169	5.7	2.6++	0.22	64
G-B	640	5.6	2.8++	0.12	
NORTHERN					
G14	216	6.0	2.7++	0.20	58
G27	84	4.8	2.8++	0.33	53
G29	123	8.4	3.5++	0.35	31
G33	91	4.9	2.3++	0.26	85
G48	52	5.9	2.9++	0.43	47
G-C	566	5.9	2.8++	0.13	
NORTH-WEST					
G11	526	6.4	3.0++	0.14	44
G12	375	7.7	3.6++	0.21	25
G26	232	8.2	4.3++	0.31	11
G43	353	8.3	3.3++	0.20	36
G-D	1486	7.4	3.4++	0.10	

SOUTH-EAST					
G01	1245	5.7	2.4++	0.08	82
G22	58	3.9	2.1+	0.29	88
G23	90	4.4	2.3++	0.26	85
G24	78	5.0	2.6++	0.32	64
G34	234	10.9	3.0++	0.25	44
G35	255	5.8	2.6++	0.18	64
G37	277	6.4	3.1++	0.20	40
G39	151	5.2	2.8++	0.24	53
G41	28	7.7	2.6+	0.53	64
G42	269	6.0	2.7++	0.18	58
G51	81	5.2	2.7++	0.32	58
G56	173	5.6	2.4++	0.20	82
G58	177	8.8	2.9++	0.26	47
G-E	3116	6.0	2.6++	0.05	
SOUTH-WEST					
G21	170	5.9	2.5++	0.21	74
G28	129	10.0	3.5++	0.33	31
G31	244	8.4	2.8++	0.20	53
G32	134	7.2	2.5++	0.25	74
G36	105	6.9	3.1++	0.33	40
G53	77	6.1	2.5++	0.32	74
G59	62	4.0	2.0+	0.28	91
G-F	921	7.0	2.7++	0.10	
WEST MIDLANDS					
G15	464	5.6	2.9++	0.14	47
G38	113	6.1	2.9++	0.29	47
G52	67	6.0	2.9++	0.38	47
G54	170	5.6	3.2++	0.26	38
G57	69	4.9	2.7++	0.35	58
G-G	883	5.6	2.9++	0.11	
YORKSHIRE AND HUMBERSIDE					
G13	161	4.0	2.0++	0.17	91
G16	378	5.9	2.6++	0.15	64
G40	151	5.8	2.8++	0.25	53
G49	125	6.2	2.4++	0.24	82
G-H	815	5.4	2.4++	0.09	
WALES					
G61	102	8.6	3.6++	0.42	25
G62	84	8.3	3.4++	0.41	35
G63	81	6.0	3.0++	0.36	44
G64	74	10.5	3.6++	0.48	25
G65	123	7.4	3.9++	0.38	19
G66	24	7.6	2.5+	0.55	74
G67	101	8.4	3.9++	0.43	19
G68	90	7.9	3.6++	0.41	25
G-I	679	7.9	3.6++	0.15	
SCOTLAND(1975-80)					
S01	41	7.2	3.1++	0.52	40
S02	109	7.6	3.2++	0.33	38
S03	124	9.9	4.1++	0.41	15
S04	62	6.0	2.9++	0.40	47
S05	205	8.7	4.0++	0.31	17
S06	35	11.2	3.5++	0.67	31
S07	59	7.2	3.8++	0.52	22
S08	579	7.5	3.9++	0.17	19
S09	44	10.0	4.3++	0.71	11
S10	6	11.0	4.3	2.09	11
S11	3	4.9	1.3	0.73	121
S12	13	14.4	6.0+	1.99	3
G-J	1280	7.9	3.8++	0.11	
NORTHERN IRELAND					
JE	85	5.1	2.8++	0.32	53
JN	40	4.3	2.5++	0.42	74
JS	16	2.4	1.4	0.36	113
JW	28	4.6	2.6+	0.53	64
G-K	169	4.3	2.5++	0.20	
G.0	10870	6.3	2.9++	0.03	
ITALIA (1975-79)					
ABRUZZI					
I66	8	1.0	0.4--	0.16	333
I67	1	0.1	0.1--	0.07	352
I68	5	0.7	0.3--	0.16	345
I69	11	1.2	0.6--	0.19	291
I-A	25	0.8	0.4--	0.08	
BASILICATA					
I76	9	0.9	0.6--	0.21	291
I77	2	0.4	0.3--	0.21	345
I-B	11	0.7	0.5--	0.16	
CALABRIA					
I78	9	0.5	0.3--	0.11	345
I79	12	0.7	0.4--	0.13	333
I80	11	0.7	0.4--	0.14	333
I-C	32	0.6	0.4--	0.07	

CAMPANIA					
I61	7	0.4	0.3--	0.10	345
I62	5	0.7	0.4--	0.18	333
I63	47	0.6	0.5--	0.07	317
I64	9	0.8	0.6--	0.20	291
I65	17	0.7	0.4--	0.11	333
I-D	85	0.6	0.4--	0.05	
EMILIA-ROMAGNA					
I33	14	1.9	0.8-	0.25	227
I34	21	2.0	0.8--	0.20	227
I35	18	1.7	0.7--	0.17	263
I36	20	1.4	0.6--	0.16	291
I37	44	1.8	0.8--	0.13	227
I38	13	1.3	0.6--	0.16	291
I39	20	2.2	1.0	0.25	179
I40	28	1.9	1.0	0.20	179
I-E	178	1.8	0.8--	0.06	
FRIULI-VENEZIA GIULIA					
I30	46	3.4	1.6	0.25	102
I31	15	3.9	2.1	0.56	88
I32	27	3.4	1.2	0.25	138
I93	19	2.8	1.5	0.38	106
I-F	107	3.3	1.5	0.16	
LAZIO					
I56	14	2.1	1.1	0.32	156
I57	10	2.8	1.1	0.37	156
I58	97	1.0	0.7--	0.07	263
I59	6	0.6	0.5--	0.20	317
I60	6	0.5	0.3--	0.12	345
I-G	133	1.1	0.7--	0.06	
LIGURIA					
I08	17	2.8	1.3	0.37	121
I09	12	1.5	0.8-	0.25	227
I10	70	2.5	1.0--	0.13	179
I11	10	1.6	0.6--	0.21	291
I-H	109	2.2	1.0--	0.10	
LOMBARDIA					
I12	50	2.5	1.3	0.19	121
I13	43	2.2	1.2	0.20	138
I14	10	2.3	1.1	0.36	156
I15	261	2.5	1.6	0.10	102
I16	36	1.6	1.1	0.19	156
I17	43	1.7	0.9--	0.15	205
I18	25	1.8	0.7--	0.14	263
I19	34	4.0	1.7	0.32	99
I20	22	2.2	0.8--	0.19	227
I-I	524	2.3	1.3	0.06	
MARCHE					
I41	15	1.8	0.7--	0.20	263
I42	17	1.5	0.8--	0.20	227
I43	11	1.5	0.7--	0.21	263
I44	15	1.7	0.8--	0.21	227
I-J	58	1.6	0.7--	0.10	
MOLISE					
I70	5	0.8	0.5--	0.24	317
I94	3	1.2	0.7	0.45	263
I-K	8	1.0	0.6--	0.21	
PIEMONTE					
I01	106	1.7	1.0--	0.10	179
I02	11	1.0	0.4--	0.13	333
I03	27	2.1	1.0	0.21	179
I04	24	1.7	0.8--	0.18	227
I05	16	2.8	1.0	0.29	179
I06	25	2.0	0.6--	0.14	291
I-L	209	1.8	0.8--	0.06	
PUGLIA					
I71	10	0.6	0.4--	0.13	333
I72	32	0.9	0.6--	0.11	291
I73	5	0.4	0.3--	0.12	345
I74	4	0.4	0.3--	0.17	345
I75	13	0.7	0.4--	0.13	333
I-M	64	0.7	0.5--	0.06	
SARDEGNA					
I90	2	0.2	0.1--	0.06	352
I91	10	1.4	1.0	0.33	179
I92	9	0.5	0.4--	0.13	333
I95	1	0.3	0.1--	0.13	352
I-N	22	0.6	0.4--	0.08	
SICILIA					
I81	14	1.3	0.8--	0.23	227
I82	36	1.2	0.8--	0.14	227
I83	17	1.0	0.5--	0.14	317
I84	11	0.9	0.6--	0.18	291
I85	7	1.0	0.8	0.32	227
I86	4	0.8	0.5--	0.25	317
I87	20	0.8	0.5--	0.12	317
I88	7	1.0	0.8	0.31	227
I89	8	0.8	0.6--	0.22	291
I-O	124	1.0	0.7--	0.06	

TOSCANA					
I45	10	1.9	0.7--	0.24	263
I46	23	2.3	0.9-	0.21	205
I47	15	2.2	0.8--	0.22	227
I48	69	2.2	1.0--	0.12	179
I49	13	1.5	0.7--	0.20	263
I50	18	1.8	0.8--	0.20	227
I51	17	2.2	1.0	0.25	179
I52	13	2.0	0.8--	0.23	227
I53	16	2.8	1.4	0.37	113
I-P	194	2.1	0.9--	0.07	
TRENTINO-ALTO ADIGE					
I21	23	2.1	1.4	0.30	113
I22	30	2.7	1.4	0.27	113
I-Q	53	2.4	1.4	0.20	
UMBRIA					
I54	23	1.6	0.8--	0.17	227
I55	4	0.7	0.4--	0.19	333
I-R	27	1.3	0.7--	0.13	
VALLE D'AOSTA					
I07	5	1.8	1.1	0.52	156
VENETO					
I23	46	2.4	1.3	0.20	121
I24	26	1.4	0.9-	0.20	205
I25	19	3.3	1.3	0.32	121
I26	39	2.2	1.3	0.23	121
I27	72	3.4	1.8+	0.23	96
I28	65	3.2	1.8	0.24	96
I29	20	3.1	1.5	0.37	106
I-T	287	2.6	1.5	0.09	
I.0	2255	1.6	0.9--	0.02	
IRELAND (1976-80)					
CONNAUGHT					
R07	14	3.4	2.0	0.55	91
R12	3	4.6	2.1	1.27	88
R16	17	6.1	2.2	0.56	87
R20	4	3.1	1.5	0.79	106
R21	7	5.2	2.7	1.09	58
R-A	45	4.4	2.1+	0.33	
LEINSTER					
R01	9	9.5	6.6+	2.39	2
R06	112	4.4	3.5++	0.34	31
R09	13	5.6	5.4++	1.53	6
R10	14	8.4	5.7++	1.67	5
R11	7	5.9	3.6	1.46	25
R14	3	4.1	2.5	1.46	74
R15	13	6.0	4.6+	1.36	10
R17	17	7.7	7.3++	1.83	1
R19	8	5.8	4.0	1.55	17
R24	9	6.1	5.2+	1.83	7
R25	20	8.4	4.3++	1.02	11
R26	9	4.3	3.7	1.32	23
R-B	234	5.3	4.1++	0.28	
MUNSTER					
R03	11	5.4	3.6	1.15	25
R04	71	7.2	4.8++	0.62	9
R08	14	4.8	3.1	0.89	40
R13	23	5.9	4.1++	0.91	15
R22	26	8.0	5.1++	1.07	8
R23	17	7.8	5.9++	1.54	4
R-C	162	6.7	4.5++	0.38	
ULSTER					
R02	3	2.4	1.3	0.79	121
R05	11	3.7	2.6	0.88	64
R18	7	5.8	3.7	1.49	23
R-D	21	3.9	2.5	0.59	
R.0	462	5.5	3.8++	0.19	
LUXEMBOURG (1971-80)					
LE	1	0.5	0.1--	0.14	352
LN	7	2.6	1.6	0.67	102
LS	40	3.0	1.6	0.27	102
L.0	48	2.7	1.4	0.22	
NEDERLAND (1976-80)					
N01	33	2.4	1.2	0.22	138
N02	43	3.0	1.4	0.24	113
N03	23	2.2	1.3	0.29	121
N04	61	2.4	1.4	0.19	113
N05	78	1.9	1.1-	0.13	156
N06	49	2.2	1.2	0.19	138
N07	155	2.6	1.3	0.11	121
N08	174	2.2	1.1--	0.09	156
N09	25	2.9	1.3	0.30	121
N10	67	1.3	1.0--	0.12	179
N11	26	1.0	0.7--	0.13	263
N.0	734	2.1	1.2--	0.05	
EEC-9					
EEC	23602	2.9	1.4	0.01	

BELGIE-BELGIQUE (1971-78)

BRUSSEL-BRUXELLES					
B21	954	24.1	14.5--	0.49	268
VLAANDEREN					
B10	1888	30.6	20.8++	0.49	116
B29	1006	28.0	19.0	0.62	149
B30	1514	35.7	23.3++	0.62	80
B40	2221	42.4	25.8++	0.57	50
B70	682	24.5	24.6++	0.96	59
B-V	7311	33.2	22.7++	0.27	
WALLONIE					
B25	224	21.8	14.6--	1.00	266
B50	1340	26.1	16.8--	0.47	203
B60	913	23.2	15.0--	0.51	253
B80	214	24.8	15.4--	1.09	237
B90	332	21.9	14.6--	0.82	266
B-W	3023	24.2	15.7--	0.29	
B.0	11288	29.4	19.4	0.19	

BR DEUTSCHLAND (1976-80)

BADEN-WURTTEMBERG					
D81	2611	31.4	22.6++	0.47	85
D82	1819	32.0	22.3++	0.55	89
D83	1256	28.5	20.0	0.60	133
D84	1092	30.4	22.6++	0.72	85
D-A	6778	30.8	22.0++	0.28	
BAYERN					
D91	3199	36.8	24.8++	0.45	57
D92	1253	53.5	36.2++	1.06	14
D93	1155	50.0	36.0++	1.10	15
D94	1222	49.5	30.8++	0.93	30
D95	1668	46.4	30.0++	0.76	31
D96	1179	41.3	28.1++	0.85	35
D97	1576	43.5	27.8++	0.73	38
D-B	11252	43.5	28.9++	0.28	
BERLIN(WEST)					
DB0	1610	37.6	20.6+	0.56	122
BREMEN					
D40	598	36.4	21.9++	0.94	93
HAMBURG					
D20	1455	37.5	21.5++	0.60	101
HESSEN					
D64	3182	30.3	20.4++	0.38	125
D66	971	34.2	19.9	0.68	135
D-F	4153	31.1	20.3++	0.33	
NIEDERSACHSEN					
D31	1340	34.3	21.3++	0.62	108
D32	1711	35.2	21.6++	0.56	99
D33	1274	36.4	23.7++	0.70	65
D34	1614	31.9	23.3++	0.61	80
D-G	5939	34.3	22.4++	0.31	
NORDRHEIN-WESTFALEN					
D51	4004	32.4	23.9++	0.39	64
D53	2683	28.6	23.4++	0.47	77
D55	1703	29.4	25.5++	0.65	52
D57	1418	33.1	23.4++	0.65	77
D59	2813	31.8	24.2++	0.48	60
D-H	12621	31.0	24.0++	0.22	
RHEINLAND-PFALZ					
D71	1073	33.0	20.8+	0.67	116
D72	343	30.6	20.9	1.19	114
D73	1487	34.5	23.5++	0.64	72
D-I	2903	33.4	22.1++	0.43	
SAARLAND					
DA0	713	27.8	18.2	0.72	160
SCHLESWIG-HOLSTEIN					
D10	2303	36.9	23.7++	0.53	65
D.0	50325	34.3	23.3++	0.11	

DANMARK (1971-80)

K15	1313	21.6	13.7--	0.39	292
K20	229	15.1	13.6--	0.91	297
K25	137	14.7	13.7--	1.19	292
K30	376	27.8	16.1--	0.87	222
K35	347	26.9	13.6--	0.77	297
K40	59	24.8	13.1--	1.81	311
K42	504	22.8	13.0--	0.60	313
K50	298	24.4	15.8--	0.94	230
K55	240	23.1	15.6--	1.03	235
K60	360	22.8	14.1--	0.77	283
K65	298	23.2	15.8--	0.94	230
K70	633	22.8	15.3--	0.63	240
K76	290	25.3	14.1--	0.87	283
K80	626	26.5	16.1--	0.67	222
K.0	5710	22.8	14.4--	0.20	

FRANCE (1971-78)

ALSACE					
F67	646	18.7	14.0--	0.57	286
F68	534	21.3	16.9--	0.77	198
F-A	1180	19.8	15.2--	0.46	
AQUITAINE					
F24	439	30.1	14.3--	0.72	278
F33	809	19.8	12.2--	0.45	328
F40	405	36.2	18.9	0.99	152
F47	226	19.9	10.7--	0.75	346
F64	605	29.3	17.2--	0.73	189
F-B	2484	25.2	14.2--	0.30	
AUVERGNE					
F03	434	29.3	14.8--	0.76	259
F15	231	34.9	19.2	1.33	145
F43	326	40.6	21.1	1.26	111
F63	457	20.1	13.3--	0.65	305
F-C	1448	27.7	15.9--	0.44	
BASSE-NORMANDIE					
F14	441	20.2	16.9--	0.82	198
F50	515	29.6	21.8+	1.00	95
F61	286	25.0	17.6	1.08	176
F-D	1242	24.5	18.9	0.55	
BOURGOGNE					
F21	366	20.4	14.0--	0.76	286
F58	306	31.3	14.8--	0.91	259
F71	707	31.5	18.6	0.74	155
F89	337	28.4	13.6--	0.80	297
F-E	1716	27.7	15.7--	0.40	
BRETAGNE					
F22	646	31.7	20.1	0.82	130
F29	1328	42.6	27.3++	0.78	41
F35	750	27.7	21.8++	0.81	95
F56	701	31.9	23.4++	0.91	77
F-F	3425	34.0	23.6++	0.42	
CENTRE					
F18	340	27.1	14.5--	0.84	268
F28	352	26.2	17.0-	0.96	196
F36	301	30.8	15.3--	0.96	240
F37	354	19.1	12.2--	0.68	328
F41	297	26.8	14.7--	0.92	263
F45	444	22.8	14.8--	0.74	259
F-G	2088	24.6	14.6--	0.34	
CHAMPAGNE-ARDENNE					
F08	218	17.5	13.6--	0.96	297
F10	236	21.0	12.9--	0.90	317
F51	401	19.1	15.2--	0.79	245
F52	166	19.5	13.3--	1.08	305
F-H	1021	19.2	13.9--	0.45	
CORSE					
F20	200	20.9	12.9--	0.95	317
FRANCHE-COMTE					
F25	307	16.3	15.4--	0.90	237
F39	280	29.5	18.1	1.14	162
F70	187	21.4	13.1--	1.01	311
F90	91	17.8	15.0--	1.61	253
F-J	865	20.5	15.5--	0.54	
HAUTE-NORMANDIE					
F27	370	22.1	16.6--	0.90	209
F76	1320	28.6	22.8++	0.65	84
F-K	1690	26.9	21.1++	0.53	
ILE-DE-FRANCE					
F75	1742	20.5	12.0--	0.30	335
F77	559	18.6	14.7--	0.65	263
F78	562	13.0	13.5--	0.58	301
F91	475	12.9	13.7--	0.64	292
F92	952	16.9	13.5--	0.44	301
F93	902	17.1	16.3--	0.56	215
F94	789	16.6	14.3--	0.52	278
F95	499	14.9	14.5--	0.67	268
F-L	6480	16.8	13.6--	0.17	
LANGUEDOC-ROUSSILLON					
F11	200	19.2	8.5--	0.66	354
F30	422	21.9	12.7--	0.64	323
F34	399	16.0	9.2--	0.49	352
F48	138	45.9	22.3	2.03	89
F66	266	23.0	11.4--	0.74	336
F-M	1425	20.6	10.9--	0.31	
LIMOUSIN					
F19	400	42.5	19.6	1.05	141
F23	189	33.0	12.8--	1.05	321
F87	525	38.4	18.9	0.88	152
F-N	1114	38.7	17.7--	0.57	
LORRAINE					
F54	580	20.3	16.6--	0.71	209
F55	194	24.1	16.0--	1.21	227
F57	759	18.7	17.4--	0.65	184
F88	326	21.0	15.0--	0.87	253
F-O	1859	20.1	16.5--	0.39	
MIDI-PYRENEES					
F09	124	22.7	9.8--	0.96	350
F12	244	22.5	11.4--	0.78	336
F31	465	15.5	10.6--	0.50	347
F32	143	20.5	10.8--	0.98	345
F46	139	23.6	10.9--	0.99	342
F65	213	24.0	13.7--	0.98	292
F81	237	17.9	9.6--	0.66	351
F82	141	19.7	11.0--	0.99	341
F-P	1706	19.3	10.8--	0.28	
NORD-PAS-DE-CALAIS					
F59	1739	17.7	14.4--	0.36	275
F62	1096	20.0	16.2--	0.50	218
F-Q	2835	18.5	15.1--	0.29	
PAYS DE LA LOIRE					
F44	669	18.6	14.7--	0.58	263
F49	545	22.2	15.7--	0.70	234
F53	335	33.1	24.7++	1.39	58
F72	510	26.5	17.9	0.82	166
F85	602	34.5	22.4++	0.96	88
F-R	2661	24.8	17.9--	0.36	
PICARDIE					
F02	518	24.4	16.9--	0.78	198
F60	519	21.3	17.7-	0.81	173
F80	503	23.8	16.1--	0.76	222
F-S	1540	23.1	16.9--	0.45	
POITOU-CHARENTES					
F16	335	25.4	14.0--	0.81	286
F17	446	23.0	12.7--	0.64	323
F79	393	29.5	16.8--	0.90	203
F86	311	22.2	12.4--	0.74	327
F-T	1485	24.8	13.8--	0.38	
PROVENCE-ALPES-COTE D'AZUR					
F04	112	25.0	12.9--	1.29	317
F05	91	23.5	14.0--	1.53	286
F06	547	17.8	8.1--	0.38	355
F13	1020	16.0	11.1--	0.36	340
F83	561	22.8	13.0--	0.57	313
F84	264	17.1	10.9--	0.70	342
F-U	2595	18.1	10.7--	0.22	
RHONE-ALPES					
F01	371	24.5	16.2--	0.87	218
F07	308	30.7	16.3--	0.99	215
F26	345	24.5	15.4--	0.87	237
F38	619	18.1	14.4--	0.60	275
F42	742	25.3	17.5--	0.66	180
F69	1004	17.9	14.9--	0.48	256
F73	216	17.8	13.3--	0.93	305
F74	266	14.8	12.7--	0.80	323
F-V	3871	20.5	15.2--	0.25	
F.0	44930	21.8	15.0--	0.07	

UNITED KINGDOM (1976-80)

EAST ANGLIA					
G25	356	20.7	15.2--	0.82	245
G46	592	29.7	16.9--	0.72	198
G55	407	22.9	14.5--	0.74	268
G-A	1355	24.7	15.7--	0.44	
EAST MIDLANDS					
G30	834	31.6	20.1	0.71	130
G44	637	25.9	18.1	0.74	162
G45	394	25.0	15.9--	0.82	229
G47	394	25.8	17.9	0.93	166
G50	807	28.2	19.1	0.69	147
G-B	3066	27.7	18.5-	0.34	
NORTHERN					
G14	1120	33.1	22.0++	0.67	91
G27	534	31.9	24.9++	1.09	53
G29	419	30.5	18.9	0.95	152
G33	566	31.8	21.1+	0.90	111
G48	250	29.3	17.9	1.16	166
G-C	2889	31.9	21.4++	0.41	
NORTH-WEST					
G11	2425	31.3	21.6++	0.45	99
G12	1340	29.9	20.8+	0.58	116
G26	710	26.4	19.0	0.73	149
G43	1302	33.1	19.9	0.57	135
G-D	5777	30.6	20.7++	0.28	

SOUTH-EAST

G01	5596	28.0	17.0--	0.23	196
G22	282	19.0	14.9--	0.90	256
G23	331	16.5	12.9--	0.72	317
G24	307	19.5	15.2--	0.88	245
G34	578	32.4	14.3--	0.64	278
G35	1111	26.5	17.7--	0.54	173
G37	987	22.4	16.5--	0.54	212
G39	636	23.0	16.8--	0.68	203
G41	119	36.9	16.9	1.66	198
G42	1102	26.1	16.4--	0.51	213
G51	328	19.6	16.3--	0.95	215
G56	599	20.6	13.3--	0.56	305
G58	465	26.2	13.0--	0.63	313
G-E	12441	25.3	16.2--	0.15	

SOUTH-WEST

G21	728	27.3	17.5--	0.67	180
G28	382	32.0	17.3-	0.93	185
G31	854	31.0	16.2--	0.59	218
G32	474	28.6	13.5--	0.66	301
G36	334	23.1	15.1--	0.85	249
G53	373	31.0	17.1-	0.91	191
G59	368	23.7	17.3-	0.93	185
G-F	3513	28.2	16.2--	0.28	

WEST MIDLANDS

G15	2300	28.5	20.1	0.43	130
G38	374	20.9	14.2--	0.75	282
G52	266	24.8	17.1-	1.08	191
G54	927	31.5	23.6++	0.80	69
G57	317	22.9	16.7--	0.96	207
G-G	4184	27.4	19.5	0.31	

YORKSHIRE AND HUMBERSIDE

G13	1228	32.0	20.8+	0.60	116
G16	1731	28.7	19.2	0.47	145
G40	721	29.2	19.6	0.74	141
G49	448	23.1	14.0--	0.69	286
G-H	4128	28.9	18.9	0.30	

WALES

G61	377	34.1	21.2	1.13	109
G62	333	35.5	20.7	1.17	120
G63	395	30.7	20.5	1.05	123
G64	296	45.2	26.0++	1.58	47
G65	534	33.9	23.7++	1.04	65
G66	106	33.4	17.9	1.81	166
G67	364	32.5	21.4	1.14	106
G68	354	33.5	20.9	1.15	114
G-I	2759	34.2	21.7++	0.42	

SCOTLAND(1975-80)

S01	132	23.7	17.5	1.56	180
S02	294	22.0	14.5--	0.87	268
S03	377	32.6	21.9+	1.16	93
S04	234	23.5	16.4--	1.09	213
S05	537	25.0	17.9	0.79	166
S06	61	21.2	12.1--	1.63	333
S07	182	22.7	16.8-	1.28	203
S08	1910	27.0	20.3+	0.48	128
S09	110	26.3	17.1	1.69	191
S10	16	30.1	19.0	4.95	149
S11	8	12.8	9.0--	3.25	353
S12	26	29.6	16.1	3.36	222
G-J	3887	25.9	18.6-	0.31	

NORTHERN IRELAND

JE	395	24.1	20.2	1.06	129
JN	189	20.9	17.6	1.33	176
JS	115	17.3	14.5--	1.41	268
JW	183	30.4	26.2++	2.03	46
G-K	882	23.1	19.5	0.69	
G.0	44881	27.6	18.2--	0.09	

ITALIA (1975-79)

ABRUZZI

I66	266	36.3	21.5	1.36	101
I67	164	24.8	17.3	1.38	185
I68	152	21.9	15.1--	1.26	249
I69	207	23.1	15.3--	1.08	240
I-A	789	26.4	17.4--	0.63	

BASILICATA

I76	220	21.4	15.1--	1.06	249
I77	97	19.2	15.6-	1.61	235
I-B	317	20.7	15.3--	0.88	

CALABRIA

I78	317	17.9	14.3--	0.82	278
I79	371	20.3	17.1-	0.91	191
I80	281	19.2	13.3--	0.82	305
I-C	969	19.1	14.9--	0.49	

CAMPANIA

I61	298	16.7	15.3--	0.90	240
I62	165	22.9	15.1--	1.21	249
I63	935	13.4	14.1--	0.46	283
I64	230	21.2	14.8--	1.01	259
I65	301	12.2	9.9--	0.58	349
I-D	1929	14.8	13.5--	0.31	

EMILIA-ROMAGNA

I33	511	73.4	39.4++	1.79	12
I34	697	71.7	38.1++	1.48	13
I35	685	69.0	42.3++	1.67	7
I36	700	49.3	33.0++	1.28	24
I37	1102	48.8	29.5++	0.91	32
I38	401	42.8	25.7++	1.31	51
I39	614	69.8	40.5++	1.67	10
I40	1097	75.9	52.3++	1.60	2
I-E	5807	60.5	36.7++	0.49	

FRIULI-VENEZIA GIULIA

I30	707	55.0	34.6++	1.33	19
I31	146	41.5	27.7++	2.39	39
I32	265	38.0	19.1	1.22	147
I93	226	34.6	23.5++	1.60	72
I-F	1344	45.0	27.4++	0.77	

LAZIO

I56	356	54.3	34.0++	1.85	22
I57	161	45.2	24.9++	2.05	53
I58	2194	24.7	22.0++	0.48	91
I59	206	19.8	18.6	1.31	155
I60	320	28.6	19.7	1.13	138
I-G	3237	26.8	22.3++	0.40	

LIGURIA

I08	197	35.5	17.9	1.34	166
I09	306	41.4	21.5	1.27	101
I10	946	36.7	20.0	0.67	133
I11	256	43.2	23.6++	1.52	69
I-H	1705	38.2	20.5+	0.51	

LOMBARDIA

I12	775	41.4	35.7++	1.35	17
I13	796	43.4	35.6++	1.31	18
I14	178	41.4	32.6++	2.48	26
I15	3726	38.2	33.0++	0.56	24
I16	962	44.9	42.2++	1.39	8
I17	1177	48.1	42.4++	1.25	6
I18	820	64.6	34.4++	1.25	21
I19	717	88.4	57.7++	2.22	1
I20	630	68.0	39.9++	1.63	11
I-I	9781	45.5	36.8++	0.38	

MARCHE

I41	554	68.4	43.4++	1.89	4
I42	403	39.1	24.9++	1.26	53
I43	391	55.2	33.4++	1.72	23
I44	331	38.7	26.9++	1.50	43
I-J	1679	49.3	31.7++	0.79	

MOLISE

I70	160	27.7	17.2	1.41	189
I94	77	33.3	19.5	2.28	143
I-K	237	29.3	17.9	1.20	

PIEMONTE

I01	1717	29.5	23.5++	0.58	72
I02	382	39.4	21.8+	1.17	95
I03	509	41.5	26.0++	1.19	47
I04	710	52.4	28.5++	1.12	33
I05	266	49.5	23.1+	1.53	83
I06	628	54.1	24.9++	1.06	53
I-L	4212	38.0	24.4++	0.39	

PUGLIA

I71	282	16.8	12.8--	0.79	321
I72	456	13.0	10.9--	0.52	342
I73	168	12.3	11.4--	0.89	336
I74	137	14.4	12.2--	1.06	328
I75	224	12.3	10.0--	0.68	348
I-M	1267	13.6	11.3--	0.32	

SARDEGNA

I90	220	21.0	15.3--	1.07	240
I91	149	21.9	13.7--	1.21	292
I92	273	15.5	13.9--	0.85	291
I95	75	19.3	12.1--	1.49	333
I-N	717	18.5	13.9--	0.54	

SICILIA

I81	206	20.0	13.0--	0.94	313
I82	456	15.9	12.2--	0.59	328
I83	397	24.2	16.0--	0.83	227
I84	193	16.2	11.2--	0.84	339
I85	140	19.4	14.5--	1.27	268
I86	120	23.8	15.8-	1.50	230
I87	551	22.7	17.1--	0.74	191
I88	174	26.4	17.6	1.37	176
I89	197	20.4	15.8--	1.15	230
I-O	2434	20.3	14.5--	0.30	

TOSCANA

I45	280	56.3	34.6++	2.12	19
I46	343	36.8	21.1	1.17	111
I47	367	57.5	32.4++	1.74	27
I48	2019	70.1	41.1++	0.94	9
I49	364	43.3	26.0++	1.39	47
I50	457	48.8	26.6++	1.29	45
I51	677	87.9	50.2++	1.98	3
I52	549	86.7	42.8++	1.89	5
I53	361	65.5	36.0++	1.93	15
I-P	5417	62.4	35.6++	0.50	

TRENTINO-ALTO ADIGE

I21	390	37.0	31.4++	1.62	29
I22	428	39.9	27.2++	1.35	42
I-Q	818	38.4	29.1++	1.04	

UMBRIA

I54	643	45.8	28.0++	1.13	36
I55	201	35.9	21.2	1.53	109
I-R	844	43.0	26.0++	0.91	

VALLE D'AOSTA

I07	97	34.0	24.2	2.50	60

VENETO

I23	562	30.2	22.5++	0.97	87
I24	365	21.0	17.5-	0.93	180
I25	235	43.5	28.3++	1.88	34
I26	518	30.2	23.5++	1.06	72
I27	518	25.3	20.4	0.91	125
I28	643	32.9	26.8++	1.07	44
I29	170	27.4	18.1	1.42	162
I-T	3011	28.8	22.3++	0.41	
I.0	46611	34.0	24.5++	0.12	

IRELAND (1976-80)

CONNAUGHT

R07	92	21.3	14.4--	1.60	275
R12	37	49.7	24.2	4.25	60
R16	96	32.8	18.3	2.01	159
R20	41	28.8	15.2	2.53	245
R21	43	30.9	17.6	2.81	176
R-A	309	28.6	16.8-	1.02	

LEINSTER

R01	26	26.3	21.4	4.26	106
R06	392	16.6	18.2	0.93	160
R09	51	20.1	23.7	3.38	65
R10	56	31.4	24.2	3.33	60
R11	40	30.5	23.5	3.86	72
R14	31	38.6	27.4	5.06	40
R15	71	33.0	31.7++	3.83	28
R17	32	13.7	13.3-	2.39	305
R19	24	16.1	12.5-	2.65	326
R24	30	19.6	14.9	2.81	256
R25	52	21.2	16.1	2.33	222
R26	40	19.1	17.8	2.90	172
R-B	845	19.6	19.1	0.67	

MUNSTER

R03	53	24.1	16.2	2.35	218
R04	217	21.8	17.7	1.24	173
R08	59	19.0	12.2--	1.68	328
R13	62	15.6	13.5--	1.75	301
R22	102	29.6	21.5	2.21	101
R23	51	23.2	18.6	2.69	155
R-C	544	21.9	16.6--	0.74	

ULSTER

R02	59	41.7	28.0+	3.82	36
R05	110	35.1	20.4	2.05	125
R18	33	25.1	18.5	3.31	158
R-D	202	34.5	22.0	1.63	
R.0	1900	22.4	18.3-	0.43	

LUXEMBOURG (1971-80)

LE	65	35.8	21.8	2.80	95
LN	96	36.3	20.7	2.21	120
LS	312	24.4	18.0	1.04	165
L.0	473	27.5	18.9	0.89	

NEDERLAND (1976-80)

N01	487	35.7	23.2++	1.09	82
N02	483	33.8	21.5+	1.03	101
N03	283	27.3	19.7	1.21	138
N04	622	24.8	19.3	0.80	144
N05	921	22.2	17.3--	0.59	185
N06	438	20.2	16.6--	0.81	209
N07	1540	26.6	19.8	0.52	137
N08	1744	23.1	16.7--	0.41	207
N09	360	42.4	23.6++	1.32	69
N10	1081	21.4	20.5	0.63	123
N11	580	21.8	19.7	0.83	138
N.0	8539	24.7	19.1	0.21	

EEC-9

EEC	214657	28.2	19.3	0.04	

BELGIE-BELGIQUE (1971-78)					
BRUSSEL-BRUXELLES					
B21	926	20.8	7.6--	0.29	209
VLAANDEREN					
B10	1322	20.9	10.6++	0.31	98
B29	740	20.2	9.8	0.39	132
B30	1066	24.6	12.0++	0.40	63
B40	1658	30.9	14.2++	0.38	38
B70	425	15.7	12.1++	0.60	60
B-V	5211	23.3	11.8++	0.18	
WALLONIE					
B25	178	16.6	7.0--	0.58	251
B50	1195	21.9	9.0	0.29	159
B60	791	18.8	7.5--	0.30	215
B80	166	18.6	7.7-	0.66	203
B90	248	15.4	6.3--	0.44	301
B-W	2578	19.5	8.0--	0.17	
B.0	8715	21.8	9.8++	0.12	
BR DEUTSCHLAND (1976-80)					
BADEN-WURTTEMBERG					
D81	2290	25.7	11.8++	0.27	70
D82	1705	27.5	11.8++	0.32	70
D83	1135	23.5	10.2++	0.33	110
D84	1053	27.3	12.7++	0.43	51
D-A	6183	26.0	11.6++	0.16	
BAYERN					
D91	3037	32.5	13.6++	0.27	42
D92	1187	45.3	19.4++	0.61	11
D93	1128	44.6	19.8++	0.64	9
D94	1209	43.3	16.4++	0.53	19
D95	1589	39.9	15.8++	0.44	24
D96	1099	35.4	15.3++	0.51	31
D97	1559	39.2	15.4++	0.43	27
D-B	10808	38.1	15.7++	0.17	
BERLIN (WEST)					
DB0	1954	36.8	10.7++	0.31	96
BREMEN					
D40	528	28.4	10.9++	0.55	88
HAMBURG					
D20	1336	29.9	10.6++	0.35	98
HESSEN					
D64	2727	24.0	10.2++	0.22	110
D66	803	25.9	9.9	0.39	127
D-F	3530	24.4	10.2++	0.19	
NIEDERSACHSEN					
D31	1258	29.3	11.5++	0.37	76
D32	1598	29.4	11.6++	0.33	73
D33	1009	27.3	11.6++	0.40	73
D34	1358	25.0	11.4++	0.34	78
D-G	5223	27.7	11.5++	0.18	
NORDRHEIN-WESTFALEN					
D51	3572	25.9	11.9++	0.22	68
D53	2403	23.8	12.1++	0.26	60
D55	1458	23.4	12.9++	0.36	50
D57	1206	25.4	11.3++	0.36	82
D59	2530	26.2	12.3++	0.27	56
D-H	11169	25.1	12.1++	0.12	
RHEINLAND-PFALZ					
D71	913	25.7	10.8++	0.40	93
D72	290	23.4	10.1	0.65	118
D73	1352	28.6	12.3++	0.37	56
D-I	2555	26.9	11.5++	0.25	
SAARLAND					
DA0	584	20.5	8.9	0.41	163
SCHLESWIG-HOLSTEIN					
D10	2022	30.0	12.0++	0.30	63
D.0	45892	28.6	12.0++	0.06	
DANMARK (1971-80)					
K15	1170	17.6	7.3--	0.24	232
K20	157	10.4	7.2--	0.60	236
K25	87	9.6	6.9--	0.77	261
K30	233	17.4	8.6	0.62	175
K35	205	16.1	6.5--	0.50	288
K40	26	11.1	4.5--	0.93	349
K42	350	15.6	7.1--	0.41	241
K50	222	18.2	9.1	0.66	156
K55	155	15.2	8.9	0.76	163
K60	241	15.1	7.5--	0.52	215
K65	149	11.9	7.0--	0.61	251
K70	406	14.4	7.3--	0.39	232
K76	182	16.3	7.7--	0.62	203
K80	393	16.8	8.4-	0.46	180
K.0	3976	15.6	7.5--	0.13	
FRANCE (1971-78)					
ALSACE					
F67	495	13.7	6.8--	0.34	267
F68	412	15.9	7.5--	0.42	215
F-A	907	14.6	7.1--	0.26	
AQUITAINE					
F24	342	22.3	7.0--	0.45	251
F33	661	15.0	5.6--	0.25	329
F40	321	27.4	9.4	0.63	145
F47	157	13.1	4.4--	0.41	350
F64	450	20.4	7.5--	0.41	215
F-B	1931	18.4	6.5--	0.17	
AUVERGNE					
F03	315	20.1	6.3--	0.42	301
F15	161	23.9	8.6	0.81	175
F43	290	34.5	12.0++	0.87	63
F63	365	15.4	6.4--	0.38	296
F-C	1131	20.8	7.6--	0.27	
BASSE-NORMANDIE					
F14	405	17.6	9.0	0.50	159
F50	490	26.3	11.9++	0.61	68
F61	203	16.8	7.4--	0.60	228
F-D	1098	20.4	9.7	0.33	
BOURGOGNE					
F21	269	14.6	6.7--	0.47	274
F58	228	22.6	7.2--	0.57	236
F71	476	20.5	7.1--	0.38	241
F89	215	17.6	6.0--	0.48	315
F-E	1188	18.6	6.8--	0.23	
BRETAGNE					
F22	660	30.6	11.4++	0.50	78
F29	978	29.4	12.2++	0.44	58
F35	661	22.7	10.8++	0.47	93
F56	544	23.6	10.8++	0.51	93
F-F	2843	26.6	11.4++	0.24	
CENTRE					
F18	278	21.6	6.5--	0.44	288
F28	225	16.8	7.6--	0.58	209
F36	199	19.9	7.2--	0.61	236
F37	268	13.6	5.6--	0.40	329
F41	199	17.3	5.9--	0.51	317
F45	344	17.4	6.7--	0.42	274
F-G	1513	17.3	6.5--	0.20	
CHAMPAGNE-ARDENNE					
F08	175	14.1	6.6--	0.57	282
F10	180	15.6	5.9--	0.51	317
F51	308	14.5	6.6--	0.42	282
F52	135	15.8	6.7--	0.67	274
F-H	798	14.8	6.4--	0.26	
CORSE					
F20	163	18.9	6.5--	0.58	288
FRANCHE-COMTE					
F25	215	11.3	6.6--	0.49	282
F39	199	20.4	7.6--	0.62	209
F70	125	14.0	5.3--	0.57	337
F90	69	13.5	6.2--	0.83	306
F-J	608	14.2	6.5--	0.30	
HAUTE-NORMANDIE					
F27	271	15.8	7.9-	0.55	193
F76	1015	21.2	10.6++	0.37	98
F-K	1286	19.8	9.8	0.31	
ILE-DE-FRANCE					
F75	1565	15.8	5.4--	0.16	334
F77	399	13.1	6.4--	0.36	296
F78	447	10.3	6.2--	0.32	306
F91	358	9.6	6.2--	0.37	306
F92	725	12.3	5.7--	0.23	327
F93	643	12.2	7.1--	0.31	241
F94	626	12.6	6.6--	0.30	282
F95	420	12.4	7.5--	0.41	215
F-L	5183	12.8	6.1--	0.09	
LANGUEDOC-ROUSSILLON					
F11	154	13.8	4.1--	0.39	354
F30	295	14.5	5.3--	0.35	337
F34	323	12.0	4.2--	0.28	352
F48	110	36.5	11.5	1.29	76
F66	193	15.4	5.6--	0.46	329
F-M	1075	14.5	5.0--	0.18	
LIMOUSIN					
F19	339	34.3	10.0	0.63	121
F23	146	24.1	5.8--	0.58	322
F87	389	26.7	8.2-	0.49	184
F-N	874	28.7	8.2--	0.33	
LORRAINE					
F54	405	13.9	7.2--	0.39	236
F55	147	17.8	7.5-	0.74	215
F57	501	12.6	7.6--	0.37	209
F88	302	18.6	7.8--	0.51	196
F-O	1355	14.5	7.5--	0.22	
MIDI-PYRENEES					
F09	93	16.6	4.8--	0.60	347
F12	165	14.5	4.9--	0.46	345
F31	318	10.0	4.6--	0.29	348
F32	112	15.9	5.5--	0.60	332
F46	108	17.7	5.4--	0.63	334
F65	174	18.6	6.8--	0.59	267
F81	174	12.6	5.0--	0.46	343
F82	90	12.0	4.2--	0.53	352
F-P	1234	13.3	5.0--	0.17	
NORD-PAS-DE-CALAIS					
F59	1361	13.3	6.6--	0.20	282
F62	821	14.3	7.0--	0.27	251
F-Q	2182	13.7	6.7--	0.16	
PAYS DE LA LOIRE					
F44	542	14.1	6.5--	0.32	288
F49	428	16.4	7.4--	0.41	228
F53	255	23.6	10.5	0.76	101
F72	328	16.3	7.1--	0.45	241
F85	424	23.0	9.1	0.51	156
F-R	1977	17.3	7.7--	0.20	
PICARDIE					
F02	358	16.7	7.0--	0.43	251
F60	303	12.5	6.1--	0.40	310
F80	379	17.2	7.1--	0.42	241
F-S	1040	15.4	6.8--	0.24	
POITOU-CHARENTES					
F16	258	18.7	6.5--	0.47	288
F17	295	14.5	5.2--	0.36	341
F79	251	18.5	7.0--	0.51	251
F86	236	16.3	6.1--	0.46	310
F-T	1040	16.7	6.1--	0.22	
PROVENCE-ALPES-COTE D'AZUR					
F04	77	17.3	5.4--	0.70	334
F05	72	18.4	7.5	1.02	215
F06	439	12.7	3.8--	0.22	355
F13	753	11.3	5.0--	0.20	343
F83	433	17.0	6.1--	0.33	310
F84	205	12.9	5.3--	0.41	337
F-U	1979	13.1	4.9--	0.13	
RHONE-ALPES					
F01	297	19.7	8.1-	0.53	188
F07	267	25.5	8.4	0.60	180
F26	270	18.4	7.1--	0.49	241
F38	503	14.5	7.1--	0.35	241
F42	684	22.2	9.0	0.39	159
F69	893	15.3	7.3--	0.27	232
F73	179	14.5	6.5--	0.54	288
F74	208	11.5	6.6--	0.50	282
F-V	3301	17.0	7.6--	0.15	
F.0	34706	16.2	6.9--	0.04	
UNITED KINGDOM (1976-80)					
EAST ANGLIA					
G25	220	13.0	6.0--	0.44	315
G46	370	17.8	7.0--	0.40	251
G55	291	16.4	7.0--	0.46	251
G-A	881	15.9	6.7--	0.25	
EAST MIDLANDS					
G30	570	20.8	9.4	0.43	145
G44	465	18.3	8.9	0.45	163
G45	250	15.5	6.8--	0.47	267
G47	217	13.8	6.7--	0.50	274
G50	483	16.2	7.5--	0.37	215
G-B	1985	17.3	8.1--	0.20	
NORTHERN					
G14	913	25.2	10.9++	0.39	88
G27	367	21.1	11.8++	0.66	70
G29	304	20.8	8.7	0.56	171
G33	424	22.8	10.5+	0.55	101
G48	169	19.0	8.3	0.69	182
G-C	2177	22.8	10.3++	0.24	
NORTH-WEST					
G11	1899	23.0	10.1++	0.25	118
G12	1090	22.5	9.8	0.33	132
G26	521	18.5	8.9	0.42	163
G43	1004	23.5	8.9	0.32	163
G-D	4514	22.4	9.6	0.16	

SOUTH-EAST

G01	4071	18.7	7.6--	0.13	209
G22	191	13.0	7.4--	0.56	228
G23	255	12.6	6.4--	0.43	296
G24	207	13.3	7.1--	0.52	241
G34	503	23.5	6.2--	0.35	306
G35	708	16.1	7.1--	0.29	241
G37	617	14.3	6.3--	0.28	301
G39	402	13.9	7.2--	0.38	236
G41	71	19.6	5.7--	0.85	327
G42	741	16.6	6.9--	0.28	261
G51	212	13.5	6.8--	0.51	267
G56	417	13.6	5.8--	0.31	322
G58	350	17.4	5.5--	0.35	332
G-E	8745	16.8	7.0--	0.08	

SOUTH-WEST

G21	587	20.5	8.0--	0.36	190
G28	275	21.3	7.8--	0.53	196
G31	573	19.6	6.7--	0.33	274
G32	361	19.5	5.8--	0.36	322
G36	210	13.8	5.8--	0.45	322
G53	242	19.1	7.5--	0.54	215
G59	204	13.2	6.5--	0.49	288
G-F	2452	18.5	6.9--	0.16	

WEST MIDLANDS

G15	1670	20.2	9.7	0.25	138
G38	284	15.4	7.0--	0.45	251
G52	173	15.6	6.9--	0.59	261
G54	544	17.9	9.2	0.42	151
G57	235	16.5	8.5	0.59	179
G-G	2906	18.5	9.0	0.18	

YORKSHIRE AND HUMBERSIDE

G13	805	20.1	9.2	0.35	151
G16	1375	21.5	9.2	0.28	151
G40	475	18.1	8.2--	0.41	184
G49	351	17.5	6.7--	0.40	274
G-H	3006	20.0	8.7--	0.17	

WALES

G61	301	25.4	10.2	0.66	110
G62	242	23.9	9.8	0.72	132
G63	269	20.0	9.2	0.61	151
G64	241	34.2	12.0++	0.89	63
G65	362	21.8	10.2	0.58	110
G66	72	22.7	9.2	1.22	151
G67	253	21.0	8.3	0.58	182
G68	253	22.1	10.0	0.68	121
G-I	1993	23.3	9.9+	0.24	

SCOTLAND(1975-80)

S01	93	16.3	7.8	0.88	196
S02	229	16.0	7.1--	0.53	241
S03	295	23.5	10.2	0.67	110
S04	188	18.1	9.1	0.72	156
S05	465	19.7	9.0	0.46	159
S06	61	19.5	7.7	1.18	203
S07	149	18.1	9.7	0.83	138
S08	1557	20.3	9.9+	0.27	127
S09	83	18.9	7.9	0.96	193
S10	7	12.8	4.4--	1.80	350
S11	9	14.7	7.9	3.03	193
S12	18	19.9	6.7	1.92	274
G-J	3154	19.6	9.2	0.18	

NORTHERN IRELAND

JE	338	20.2	11.2++	0.64	85
JN	120	13.0	7.3--	0.72	232
JS	60	8.8	5.2--	0.73	341
JW	159	25.9	15.4++	1.30	27
G-K	677	17.4	9.9	0.41	
G.0	32490	19.0	8.3--	0.05	

ITALIA (1975-79)

ABRUZZI

I66	194	25.2	11.6++	0.89	73
I67	114	17.0	9.4	0.93	145
I68	135	18.7	10.5	0.96	101
I69	139	15.0	7.5--	0.68	215
I-A	582	18.8	9.6	0.43	

BASILICATA

I76	169	16.2	9.7	0.79	138
I77	53	10.5	7.4	1.05	228
I-B	222	14.4	9.0	0.64	

CALABRIA

I78	227	12.6	7.8--	0.55	196
I79	223	12.1	7.5--	0.54	215
I80	174	11.7	6.4--	0.53	296
I-C	624	12.1	7.2--	0.31	

CAMPANIA

I61	168	9.2	6.8--	0.54	267
I62	102	13.8	7.6-	0.80	209
I63	642	8.8	6.8--	0.28	267
I64	121	11.0	6.3--	0.60	301
I65	199	7.9	5.3--	0.39	337
I-D	1232	9.1	6.5--	0.19	

EMILIA-ROMAGNA

I33	316	43.7	17.6++	1.07	15
I34	524	51.1	19.7++	0.93	10
I35	449	43.6	19.9++	1.00	8
I36	450	30.6	14.7++	0.73	36
I37	891	36.6	16.2++	0.58	21
I38	269	27.0	12.1++	0.78	60
I39	450	48.8	21.4++	1.09	5
I40	812	54.4	28.8++	1.06	1
I-E	4161	41.2	18.6++	0.31	

FRIULI-VENEZIA GIULIA

I30	483	35.6	15.1++	0.74	34
I31	110	28.8	12.5+	1.28	53
I32	196	24.5	8.7	0.69	171
I93	195	28.3	13.2++	1.04	48
I-F	984	30.5	12.6++	0.44	

LAZIO

I56	242	36.5	18.3++	1.24	12
I57	102	28.3	12.2+	1.31	58
I58	1571	16.7	11.1++	0.29	86
I59	112	10.8	8.2	0.79	184
I60	225	19.8	10.4	0.74	106
I-G	2252	17.8	11.3++	0.25	

LIGURIA

I08	162	27.0	9.8	0.83	132
I09	184	23.3	9.3	0.74	148
I10	744	26.3	9.9	0.39	127
I11	201	31.6	11.3+	0.87	82
I-H	1291	26.6	9.9+	0.30	

LOMBARDIA

I12	571	28.6	16.4++	0.72	19
I13	554	28.3	16.0++	0.72	23
I14	108	24.7	14.0++	1.43	41
I15	2643	25.4	15.5++	0.32	25
I16	688	31.0	20.0++	0.79	7
I17	778	30.6	18.3++	0.68	12
I18	471	34.8	13.3++	0.67	47
I19	480	55.9	25.1++	1.24	3
I20	371	37.9	16.1++	0.90	22
I-I	6664	29.3	16.5++	0.21	

MARCHE

I41	315	38.0	17.6++	1.05	15
I42	303	27.5	13.0++	0.80	49
I43	275	37.1	17.3++	1.11	17
I44	255	28.6	15.2++	1.00	32
I-J	1148	32.2	15.5++	0.49	

MOLISE

I70	125	20.8	10.9	1.05	88
I94	68	28.3	12.6+	1.64	52
I-K	193	22.9	11.4+	0.89	

PIEMONTE

I01	1255	20.6	11.4++	0.34	78
I02	295	27.9	10.2	0.66	110
I03	336	25.6	11.1++	0.66	86
I04	491	35.8	14.9++	0.73	35
I05	188	33.4	11.4+	0.92	78
I06	378	30.5	10.5	0.62	101
I-L	2943	25.3	11.5++	0.23	

PUGLIA

I71	206	12.0	8.0-	0.58	190
I72	323	8.9	5.9--	0.35	317
I73	110	7.9	5.8--	0.57	322
I74	88	8.9	6.1--	0.67	310
I75	143	7.4	4.9--	0.43	345
I-M	870	9.0	6.1--	0.22	

SARDEGNA

I90	132	12.4	6.9--	0.64	261
I91	120	17.4	10.0	0.98	121
I92	196	11.0	8.1-	0.60	188
I95	45	11.6	5.9--	0.98	317
I-N	493	12.6	7.8--	0.37	

SICILIA

I81	131	12.3	6.5--	0.61	288
I82	307	10.3	6.3--	0.38	301
I83	255	14.7	7.7--	0.51	203
I84	116	9.7	6.4--	0.63	296
I85	102	13.9	9.3	0.96	148
I86	89	17.3	10.2	1.14	110
I87	400	16.0	9.8	0.51	132
I88	105	15.4	8.7	0.89	171
I89	101	10.4	6.8--	0.70	267
I-O	1606	13.0	7.7--	0.20	

TOSCANA

I45	191	36.1	15.4++	1.22	27
I46	262	26.0	10.2	0.70	110
I47	254	37.6	15.4++	1.05	27
I48	1475	47.7	20.7++	0.58	6
I49	279	31.6	13.4++	0.86	45
I50	279	28.4	12.0++	0.78	63
I51	456	57.8	25.2++	1.27	2
I52	382	58.4	22.4++	1.25	4
I53	213	37.9	17.2++	1.24	18
I-P	3791	41.3	17.5++	0.31	

TRENTINO-ALTO ADIGE

I21	259	23.8	15.5++	1.00	25
I22	286	25.5	12.4++	0.79	54
I-Q	545	24.7	13.8++	0.63	

UMBRIA

I54	435	30.2	14.2++	0.72	38
I55	122	21.1	10.0	0.95	121
I-R	557	27.6	13.0++	0.58	

VALLE D'AOSTA

I07	48	16.9	9.6	1.45	142

VENETO

I23	377	19.3	10.3	0.56	109
I24	250	13.8	8.0-	0.53	190
I25	181	31.0	13.6++	1.11	42
I26	303	16.9	8.9	0.55	163
I27	401	18.7	10.4+	0.54	106
I28	379	18.6	10.5+	0.57	101
I29	106	16.4	7.7-	0.80	203
I-T	1997	18.2	9.8+	0.23	
I.0	32203	22.4	12.0++	0.07	

IRELAND (1976-80)

CONNAUGHT

R07	51	12.5	7.8	1.20	196
R12	17	26.2	9.3	2.34	148
R16	54	19.4	9.8	1.53	132
R20	21	16.3	7.8	1.79	196
R21	44	32.8	15.2+	2.54	32
R-A	187	18.5	9.5	0.77	

LEINSTER

R01	24	25.4	17.9+	3.88	14
R06	343	13.4	9.6	0.55	142
R09	14	6.0	6.1	1.67	310
R10	34	20.3	13.6	2.44	42
R11	19	16.0	8.8	2.12	170
R14	9	12.2	5.9	2.14	317
R15	40	18.6	14.1+	2.33	40
R17	25	11.4	8.9	1.84	163
R19	13	9.4	6.9	2.03	261
R24	28	19.1	11.3	2.24	82
R25	29	12.2	8.2	1.61	184
R26	20	9.5	6.7	1.62	274
R-B	598	13.6	9.6	0.41	

MUNSTER

R03	27	13.2	8.6	1.80	175
R04	167	17.0	10.1	0.84	118
R08	39	13.4	6.9-	1.15	261
R13	59	15.1	9.7	1.35	138
R22	57	17.6	10.9	1.51	88
R23	39	18.0	12.4	2.13	54
R-C	388	16.1	9.8	0.53	

ULSTER

R02	37	29.1	14.3	2.58	37
R05	60	20.2	9.9	1.45	127
R18	21	17.4	10.9	2.65	88
R-D	118	21.7	11.2	1.16	
R.0	1291	15.4	9.8	0.29	

LUXEMBOURG (1971-80)

LE	43	22.4	10.0	1.65	121
LN	79	29.9	13.4+	1.63	45
LS	225	16.7	8.7	0.61	171
L.0	347	19.3	9.6	0.55	

NEDERLAND (1976-80)

N01	269	19.6	9.5	0.64	144
N02	304	21.2	10.7+	0.68	96
N03	153	14.9	8.6	0.75	175
N04	325	13.0	7.5--	0.44	215
N05	562	13.4	7.8--	0.35	196
N06	298	13.3	7.5--	0.47	215
N07	936	15.7	7.7--	0.27	203
N08	1084	14.0	7.0--	0.23	251
N09	197	23.1	9.9	0.77	127
N10	715	14.3	10.4++	0.40	106
N11	395	14.9	10.0	0.53	121
N.0	5238	15.0	8.3--	0.12	

EEC-9

EEC	164858	20.6	9.3	0.03	

BELGIE-BELGIQUE (1971-78)					
BRUSSEL-BRUXELLES					
B21	1367	34.6	20.6	0.58	175
VLAANDEREN					
B10	1981	32.1	21.9++	0.50	114
B29	1119	31.1	20.9	0.64	159
B30	1353	31.9	21.1	0.60	146
B40	1912	36.5	22.5++	0.53	87
B70	543	19.5	19.6	0.85	213
B-V	6908	31.4	21.5++	0.27	
WALLONIE					
B25	312	30.4	20.6	1.20	175
B50	1537	30.0	19.1-	0.50	237
B60	1062	27.0	17.5--	0.55	289
B80	231	26.8	17.1--	1.16	293
B90	413	27.2	18.4	0.93	263
B-W	3555	28.5	18.5--	0.32	
B.0	11830	30.8	20.4	0.19	
BR DEUTSCHLAND (1976-80)					
BADEN-WURTTEMBERG					
D81	2646	31.8	22.8++	0.47	81
D82	1981	34.9	24.5++	0.58	31
D83	1376	31.2	22.1++	0.63	104
D84	977	27.2	19.9	0.67	200
D-A	6980	31.7	22.7++	0.29	
BAYERN					
D91	2715	31.2	21.1+	0.42	146
D92	794	33.9	23.1++	0.85	64
D93	882	38.1	27.7++	0.97	6
D94	1043	42.3	26.3++	0.85	9
D95	1477	41.1	26.7++	0.72	8
D96	1052	36.9	25.6++	0.82	16
D97	1302	36.0	23.4++	0.68	52
D-B	9265	35.8	24.0++	0.26	
BERLIN(WEST)					
DB0	1820	42.6	22.5++	0.58	87
BREMEN					
D40	637	38.7	23.3++	0.97	56
HAMBURG					
D20	1511	39.0	21.5+	0.59	129
HESSEN					
D64	3732	35.5	23.9++	0.41	46
D66	1063	37.5	22.1++	0.72	104
D-F	4795	35.9	23.5++	0.36	
NIEDERSACHSEN					
D31	1396	35.8	22.2++	0.63	101
D32	1808	37.2	22.2++	0.56	101
D33	1190	34.0	22.0++	0.68	110
D34	1577	31.2	22.3++	0.59	95
D-G	5971	34.5	22.2++	0.30	
NORDRHEIN-WESTFALEN					
D51	4112	33.3	24.6++	0.40	29
D53	2696	28.7	23.1++	0.46	64
D55	1636	28.2	24.3++	0.63	33
D57	1386	32.3	22.9++	0.64	73
D59	2998	33.9	25.6++	0.49	16
D-H	12828	31.6	24.2++	0.22	
RHEINLAND-PFALZ					
D71	1208	37.1	23.3++	0.71	56
D72	380	33.9	22.5	1.21	87
D73	1593	37.0	25.2++	0.67	20
D-I	3181	36.6	24.1++	0.45	
SAARLAND					
DA0	906	35.4	22.9++	0.80	73
SCHLESWIG-HOLSTEIN					
D10	1925	30.9	19.6	0.48	213
D.0	49819	34.0	22.9++	0.11	
DANMARK (1971-80)					
K15	2439	40.1	25.2++	0.52	20
K20	419	27.7	25.1++	1.25	24
K25	252	27.1	25.4++	1.62	19
K30	578	42.7	24.6++	1.07	29
K35	551	42.8	22.1	0.99	104
K40	86	36.2	18.1	2.06	276
K42	867	39.1	22.3++	0.78	95
K50	370	30.2	19.8	1.06	208
K55	348	33.4	23.2+	1.28	62
K60	535	33.9	21.0	0.94	152
K65	396	30.9	21.5	1.12	129
K70	911	32.8	22.1++	0.76	104
K76	414	36.2	20.8	1.07	166
K80	779	33.0	20.5	0.76	179
K.0	8945	35.7	22.8++	0.25	

FRANCE (1971-78)					
ALSACE					
F67	1009	29.2	21.6+	0.71	124
F68	736	29.4	23.3++	0.90	56
F-A	1745	29.3	22.3++	0.56	
AQUITAINE					
F24	737	50.6	24.3++	0.95	33
F33	1437	35.2	21.6+	0.59	124
F40	458	40.9	22.3	1.11	95
F47	464	40.8	20.6	1.01	175
F64	608	29.4	16.5--	0.70	304
F-B	3704	37.6	21.0+	0.36	
AUVERGNE					
F03	575	38.8	19.9	0.89	200
F15	241	36.4	20.5	1.40	179
F43	322	40.1	21.7	1.30	122
F63	679	29.8	20.2	0.81	190
F-C	1817	34.8	20.4	0.50	
BASSE-NORMANDIE					
F14	490	22.4	18.9	0.87	247
F50	443	25.5	18.4-	0.91	263
F61	310	27.1	19.5	1.15	219
F-D	1243	24.5	18.8-	0.55	
BOURGOGNE					
F21	533	29.7	20.7	0.93	172
F58	426	43.5	20.9	1.09	159
F71	873	38.9	23.0++	0.83	69
F89	466	39.3	20.2	1.03	190
F-E	2298	37.1	21.5++	0.48	
BRETAGNE					
F22	765	37.5	24.2++	0.91	39
F29	948	30.4	19.9	0.67	200
F35	699	25.9	20.3	0.79	186
F56	691	31.4	23.0++	0.90	69
F-F	3103	30.8	21.6++	0.40	
CENTRE					
F18	498	39.7	21.5	1.03	129
F28	380	28.3	18.4	0.99	263
F36	363	37.2	18.6	1.06	258
F37	579	31.2	20.1	0.87	193
F41	397	35.8	19.9	1.07	200
F45	577	29.7	19.4	0.85	222
F-G	2794	32.9	19.7	0.39	
CHAMPAGNE-ARDENNE					
F08	337	27.1	20.1	1.14	193
F10	321	28.6	17.7-	1.05	285
F51	492	23.4	19.2	0.89	230
F52	226	26.6	18.5	1.28	260
F-H	1376	25.9	18.9-	0.53	
CORSE					
F20	117	12.2	7.5--	0.72	351
FRANCHE-COMTE					
F25	420	22.3	21.2	1.06	142
F39	292	30.7	18.5	1.14	260
F70	274	31.4	19.4	1.24	222
F90	125	24.5	20.4	1.88	183
F-J	1111	26.4	19.8	0.62	
HAUTE-NORMANDIE					
F27	398	23.8	17.4--	0.91	290
F76	972	21.1	16.7--	0.55	301
F-K	1370	21.8	16.9--	0.47	
ILE-DE-FRANCE					
F75	2986	35.1	20.2	0.38	190
F77	798	26.5	21.0	0.77	152
F78	789	18.3	18.5--	0.67	260
F91	626	17.0	18.2--	0.74	271
F92	1374	24.4	19.3	0.53	228
F93	1142	21.6	20.8	0.63	166
F94	1067	22.5	19.4	0.61	222
F95	659	19.7	19.3	0.77	228
F-L	9441	24.5	19.7-	0.21	
LANGUEDOC-ROUSSILLON					
F11	378	36.3	16.2--	0.92	306
F30	609	31.6	18.3-	0.77	267
F34	728	29.2	16.3--	0.64	305
F48	114	37.9	18.3	1.81	267
F66	421	36.4	17.0--	0.88	297
F-M	2250	32.5	17.0--	0.38	
LIMOUSIN					
F19	448	47.6	22.4+	1.13	92
F23	270	47.1	19.1	1.31	237
F87	589	43.1	21.6	0.95	124
F-N	1307	45.4	21.2	0.63	

LORRAINE					
F54	725	25.4	20.3	0.78	186
F55	278	34.6	22.0	1.40	110
F57	841	20.8	19.2	0.68	230
F88	463	29.8	20.9	1.01	159
F-O	2307	24.9	20.2	0.43	
MIDI-PYRENEES					
F09	202	36.9	14.7--	1.13	310
F12	446	41.2	20.3	1.03	186
F31	904	30.1	19.7	0.68	210
F32	292	41.9	20.9	1.33	159
F46	266	45.2	21.9	1.45	114
F65	324	36.5	21.0	1.21	152
F81	516	39.0	20.0	0.93	197
F82	286	39.9	21.5	1.35	129
F-P	3236	36.6	19.9	0.37	
NORD-PAS-DE-CALAIS					
F59	2813	28.6	23.1++	0.45	64
F62	1529	27.9	21.9++	0.58	114
F-Q	4342	28.3	22.7++	0.36	
PAYS DE LA LOIRE					
F44	794	22.0	17.9--	0.65	282
F49	602	24.5	17.3--	0.73	292
F53	305	30.1	21.8	1.29	119
F72	500	26.0	18.0--	0.83	278
F85	578	33.1	21.5	0.94	129
F-R	2779	25.9	18.9--	0.37	
PICARDIE					
F02	647	30.5	21.2	0.88	142
F60	566	23.2	19.2	0.84	230
F80	572	27.1	18.2-	0.80	271
F-S	1785	26.7	19.5	0.48	
POITOU-CHARENTES					
F16	482	36.6	21.5	1.03	129
F17	678	35.0	19.6	0.79	213
F79	472	35.4	20.9	1.02	159
F86	483	34.4	20.1	0.96	193
F-T	2115	35.3	20.4	0.47	
PROVENCE-ALPES-COTE D'AZUR					
F04	128	28.5	14.6--	1.36	311
F05	120	30.9	17.8	1.68	283
F06	689	22.4	10.0--	0.42	332
F13	1299	20.3	14.0--	0.40	315
F83	713	29.0	16.6--	0.65	303
F84	420	27.1	17.4--	0.88	290
F-U	3369	23.5	13.8--	0.25	
RHONE-ALPES					
F01	375	24.8	17.0--	0.92	297
F07	364	36.3	20.3	1.13	186
F26	423	30.0	19.0	0.97	241
F38	841	24.6	19.4	0.69	222
F42	971	33.2	22.9++	0.76	73
F69	1416	25.2	20.8	0.57	166
F73	313	25.7	18.7	1.09	256
F74	354	19.7	16.7--	0.91	301
F-V	5057	26.8	19.8	0.29	
F.0	58666	28.5	19.4--	0.08	
UNITED KINGDOM (1976-80)					
EAST ANGLIA					
G25	445	25.9	19.7	0.96	210
G46	683	34.3	19.9	0.79	200
G55	568	32.0	21.2	0.92	142
G-A	1696	30.9	20.3	0.51	
EAST MIDLANDS					
G30	851	32.3	20.9	0.74	159
G44	667	27.1	19.2	0.77	230
G45	627	39.8	25.5++	1.06	18
G47	451	29.5	21.1	1.02	146
G50	908	31.7	21.5	0.73	129
G-B	3504	31.7	21.4++	0.37	
NORTHERN					
G14	1296	38.3	25.7++	0.73	14
G27	518	31.0	24.3++	1.08	33
G29	528	38.5	23.7++	1.06	47
G33	609	34.2	23.0++	0.95	69
G48	283	33.2	20.1	1.23	193
G-C	3234	35.7	24.0++	0.43	
NORTH-WEST					
G11	2585	33.3	23.3++	0.47	56
G12	1569	35.1	24.7++	0.64	28
G26	801	29.7	22.5++	0.82	87
G43	1438	36.5	22.0++	0.60	110
G-D	6393	33.9	23.2++	0.30	

Area	Cases	Crude	ASR	SE	Rank
SOUTH-EAST					
G01	5666	28.4	17.6--	0.24	287
G22	396	26.6	21.5	1.11	129
G23	499	24.8	19.6	0.89	213
G24	398	25.3	19.7	1.00	210
G34	791	44.4	19.2	0.75	230
G35	1279	30.5	20.8	0.60	166
G37	1253	28.5	21.0	0.61	152
G39	697	25.2	18.8	0.73	254
G41	168	52.1	23.0	1.91	69
G42	1317	31.2	20.0	0.57	197
G51	472	28.2	24.5++	1.21	31
G56	799	27.5	18.2--	0.67	271
G58	663	37.4	18.9	0.78	247
G-E	14398	29.3	19.0--	0.16	
SOUTH-WEST					
G21	805	30.2	19.4	0.71	222
G28	424	35.5	19.0	0.97	241
G31	1039	37.7	19.9	0.66	200
G32	712	43.0	20.5	0.82	179
G36	460	31.8	20.7	0.99	172
G53	403	33.4	19.1	0.99	237
G59	459	29.6	21.8	1.05	119
G-F	4302	34.5	20.0	0.32	
WEST MIDLANDS					
G15	2588	32.1	22.9++	0.46	73
G38	562	31.4	21.5	0.93	129
G52	339	31.6	22.3	1.26	95
G54	880	29.9	22.3++	0.77	95
G57	420	30.3	22.8+	1.15	81
G-G	4789	31.4	22.6++	0.34	
YORKSHIRE AND HUMBERSIDE					
G13	1370	35.7	23.6++	0.65	48
G16	1855	30.8	20.6	0.49	175
G40	816	33.0	22.1+	0.79	104
G49	642	33.1	20.4	0.84	183
G-H	4683	32.8	21.6++	0.32	
WALES					
G61	439	39.7	24.8++	1.23	27
G62	368	39.2	23.6++	1.27	48
G63	431	33.5	22.6+	1.12	85
G64	259	39.5	22.9	1.50	73
G65	496	31.5	22.1	1.02	104
G66	118	37.2	20.9	2.04	159
G67	349	31.1	21.0	1.14	152
G68	427	40.4	26.3++	1.32	9
G-I	2887	35.8	23.2++	0.45	
SCOTLAND(1975-80)					
S01	227	40.8	28.7++	1.95	3
S02	472	35.3	23.4++	1.11	52
S03	438	37.9	25.0++	1.24	25
S04	279	28.0	19.9	1.22	200
S05	620	28.8	21.0	0.87	152
S06	120	41.8	22.9	2.18	73
S07	217	27.1	19.0	1.32	241
S08	2264	32.0	24.3++	0.53	33
S09	136	32.5	21.1	1.87	146
S10	7	13.2	6.2--	2.42	352
S11	15	24.0	18.3	4.91	267
S12	29	33.0	14.1-	2.71	314
G-J	4824	32.2	23.1++	0.34	
NORTHERN IRELAND					
JE	465	28.3	23.5++	1.14	51
JN	235	26.0	21.9	1.50	114
JS	114	17.2	14.4--	1.42	313
JW	184	30.6	25.9++	2.00	13
G-K	998	26.2	21.9+	0.73	
G.0	51708	31.8	21.2++	0.10	
ITALIA (1975-79)					
ABRUZZI					
I66	157	21.4	13.0--	1.07	318
I67	122	18.4	12.2--	1.13	321
I68	124	17.8	12.9--	1.20	319
I69	156	17.4	11.4--	0.94	324
I-A	559	18.7	12.3--	0.53	
BASILICATA					
I76	115	11.2	8.2--	0.79	350
I77	70	13.9	11.3--	1.38	327
I-B	185	12.1	9.1--	0.69	
CALABRIA					
I78	188	10.6	8.8--	0.66	344
I79	195	10.7	8.9--	0.65	342
I80	180	12.3	8.7--	0.67	345
I-C	563	11.1	8.8--	0.38	
CAMPANIA					
I61	167	9.3	8.7--	0.68	345
I62	100	13.9	9.2--	0.95	340
I63	879	12.6	13.2--	0.45	317
I64	128	11.8	8.4--	0.77	349
I65	256	10.4	8.5--	0.54	348
I-D	1530	11.7	10.7--	0.28	
EMILIA-ROMAGNA					
I33	274	39.3	21.3	1.33	140
I34	420	43.2	23.1+	1.16	64
I35	343	34.6	21.3	1.20	140
I36	480	33.8	22.6+	1.06	85
I37	839	37.1	22.9++	0.81	73
I38	342	36.5	22.2	1.22	101
I39	301	34.2	20.5	1.21	179
I40	442	30.6	21.0	1.02	152
I-E	3441	35.8	22.0++	0.38	
FRIULI-VENEZIA GIULIA					
I30	357	27.8	16.9--	0.91	300
I31	106	30.2	20.0	2.03	197
I32	313	44.9	23.3+	1.39	56
I93	179	27.4	18.4	1.40	263
I-F	955	32.0	19.2	0.64	
LAZIO					
I56	214	32.6	19.8	1.38	208
I57	99	27.8	14.6--	1.54	311
I58	1860	20.9	18.9--	0.45	247
I59	141	13.6	12.6--	1.07	320
I60	183	16.4	11.2--	0.85	328
I-G	2497	20.7	17.3--	0.35	
LIGURIA					
I08	193	34.8	18.3	1.39	267
I09	334	45.2	24.1++	1.36	40
I10	1056	40.9	22.3++	0.71	95
I11	241	40.7	22.0	1.46	110
I-H	1824	40.9	22.1++	0.53	
LOMBARDIA					
I12	631	33.7	30.7++	1.31	2
I13	538	29.3	24.9++	1.14	26
I14	88	20.5	16.0-	1.73	307
I15	2850	29.2	25.7++	0.50	14
I16	432	20.2	19.0	0.93	241
I17	515	21.1	18.7	0.84	256
I18	554	43.6	22.8+	1.01	81
I19	253	31.2	20.7	1.35	172
I20	265	28.6	17.7-	1.12	285
I-I	6126	28.5	23.4++	0.31	
MARCHE					
I41	233	28.7	18.0	1.20	278
I42	353	34.2	21.9	1.19	114
I43	207	29.2	17.8	1.26	283
I44	186	21.8	14.8--	1.11	309
I-J	979	28.8	18.4--	0.60	
MOLISE					
I70	91	15.8	9.4--	1.01	339
I94	39	16.8	10.7--	1.80	329
I-K	130	16.1	9.7--	0.88	
PIEMONTE					
I01	1672	28.7	23.2++	0.59	62
I02	352	36.3	19.2	1.06	230
I03	446	36.4	23.1++	1.13	64
I04	473	34.9	18.6	0.89	258
I05	253	47.1	21.2	1.44	142
I06	613	52.8	24.0++	1.02	43
I-L	3809	34.4	22.0++	0.37	
PUGLIA					
I71	287	17.1	13.3--	0.81	316
I72	474	13.5	11.4--	0.54	324
I73	140	10.2	9.6--	0.82	337
I74	109	11.5	9.8--	0.95	335
I75	222	12.2	10.2--	0.70	331
I-M	1232	13.2	11.1--	0.32	
SARDEGNA					
I90	146	13.9	9.9--	0.85	333
I91	81	11.9	8.6--	1.03	347
I92	187	10.6	9.5--	0.70	338
I95	42	10.8	6.2--	1.04	352
I-N	456	11.8	8.9--	0.43	
SICILIA					
I81	140	13.6	9.0--	0.79	341
I82	456	15.9	12.0--	0.58	322
I83	225	13.7	8.9--	0.61	342
I84	97	8.1	6.1--	0.64	354
I85	93	12.9	9.9--	1.06	333
I86	46	9.1	6.0--	0.92	355
I87	339	13.9	10.6--	0.59	330
I88	108	16.4	11.4--	1.13	324
I89	118	12.2	9.7--	0.91	336
I-O	1622	13.5	9.8--	0.25	
TOSCANA					
I45	152	30.6	18.8	1.56	254
I46	298	32.0	18.2	1.09	271
I47	251	39.3	22.4	1.46	92
I48	1029	35.7	21.1	0.68	146
I49	349	41.5	26.0++	1.43	12
I50	365	39.0	21.5	1.16	129
I51	289	37.5	21.6	1.31	124
I52	311	49.1	23.6+	1.38	48
I53	272	49.3	27.7++	1.72	6
I-P	3316	38.2	21.9++	0.39	
TRENTINO-ALTO ADIGE					
I21	219	20.8	17.6-	1.22	287
I22	294	27.4	19.2	1.15	230
I-Q	513	24.1	18.4-	0.84	
UMBRIA					
I54	418	29.8	18.2-	0.92	271
I55	179	31.9	18.9	1.43	247
I-R	597	30.4	18.4-	0.77	
VALLE D'AOSTA					
I07	90	31.6	21.7	2.31	122
VENETO					
I23	451	24.2	18.1-	0.87	276
I24	392	22.6	18.9	0.97	247
I25	149	27.6	18.0	1.52	278
I26	367	21.4	17.1--	0.92	293
I27	494	24.2	19.6	0.90	213
I28	456	23.4	18.9	0.90	247
I29	183	29.5	19.6	1.49	213
I-T	2492	23.8	18.6--	0.38	
I.0	32916	24.0	17.4--	0.10	
IRELAND (1976-80)					
CONNAUGHT					
R07	138	31.9	19.5	1.77	219
R12	41	55.1	24.1	4.13	40
R16	130	44.5	24.0	2.29	43
R20	59	41.4	24.0	3.44	43
R21	57	41.0	23.4	3.27	52
R-A	425	39.3	22.3	1.16	
LEINSTER					
R01	27	27.4	23.3	4.62	56
R06	550	23.3	26.2++	1.15	11
R09	54	21.3	25.2	3.51	20
R10	35	19.6	15.0-	2.62	308
R11	35	26.7	20.4	3.53	183
R14	16	19.9	11.9--	3.10	323
R15	71	33.0	31.1++	3.80	1
R17	44	18.8	17.1	2.63	293
R19	49	32.9	25.2	3.69	20
R24	41	26.8	21.6	3.44	124
R25	65	26.5	19.4	2.53	222
R26	48	22.9	22.4	3.30	92
R-B	1035	24.0	23.6++	0.75	
MUNSTER					
R03	58	26.4	17.1	2.39	293
R04	342	34.3	28.3++	1.58	4
R08	116	37.3	24.1	2.37	40
R13	111	28.0	23.4	2.28	52
R22	96	27.9	19.9	2.12	200
R23	56	25.5	22.8	3.13	81
R-C	779	31.3	24.1++	0.89	
ULSTER					
R02	44	31.1	19.0	3.05	241
R05	113	36.1	20.8	2.06	166
R18	47	35.8	24.3	3.71	33
R-D	204	34.8	21.1	1.56	
R.0	2443	28.9	23.2++	0.48	
LUXEMBOURG (1971-80)					
LE	83	45.7	28.2+	3.25	5
LN	111	42.0	24.3	2.44	33
LS	399	31.3	22.9+	1.18	73
L.0	593	34.4	23.6++	1.00	
NEDERLAND (1976-80)					
N01	443	32.5	21.1	1.05	146
N02	422	29.6	19.1	0.98	237
N03	331	31.9	22.5	1.27	87
N04	694	27.7	21.5	0.84	129
N05	1012	24.4	19.0	0.61	241
N06	508	23.5	19.5	0.88	219
N07	1472	25.4	18.9--	0.50	247
N08	1887	25.0	18.0--	0.43	278
N09	251	29.5	17.0--	1.14	297
N10	1164	23.0	21.8+	0.65	119
N11	603	22.7	20.8	0.86	166
N.0	8787	25.4	19.6--	0.21	
EEC-9					
EEC	225707	29.7	20.2	0.04	

BELGIE-BELGIQUE (1971-78)

BRUSSEL-BRUXELLES					
B21	1904	42.7	16.0	0.42	140
VLAANDEREN					
B10	1967	31.2	16.5++	0.40	119
B29	1215	33.2	17.9++	0.55	60
B30	1508	34.8	18.1++	0.51	52
B40	1999	37.2	18.3++	0.45	47
B70	566	21.0	16.9+	0.73	96
B-V	7255	32.4	17.6++	0.22	
WALLONIE					
B25	387	36.1	17.0+	0.95	90
B50	1924	35.3	15.3	0.39	158
B60	1424	33.8	14.5	0.43	198
B80	305	34.1	15.2	0.95	164
B90	531	33.0	13.9	0.66	221
B-W	4571	34.5	15.0	0.25	
B.0	13730	34.3	16.5++	0.15	

BR DEUTSCHLAND (1976-80)

BADEN-WURTTEMBERG					
D81	2932	32.9	15.8+	0.32	146
D82	2352	37.9	17.1++	0.39	87
D83	1495	30.9	14.6	0.42	192
D84	1017	26.4	13.0--	0.45	250
D-A	7796	32.7	15.5	0.19	
BAYERN					
D91	3104	33.2	14.7	0.29	184
D92	935	35.7	16.6+	0.59	109
D93	944	37.3	17.8++	0.63	65
D94	1183	42.3	17.7++	0.57	70
D95	1642	41.2	17.8++	0.49	65
D96	1125	36.3	17.0++	0.55	90
D97	1357	34.1	14.8	0.44	180
D-B	10290	36.3	16.2++	0.18	
BERLIN(WEST)					
DB0	3303	62.2	18.3++	0.40	47
BREMEN					
D40	955	51.4	19.9++	0.72	15
HAMBURG					
D20	2197	49.2	17.2++	0.43	81
HESSEN					
D64	4788	42.2	18.7++	0.30	39
D66	1297	41.8	16.7++	0.52	103
D-F	6085	42.1	18.2++	0.26	
NIEDERSACHSEN					
D31	1786	41.6	16.6++	0.44	109
D32	2470	45.5	18.1++	0.41	52
D33	1477	40.0	17.6++	0.51	72
D34	2089	38.5	19.0++	0.46	30
D-G	7822	41.5	17.9++	0.23	
NORDRHEIN-WESTFALEN					
D51	5735	41.6	19.6++	0.28	19
D53	3775	37.4	19.1++	0.33	26
D55	2191	35.1	19.5++	0.44	21
D57	1895	39.9	18.6++	0.47	41
D59	3741	38.7	18.8++	0.33	34
D-H	17337	38.9	19.2++	0.16	
RHEINLAND-PFALZ					
D71	1564	44.0	19.1++	0.53	26
D72	505	40.7	18.5++	0.90	43
D73	2026	42.9	19.0++	0.47	30
D-I	4095	43.0	19.0++	0.33	
SAARLAND					
DA0	1064	37.4	17.4++	0.58	76
SCHLESWIG-HOLSTEIN					
D10	2700	40.1	16.3++	0.36	127
D.0	63644	39.6	17.4++	0.08	

DANMARK (1971-80)

K15	2954	44.4	18.9++	0.38	33
K20	400	26.6	19.0++	1.00	30
K25	275	30.2	23.9++	1.50	4
K30	527	39.4	19.8++	0.93	16
K35	497	39.0	17.2+	0.85	81
K40	95	40.5	19.3	2.19	24
K42	783	35.0	16.6+	0.64	109
K50	401	32.8	17.3+	0.93	78
K55	324	31.8	19.4++	1.14	22
K60	591	37.1	19.8++	0.88	16
K65	335	26.8	17.2+	0.99	81
K70	914	32.4	17.9++	0.63	60
K76	391	34.9	17.2+	0.94	81
K80	739	31.5	16.8+	0.66	100
K.0	9226	36.2	18.3++	0.21	

FRANCE (1971-78)

ALSACE					
F67	919	25.4	13.6--	0.50	227
F68	694	26.8	13.3--	0.57	239
F-A	1613	26.0	13.5--	0.37	
AQUITAINE					
F24	656	42.9	14.7	0.69	184
F33	1595	36.2	14.9	0.44	176
F40	468	39.9	14.8	0.82	180
F47	447	37.4	14.4	0.80	202
F64	628	28.4	10.6--	0.49	310
F-B	3794	36.1	13.9--	0.27	
AUVERGNE					
F03	629	40.2	14.2	0.68	211
F15	239	35.4	12.6--	0.95	266
F43	314	37.4	13.0-	0.88	250
F63	698	29.5	13.0--	0.56	250
F-C	1880	34.5	13.4--	0.36	
BASSE-NORMANDIE					
F14	575	25.0	12.4--	0.58	275
F50	536	28.8	13.0--	0.63	250
F61	350	28.9	13.0--	0.79	250
F-D	1461	27.2	12.8--	0.38	
BOURGOGNE					
F21	482	26.1	12.5--	0.65	269
F58	431	42.6	14.3	0.85	206
F71	721	31.1	12.0--	0.52	290
F89	439	36.0	13.0--	0.75	250
F-E	2073	32.4	12.7--	0.33	
BRETAGNE					
F22	773	35.9	14.2	0.59	211
F29	963	29.0	12.3--	0.45	281
F35	862	29.5	15.2	0.58	164
F56	799	34.7	16.2	0.64	133
F-F	3397	31.8	14.2--	0.28	
CENTRE					
F18	459	35.7	13.3--	0.73	239
F28	387	28.9	13.7	0.81	224
F36	392	39.3	13.2-	0.81	245
F37	536	27.3	11.9--	0.61	292
F41	400	34.8	12.9--	0.80	259
F45	572	28.9	12.9--	0.62	259
F-G	2746	31.5	12.9--	0.29	
CHAMPAGNE-ARDENNE					
F08	360	29.0	15.0	0.90	170
F10	358	31.1	12.2--	0.75	284
F51	541	25.4	13.4--	0.66	234
F52	238	27.8	13.5	1.00	230
F-H	1497	27.8	13.5--	0.40	
CORSE					
F20	155	18.0	7.1--	0.66	344
FRANCHE-COMTE					
F25	398	21.0	12.3--	0.67	281
F39	297	30.5	13.2-	0.88	245
F70	262	29.4	12.4--	0.91	275
F90	153	29.9	14.7	1.33	184
F-J	1110	26.0	12.8--	0.43	
HAUTE-NORMANDIE					
F27	404	23.6	11.4--	0.65	302
F76	1162	24.2	12.4--	0.41	275
F-K	1566	24.1	12.1--	0.34	
ILE-DE-FRANCE					
F75	3608	36.5	13.2--	0.26	245
F77	782	25.7	13.4--	0.55	234
F78	835	19.3	12.7--	0.49	265
F91	676	18.2	12.5--	0.54	269
F92	1563	26.5	12.9--	0.36	259
F93	1235	23.4	14.2-	0.44	211
F94	1166	23.5	12.6--	0.42	266
F95	647	19.1	12.1--	0.53	285
F-L	10512	26.0	13.0--	0.14	
LANGUEDOC-ROUSSILLON					
F11	335	29.9	10.1--	0.68	317
F30	602	29.7	11.6--	0.55	299
F34	746	27.7	10.6--	0.46	310
F48	88	29.2	10.6--	1.39	310
F66	411	32.9	12.1--	0.68	285
F-M	2182	29.5	11.0--	0.28	
LIMOUSIN					
F19	377	38.2	12.8--	0.78	264
F23	298	49.2	12.5--	0.95	269
F87	593	40.7	14.3	0.71	206
F-N	1268	41.6	13.4--	0.46	
LORRAINE					
F54	690	23.7	12.5--	0.52	269
F55	240	29.1	13.0-	1.00	250
F57	748	18.8	12.1--	0.47	285
F88	516	31.7	14.6	0.73	192
F-O	2194	23.5	12.8--	0.30	
MIDI-PYRENEES					
F09	155	27.6	8.7--	0.87	332
F12	395	34.6	12.3--	0.75	281
F31	905	28.4	13.4--	0.51	234
F32	245	34.9	11.9--	0.88	292
F46	232	38.1	12.4--	0.97	275
F65	338	36.2	13.9	0.89	221
F81	457	33.0	12.4--	0.68	275
F82	258	34.3	13.0-	0.96	250
F-P	2985	32.2	12.6--	0.27	
NORD-PAS-DE-CALAIS					
F59	3205	31.3	16.6++	0.33	109
F62	1818	31.6	16.6++	0.43	109
F-Q	5023	31.4	16.6++	0.26	
PAYS DE LA LOIRE					
F44	912	23.7	12.1--	0.45	285
F49	758	29.0	13.6--	0.57	227
F53	282	26.1	11.6--	0.78	299
F72	513	25.4	11.1--	0.56	304
F85	592	32.1	14.3	0.69	206
F-R	3057	26.8	12.6--	0.26	
PICARDIE					
F02	680	31.7	15.2	0.68	164
F60	599	24.7	13.3--	0.62	239
F80	679	30.9	14.1	0.62	216
F-S	1958	28.9	14.2--	0.37	
POITOU-CHARENTES					
F16	469	33.9	13.5-	0.74	230
F17	735	36.2	14.6	0.64	192
F79	429	31.6	12.9--	0.73	259
F86	526	36.3	14.7	0.76	184
F-T	2159	34.7	14.0--	0.36	
PROVENCE-ALPES-COTE D'AZUR					
F04	114	25.6	10.1--	1.11	317
F05	100	25.6	11.1--	1.29	304
F06	745	21.6	6.9--	0.30	349
F13	1566	23.5	10.9--	0.31	307
F83	747	29.3	11.7--	0.49	298
F84	414	26.0	12.0--	0.67	290
F-U	3686	24.4	10.0--	0.19	
RHONE-ALPES					
F01	393	26.1	11.8--	0.69	295
F07	368	35.1	13.3-	0.83	239
F26	396	27.0	12.5--	0.72	269
F38	806	23.2	11.8--	0.47	295
F42	1066	34.6	14.9	0.52	176
F69	1603	27.4	14.3-	0.40	206
F73	326	26.4	13.3-	0.83	239
F74	364	20.2	11.4--	0.65	302
F-V	5322	27.3	13.3--	0.21	
F.0	61638	28.7	13.0--	0.06	

UNITED KINGDOM (1976-80)

EAST ANGLIA					
G25	450	26.6	13.9	0.72	221
G46	793	38.2	16.6+	0.67	109
G55	597	33.7	14.5	0.66	198
G-A	1840	33.2	15.2	0.39	
EAST MIDLANDS					
G30	903	32.9	15.3	0.55	158
G44	828	32.6	16.2	0.62	133
G45	636	39.5	18.0++	0.78	57
G47	514	32.8	16.7	0.81	103
G50	999	33.5	16.3+	0.56	127
G-B	3880	33.9	16.4++	0.29	
NORTHERN					
G14	1413	39.0	17.8++	0.52	65
G27	551	31.7	18.3++	0.83	47
G29	579	39.6	16.9+	0.78	96
G33	619	33.3	15.8	0.68	146
G48	306	34.5	16.8	1.06	100
G-C	3468	36.2	17.2++	0.32	
NORTH-WEST					
G11	3089	37.4	17.3++	0.34	78
G12	1860	38.4	17.9++	0.46	60
G26	919	32.7	17.0++	0.60	90
G43	1728	40.4	16.5++	0.45	119
G-D	7596	37.6	17.2++	0.22	

SOUTH-EAST					
G01	7612	34.9	14.6--	0.19	192
G22	400	27.2	16.1	0.85	136
G23	553	27.3	15.0	0.69	170
G24	458	29.4	16.1	0.80	136
G34	1266	59.2	16.6+	0.58	109
G35	1423	32.4	15.0	0.44	170
G37	1498	34.7	16.6++	0.47	109
G39	888	30.6	16.3+	0.58	127
G41	175	48.4	15.5	1.35	152
G42	1726	38.6	17.0++	0.46	90
G51	486	31.0	16.3	0.80	127
G56	1134	37.0	16.5+	0.53	119
G58	943	46.8	16.1	0.63	136
G-E	18562	35.6	15.5++	0.13	
SOUTH-WEST					
G21	1020	35.7	15.2	0.54	164
G28	579	44.8	17.8++	0.83	65
G31	1280	43.8	16.0	0.52	140
G32	815	44.1	14.5	0.61	198
G36	557	36.7	16.2	0.76	133
G53	511	40.4	16.7	0.83	103
G59	478	31.0	16.1	0.79	136
G-F	5240	39.6	15.8++	0.25	
WEST MIDLANDS					
G15	2757	33.4	16.4++	0.34	123
G38	604	32.7	15.9	0.70	144
G52	353	31.8	14.7	0.88	184
G54	951	31.4	17.0++	0.59	90
G57	470	33.0	17.7++	0.87	70
G-G	5135	32.8	16.5++	0.25	
YORKSHIRE AND HUMBERSIDE					
G13	1357	33.9	16.4+	0.48	123
G16	2192	34.2	15.4	0.37	157
G40	930	35.5	16.8++	0.60	100
G49	718	35.9	15.1	0.64	168
G-H	5197	34.6	15.8++	0.24	
WALES					
G61	499	42.1	18.0++	0.92	57
G62	406	40.2	17.2+	0.95	81
G63	433	32.2	15.5	0.80	152
G64	337	47.9	18.8++	1.18	34
G65	508	30.7	15.3	0.73	158
G66	129	40.8	18.0	1.75	57
G67	373	31.0	14.1	0.81	216
G68	425	37.1	17.1+	0.91	87
G-I	3110	36.3	16.5++	0.33	
SCOTLAND(1975-80)					
S01	247	43.2	22.3++	1.57	5
S02	589	41.2	19.1++	0.87	26
S03	555	44.3	18.8++	0.90	34
S04	381	36.6	17.5+	0.97	74
S05	846	35.8	16.9++	0.63	96
S06	148	47.4	16.6	1.56	109
S07	311	37.7	21.1++	1.27	9
S08	2811	36.6	18.6++	0.38	41
S09	165	37.5	18.1	1.52	52
S10	14	25.6	9.8	2.84	322
S11	26	42.6	18.8	4.30	34
S12	46	50.9	18.3	3.24	47
G-J	6139	38.1	18.5++	0.26	
NORTHERN IRELAND					
JE	614	36.6	20.9++	0.90	10
JN	230	24.9	15.0	1.06	170
JS	123	18.1	10.3--	1.01	316
JW	230	37.5	21.5++	1.52	8
G-K	1197	30.7	17.7++	0.55	
G.0	61364	35.8	16.3++	0.07	
ITALIA (1975-79)					
ABRUZZI					
I66	142	18.5	9.0--	0.81	329
I67	86	12.8	6.4--	0.76	352
I68	174	24.1	14.1	1.13	216
I69	151	16.3	7.9--	0.69	336
I-A	553	17.9	9.2--	0.42	
BASILICATA					
I76	121	11.6	7.5--	0.72	340
I77	48	9.5	6.3--	0.94	354
I-B	169	10.9	7.1--	0.57	
CALABRIA					
I78	174	9.6	6.6--	0.53	351
I79	187	10.2	6.9--	0.54	349
I80	180	12.1	7.0--	0.56	347
I-C	541	10.5	6.8--	0.31	
CAMPANIA					
I61	186	10.2	7.8--	0.59	337
I62	89	12.1	7.1--	0.80	344
I63	993	13.6	10.7--	0.35	308
I64	141	12.8	7.7--	0.69	338
I65	280	11.1	7.4--	0.46	341
I-D	1689	12.5	9.1--	0.23	
EMILIA-ROMAGNA					
I33	247	34.1	14.4	1.01	202
I34	355	34.7	14.6	0.84	192
I35	321	31.2	15.5	0.91	152
I36	458	31.1	16.4	0.81	123
I37	852	35.0	16.3	0.59	127
I38	329	33.0	15.8	0.92	146
I39	313	34.0	16.0	0.98	140
I40	440	29.5	15.8	0.79	146
I-E	3315	32.8	15.7	0.29	
FRIULI-VENEZIA GIULIA					
I30	331	24.4	11.0--	0.66	306
I31	101	26.4	12.5-	1.34	269
I32	316	39.5	14.5	0.89	198
I93	139	20.2	10.5--	0.96	313
I-F	887	27.5	12.1--	0.44	
LAZIO					
I56	190	28.7	15.7	1.18	150
I57	69	19.1	9.2--	1.21	327
I58	1874	19.9	13.5--	0.32	230
I59	131	12.6	10.1--	0.90	317
I60	168	14.8	8.3--	0.68	334
I-G	2432	19.3	12.6--	0.26	
LIGURIA					
I08	203	33.9	13.4	1.02	234
I09	315	39.9	16.7	1.01	103
I10	1229	43.4	18.1++	0.56	52
I11	265	41.7	16.7	1.13	103
I-H	2012	41.4	17.1++	0.41	
LOMBARDIA					
I12	616	30.8	18.7++	0.79	39
I13	545	27.9	16.3	0.74	127
I14	93	21.3	11.9-	1.31	292
I15	2966	28.5	17.9++	0.34	60
I16	501	22.6	14.9	0.69	176
I17	545	21.4	13.4--	0.60	234
I18	556	41.1	17.0+	0.80	90
I19	273	31.8	14.7	0.96	184
I20	291	29.8	13.7	0.88	224
I-I	6386	28.1	16.5++	0.22	
MARCHE					
I41	221	26.6	13.6	0.98	227
I42	342	31.1	14.7	0.85	184
I43	224	30.3	14.0	0.99	220
I44	212	23.8	13.2-	0.95	245
I-J	999	28.1	14.0-	0.47	
MOLISE					
I70	106	17.7	9.1--	0.96	328
I94	37	15.4	7.2--	1.29	342
I-K	143	17.0	8.5--	0.77	
PIEMONTE					
I01	1671	27.5	16.0+	0.41	140
I02	438	41.4	15.7	0.84	150
I03	464	35.3	16.5	0.84	119
I04	434	31.6	14.1	0.74	216
I05	252	44.8	16.4	1.18	123
I06	521	42.1	15.5	0.78	152
I-L	3780	32.5	15.6	0.27	
PUGLIA					
I71	278	16.2	10.7--	0.68	308
I72	508	14.0	9.7--	0.45	324
I73	170	12.2	9.4--	0.74	326
I74	125	12.6	8.9--	0.83	330
I75	200	10.4	7.2--	0.53	342
I-M	1281	13.3	9.3--	0.27	
SARDEGNA					
I90	170	16.0	10.0--	0.83	320
I91	92	13.3	8.6--	0.97	333
I92	207	11.7	8.9--	0.64	330
I95	57	14.7	8.3--	1.21	334
I-N	526	13.4	9.0--	0.42	
SICILIA					
I81	155	14.5	7.7--	0.68	338
I82	463	15.5	10.0--	0.49	320
I83	227	13.1	7.0--	0.50	347
I84	107	9.0	5.8--	0.58	355
I85	77	10.5	7.1--	0.85	344
I86	51	9.9	6.4--	0.93	352
I87	360	14.4	9.6--	0.53	325
I88	120	17.6	9.8--	0.93	322
I89	151	15.6	10.5--	0.89	313
I-O	1711	13.8	8.5--	0.22	
TOSCANA					
I45	156	29.5	12.9	1.17	259
I46	316	31.4	13.0--	0.81	250
I47	228	33.7	14.4	1.04	202
I48	1158	37.5	16.9++	0.54	96
I49	353	39.9	17.8++	1.01	65
I50	345	35.1	15.3	0.90	158
I51	222	28.1	12.4--	0.91	275
I52	296	45.2	18.8++	1.24	34
I53	224	39.9	19.1++	1.35	26
I-P	3298	35.9	15.8+	0.30	
TRENTINO-ALTO ADIGE					
I21	245	22.6	15.0	1.00	170
I22	269	24.0	12.1--	0.80	285
I-Q	514	23.3	13.4--	0.63	
UMBRIA					
I54	422	29.3	14.2	0.74	211
I55	158	27.3	13.2	1.11	245
I-R	580	28.7	14.0	0.62	
VALLE D'AOSTA					
I07	74	26.1	15.0	1.83	170
VENETO					
I23	453	23.2	13.3--	0.66	239
I24	349	19.2	11.5--	0.65	301
I25	152	26.0	11.8--	1.05	295
I26	334	18.7	10.4--	0.61	315
I27	545	25.4	14.6	0.66	192
I28	473	23.2	13.5-	0.65	230
I29	157	24.3	12.6-	1.08	266
I-T	2463	22.5	12.7--	0.27	
I.0	33353	23.3	13.0--	0.08	
IRELAND (1976-80)					
CONNAUGHT					
R07	101	24.8	15.3	1.66	158
R12	37	57.1	24.7+	4.52	2
R16	96	34.6	17.3	2.02	78
R20	58	45.1	24.9++	3.78	1
R21	54	40.3	19.2	2.81	25
R-A	346	34.2	18.4++	1.10	
LEINSTER					
R01	20	21.1	14.8	3.59	180
R06	603	23.6	18.1++	0.78	52
R09	37	15.9	14.4	2.44	202
R10	44	26.3	17.1	2.73	87
R11	33	27.8	17.2	3.22	81
R14	22	29.9	19.4	4.44	22
R15	70	32.5	24.3++	3.01	3
R17	48	21.8	18.4	2.80	46
R19	39	28.3	20.4	3.55	13
R24	40	27.3	18.5	3.08	43
R25	67	28.2	18.2	2.43	51
R26	63	30.0	22.2+	2.98	6
R-B	1086	24.6	18.4++	0.59	
MUNSTER					
R03	55	26.8	15.3	2.22	158
R04	311	31.6	19.8++	1.22	16
R08	106	36.4	20.7+	2.25	11
R13	112	28.7	18.5	1.86	43
R22	102	31.5	20.7+	2.23	11
R23	72	33.2	22.1+	2.88	7
R-C	758	31.4	19.6++	0.77	
ULSTER					
R02	43	33.8	17.4	2.83	76
R05	93	31.4	17.6	1.97	72
R18	37	30.7	19.6	3.40	19
R-D	173	31.8	17.9	1.46	
R.0	2363	28.2	18.7++	0.41	
LUXEMBOURG (1971-80)					
LE	61	31.8	13.7	1.91	224
LN	113	42.7	20.3+	2.06	14
LS	380	28.3	14.8	0.80	180
L.0	554	30.8	15.5	0.70	
NEDERLAND (1976-80)					
N01	425	31.0	15.9	0.85	144
N02	397	27.7	14.2	0.79	211
N03	262	25.5	14.3	0.94	206
N04	667	26.7	16.7+	0.69	103
N05	1133	27.1	16.6++	0.53	109
N06	595	26.6	14.9	0.66	176
N07	1693	28.4	14.7	0.39	184
N08	2259	29.1	15.1	0.34	168
N09	278	32.7	15.5	1.01	152
N10	1167	23.4	17.5++	0.53	74
N11	681	25.8	17.9++	0.71	60
N.0	9557	27.3	15.8++	0.17	
EEC-9					
EEC	255429	31.9	15.2	0.03	

BELGIE-BELGIQUE (1971-78)

BRUSSEL-BRUXELLES					
B21	151	3.8	2.2++	0.19	41
VLAANDEREN					
B10	222	3.6	2.4++	0.17	31
B29	89	2.5	1.7	0.18	77
B30	47	1.1	0.8--	0.12	298
B40	106	2.0	1.2--	0.12	157
B70	56	2.0	2.0	0.27	50
B-V	520	2.4	1.6	0.07	
WALLONIE					
B25	19	1.9	1.2	0.29	157
B50	95	1.9	1.2-	0.13	157
B60	145	3.7	2.4++	0.21	31
B80	34	3.9	2.5+	0.45	25
B90	79	5.2	3.4++	0.39	2
B-W	372	3.0	1.9++	0.10	
B.0	1043	2.7	1.8++	0.06	

BR DEUTSCHLAND (1976-80)

BADEN-WURTTEMBERG					
D81	325	3.9	2.9++	0.17	13
D82	276	4.9	3.4++	0.21	2
D83	140	3.2	2.1++	0.19	46
D84	132	3.7	2.8++	0.26	17
D-A	873	4.0	2.8++	0.10	
BAYERN					
D91	296	3.4	2.3++	0.14	39
D92	63	2.7	1.9	0.25	54
D93	72	3.1	2.3++	0.28	39
D94	105	4.3	2.5++	0.26	25
D95	149	4.1	2.6++	0.22	21
D96	98	3.4	2.4++	0.25	31
D97	141	3.9	2.5++	0.22	25
D-B	924	3.6	2.4++	0.08	
BERLIN(WEST)					
DB0	249	5.8	3.0++	0.21	9
BREMEN					
D40	57	3.5	2.1+	0.30	46
HAMBURG					
D20	175	4.5	2.5++	0.20	25
HESSEN					
D64	407	3.9	2.6++	0.14	21
D66	145	5.1	3.0++	0.27	9
D-F	552	4.1	2.7++	0.12	
NIEDERSACHSEN					
D31	229	5.9	3.5++	0.25	1
D32	259	5.3	3.1++	0.21	4
D33	146	4.2	2.6++	0.23	21
D34	218	4.3	3.1++	0.22	4
D-G	852	4.9	3.1++	0.11	
NORDRHEIN-WESTFALEN					
D51	477	3.9	2.9++	0.14	13
D53	311	3.3	2.7++	0.16	18
D55	196	3.4	3.0++	0.23	9
D57	182	4.2	3.0++	0.23	9
D59	314	3.6	2.7++	0.16	18
D-H	1480	3.6	2.8++	0.08	
RHEINLAND-PFALZ					
D71	158	4.9	3.1++	0.26	4
D72	51	4.6	3.1++	0.45	4
D73	193	4.5	3.1++	0.23	4
D-I	402	4.6	3.1++	0.16	
SAARLAND					
DA0	95	3.7	2.4++	0.25	31
SCHLESWIG-HOLSTEIN					
D10	191	3.1	1.9++	0.15	54
D.0	5850	4.0	2.7++	0.04	

DANMARK (1971-80)

K15	196	3.2	2.0++	0.15	50
K20	27	1.8	1.7	0.32	77
K25	9	1.0	0.9-	0.31	270
K30	40	3.0	1.8	0.29	64
K35	44	3.4	1.9	0.31	54
K40	5	2.1	1.1	0.50	188
K42	72	3.3	1.8	0.22	64
K50	36	2.9	1.8	0.31	64
K55	17	1.6	1.2	0.31	157
K60	41	2.6	1.7	0.27	77
K65	29	2.3	1.6	0.30	86
K70	95	3.4	2.4++	0.25	31
K76	23	2.0	1.1	0.25	188
K80	58	2.5	1.5	0.20	103
K.0	692	2.8	1.8++	0.07	

FRANCE (1971-78)

ALSACE					
F67	81	2.3	1.8	0.21	64
F68	57	2.3	2.0	0.27	50
F-A	138	2.3	1.9	0.16	
AQUITAINE					
F24	38	2.6	1.3	0.23	130
F33	60	1.5	0.9--	0.12	270
F40	12	1.1	0.5--	0.16	336
F47	13	1.1	0.5--	0.15	336
F64	40	1.9	1.1-	0.18	188
F-B	163	1.7	0.9--	0.08	
AUVERGNE					
F03	32	2.2	1.0--	0.19	225
F15	15	2.3	1.7	0.45	77
F43	16	2.0	1.0	0.28	225
F63	31	1.4	1.0--	0.19	225
F-C	94	1.8	1.1--	0.12	
BASSE-NORMANDIE					
F14	29	1.3	1.1-	0.21	188
F50	18	1.0	0.8--	0.19	298
F61	12	1.0	0.7--	0.22	316
F-D	59	1.2	0.9--	0.12	
BOURGOGNE					
F21	37	2.1	1.5	0.25	103
F58	33	3.4	1.4	0.27	117
F71	49	2.2	1.3	0.20	130
F89	23	1.9	1.0-	0.24	225
F-E	142	2.3	1.3	0.12	
BRETAGNE					
F22	29	1.4	0.9--	0.18	270
F29	42	1.3	0.8--	0.14	298
F35	24	0.9	0.7--	0.14	316
F56	31	1.4	1.0--	0.18	225
F-F	126	1.3	0.9--	0.08	
CENTRE					
F18	22	1.8	1.0--	0.22	225
F28	16	1.2	0.8--	0.21	298
F36	20	2.0	1.1	0.26	188
F37	33	1.8	1.2	0.22	157
F41	24	2.2	1.2	0.26	157
F45	38	2.0	1.3	0.22	130
F-G	153	1.8	1.1--	0.09	
CHAMPAGNE-ARDENNE					
F08	19	1.5	1.1	0.26	188
F10	19	1.7	1.0-	0.24	225
F51	38	1.8	1.5	0.25	103
F52	17	2.0	1.4	0.35	117
F-H	93	1.7	1.3-	0.14	
CORSE					
F20	14	1.5	1.0	0.28	225
FRANCHE-COMTE					
F25	26	1.4	1.3	0.27	130
F39	14	1.5	0.9--	0.25	270
F70	10	1.1	0.7--	0.22	316
F90	8	1.6	1.3	0.47	130
F-J	58	1.4	1.1--	0.14	
HAUTE-NORMANDIE					
F27	34	2.0	1.5	0.26	103
F76	63	1.4	1.0--	0.14	225
F-K	97	1.5	1.2--	0.12	
ILE-DE-FRANCE					
F75	146	1.7	1.0--	0.08	225
F77	53	1.8	1.4	0.19	117
F78	40	0.9	1.0--	0.16	225
F91	41	1.1	1.2	0.19	157
F92	80	1.4	1.1--	0.12	188
F93	64	1.2	1.1--	0.15	188
F94	59	1.2	1.1--	0.14	188
F95	30	0.9	0.9--	0.17	270
F-L	513	1.3	1.1--	0.05	
LANGUEDOC-ROUSSILLON					
F11	25	2.4	1.1	0.24	188
F30	40	2.1	1.2	0.20	157
F34	49	2.0	1.0--	0.15	225
F48	2	0.7	0.4--	0.32	347
F66	20	1.7	0.7--	0.17	316
F-M	136	2.0	1.0--	0.09	
LIMOUSIN					
F19	18	1.9	1.1	0.27	188
F23	13	2.3	0.9-	0.27	270
F87	35	2.6	1.3	0.22	130
F-N	66	2.3	1.1--	0.15	
LORRAINE					
F54	66	2.3	1.8	0.23	64
F55	12	1.5	1.1	0.34	188
F57	80	2.0	1.9	0.22	54
F88	23	1.5	1.1	0.25	188
F-O	181	2.0	1.6	0.12	
MIDI-PYRENEES					
F09	14	2.6	1.2	0.37	157
F12	17	1.6	0.7--	0.18	316
F31	40	1.3	0.8--	0.14	298
F32	9	1.3	0.5--	0.19	336
F46	12	2.0	1.1	0.33	188
F65	13	1.5	0.8--	0.25	298
F81	25	1.9	1.1	0.24	188
F82	8	1.1	0.6--	0.23	329
F-P	138	1.6	0.9--	0.08	
NORD-PAS-DE-CALAIS					
F59	148	1.5	1.3--	0.11	130
F62	98	1.8	1.5	0.15	103
F-Q	246	1.6	1.3-	0.09	
PAYS DE LA LOIRE					
F44	28	0.8	0.6--	0.12	329
F49	36	1.5	1.1-	0.19	188
F53	18	1.8	1.2	0.29	157
F72	24	1.2	0.8--	0.18	298
F85	10	0.6	0.3--	0.11	351
F-R	116	1.1	0.8--	0.07	
PICARDIE					
F02	31	1.5	0.9--	0.18	270
F60	29	1.2	1.0--	0.19	225
F80	29	1.4	1.0--	0.19	225
F-S	89	1.3	1.0--	0.11	
POITOU-CHARENTES					
F16	18	1.4	0.9--	0.21	270
F17	31	1.6	0.9--	0.17	270
F79	21	1.6	1.0--	0.22	225
F86	26	1.9	1.1-	0.22	188
F-T	96	1.6	0.9--	0.10	
PROVENCE-ALPES-COTE D'AZUR					
F04	9	2.0	1.2	0.43	157
F05	6	1.5	1.0	0.41	225
F06	47	1.5	0.7--	0.11	316
F13	110	1.7	1.1--	0.11	188
F83	58	2.4	1.4	0.19	117
F84	23	1.5	1.0-	0.22	225
F-U	253	1.8	1.0--	0.07	
RHONE-ALPES					
F01	16	1.1	0.7--	0.19	316
F07	18	1.8	1.0-	0.26	225
F26	23	1.6	1.0-	0.22	225
F38	38	1.1	0.9--	0.14	270
F42	51	1.7	1.2-	0.17	157
F69	69	1.2	1.0--	0.12	225
F73	25	2.1	1.5	0.31	103
F74	18	1.0	0.9--	0.21	270
F-V	258	1.4	1.0--	0.06	
F.0	3229	1.6	1.1--	0.02	

UNITED KINGDOM (1976-80)

EAST ANGLIA					
G25	21	1.2	0.9--	0.21	270
G46	20	1.0	0.5--	0.13	336
G55	33	1.9	1.2	0.22	157
G-A	74	1.3	0.9--	0.10	
EAST MIDLANDS					
G30	45	1.7	1.0--	0.16	225
G44	35	1.4	1.0--	0.18	225
G45	20	1.3	0.8--	0.18	298
G47	27	1.8	1.3	0.25	130
G50	47	1.6	1.1-	0.17	188
G-B	174	1.6	1.0--	0.08	
NORTHERN					
G14	58	1.7	1.1--	0.15	188
G27	37	2.2	1.7	0.29	77
G29	27	2.0	1.2	0.24	157
G33	49	2.8	1.8	0.26	64
G48	12	1.4	0.8--	0.23	298
G-C	183	2.0	1.3-	0.10	
NORTH-WEST					
G11	115	1.5	1.0--	0.10	225
G12	76	1.7	1.2--	0.14	157
G26	44	1.6	1.2	0.19	157
G43	94	2.4	1.5	0.16	103
G-D	329	1.7	1.2--	0.07	

SOUTH-EAST					
G01	417	2.1	1.3--	0.07	130
G22	28	1.9	1.5	0.29	103
G23	27	1.3	1.0-	0.20	225
G24	33	2.1	1.7	0.30	77
G34	35	2.0	0.8--	0.15	298
G35	70	1.7	1.2--	0.14	157
G37	63	1.4	1.1--	0.14	188
G39	39	1.4	1.1--	0.17	188
G41	4	1.2	0.5--	0.25	336
G42	66	1.6	1.0--	0.12	225
G51	23	1.4	1.0-	0.21	225
G56	29	1.0	0.6--	0.11	329
G58	31	1.7	1.0--	0.19	225
G-E	865	1.8	1.2--	0.04	
SOUTH-WEST					
G21	39	1.5	1.0--	0.16	225
G28	27	2.3	1.2	0.24	157
G31	45	1.6	0.9--	0.15	270
G32	32	1.9	0.9--	0.17	270
G36	18	1.2	0.8--	0.20	298
G53	28	2.3	1.4	0.27	117
G59	19	1.2	0.9--	0.21	270
G-F	208	1.7	1.0--	0.07	
WEST MIDLANDS					
G15	132	1.6	1.2--	0.10	157
G38	23	1.3	0.9--	0.18	270
G52	12	1.1	0.8--	0.25	298
G54	46	1.6	1.1-	0.17	188
G57	24	1.7	1.3	0.27	130
G-G	237	1.6	1.1--	0.07	
YORKSHIRE AND HUMBERSIDE					
G13	67	1.7	1.1--	0.14	188
G16	116	1.9	1.3	0.12	130
G40	37	1.5	1.0--	0.17	225
G49	40	2.1	1.3	0.21	130
G-H	260	1.8	1.2--	0.08	
WALES					
G61	12	1.1	0.6--	0.19	329
G62	14	1.5	0.9--	0.25	270
G63	26	2.0	1.3	0.27	130
G64	11	1.7	1.2	0.38	157
G65	23	1.5	1.1-	0.23	188
G66	4	1.3	0.8	0.45	298
G67	23	2.1	1.3	0.29	130
G68	19	1.8	1.2	0.27	157
G-I	132	1.6	1.1--	0.10	
SCOTLAND (1975-80)					
S01	11	2.0	1.6	0.48	86
S02	19	1.4	0.9--	0.22	270
S03	10	0.9	0.7--	0.22	316
S04	12	1.2	0.8--	0.23	298
S05	32	1.5	1.0--	0.19	225
S06	5	1.7	1.3	0.59	130
S07	12	1.5	1.0	0.29	225
S08	112	1.6	1.2--	0.12	157
S09	16	3.8	2.5	0.65	25
S10	2	3.8	1.6	1.13	86
S11	2	3.2	1.9	1.32	54
S12	3	3.4	1.3	0.79	130
G-J	236	1.6	1.1--	0.07	
NORTHERN IRELAND					
JE	25	1.5	1.4	0.29	117
JN	15	1.7	1.3	0.35	130
JS	7	1.1	0.9-	0.33	270
JW	7	1.2	1.0	0.38	225
G-K	54	1.4	1.2	0.17	
G.0	2752	1.7	1.1--	0.02	
ITALIA (1975-79)					
ABRUZZI					
I66	14	1.9	1.3	0.35	130
I67	10	1.5	1.1	0.35	188
I68	11	1.6	1.1	0.33	188
I69	16	1.8	1.1	0.29	188
I-A	51	1.7	1.1-	0.16	
BASILICATA					
I76	9	0.9	0.7--	0.24	316
I77	10	2.0	1.8	0.57	64
I-B	19	1.2	1.0-	0.24	
CALABRIA					
I78	9	0.5	0.4--	0.15	347
I79	23	1.3	1.0-	0.22	225
I80	15	1.0	0.7--	0.19	316
I-C	47	0.9	0.7--	0.11	
CAMPANIA					
I61	12	0.7	0.6--	0.18	329
I62	3	0.4	0.3--	0.15	351
I63	63	0.9	1.0--	0.12	225
I64	6	0.6	0.4--	0.18	347
I65	30	1.2	1.0--	0.18	225
I-D	114	0.9	0.8--	0.08	
EMILIA-ROMAGNA					
I33	19	2.7	1.6	0.37	86
I34	14	1.4	0.7--	0.20	316
I35	23	2.3	1.5	0.34	103
I36	26	1.8	1.2	0.25	157
I37	62	2.7	1.6	0.21	86
I38	27	2.9	1.7	0.33	77
I39	20	2.3	1.3	0.30	130
I40	37	2.6	1.8	0.29	64
I-E	228	2.4	1.4	0.10	
FRIULI-VENEZIA GIULIA					
I30	20	1.6	1.0-	0.23	225
I31	8	2.3	1.4	0.50	117
I32	28	4.0	1.9	0.38	54
I93	16	2.4	1.8	0.45	64
I-F	72	2.4	1.5	0.18	
LAZIO					
I56	13	2.0	1.2	0.34	157
I57	11	3.1	1.6	0.50	86
I58	173	1.9	1.7	0.13	77
I59	14	1.3	1.2	0.32	157
I60	13	1.2	0.8--	0.22	298
I-G	224	1.9	1.5	0.10	
LIGURIA					
I08	25	4.5	2.2	0.46	41
I09	19	2.6	1.4	0.35	117
I10	76	2.9	1.6	0.19	86
I11	13	2.2	1.0	0.29	225
I-H	133	3.0	1.6	0.14	
LOMBARDIA					
I12	33	1.8	1.5	0.28	103
I13	21	1.1	0.9--	0.21	270
I14	5	1.2	0.9	0.39	270
I15	175	1.8	1.6	0.12	86
I16	34	1.6	1.4	0.25	117
I17	38	1.6	1.3	0.21	130
I18	37	2.9	1.6	0.28	86
I19	12	1.5	1.0	0.29	225
I20	19	2.1	1.3	0.32	130
I-I	374	1.7	1.4	0.07	
MARCHE					
I41	24	3.0	1.8	0.36	64
I42	19	1.8	1.1	0.25	188
I43	13	1.8	1.2	0.33	157
I44	11	1.3	1.0	0.29	225
I-J	67	2.0	1.2	0.15	
MOLISE					
I70	14	2.4	1.6	0.46	86
I94	2	0.9	0.5--	0.33	336
I-K	16	2.0	1.3	0.34	
PIEMONTE					
I01	118	2.0	1.6	0.15	86
I02	21	2.2	1.3	0.30	130
I03	19	1.5	1.1	0.25	188
I04	28	2.1	1.1	0.22	188
I05	17	3.2	1.6	0.41	86
I06	29	2.5	1.1	0.22	188
I-L	232	2.1	1.4	0.09	
PUGLIA					
I71	22	1.3	1.0-	0.23	225
I72	41	1.2	0.9--	0.15	270
I73	16	1.2	1.1	0.28	188
I74	15	1.6	1.3	0.35	130
I75	17	0.9	0.8--	0.19	298
I-M	111	1.2	1.0--	0.09	
SARDEGNA					
I90	15	1.4	1.1	0.30	188
I91	13	1.9	1.4	0.42	117
I92	20	1.1	1.0-	0.23	225
I95	11	2.8	1.5	0.48	103
I-N	59	1.5	1.2-	0.16	
SICILIA					
I81	13	1.3	0.9-	0.26	270
I82	20	0.7	0.5--	0.13	336
I83	14	0.9	0.5--	0.14	336
I84	16	1.3	0.9--	0.23	270
I85	11	1.5	1.4	0.44	117
I86	6	1.2	0.7-	0.32	316
I87	19	0.8	0.6--	0.15	329
I88	18	2.7	1.9	0.45	54
I89	12	1.2	1.0	0.30	225
I-O	129	1.1	0.8--	0.07	
TOSCANA					
I45	17	3.4	2.0	0.51	50
I46	28	3.0	1.8	0.34	64
I47	15	2.3	1.3	0.35	130
I48	64	2.2	1.3	0.17	130
I49	15	1.8	1.2	0.32	157
I50	23	2.5	1.5	0.32	103
I51	12	1.6	0.8--	0.22	298
I52	11	1.7	0.8--	0.25	298
I53	11	2.0	1.0	0.32	225
I-P	196	2.3	1.3--	0.09	
TRENTINO-ALTO ADIGE					
I21	26	2.5	2.2	0.44	41
I22	17	1.6	1.0-	0.25	225
I-Q	43	2.0	1.5	0.24	
UMBRIA					
I54	23	1.6	0.9--	0.19	270
I55	13	2.3	1.3	0.37	130
I-R	36	1.8	1.0--	0.17	
VALLE D'AOSTA					
I07	9	3.2	2.2	0.72	41
VENETO					
I23	36	1.9	1.4	0.24	117
I24	24	1.4	1.1	0.23	188
I25	13	2.4	1.6	0.44	86
I26	33	1.9	1.5	0.27	103
I27	36	1.8	1.4	0.24	117
I28	44	2.3	1.8	0.28	64
I29	15	2.4	1.6	0.43	86
I-T	201	1.9	1.5	0.11	
I.0	2361	1.7	1.2--	0.03	
IRELAND (1976-80)					
CONNAUGHT					
R07	13	3.0	1.9	0.55	54
R12	2	2.7	1.3	0.99	130
R16	5	1.7	0.9	0.40	270
R20	7	4.9	2.6	1.00	21
R21	1	0.7	0.4--	0.37	347
R-A	28	2.6	1.5	0.29	
LEINSTER					
R01	0	0.0	0.0--	0.00	353
R06	23	1.0	1.1-	0.22	188
R09	3	1.2	1.2	0.71	157
R10	2	1.1	0.7	0.52	316
R11	3	2.3	1.7	0.99	77
R14	0	0.0	0.0--	0.00	353
R15	0	0.0	0.0--	0.00	353
R17	3	1.3	1.2	0.73	157
R19	3	2.0	1.6	0.95	86
R24	1	0.7	0.5-	0.46	336
R25	7	2.9	2.5	0.95	25
R26	2	1.0	0.9	0.67	270
R-B	47	1.1	1.1--	0.16	
MUNSTER					
R03	2	0.9	0.6-	0.40	329
R04	13	1.3	1.1	0.32	188
R08	6	1.9	1.2	0.51	157
R13	7	1.8	1.5	0.55	103
R22	6	1.7	1.2	0.50	157
R23	2	0.9	0.9	0.62	270
R-C	36	1.4	1.1-	0.19	
ULSTER					
R02	1	0.7	0.5	0.53	336
R05	2	0.6	0.5--	0.33	336
R18	3	2.3	1.6	1.00	86
R-D	6	1.0	0.7--	0.31	
R.0	117	1.4	1.1--	0.11	
LUXEMBOURG (1971-80)					
LE	7	3.9	1.9	0.75	54
LN	4	1.5	1.0	0.52	225
LS	40	3.1	2.1	0.34	46
L.0	51	3.0	1.9	0.27	
NEDERLAND (1976-80)					
N01	49	3.6	2.4+	0.36	31
N02	51	3.6	2.4+	0.35	31
N03	28	2.7	1.9	0.37	54
N04	93	3.7	2.9++	0.30	13
N05	128	3.1	2.4++	0.22	31
N06	58	2.7	2.2+	0.29	41
N07	162	2.8	2.1++	0.17	46
N08	194	2.6	1.8+	0.13	64
N09	24	2.8	1.6	0.33	86
N10	149	2.9	2.9++	0.24	13
N11	77	2.9	2.7++	0.31	18
N.0	1013	2.9	2.3++	0.07	
EEC-9					
EEC	17108	2.2	1.5	0.01	

BELGIE-BELGIQUE (1971-78)

BRUSSEL-BRUXELLES

B21	299	6.7	2.5	0.16	76

VLAANDEREN

B10	400	6.3	3.3++	0.17	45
B29	152	4.1	2.0-	0.17	125
B30	152	3.5	1.8--	0.16	146
B40	241	4.5	2.2	0.16	101
B70	116	4.3	3.4++	0.33	43
B-V	1061	4.7	2.5	0.08	

WALLONIE

B25	65	6.1	3.1	0.42	49
B50	200	3.7	1.7--	0.14	160
B60	269	6.4	2.7	0.18	65
B80	43	4.8	2.4	0.38	82
B90	98	6.1	2.7	0.30	65
B-W	675	5.1	2.3	0.10	
B.0	2035	5.1	2.4	0.06	

BR DEUTSCHLAND (1976-80)

BADEN-WURTTEMBERG

D81	900	10.1	4.7++	0.17	17
D82	835	13.5	6.2++	0.24	2
D83	548	11.3	5.2++	0.24	12
D84	372	9.7	4.7++	0.27	17
D-A	2655	11.2	5.2++	0.11	

BAYERN

D91	740	7.9	3.6++	0.15	37
D92	162	6.2	2.9	0.25	60
D93	206	8.1	3.9++	0.29	31
D94	277	9.9	4.0++	0.27	30
D95	383	9.6	3.8++	0.21	34
D96	275	8.9	4.1++	0.27	28
D97	384	9.7	4.1++	0.23	28
D-B	2427	8.6	3.8++	0.08	

BERLIN(WEST)

DB0	1077	20.3	5.7++	0.21	6

BREMEN

D40	179	9.6	3.6++	0.30	37

HAMBURG

D20	516	11.6	3.9++	0.20	31

HESSEN

D64	1329	11.7	5.1++	0.16	13
D66	454	14.6	5.8++	0.30	5
D-F	1783	12.3	5.3++	0.14	

NIEDERSACHSEN

D31	591	13.8	5.4++	0.25	8
D32	729	13.4	5.0++	0.21	15
D33	404	10.9	4.6++	0.25	20
D34	583	10.7	5.0++	0.23	15
D-G	2307	12.2	5.0++	0.12	

NORDRHEIN-WESTFALEN

D51	1579	11.4	5.3++	0.14	10
D53	930	9.2	4.6++	0.16	20
D55	641	10.3	5.5++	0.23	7
D57	565	11.9	5.3++	0.24	10
D59	1112	11.5	5.4++	0.17	8
D-H	4827	10.8	5.2++	0.08	

RHEINLAND-PFALZ

D71	568	16.0	6.9++	0.32	1
D72	171	13.8	6.2++	0.52	2
D73	623	13.2	6.0++	0.26	4
D-I	1362	14.3	6.3++	0.19	

SAARLAND

DA0	303	10.6	4.7++	0.29	17

SCHLESWIG-HOLSTEIN

D10	595	8.8	3.6++	0.17	37
D.0	18031	11.2	4.9++	0.04	

DANMARK (1971-80)

K15	397	6.0	2.4	0.13	82
K20	60	4.0	3.1	0.42	49
K25	31	3.4	2.3	0.44	93
K30	84	6.3	3.1	0.36	49
K35	93	7.3	3.1	0.35	49
K40	14	6.0	2.6	0.72	71
K42	131	5.9	2.7	0.26	65
K50	79	6.5	3.3+	0.40	45
K55	38	3.7	2.2	0.37	101
K60	75	4.7	2.5	0.32	76
K65	49	3.9	2.5	0.38	76
K70	174	6.2	3.3++	0.27	45
K76	51	4.6	2.2	0.34	101
K80	109	4.7	2.4	0.24	82
K.0	1385	5.4	2.7++	0.08	

FRANCE (1971-78)

ALSACE

F67	258	7.1	3.7++	0.25	35
F68	210	8.1	4.3++	0.33	26
F-A	468	7.5	4.0++	0.20	

AQUITAINE

F24	52	3.4	1.4--	0.22	213
F33	90	2.0	0.8--	0.10	339
F40	21	1.8	0.6--	0.15	347
F47	30	2.5	1.0--	0.21	309
F64	59	2.7	1.1--	0.16	288
F-B	252	2.4	1.0--	0.07	

AUVERGNE

F03	88	5.6	2.0	0.26	125
F15	22	3.3	1.4--	0.35	213
F43	31	3.7	1.1--	0.24	288
F63	68	2.9	1.4--	0.18	213
F-C	209	3.8	1.5--	0.12	

BASSE-NORMANDIE

F14	61	2.7	1.4--	0.20	213
F50	27	1.4	0.6--	0.13	347
F61	34	2.8	1.4--	0.26	213
F-D	122	2.3	1.1--	0.11	

BOURGOGNE

F21	103	5.6	2.6	0.29	71
F58	69	6.8	2.4	0.35	82
F71	114	4.9	1.9-	0.21	137
F89	61	5.0	1.9	0.29	137
F-E	347	5.4	2.2	0.14	

BRETAGNE

F22	84	3.9	1.7--	0.22	160
F29	99	3.0	1.4--	0.16	213
F35	55	1.9	0.9--	0.13	323
F56	64	2.8	1.5--	0.21	190
F-F	302	2.8	1.4--	0.09	

CENTRE

F18	55	4.3	1.9	0.29	137
F28	44	3.3	1.4--	0.23	213
F36	46	4.6	1.8-	0.30	146
F37	82	4.2	1.9-	0.23	137
F41	36	3.1	1.6--	0.30	172
F45	67	3.4	1.6--	0.22	172
F-G	330	3.8	1.7--	0.11	

CHAMPAGNE-ARDENNE

F08	46	3.7	2.1	0.35	115
F10	56	4.9	2.3	0.34	93
F51	77	3.6	2.0	0.25	125
F52	48	5.6	2.8	0.46	62
F-H	227	4.2	2.2	0.17	

CORSE

F20	32	3.7	1.4--	0.27	213

FRANCHE-COMTE

F25	42	2.2	1.6--	0.26	172
F39	45	4.6	2.4	0.41	82
F70	41	4.6	2.3	0.40	93
F90	19	3.7	2.3	0.58	93
F-J	147	3.4	2.0-	0.18	

HAUTE-NORMANDIE

F27	41	2.4	1.2--	0.22	263
F76	130	2.7	1.4--	0.14	213
F-K	171	2.6	1.3--	0.11	

ILE-DE-FRANCE

F75	299	3.0	1.1--	0.07	288
F77	94	3.1	1.7--	0.20	160
F78	82	1.9	1.2--	0.15	263
F91	64	1.7	1.3--	0.18	240
F92	131	2.2	1.1--	0.10	288
F93	106	2.0	1.3--	0.13	240
F94	103	2.1	1.1--	0.13	288
F95	67	2.0	1.3--	0.17	240
F-L	946	2.3	1.2--	0.04	

LANGUEDOC-ROUSSILLON

F11	36	3.2	1.1--	0.23	288
F30	71	3.5	1.5--	0.20	190
F34	76	2.8	1.0--	0.14	309
F48	9	3.0	1.2-	0.48	263
F66	39	3.1	1.3--	0.23	240
F-M	231	3.1	1.2--	0.09	

LIMOUSIN

F19	41	4.1	1.6--	0.28	172
F23	33	5.4	1.8	0.42	146
F87	92	6.3	2.2	0.26	101
F-N	166	5.4	1.9--	0.17	

LORRAINE

F54	127	4.4	2.4	0.23	82
F55	44	5.3	2.4	0.43	82
F57	182	4.6	3.0+	0.23	58
F88	58	3.6	1.7--	0.25	160
F-O	411	4.4	2.5	0.13	

MIDI-PYRENEES

F09	18	3.2	1.1--	0.33	288
F12	36	3.2	1.3--	0.26	240
F31	56	1.8	1.0--	0.15	309
F32	18	2.6	0.9--	0.26	323
F46	18	3.0	1.1--	0.29	288
F65	26	2.8	1.1--	0.26	288
F81	32	2.3	0.9--	0.18	323
F82	17	2.3	0.9--	0.25	323
F-P	221	2.4	1.0--	0.08	

NORD-PAS-DE-CALAIS

F59	423	4.1	2.2	0.12	101
F62	263	4.6	2.5	0.17	76
F-Q	686	4.3	2.3	0.10	

PAYS DE LA LOIRE

F44	74	1.9	1.0--	0.13	309
F49	80	3.1	1.8--	0.23	146
F53	15	1.4	0.7--	0.21	343
F72	38	1.9	1.1--	0.19	288
F85	43	2.3	1.1--	0.18	288
F-R	250	2.2	1.2--	0.08	

PICARDIE

F02	64	3.0	1.6--	0.22	172
F60	85	3.5	2.1	0.25	115
F80	97	4.4	2.3	0.27	93
F-S	246	3.6	2.0--	0.14	

POITOU-CHARENTES

F16	42	3.0	1.3--	0.23	240
F17	53	2.6	1.1--	0.17	288
F79	61	4.5	2.2	0.32	101
F86	78	5.4	2.4	0.32	82
F-T	234	3.8	1.7--	0.13	

PROVENCE-ALPES-COTE D'AZUR

F04	17	3.8	1.5-	0.40	190
F05	24	6.1	2.5	0.58	76
F06	89	2.6	0.9--	0.11	323
F13	144	2.2	1.0--	0.09	309
F83	96	3.8	1.5--	0.18	190
F84	46	2.9	1.2--	0.20	263
F-U	416	2.8	1.1--	0.06	

RHONE-ALPES

F01	43	2.9	1.4--	0.25	213
F07	52	5.0	2.0	0.34	125
F26	46	3.1	1.2--	0.20	263
F38	114	3.3	1.6--	0.17	172
F42	154	5.0	2.3	0.21	93
F69	221	3.8	2.1-	0.16	115
F73	35	2.8	1.5--	0.28	190
F74	40	2.2	1.3--	0.23	240
F-V	705	3.6	1.8--	0.08	
F.0	7119	3.3	1.6--	0.02	

UNITED KINGDOM (1976-80)

EAST ANGLIA

G25	38	2.3	1.2--	0.22	263
G46	54	2.6	1.1--	0.16	288
G55	44	2.5	1.2--	0.20	263
G-A	136	2.5	1.1--	0.11	

EAST MIDLANDS

G30	74	2.7	1.2--	0.16	263
G44	68	2.7	1.3--	0.17	240
G45	46	2.9	1.4--	0.22	213
G47	59	3.8	1.8-	0.26	146
G50	98	3.3	1.5--	0.16	190
G-B	345	3.0	1.4--	0.08	

NORTHERN

G14	80	2.2	1.0--	0.12	309
G27	48	2.8	1.6--	0.24	172
G29	45	3.1	1.3--	0.21	240
G33	60	3.2	1.6--	0.22	172
G48	35	3.9	2.0	0.36	125
G-C	268	2.8	1.3--	0.09	

NORTH-WEST

G11	210	2.5	1.2--	0.09	263
G12	118	2.4	1.2--	0.12	263
G26	60	2.1	1.1--	0.15	288
G43	148	3.5	1.5--	0.14	190
G-D	536	2.7	1.3--	0.06	

SOUTH-EAST

G01	591	2.7	1.2--	0.05	263
G22	32	2.2	1.2--	0.23	263
G23	35	1.7	0.9--	0.17	323
G24	28	1.8	0.9--	0.19	323
G34	80	3.7	1.2--	0.17	263
G35	90	2.0	0.9--	0.11	323
G37	83	1.9	0.9--	0.11	323
G39	54	1.9	1.0--	0.15	309
G41	14	3.9	1.4-	0.46	213
G42	115	2.6	1.2--	0.13	263
G51	44	2.8	1.3--	0.21	240
G56	72	2.4	1.0--	0.12	309
G58	53	2.6	0.9--	0.16	323
G-E	1291	2.5	1.1--	0.03	

SOUTH-WEST

G21	75	2.6	1.1--	0.14	288
G28	32	2.5	1.2--	0.23	263
G31	78	2.7	1.1--	0.14	288
G32	65	3.5	1.1--	0.15	288
G36	39	2.6	1.2--	0.21	263
G53	36	2.8	1.3--	0.25	240
G59	33	2.1	1.1--	0.21	288
G-F	358	2.7	1.1--	0.07	

WEST MIDLANDS

G15	239	2.9	1.5--	0.10	190
G38	50	2.7	1.3--	0.20	240
G52	36	3.2	1.4--	0.26	213
G54	96	3.2	1.7--	0.18	160
G57	35	2.5	1.2--	0.22	263
G-G	456	2.9	1.5--	0.07	

YORKSHIRE AND HUMBERSIDE

G13	124	3.1	1.5--	0.15	190
G16	170	2.7	1.2--	0.10	263
G40	59	2.3	1.1--	0.15	288
G49	65	3.2	1.3--	0.19	240
G-H	418	2.8	1.3--	0.07	

WALES

G61	26	2.2	0.9--	0.19	323
G62	24	2.4	0.8--	0.18	339
G63	39	2.9	1.4--	0.24	213
G64	27	3.8	1.8	0.40	146
G65	42	2.5	1.2--	0.19	263
G66	9	2.8	1.4-	0.48	213
G67	33	2.7	1.3--	0.24	240
G68	36	3.1	1.5--	0.26	190
G-I	236	2.8	1.2--	0.09	

SCOTLAND(1975-80)

S01	12	2.1	1.0--	0.31	309
S02	48	3.4	1.5--	0.23	190
S03	33	2.6	1.1--	0.22	288
S04	30	2.9	1.4--	0.28	213
S05	67	2.8	1.4--	0.19	213
S06	10	3.2	1.3-	0.50	240
S07	23	2.8	1.5--	0.34	190
S08	238	3.1	1.6--	0.11	172
S09	16	3.6	1.9	0.52	137
S10	1	1.8	1.0	0.95	309
S11	4	6.5	2.0	1.02	125
S12	3	3.3	0.9--	0.53	323
G-J	485	3.0	1.5--	0.07	

NORTHERN IRELAND

JE	40	2.4	1.3--	0.22	240
JN	15	1.6	1.0--	0.27	309
JS	6	0.9	0.4--	0.20	353
JW	18	2.9	1.7	0.42	160
G-K	79	2.0	1.1--	0.14	
G.0	4608	2.7	1.2--	0.02	

ITALIA (1975-79)

ABRUZZI

I66	34	4.4	2.1	0.37	115
I67	21	3.1	1.7	0.40	160
I68	24	3.3	2.1	0.45	115
I69	33	3.6	2.0	0.36	125
I-A	112	3.6	2.0-	0.20	

BASILICATA

I76	15	1.4	1.0--	0.27	309
I77	10	2.0	1.4-	0.48	213
I-B	25	1.6	1.2--	0.24	

CALABRIA

I78	28	1.5	1.1--	0.22	288
I79	37	2.0	1.5--	0.25	190
I80	22	1.5	0.9--	0.19	323
I-C	87	1.7	1.2--	0.13	

CAMPANIA

I61	32	1.7	1.4--	0.25	213
I62	22	3.0	1.9	0.42	137
I63	190	2.6	2.1	0.16	115
I64	19	1.7	0.9--	0.23	323
I65	58	2.3	1.6--	0.22	172
I-D	321	2.4	1.8--	0.10	

EMILIA-ROMAGNA

I33	22	3.0	1.4--	0.31	213
I34	46	4.5	1.8-	0.28	146
I35	31	3.0	1.5--	0.27	190
I36	46	3.1	1.5--	0.24	190
I37	81	3.3	1.5--	0.18	190
I38	31	3.1	1.4--	0.26	213
I39	32	3.5	1.6--	0.30	172
I40	59	4.0	2.2	0.30	101
I-E	348	3.4	1.6--	0.09	

FRIULI-VENEZIA GIULIA

I30	36	2.7	1.2--	0.21	263
I31	40	10.5	5.1++	0.86	13
I32	78	9.8	3.4+	0.42	43
I93	21	3.1	1.4--	0.33	213
I-F	175	5.4	2.3	0.19	

LAZIO

I56	37	5.6	3.1	0.53	49
I57	15	4.2	2.0	0.53	125
I58	350	3.7	2.5	0.14	76
I59	30	2.9	2.3	0.42	93
I60	24	2.1	1.3--	0.27	240
I-G	456	3.6	2.4	0.11	

LIGURIA

I08	19	3.2	1.5-	0.36	190
I09	48	6.1	2.6	0.41	71
I10	179	6.3	2.7	0.22	65
I11	39	6.1	2.6	0.44	71
I-H	285	5.9	2.5	0.16	

LOMBARDIA

I12	66	3.3	2.1	0.27	115
I13	60	3.1	1.8-	0.25	146
I14	14	3.2	2.2	0.61	101
I15	360	3.5	2.2-	0.12	101
I16	49	2.2	1.4--	0.21	213
I17	77	3.0	1.9-	0.23	137
I18	48	3.5	1.5--	0.23	190
I19	24	2.8	1.2--	0.26	263
I20	42	4.3	2.0	0.33	125
I-I	740	3.3	1.9--	0.07	

MARCHE

I41	21	2.5	1.3--	0.29	240
I42	42	3.8	1.8-	0.29	146
I43	21	2.8	1.6-	0.37	172
I44	11	1.2	0.7--	0.22	343
I-J	95	2.7	1.4--	0.15	

MOLISE

I70	21	3.5	1.6-	0.38	172
I94	5	2.1	1.4	0.65	213
I-K	26	3.1	1.6-	0.33	

PIEMONTE

I01	230	3.8	2.2	0.15	101
I02	37	3.5	1.4--	0.25	213
I03	70	5.3	2.6	0.34	71
I04	64	4.7	2.2	0.30	101
I05	27	4.8	2.1	0.44	115
I06	58	4.7	1.7--	0.25	160
I-L	486	4.2	2.1--	0.10	

PUGLIA

I71	46	2.7	1.8-	0.28	146
I72	74	2.0	1.5--	0.18	190
I73	33	2.4	1.8	0.33	146
I74	21	2.1	1.6-	0.36	172
I75	39	2.0	1.3--	0.22	240
I-M	213	2.2	1.6--	0.11	

SARDEGNA

I90	24	2.3	1.5--	0.33	190
I91	15	2.2	1.2--	0.34	263
I92	30	1.7	1.3--	0.25	240
I95	6	1.5	0.5--	0.22	351
I-N	75	1.9	1.3--	0.16	

SICILIA

I81	14	1.3	0.9--	0.26	323
I82	40	1.3	1.0--	0.17	309
I83	20	1.2	0.6--	0.13	347
I84	11	0.9	0.7--	0.21	343
I85	4	0.5	0.4--	0.20	353
I86	7	1.4	0.9--	0.36	323
I87	50	2.0	1.4--	0.21	213
I88	24	3.5	2.2	0.45	101
I89	24	2.5	1.7	0.36	160
I-O	194	1.6	1.1--	0.08	

TOSCANA

I45	16	3.0	1.3--	0.35	240
I46	52	5.2	2.1	0.32	115
I47	39	5.8	2.4	0.41	82
I48	125	4.0	1.8--	0.17	146
I49	52	5.9	2.7	0.39	65
I50	34	3.5	1.6--	0.28	172
I51	31	3.9	1.9	0.37	137
I52	19	2.9	1.0--	0.25	309
I53	19	3.4	1.6-	0.38	172
I-P	387	4.2	1.8--	0.10	

TRENTINO-ALTO ADIGE

I21	51	4.7	3.1	0.45	49
I22	65	5.8	2.9	0.39	60
I-Q	116	5.3	3.0+	0.29	

UMBRIA

I54	47	3.3	1.6--	0.24	172
I55	22	3.8	1.7	0.38	160
I-R	69	3.4	1.6--	0.20	

VALLE D'AOSTA

I07	8	2.8	1.5	0.55	190

VENETO

I23	81	4.2	2.4	0.28	82
I24	56	3.1	1.8-	0.26	146
I25	22	3.8	1.9	0.42	137
I26	70	3.9	2.2	0.28	101
I27	74	3.5	2.0	0.24	125
I28	67	3.3	2.0	0.26	125
I29	28	4.3	2.3	0.45	93
I-T	398	3.6	2.1--	0.11	
I.0	4616	3.2	1.8--	0.03	

IRELAND (1976-80)

CONNAUGHT

R07	19	4.7	3.5	0.85	41
R12	2	3.1	1.4	1.10	213
R16	18	6.5	3.3	0.87	45
R20	4	3.1	2.1	1.07	115
R21	6	4.5	2.8	1.17	62
R-A	49	4.8	3.0	0.46	

LEINSTER

R01	1	1.1	0.8-	0.76	339
R06	59	2.3	1.8--	0.24	146
R09	3	1.3	1.5	0.89	190
R10	3	1.8	1.3	0.72	240
R11	2	1.7	1.2	0.88	263
R14	1	1.4	0.8	0.82	339
R15	1	0.5	0.3--	0.32	355
R17	5	2.3	2.0	0.92	125
R19	2	1.5	1.3	0.94	240
R24	2	1.4	0.5--	0.35	351
R25	9	3.8	2.4	0.87	82
R26	3	1.4	0.6--	0.36	347
R-B	91	2.1	1.5--	0.17	

MUNSTER

R03	2	1.0	0.7--	0.58	343
R04	40	4.1	3.0	0.50	58
R08	5	1.7	1.2	0.61	263
R13	9	2.3	1.7	0.58	160
R22	13	4.0	2.7	0.78	65
R23	6	2.8	1.6	0.67	172
R-C	75	3.1	2.2	0.27	

ULSTER

R02	3	2.4	1.5	0.89	190
R05	6	2.0	1.7	0.76	160
R18	6	5.0	3.9	1.69	31
R-D	15	2.8	2.2	0.60	
R.0	230	2.7	2.0--	0.14	

LUXEMBOURG (1971-80)

LE	12	6.3	3.1	0.99	49
LN	8	3.0	1.2--	0.44	263
LS	58	4.3	2.2	0.31	101
L.0	78	4.3	2.1	0.26	

NEDERLAND (1976-80)

N01	118	8.6	4.5++	0.46	23
N02	120	8.4	4.2++	0.41	27
N03	80	7.8	4.5++	0.54	23
N04	187	7.5	4.6++	0.35	20
N05	310	7.4	4.4++	0.27	25
N06	134	6.0	3.5++	0.32	41
N07	360	6.0	3.1++	0.18	49
N08	471	6.1	3.1++	0.15	49
N09	46	5.4	2.8	0.45	62
N10	245	4.9	3.6++	0.24	37
N11	147	5.6	3.7++	0.32	35
N.0	2218	6.3	3.6++	0.08	

EEC-9

EEC	40320	5.0	2.4	0.01	

BELGIE-BELGIQUE (1971-78)

BRUSSEL-BRUXELLES					
B21	501	12.7	8.0+	0.37	114
VLAANDEREN					
B10	661	10.7	7.4	0.29	155
B29	316	8.8	6.1--	0.35	252
B30	463	10.9	7.6	0.37	144
B40	547	10.4	6.8	0.30	193
B70	152	5.5	5.5--	0.45	290
B-V	2139	9.7	6.9-	0.15	
WALLONIE					
B25	109	10.6	7.6	0.74	144
B50	594	11.6	7.8	0.33	126
B60	411	10.4	7.0	0.35	181
B80	115	13.3	8.6	0.83	72
B90	186	12.3	8.7+	0.65	69
B-W	1415	11.3	7.7+	0.21	
B.0	4055	10.5	7.3	0.12	

BR DEUTSCHLAND (1976-80)

BADEN-WURTTEMBERG					
D81	805	9.7	7.3	0.27	164
D82	653	11.5	8.4++	0.35	79
D83	387	8.8	6.4-	0.34	228
D84	328	9.1	7.2	0.42	170
D-A	2173	9.9	7.4	0.17	
BAYERN					
D91	918	10.5	7.7	0.26	135
D92	270	11.5	8.6++	0.55	72
D93	278	12.0	9.0++	0.56	50
D94	301	12.2	7.8	0.47	126
D95	417	11.6	7.8	0.40	126
D96	328	11.5	8.3+	0.48	90
D97	463	12.8	8.9++	0.43	61
D-B	2975	11.5	8.1++	0.16	
BERLIN(WEST)					
DB0	594	13.9	8.5++	0.38	77
BREMEN					
D40	172	10.5	6.5	0.53	221
HAMBURG					
D20	543	14.0	8.0+	0.37	114
HESSEN					
D64	1147	10.9	7.7+	0.24	135
D66	343	12.1	7.5	0.43	151
D-F	1490	11.2	7.6+	0.21	
NIEDERSACHSEN					
D31	366	9.4	6.1--	0.34	252
D32	499	10.3	6.6-	0.31	210
D33	376	10.7	7.1	0.39	177
D34	459	9.1	6.9	0.34	188
D-G	1700	9.8	6.7--	0.17	
NORDRHEIN-WESTFALEN					
D51	1310	10.6	8.1++	0.23	105
D53	874	9.3	7.6	0.26	144
D55	529	9.1	8.0+	0.36	114
D57	402	9.4	6.7	0.35	203
D59	874	9.9	7.6	0.27	144
D-H	3989	9.8	7.7++	0.13	
RHEINLAND-PFALZ					
D71	328	10.1	6.6	0.39	210
D72	127	11.3	8.1	0.75	105
D73	480	11.1	7.7	0.37	135
D-I	935	10.8	7.3	0.25	
SAARLAND					
DA0	233	9.1	6.3-	0.43	234
SCHLESWIG-HOLSTEIN					
D10	621	10.0	6.6-	0.28	210
D.0	15425	10.5	7.5++	0.06	

DANMARK (1971-80)

K15	1078	17.7	11.4++	0.35	6
K20	179	11.8	10.7++	0.81	12
K25	81	8.7	8.4	0.94	79
K30	186	13.7	8.4	0.64	79
K35	223	17.3	9.7++	0.69	29
K40	37	15.6	8.8	1.53	65
K42	314	14.2	8.2+	0.48	102
K50	180	14.7	9.9++	0.75	22
K55	139	13.4	9.6++	0.84	34
K60	225	14.3	9.3++	0.65	39
K65	133	10.4	7.4	0.67	155
K70	325	11.7	8.1	0.46	105
K76	135	11.8	6.9	0.62	188
K80	337	14.3	9.0++	0.51	50
K.0	3572	14.3	9.4++	0.16	

FRANCE (1971-78)

ALSACE					
F67	332	9.6	7.7	0.44	135
F68	225	9.0	7.4	0.52	155
F-A	557	9.4	7.6	0.33	
AQUITAINE					
F24	158	10.8	5.5--	0.47	290
F33	391	9.6	6.3--	0.33	234
F40	167	14.9	8.8+	0.72	65
F47	93	8.2	4.6--	0.51	314
F64	185	8.9	5.5--	0.42	290
F-B	994	10.1	6.1--	0.20	
AUVERGNE					
F03	181	12.2	6.4	0.51	228
F15	77	11.6	6.9	0.85	188
F43	111	13.8	7.3	0.74	164
F63	238	10.5	7.5	0.50	151
F-C	607	11.6	7.1	0.30	
BASSE-NORMANDIE					
F14	189	8.7	7.5	0.56	151
F50	154	8.8	6.8	0.57	193
F61	115	10.0	7.2	0.69	170
F-D	458	9.0	7.2	0.34	
BOURGOGNE					
F21	155	8.6	6.2-	0.52	242
F58	145	14.8	8.4	0.78	79
F71	235	10.5	6.3-	0.44	234
F89	141	11.9	6.4	0.59	228
F-E	676	10.9	6.7-	0.27	
BRETAGNE					
F22	182	8.9	5.9--	0.45	266
F29	373	12.0	8.1+	0.43	105
F35	161	6.0	4.6--	0.37	314
F56	183	8.3	6.2-	0.47	242
F-F	899	8.9	6.3--	0.22	
CENTRE					
F18	156	12.4	6.9	0.59	188
F28	121	9.0	6.6	0.62	210
F36	116	11.9	6.0-	0.61	258
F37	158	8.5	5.8--	0.48	273
F41	105	9.5	5.4--	0.57	296
F45	178	9.2	6.1-	0.48	252
F-G	834	9.8	6.1--	0.23	
CHAMPAGNE-ARDENNE					
F08	97	7.8	5.8-	0.62	273
F10	85	7.6	5.0--	0.57	306
F51	148	7.0	5.9--	0.50	266
F52	59	6.9	5.1--	0.69	303
F-H	389	7.3	5.5--	0.29	
CORSE					
F20	71	7.4	4.6--	0.57	314
FRANCHE-COMTE					
F25	146	7.8	7.4	0.63	155
F39	85	8.9	5.8-	0.66	273
F70	85	9.7	6.1	0.69	252
F90	36	7.0	6.2	1.05	242
F-J	352	8.4	6.5	0.36	
HAUTE-NORMANDIE					
F27	165	9.9	7.7	0.62	135
F76	454	9.9	8.1+	0.39	105
F-K	619	9.9	8.0+	0.33	
ILE-DE-FRANCE					
F75	916	10.8	6.5--	0.22	221
F77	224	7.4	6.0--	0.42	258
F78	240	5.6	5.8--	0.38	273
F91	223	6.1	6.7	0.46	203
F92	453	8.1	6.5-	0.31	221
F93	401	7.6	7.2	0.37	170
F94	364	7.7	6.8	0.36	193
F95	215	6.4	6.5	0.45	221
F-L	3036	7.9	6.5--	0.12	
LANGUEDOC-ROUSSILLON					
F11	128	12.3	5.9-	0.57	266
F30	194	10.1	6.2-	0.46	242
F34	250	10.0	6.1--	0.41	252
F48	37	12.3	6.2	1.09	242
F66	130	11.2	5.6--	0.52	283
F-M	739	10.7	6.0--	0.23	
LIMOUSIN					
F19	85	9.0	4.5--	0.53	318
F23	83	14.5	6.6	0.81	210
F87	146	10.7	5.6--	0.49	283
F-N	314	10.9	5.4--	0.33	
LORRAINE					
F54	210	7.4	6.0--	0.43	258
F55	68	8.5	6.0	0.77	258
F57	285	7.0	6.6	0.40	210
F88	134	8.6	6.4	0.58	228
F-O	697	7.5	6.3--	0.24	
MIDI-PYRENEES					
F09	57	10.4	5.1--	0.75	303
F12	117	10.8	5.5--	0.54	290
F31	280	9.3	6.4-	0.39	228
F32	67	9.6	5.4--	0.70	296
F46	72	12.2	6.7	0.84	203
F65	92	10.4	6.2	0.68	242
F81	112	8.5	4.6--	0.46	314
F82	74	10.3	5.4--	0.67	296
F-P	871	9.8	5.7--	0.20	
NORD-PAS-DE-CALAIS					
F59	864	8.8	7.3	0.26	164
F62	453	8.3	6.8	0.32	193
F-Q	1317	8.6	7.1	0.20	
PAYS DE LA LOIRE					
F44	221	6.1	5.0--	0.34	306
F49	186	7.6	5.9--	0.45	266
F53	78	7.7	5.8-	0.67	273
F72	153	8.0	5.6--	0.47	283
F85	167	9.6	6.6	0.53	210
F-R	805	7.5	5.7--	0.21	
PICARDIE					
F02	195	9.2	6.8	0.51	193
F60	188	7.7	6.7	0.51	203
F80	169	8.0	5.8--	0.47	273
F-S	552	8.3	6.4--	0.29	
POITOU-CHARENTES					
F16	115	8.7	5.0--	0.49	306
F17	207	10.7	6.3-	0.46	234
F79	128	9.6	5.9-	0.55	266
F86	137	9.8	6.0-	0.54	258
F-T	587	9.8	5.8--	0.25	
PROVENCE-ALPES-COTE D'AZUR					
F04	38	8.5	4.5--	0.78	318
F05	47	12.1	7.5	1.14	151
F06	250	8.1	4.0--	0.28	327
F13	527	8.2	5.9--	0.26	266
F83	275	11.2	6.7	0.42	203
F84	131	8.5	5.6--	0.51	283
F-U	1268	8.9	5.5--	0.16	
RHONE-ALPES					
F01	151	10.0	6.8	0.58	193
F07	114	11.4	6.8	0.68	193
F26	156	11.1	7.0	0.59	181
F38	275	8.1	6.7	0.41	203
F42	316	10.8	7.4	0.43	155
F69	503	9.0	7.7	0.35	135
F73	116	9.5	7.2	0.68	170
F74	138	7.7	6.6	0.58	210
F-V	1769	9.4	7.2	0.17	
F.0	18411	8.9	6.4--	0.05	

UNITED KINGDOM (1976-80)

EAST ANGLIA					
G25	172	10.0	7.4	0.58	155
G46	242	12.1	7.2	0.48	170
G55	224	12.6	8.3	0.57	90
G-A	638	11.6	7.6	0.31	
EAST MIDLANDS					
G30	311	11.8	7.6	0.44	144
G44	217	8.8	6.1-	0.43	252
G45	225	14.3	9.2++	0.63	42
G47	168	11.0	7.9	0.62	123
G50	377	13.2	9.0++	0.47	50
G-B	1298	11.7	7.9++	0.22	
NORTHERN					
G14	409	12.1	8.3+	0.42	90
G27	192	11.5	9.0++	0.66	50
G29	175	12.7	8.4	0.65	79
G33	244	13.7	9.1++	0.60	46
G48	136	16.0	10.2++	0.90	18
G-C	1156	12.7	8.8++	0.26	
NORTH-WEST					
G11	998	12.9	9.0++	0.29	50
G12	600	13.4	9.6++	0.40	34
G26	257	9.5	7.1	0.46	177
G43	483	12.3	7.4	0.35	155
G-D	2338	12.4	8.5++	0.18	

SOUTH-EAST					
G01	2609	13.1	8.2++	0.16	102
G22	154	10.4	8.3	0.68	90
G23	202	10.1	8.0	0.57	114
G24	141	9.0	7.0	0.59	181
G34	369	20.7	9.0++	0.51	50
G35	485	11.6	7.8	0.36	126
G37	471	10.7	7.8	0.37	126
G39	299	10.8	8.3+	0.49	90
G41	55	17.1	7.9	1.13	123
G42	541	12.8	8.1+	0.36	105
G51	137	8.2	7.0	0.63	181
G56	351	12.1	8.0	0.44	114
G58	268	15.1	8.0	0.52	114
G-E	6082	12.4	8.1++	0.11	

SOUTH-WEST					
G21	337	12.6	8.1+	0.45	105
G28	174	14.6	8.3	0.66	90
G31	418	15.2	8.0	0.41	114
G32	281	17.0	8.3+	0.53	90
G36	165	11.4	7.3	0.58	164
G53	155	12.9	7.6	0.64	144
G59	176	11.4	8.3	0.64	90
G-F	1706	13.7	8.0++	0.20	

WEST MIDLANDS					
G15	952	11.8	8.3++	0.27	90
G38	184	10.3	7.0	0.53	181
G52	122	11.4	7.8	0.73	126
G54	332	11.3	8.6++	0.48	72
G57	148	10.7	7.8	0.66	126
G-G	1738	11.4	8.1++	0.20	

YORKSHIRE AND HUMBERSIDE					
G13	471	12.3	8.4++	0.40	79
G16	734	12.2	8.1++	0.31	105
G40	313	12.7	9.0++	0.52	50
G49	273	14.1	8.8++	0.55	65
G-H	1791	12.6	8.4++	0.20	

WALES					
G61	147	13.3	8.2	0.70	102
G62	134	14.3	8.3	0.74	90
G63	168	13.1	8.9+	0.70	61
G64	114	17.4	10.5++	1.03	15
G65	209	13.3	9.7++	0.69	29
G66	47	14.8	8.8	1.35	65
G67	177	15.8	10.8++	0.83	11
G68	141	13.3	8.4	0.73	79
G-I	1137	14.1	9.2++	0.28	

SCOTLAND(1975-80)					
S01	67	12.0	8.4	1.05	79
S02	151	11.3	7.8	0.65	126
S03	168	14.5	9.8++	0.78	25
S04	125	12.5	9.3+	0.85	39
S05	277	12.9	9.0++	0.56	50
S06	52	18.1	9.9	1.41	22
S07	83	10.4	7.4	0.83	155
S08	830	11.7	8.7++	0.31	69
S09	47	11.2	7.3	1.10	164
S10	9	16.9	12.1	4.14	4
S11	3	4.8	3.1-	1.89	340
S12	18	20.5	11.1	2.82	9
G-J	1830	12.2	8.7++	0.21	

NORTHERN IRELAND					
JE	195	11.9	9.9++	0.73	22
JN	94	10.4	8.9	0.96	61
JS	51	7.7	6.6	0.97	210
JW	65	10.8	9.0	1.15	50
G-K	405	10.6	8.9++	0.46	
G.0	20119	12.4	8.3++	0.06	

ITALIA (1975-79)

ABRUZZI					
I66	52	7.1	4.5--	0.65	318
I67	38	5.7	3.9--	0.65	328
I68	42	6.0	4.4--	0.69	321
I69	48	5.4	3.7--	0.55	330
I-A	180	6.0	4.1--	0.31	

BASILICATA					
I76	35	3.4	2.7--	0.46	346
I77	15	3.0	2.5--	0.65	347
I-B	50	3.3	2.6--	0.38	

CALABRIA					
I78	70	3.9	3.5--	0.42	333
I79	78	4.3	3.6--	0.42	331
I80	57	3.9	3.1--	0.42	340
I-C	205	4.0	3.4--	0.24	

CAMPANIA					
I61	41	2.3	2.2--	0.34	353
I62	26	3.6	2.5--	0.51	347
I63	207	3.0	3.2--	0.22	338
I64	31	2.9	2.2--	0.41	353
I65	71	2.9	2.4--	0.29	351
I-D	376	2.9	2.7--	0.14	

EMILIA-ROMAGNA					
I33	82	11.8	6.6	0.74	210
I34	156	16.0	9.0+	0.74	50
I35	129	13.0	8.6	0.78	72
I36	134	9.4	6.5	0.58	221
I37	280	12.4	7.7	0.47	135
I38	116	12.4	7.8	0.73	126
I39	102	11.6	7.2	0.72	170
I40	158	10.9	7.7	0.62	135
I-E	1157	12.0	7.6	0.23	

FRIULI-VENEZIA GIULIA					
I30	197	15.3	9.8++	0.71	25
I31	47	13.4	8.5	1.25	77
I32	110	15.8	8.3	0.83	90
I93	105	16.1	11.4++	1.13	6
I-F	459	15.4	9.5++	0.46	

LAZIO					
I56	38	5.8	3.4--	0.57	334
I57	27	7.6	4.4--	0.90	321
I58	623	7.0	6.3--	0.26	234
I59	55	5.3	4.9--	0.67	310
I60	58	5.2	3.6--	0.48	331
I-G	801	6.6	5.5--	0.20	

LIGURIA					
I08	54	9.7	5.6-	0.80	283
I09	71	9.6	5.4--	0.66	296
I10	254	9.8	5.7--	0.37	281
I11	61	10.3	5.8	0.77	273
I-H	440	9.9	5.6--	0.28	

LOMBARDIA					
I12	176	9.4	8.1	0.63	105
I13	188	10.2	8.3	0.62	90
I14	27	6.3	5.3	1.02	301
I15	1047	10.7	9.2++	0.29	42
I16	241	11.3	10.6++	0.69	13
I17	259	10.6	9.5++	0.60	36
I18	161	12.7	7.3	0.59	164
I19	142	17.5	11.5++	0.99	5
I20	83	9.0	5.2--	0.59	302
I-I	2324	10.8	8.8++	0.19	

MARCHE					
I41	70	8.6	5.5-	0.68	290
I42	98	9.5	6.2	0.64	242
I43	63	8.9	5.6-	0.73	283
I44	50	5.9	4.1--	0.58	326
I-J	281	8.3	5.4--	0.33	

MOLISE					
I70	28	4.9	3.0--	0.58	342
I94	10	4.3	2.3--	0.75	352
I-K	38	4.7	2.8--	0.47	

PIEMONTE					
I01	457	7.8	6.4--	0.31	228
I02	107	11.0	6.2	0.62	242
I03	129	10.5	6.8	0.61	193
I04	117	8.6	5.0--	0.48	306
I05	58	10.8	5.5-	0.77	290
I06	136	11.7	6.3	0.58	234
I-L	1004	9.1	6.1--	0.20	

PUGLIA					
I71	66	3.9	3.3--	0.41	337
I72	155	4.4	3.8--	0.31	329
I73	45	3.3	3.2--	0.48	338
I74	33	3.5	3.0--	0.53	342
I75	74	4.1	3.4--	0.40	334
I-M	373	4.0	3.5--	0.18	

SARDEGNA					
I90	106	10.1	7.6	0.77	144
I91	52	7.6	4.7--	0.71	312
I92	120	6.8	6.3	0.58	234
I95	33	8.5	4.7--	0.89	312
I-N	311	8.0	6.2--	0.36	

SICILIA					
I81	50	4.8	3.4--	0.50	334
I82	104	3.6	2.8--	0.28	345
I83	46	2.8	2.1--	0.32	355
I84	47	3.9	2.9--	0.44	344
I85	23	3.2	2.5--	0.53	347
I86	18	3.6	2.5--	0.61	347
I87	128	5.3	4.4--	0.40	321
I88	37	5.6	4.2--	0.72	324
I89	50	5.2	4.2--	0.61	324
I-O	503	4.2	3.2--	0.15	

TOSCANA					
I45	42	8.5	5.4-	0.85	296
I46	108	11.6	7.4	0.74	155
I47	74	11.6	6.8	0.82	193
I48	283	9.8	6.0--	0.37	258
I49	84	10.0	6.5	0.73	221
I50	109	11.6	6.9	0.69	188
I51	82	10.6	6.3	0.71	234
I52	73	11.5	6.0	0.73	258
I53	52	9.4	5.6-	0.80	283
I-P	907	10.5	6.3--	0.22	

TRENTINO-ALTO ADIGE					
I21	111	10.5	9.1+	0.87	46
I22	136	12.7	9.0+	0.79	50
I-Q	247	11.6	9.0++	0.59	

UMBRIA					
I54	137	9.8	6.2-	0.53	242
I55	55	9.8	5.7	0.78	281
I-R	192	9.8	6.0--	0.44	

VALLE D'AOSTA					
I07	21	7.4	5.1	1.12	303

VENETO					
I23	172	9.2	7.0	0.54	181
I24	142	8.2	6.8	0.57	193
I25	76	14.1	9.1	1.06	46
I26	199	11.6	9.2++	0.67	42
I27	239	11.7	9.7++	0.64	29
I28	156	8.0	6.7	0.54	203
I29	78	12.6	8.4	0.97	79
I-T	1062	10.1	8.0++	0.25	
I.0	10931	8.0	5.9--	0.06	

IRELAND (1976-80)

CONNAUGHT					
R07	46	10.6	6.6	1.03	210
R12	15	20.2	10.6	2.94	13
R16	32	10.9	5.8	1.12	273
R20	21	14.7	8.4	2.11	79
R21	18	12.9	7.7	1.95	135
R-A	132	12.2	7.1	0.66	

LEINSTER					
R01	16	16.2	15.8+	4.07	1
R06	206	8.7	9.7++	0.68	29
R09	21	8.3	9.8	2.17	25
R10	28	15.7	12.2+	2.38	2
R11	21	16.0	12.2	2.74	2
R14	9	11.2	5.9	2.01	266
R15	20	9.3	8.9	2.02	61
R17	15	6.4	6.2	1.63	242
R19	12	8.1	6.0	1.78	258
R24	16	10.5	7.9	2.06	123
R25	24	9.8	7.2	1.55	170
R26	15	7.1	6.5	1.71	221
R-B	403	9.3	9.2++	0.46	

MUNSTER					
R03	34	15.5	10.5	1.86	15
R04	111	11.1	9.1+	0.89	46
R08	49	15.8	10.2	1.53	18
R13	49	12.4	10.3+	1.50	17
R22	38	11.0	8.0	1.33	114
R23	28	12.7	11.0	2.13	10
R-C	309	12.4	9.5++	0.55	

ULSTER					
R02	23	16.3	9.7	2.07	29
R05	25	8.0	4.8-	1.01	311
R18	16	12.2	8.7	2.33	69
R-D	64	10.9	6.8	0.90	
R.0	908	10.7	8.7++	0.30	

LUXEMBOURG (1971-80)

LE	28	15.4	10.1	1.99	21
LN	42	15.9	9.4	1.51	37
LS	116	9.1	7.0	0.66	181
L.0	186	10.8	7.7	0.58	

NEDERLAND (1976-80)

N01	158	11.6	8.4	0.69	79
N02	190	13.3	9.3++	0.71	39
N03	98	9.5	7.1	0.74	177
N04	249	9.9	8.0	0.52	114
N05	473	11.4	9.4++	0.44	37
N06	284	13.1	11.2++	0.67	8
N07	767	13.2	10.2++	0.37	18
N08	992	13.2	9.8++	0.32	25
N09	110	13.0	8.6	0.85	72
N10	481	9.5	9.2++	0.43	42
N11	212	8.0	7.1	0.49	177
N.0	4014	11.6	9.3++	0.15	

EEC-9

EEC	77621	10.2	7.2	0.03	

BELGIE-BELGIQUE (1971-78)

BRUSSEL-BRUXELLES					
B21	428	9.6	3.8-	0.21	190
VLAANDEREN					
B10	528	8.4	4.4	0.20	150
B29	248	6.8	3.6-	0.24	208
B30	385	8.9	4.5	0.25	140
B40	453	8.4	4.1	0.21	176
B70	117	4.3	3.5	0.34	224
B-V	1731	7.7	4.1	0.11	
WALLONIE					
B25	73	6.8	3.2-	0.41	250
B50	498	9.1	4.2	0.21	167
B60	334	7.9	3.6--	0.22	208
B80	88	9.8	4.6	0.54	129
B90	168	10.5	4.7	0.40	120
B-W	1161	8.8	4.0	0.13	
B.0	3320	8.3	4.0-	0.08	

BR DEUTSCHLAND (1976-80)

BADEN-WURTTEMBERG					
D81	845	9.5	4.7++	0.18	120
D82	665	10.7	4.9++	0.21	97
D83	458	9.5	4.6	0.23	129
D84	348	9.0	4.6	0.27	129
D-A	2316	9.7	4.7++	0.11	
BAYERN					
D91	939	10.0	4.6+	0.17	129
D92	298	11.4	5.6++	0.35	39
D93	261	10.3	4.8	0.32	109
D94	292	10.4	4.2	0.27	167
D95	377	9.5	4.0	0.23	184
D96	318	10.3	4.6	0.28	129
D97	438	11.0	4.9++	0.26	97
D-B	2923	10.3	4.6++	0.09	
BERLIN(WEST)					
DB0	876	16.5	5.3++	0.22	60
BREMEN					
D40	180	9.7	4.0	0.34	184
HAMBURG					
D20	627	14.0	5.0++	0.23	86
HESSEN					
D64	1255	11.1	4.9++	0.15	97
D66	343	11.0	4.5	0.28	140
D-F	1598	11.1	4.8++	0.13	
NIEDERSACHSEN					
D31	481	11.2	4.8+	0.25	109
D32	630	11.6	4.6+	0.21	129
D33	368	10.0	4.4	0.25	150
D34	491	9.0	4.5	0.22	140
D-G	1970	10.4	4.6++	0.12	
NORDRHEIN-WESTFALEN					
D51	1404	10.2	4.8++	0.14	109
D53	929	9.2	4.7++	0.17	120
D55	486	7.8	4.3	0.21	162
D57	444	9.4	4.4	0.22	150
D59	951	9.8	4.8++	0.17	109
D-H	4214	9.5	4.7++	0.08	
RHEINLAND-PFALZ					
D71	383	10.8	4.7+	0.27	120
D72	125	10.1	4.3	0.41	162
D73	436	9.2	4.2	0.22	167
D-I	944	9.9	4.4	0.16	
SAARLAND					
DA0	235	8.3	3.7	0.26	200
SCHLESWIG-HOLSTEIN					
D10	767	11.4	4.8++	0.19	109
D.0	16650	10.4	4.7++	0.04	

DANMARK (1971-80)

K15	1132	17.0	7.3++	0.24	5
K20	148	9.8	6.9++	0.60	12
K25	60	6.6	5.3	0.71	60
K30	147	11.0	5.5++	0.49	46
K35	177	13.9	6.4++	0.52	20
K40	24	10.2	5.2	1.17	76
K42	279	12.5	6.2++	0.41	25
K50	111	9.1	4.8	0.49	109
K55	101	9.9	6.2++	0.65	25
K60	185	11.6	6.4++	0.50	20
K65	88	7.0	4.5	0.50	140
K70	323	11.4	6.5++	0.38	17
K76	111	9.9	5.0	0.51	86
K80	280	11.9	6.5++	0.41	17
K.0	3166	12.4	6.4++	0.12	

FRANCE (1971-78)

ALSACE					
F67	212	5.9	3.0--	0.22	268
F68	178	6.9	3.6-	0.30	208
F-A	390	6.3	3.2--	0.18	
AQUITAINE					
F24	131	8.6	3.0--	0.31	268
F33	299	6.8	2.7--	0.18	293
F40	89	7.6	2.7--	0.34	293
F47	90	7.5	2.9--	0.35	276
F64	171	7.7	3.2--	0.28	250
F-B	780	7.4	2.9--	0.12	
AUVERGNE					
F03	178	11.4	3.7	0.34	200
F15	80	11.9	4.8	0.62	109
F43	96	11.4	3.8	0.45	190
F63	198	8.4	3.8	0.31	190
F-C	552	10.1	3.9	0.20	
BASSE-NORMANDIE					
F14	133	5.8	3.0--	0.29	268
F50	113	6.1	2.7--	0.28	293
F61	88	7.3	3.6	0.44	208
F-D	334	6.2	3.0--	0.19	
BOURGOGNE					
F21	140	7.6	3.8	0.36	190
F58	108	10.7	3.3-	0.39	245
F71	174	7.5	3.0--	0.26	268
F89	124	10.2	3.3-	0.37	245
F-E	546	8.5	3.3--	0.17	
BRETAGNE					
F22	136	6.3	2.5--	0.24	305
F29	249	7.5	3.4--	0.24	233
F35	135	4.6	2.5--	0.24	305
F56	120	5.2	2.3--	0.23	316
F-F	640	6.0	2.7--	0.12	
CENTRE					
F18	126	9.8	3.6	0.38	208
F28	96	7.2	3.8	0.44	190
F36	94	9.4	3.0--	0.37	268
F37	145	7.4	3.6	0.35	208
F41	88	7.6	2.8--	0.37	284
F45	147	7.4	3.5-	0.33	224
F-G	696	8.0	3.4--	0.15	
CHAMPAGNE-ARDENNE					
F08	66	5.3	2.5--	0.35	305
F10	97	8.4	3.3-	0.39	245
F51	113	5.3	2.8--	0.29	284
F52	53	6.2	2.6--	0.39	300
F-H	329	6.1	2.8--	0.18	
CORSE					
F20	54	6.3	2.2--	0.35	320
FRANCHE-COMTE					
F25	93	4.9	3.2--	0.35	250
F39	66	6.8	2.8--	0.39	284
F70	52	5.8	2.3--	0.37	316
F90	26	5.1	2.5--	0.56	305
F-J	237	5.5	2.8--	0.20	
HAUTE-NORMANDIE					
F27	109	6.4	3.6	0.39	208
F76	326	6.8	3.7-	0.23	200
F-K	435	6.7	3.7--	0.20	
ILE-DE-FRANCE					
F75	876	8.9	3.4--	0.13	233
F77	170	5.6	3.2--	0.28	250
F78	183	4.2	2.8--	0.23	284
F91	187	5.0	3.6-	0.29	208
F92	391	6.6	3.5--	0.19	224
F93	240	4.5	2.9--	0.20	276
F94	306	6.2	3.5--	0.22	224
F95	157	4.6	3.1--	0.27	260
F-L	2510	6.2	3.3--	0.07	
LANGUEDOC-ROUSSILLON					
F11	84	7.5	2.5--	0.33	305
F30	157	7.7	3.2--	0.29	250
F34	185	6.9	2.5--	0.21	305
F48	33	10.9	4.3	0.96	162
F66	97	7.8	2.9--	0.34	276
F-M	556	7.5	2.8--	0.14	
LIMOUSIN					
F19	88	8.9	2.9--	0.37	276
F23	67	11.1	3.4	0.51	233
F87	107	7.4	2.6--	0.31	300
F-N	262	8.6	2.9--	0.22	
LORRAINE					
F54	149	5.1	2.8--	0.25	284
F55	56	6.8	3.6	0.56	208
F57	182	4.6	2.9--	0.23	276
F88	89	5.5	2.6--	0.32	300
F-O	476	5.1	2.8--	0.14	
MIDI-PYRENEES					
F09	38	6.8	2.1--	0.41	324
F12	91	8.0	3.1--	0.38	260
F31	201	6.3	3.1--	0.24	260
F32	52	7.4	2.6--	0.42	300
F46	58	9.5	2.9--	0.45	276
F65	66	7.1	2.7--	0.38	293
F81	95	6.9	2.7--	0.32	293
F82	46	6.1	2.1--	0.35	324
F-P	647	7.0	2.8--	0.13	
NORD-PAS-DE-CALAIS					
F59	653	6.4	3.5--	0.15	224
F62	403	7.0	3.7-	0.20	200
F-Q	1056	6.6	3.6--	0.12	
PAYS DE LA LOIRE					
F44	214	5.6	2.7--	0.21	293
F49	170	6.5	3.1--	0.28	260
F53	70	6.5	3.0--	0.41	268
F72	132	6.5	3.1--	0.31	260
F85	140	7.6	3.3--	0.32	245
F-R	726	6.4	3.0--	0.13	
PICARDIE					
F02	147	6.9	3.4--	0.32	233
F60	149	6.1	3.5-	0.33	224
F80	154	7.0	3.4-	0.31	233
F-S	450	6.6	3.4--	0.19	
POITOU-CHARENTES					
F16	75	5.4	2.0--	0.27	330
F17	169	8.3	3.6	0.32	208
F79	93	6.9	2.8--	0.33	284
F86	119	8.2	3.4-	0.37	233
F-T	456	7.3	3.0--	0.16	
PROVENCE-ALPES-COTE D'AZUR					
F04	24	5.4	2.0--	0.44	330
F05	23	5.9	2.9	0.70	276
F06	233	6.8	2.3--	0.18	316
F13	401	6.0	2.9--	0.16	276
F83	202	7.9	3.2--	0.25	250
F84	94	5.9	2.8--	0.33	284
F-U	977	6.5	2.8--	0.10	
RHONE-ALPES					
F01	120	8.0	4.1	0.43	176
F07	110	10.5	3.6	0.39	208
F26	131	8.9	3.8	0.37	190
F38	226	6.5	3.4--	0.25	233
F42	249	8.1	3.5--	0.25	224
F69	357	6.1	3.1--	0.18	260
F73	84	6.8	3.3-	0.41	245
F74	102	5.7	3.4-	0.36	233
F-V	1379	7.1	3.4--	0.10	
F.0	14488	6.7	3.1--	0.03	

UNITED KINGDOM (1976-80)

EAST ANGLIA					
G25	166	9.8	5.2+	0.44	76
G46	249	12.0	5.3++	0.38	60
G55	207	11.7	5.0+	0.39	86
G-A	622	11.2	5.2++	0.23	
EAST MIDLANDS					
G30	316	11.5	5.3++	0.32	60
G44	240	9.4	4.6	0.32	129
G45	180	11.2	5.4++	0.44	53
G47	146	9.3	4.9	0.43	97
G50	351	11.8	5.8++	0.33	34
G-B	1233	10.8	5.2++	0.16	
NORTHERN					
G14	374	10.3	4.9+	0.27	97
G27	142	8.2	4.9	0.44	97
G29	178	12.2	5.6++	0.47	39
G33	183	9.9	4.8	0.38	109
G48	92	10.4	4.7	0.54	120
G-C	969	10.1	5.0++	0.17	
NORTH-WEST					
G11	899	10.9	5.2++	0.19	76
G12	567	11.7	5.5++	0.25	46
G26	230	8.2	4.2	0.30	167
G43	526	12.3	4.9++	0.24	97
G-D	2222	11.0	5.1++	0.12	

SOUTH-EAST

G01	2378	10.9	4.8++	0.11	109
G22	115	7.8	4.7	0.47	120
G23	184	9.1	5.3++	0.41	60
G24	139	8.9	5.3+	0.48	60
G34	370	17.3	5.3++	0.33	60
G35	439	10.0	4.9++	0.25	97
G37	424	9.8	4.6	0.25	129
G39	266	9.2	5.1++	0.33	80
G41	67	18.5	6.8++	0.94	13
G42	510	11.4	5.1++	0.25	80
G51	162	10.3	5.6++	0.47	39
G56	339	11.1	5.1++	0.30	80
G58	288	14.3	5.0+	0.35	86
G-E	5681	10.9	5.0++	0.07	

SOUTH-WEST

G21	309	10.8	4.9+	0.31	97
G28	145	11.2	4.7	0.45	120
G31	421	14.4	5.4++	0.31	53
G32	254	13.7	4.4	0.32	150
G36	177	11.7	5.3++	0.44	60
G53	146	11.5	4.4	0.41	150
G59	152	9.9	5.3+	0.46	60
G-F	1604	12.1	5.0++	0.14	

WEST MIDLANDS

G15	820	9.9	5.0++	0.19	86
G38	198	10.7	5.0+	0.38	86
G52	114	10.3	4.9	0.50	97
G54	296	9.8	5.3++	0.33	60
G57	129	9.1	4.5	0.43	140
G-G	1557	9.9	5.0++	0.14	

YORKSHIRE AND HUMBERSIDE

G13	351	8.8	4.3	0.25	162
G16	726	11.3	5.3++	0.22	60
G40	291	11.1	5.5++	0.35	46
G49	268	13.4	5.5++	0.37	46
G-H	1636	10.9	5.1++	0.14	

WALES

G61	129	10.9	4.5	0.45	140
G62	116	11.5	5.0	0.51	86
G63	140	10.4	5.3+	0.48	60
G64	74	10.5	3.9	0.50	188
G65	146	8.8	4.6	0.41	129
G66	30	9.5	4.4	0.87	150
G67	136	11.3	5.2+	0.50	76
G68	158	13.8	6.6++	0.56	15
G-I	929	10.8	5.0++	0.18	

SCOTLAND (1975-80)

S01	62	10.8	5.5	0.76	46
S02	178	12.5	5.8++	0.47	34
S03	171	13.6	5.8++	0.49	34
S04	124	11.9	6.1++	0.59	28
S05	281	11.9	5.6++	0.37	39
S06	43	13.8	5.5	0.92	46
S07	84	10.2	6.1++	0.70	28
S08	814	10.6	5.6++	0.21	39
S09	46	10.5	4.6	0.75	129
S10	9	16.5	7.2	2.56	6
S11	2	3.3	1.0--	0.75	355
S12	15	16.6	5.4	1.65	53
G-J	1829	11.3	5.6++	0.14	

NORTHERN IRELAND

JE	171	10.2	5.9++	0.48	32
JN	80	8.7	4.7	0.57	120
JS	40	5.9	4.1	0.68	176
JW	68	11.1	7.0++	0.90	9
G-K	359	9.2	5.5++	0.31	
G.0	18641	10.9	5.1++	0.04	

ITALIA (1975-79)

ABRUZZI

I66	34	4.4	2.2--	0.40	320
I67	39	5.8	3.0-	0.51	268
I68	27	3.7	2.1--	0.42	324
I69	40	4.3	2.2--	0.36	320
I-A	140	4.5	2.3--	0.21	

BASILICATA

I76	29	2.8	1.8--	0.35	340
I77	9	1.8	1.3--	0.43	352
I-B	38	2.5	1.6--	0.28	

CALABRIA

I78	46	2.5	1.6--	0.25	346
I79	59	3.2	1.9--	0.27	334
I80	61	4.1	2.5--	0.34	305
I-C	166	3.2	2.0--	0.16	

CAMPANIA

I61	38	2.1	1.6--	0.26	346
I62	26	3.5	2.1--	0.44	324
I63	162	2.2	1.8--	0.15	340
I64	33	3.0	1.9--	0.36	334
I65	50	2.0	1.3--	0.20	352
I-D	309	2.3	1.7--	0.10	

EMILIA-ROMAGNA

I33	64	8.8	4.2	0.62	167
I34	105	10.2	4.2	0.44	167
I35	77	7.5	3.7	0.44	200
I36	110	7.5	3.8	0.38	190
I37	226	9.3	4.4	0.30	150
I38	107	10.7	5.0	0.51	86
I39	71	7.7	3.6	0.46	208
I40	99	6.6	3.7	0.39	200
I-E	859	8.5	4.1	0.15	

FRIULI-VENEZIA GIULIA

I30	157	11.6	5.3+	0.46	60
I31	46	12.0	5.1	0.80	80
I32	103	12.9	5.0	0.62	86
I93	78	11.3	6.0+	0.74	31
I-F	384	11.9	5.3++	0.30	

LAZIO

I56	32	4.8	2.4--	0.45	312
I57	14	3.9	1.9--	0.54	334
I58	502	5.3	3.6--	0.17	208
I59	24	2.3	1.8--	0.38	340
I60	35	3.1	1.8--	0.33	340
I-G	607	4.8	3.1--	0.13	

LIGURIA

I08	60	10.0	4.2	0.59	167
I09	68	8.6	3.6	0.46	208
I10	252	8.9	3.8	0.26	190
I11	53	8.3	3.2	0.50	250
I-H	433	8.9	3.8-	0.19	

LOMBARDIA

I12	129	6.5	4.0	0.37	184
I13	152	7.8	4.5	0.39	140
I14	31	7.1	4.1	0.78	176
I15	791	7.6	4.7++	0.17	120
I16	155	7.0	4.5	0.38	140
I17	211	8.3	5.0+	0.36	86
I18	134	9.9	4.1	0.39	176
I19	93	10.8	5.3	0.58	60
I20	80	8.2	3.4	0.42	233
I-I	1776	7.8	4.5++	0.11	

MARCHE

I41	47	5.7	3.0-	0.47	268
I42	70	6.4	3.2-	0.41	250
I43	36	4.9	2.4--	0.43	312
I44	27	3.0	1.5--	0.31	350
I-J	180	5.1	2.6--	0.20	

MOLISE

I70	18	3.0	1.3--	0.33	352
I94	9	3.7	1.6--	0.56	346
I-K	27	3.2	1.4--	0.29	

PIEMONTE

I01	410	6.7	4.0	0.20	184
I02	78	7.4	2.8--	0.34	284
I03	93	7.1	3.1--	0.34	260
I04	83	6.0	2.6--	0.31	300
I05	52	9.2	3.8	0.59	190
I06	122	9.9	3.4-	0.34	233
I-L	838	7.2	3.5--	0.13	

PUGLIA

I71	50	2.9	2.0--	0.30	330
I72	118	3.3	2.4--	0.23	312
I73	39	2.8	2.2--	0.36	320
I74	26	2.6	1.9--	0.38	334
I75	61	3.2	2.1--	0.28	324
I-M	294	3.0	2.2--	0.13	

SARDEGNA

I90	59	5.5	3.4	0.48	233
I91	43	6.2	3.7	0.62	200
I92	85	4.8	3.7	0.42	200
I95	24	6.2	3.9	0.85	188
I-N	211	5.4	3.6-	0.26	

SICILIA

I81	38	3.6	1.8--	0.31	340
I82	94	3.1	2.1--	0.22	324
I83	47	2.7	1.5--	0.23	350
I84	43	3.6	2.3--	0.36	316
I85	25	3.4	2.4--	0.50	312
I86	13	2.5	1.6--	0.47	346
I87	65	2.6	1.8--	0.24	340
I88	23	3.4	2.0--	0.44	330
I89	26	2.7	1.9--	0.40	334
I-O	374	3.0	1.9--	0.10	

TOSCANA

I45	35	6.6	2.8--	0.49	284
I46	70	7.0	2.7--	0.34	293
I47	52	7.7	3.1-	0.46	260
I48	254	8.2	3.6-	0.25	208
I49	81	9.2	4.4	0.52	150
I50	71	7.2	3.2--	0.39	250
I51	65	8.2	4.1	0.55	176
I52	65	9.9	3.8	0.52	190
I53	39	6.9	3.5	0.58	224
I-P	732	8.0	3.5--	0.14	

TRENTINO-ALTO ADIGE

I21	97	8.9	5.8+	0.61	34
I22	106	9.4	4.8	0.50	109
I-Q	203	9.2	5.2++	0.39	

UMBRIA

I54	89	6.2	3.2--	0.35	250
I55	37	6.4	3.4	0.57	233
I-R	126	6.2	3.2--	0.30	

VALLE D'AOSTA

I07	27	9.5	5.3	1.09	60

VENETO

I23	142	7.3	4.1	0.36	176
I24	121	6.7	4.1	0.39	176
I25	55	9.4	4.4	0.63	150
I26	139	7.8	4.4	0.39	150
I27	180	8.4	4.8	0.38	109
I28	156	7.6	4.3	0.36	162
I29	71	11.0	5.6+	0.70	39
I-T	864	7.9	4.4	0.16	
I.0	8588	6.0	3.4--	0.04	

IRELAND (1976-80)

CONNAUGHT

R07	29	7.1	4.5	0.89	140
R12	7	10.8	4.4	1.77	150
R16	28	10.1	4.9	0.97	97
R20	12	9.3	4.5	1.45	140
R21	18	13.4	5.5	1.35	46
R-A	94	9.3	4.8	0.53	

LEINSTER

R01	7	7.4	6.4	2.46	20
R06	191	7.5	5.8++	0.44	34
R09	16	6.9	6.8	1.74	13
R10	20	12.0	7.5	1.77	4
R11	13	11.0	7.2	2.05	6
R14	7	9.5	6.2	2.63	25
R15	14	6.5	5.1	1.42	80
R17	19	8.6	7.2	1.72	6
R19	15	10.9	8.3	2.26	2
R24	18	12.3	7.7	1.90	3
R25	17	7.2	4.2	1.11	167
R26	14	6.7	4.6	1.30	129
R-B	351	8.0	6.0++	0.34	

MUNSTER

R03	24	11.7	7.0	1.52	9
R04	98	10.0	6.3++	0.68	23
R08	33	11.3	7.0+	1.30	9
R13	50	12.8	8.5++	1.27	1
R22	34	10.5	6.5	1.22	17
R23	23	10.6	6.6	1.51	15
R-C	262	10.9	6.8++	0.45	

ULSTER

R02	9	7.1	4.2	1.46	167
R05	26	8.8	6.1	1.27	28
R18	7	5.8	3.5	1.40	224
R-D	42	7.7	5.1	0.83	
R.0	749	8.9	6.0++	0.23	

LUXEMBOURG (1971-80)

LE	18	9.4	3.6	0.89	208
LN	15	5.7	1.9--	0.63	334
LS	111	8.3	4.4	0.44	150
L.0	144	8.0	3.9	0.35	

NEDERLAND (1976-80)

N01	133	9.7	5.4+	0.51	53
N02	134	9.3	5.1	0.48	80
N03	77	7.5	5.0	0.60	86
N04	203	8.1	5.4++	0.40	53
N05	329	7.9	4.9+	0.28	97
N06	207	9.3	5.4++	0.41	53
N07	696	11.7	6.3++	0.26	23
N08	775	10.0	5.3++	0.21	60
N09	90	10.6	5.4+	0.63	53
N10	389	7.8	5.9++	0.31	32
N11	209	7.9	5.6++	0.40	39
N.0	3242	9.3	5.5++	0.10	

EEC-9

EEC	68988	8.6	4.2	0.02	

BELGIE-BELGIQUE (1971-78)

BRUSSEL-BRUXELLES					
B21	331	8.4	5.3	0.30	153
VLAANDEREN					
B10	326	5.3	3.7--	0.21	186
B29	226	6.3	4.5--	0.30	167
B30	211	5.0	3.6--	0.26	189
B40	348	6.6	4.4--	0.25	170
B70	108	3.9	3.9--	0.38	184
B-V	1219	5.5	4.0--	0.12	
WALLONIE					
B25	77	7.5	5.5	0.64	147
B50	440	8.6	5.9	0.29	138
B60	308	7.8	5.2	0.30	154
B80	62	7.2	4.9	0.64	160
B90	97	6.4	4.6-	0.47	165
B-W	984	7.9	5.4	0.18	
B.0	2534	6.6	4.6--	0.09	

BR DEUTSCHLAND (1976-80)

BADEN-WURTTEMBERG					
D81	201	2.4	1.8--	0.13	268
D82	199	3.5	2.6--	0.19	221
D83	143	3.2	2.4--	0.21	231
D84	86	2.4	1.8--	0.20	268
D-A	629	2.9	2.1--	0.09	
BAYERN					
D91	265	3.0	2.2--	0.14	242
D92	85	3.6	2.7--	0.30	217
D93	84	3.6	2.7--	0.30	217
D94	94	3.8	2.6--	0.28	221
D95	129	3.6	2.5--	0.23	227
D96	94	3.3	2.5--	0.27	227
D97	139	3.8	2.6--	0.23	221
D-B	890	3.4	2.5--	0.09	
BERLIN(WEST)					
DB0	211	4.9	3.0--	0.23	206
BREMEN					
D40	57	3.5	2.3--	0.32	236
HAMBURG					
D20	123	3.2	1.8--	0.17	268
HESSEN					
D64	352	3.3	2.3--	0.13	236
D66	75	2.6	1.6--	0.20	287
D-F	427	3.2	2.2--	0.11	
NIEDERSACHSEN					
D31	117	3.0	2.0--	0.19	249
D32	181	3.7	2.3--	0.19	236
D33	67	1.9	1.2--	0.16	325
D34	133	2.6	1.9--	0.17	257
D-G	498	2.9	1.9--	0.09	
NORDRHEIN-WESTFALEN					
D51	530	4.3	3.2--	0.14	200
D53	314	3.3	2.7--	0.16	217
D55	176	3.0	2.6--	0.20	221
D57	138	3.2	2.4--	0.21	231
D59	330	3.7	2.8--	0.16	212
D-H	1488	3.7	2.8--	0.08	
RHEINLAND-PFALZ					
D71	140	4.3	2.8--	0.25	212
D72	73	6.5	4.4-	0.53	170
D73	200	4.6	3.3--	0.24	198
D-I	413	4.8	3.3--	0.17	
SAARLAND					
DA0	129	5.0	3.4--	0.31	195
SCHLESWIG-HOLSTEIN					
D10	153	2.5	1.6--	0.13	287
D.0	5018	3.4	2.4--	0.04	

DANMARK (1971-80)

K15	308	5.1	3.3--	0.19	198
K20	30	2.0	1.8--	0.33	268
K25	20	2.2	2.2--	0.48	242
K30	39	2.9	1.9--	0.32	257
K35	32	2.5	1.4--	0.27	304
K40	4	1.7	1.0--	0.52	344
K42	45	2.0	1.2--	0.19	325
K50	16	1.3	0.9--	0.24	347
K55	18	1.7	1.2--	0.30	325
K60	29	1.8	1.3--	0.24	318
K65	19	1.5	1.1--	0.25	337
K70	55	2.0	1.4--	0.19	304
K76	16	1.4	0.9--	0.23	347
K80	38	1.6	1.0--	0.18	344
K.0	669	2.7	1.8--	0.07	

FRANCE (1971-78)

ALSACE					
F67	394	11.4	10.1++	0.52	75
F68	327	13.1	11.3++	0.65	50
F-A	721	12.1	10.6++	0.41	
AQUITAINE					
F24	334	22.9	13.6++	0.79	14
F33	802	19.7	14.0++	0.51	10
F40	223	19.9	12.7++	0.90	26
F47	185	16.3	10.4++	0.80	68
F64	309	14.9	9.9++	0.59	82
F-B	1853	18.8	12.5++	0.30	
AUVERGNE					
F03	230	15.5	10.2++	0.70	72
F15	139	21.0	12.2++	1.09	32
F43	133	16.6	10.2++	0.94	72
F63	380	16.7	12.8++	0.68	23
F-C	882	16.9	11.5++	0.41	
BASSE-NORMANDIE					
F14	247	11.3	10.3++	0.67	71
F50	293	16.8	12.8++	0.77	23
F61	154	13.4	10.8++	0.90	61
F-D	694	13.7	11.3++	0.44	
BOURGOGNE					
F21	194	10.8	8.7++	0.64	104
F58	197	20.1	13.1++	1.00	19
F71	299	13.3	9.4++	0.57	95
F89	175	14.8	9.7++	0.79	87
F-E	865	13.9	9.9++	0.35	
BRETAGNE					
F22	428	21.0	15.3++	0.76	5
F29	725	23.2	17.7++	0.67	1
F35	406	15.0	12.5++	0.63	29
F56	461	20.9	16.7++	0.79	2
F-F	2020	20.1	15.7++	0.36	
CENTRE					
F18	214	17.1	11.2++	0.81	52
F28	165	12.3	9.3++	0.76	98
F36	160	16.4	10.0++	0.85	78
F37	275	14.8	11.1++	0.70	55
F41	173	15.6	11.0++	0.89	58
F45	239	12.3	9.6++	0.65	89
F-G	1226	14.5	10.4++	0.31	
CHAMPAGNE-ARDENNE					
F08	180	14.5	12.7++	0.97	26
F10	164	14.6	11.2++	0.92	52
F51	255	12.1	10.8++	0.69	61
F52	126	14.8	11.4++	1.05	48
F-H	725	13.6	11.4++	0.44	
CORSE					
F20	82	8.6	5.9	0.67	138
FRANCHE-COMTE					
F25	225	12.0	11.7++	0.79	42
F39	154	16.2	11.1++	0.94	55
F70	110	12.6	9.8++	0.99	86
F90	85	16.6	15.1++	1.66	6
F-J	574	13.6	11.5++	0.49	
HAUTE-NORMANDIE					
F27	246	14.7	12.7++	0.83	26
F76	687	14.9	13.1++	0.51	19
F-K	933	14.9	13.0++	0.43	
ILE-DE-FRANCE					
F75	1377	16.2	10.9++	0.30	59
F77	406	13.5	12.1++	0.62	35
F78	479	11.1	11.6++	0.54	45
F91	399	10.8	11.9++	0.61	39
F92	849	15.1	12.4++	0.43	30
F93	889	16.8	16.1++	0.55	3
F94	737	15.5	14.1++	0.53	8
F95	461	13.8	13.9++	0.66	11
F-L	5597	14.5	12.6++	0.17	
LANGUEDOC-ROUSSILLON					
F11	193	18.5	9.5++	0.75	93
F30	338	17.6	11.7++	0.66	42
F34	385	15.5	10.0++	0.53	78
F48	60	20.0	12.2++	1.66	32
F66	179	15.5	9.1++	0.73	100
F-M	1155	16.7	10.3++	0.32	
LIMOUSIN					
F19	183	19.5	11.5++	0.90	46
F23	147	25.7	13.4++	1.21	16
F87	242	17.7	10.8++	0.74	61
F-N	572	19.9	11.6++	0.52	
LORRAINE					
F54	406	14.2	12.4++	0.63	30
F55	143	17.8	13.8++	1.20	12
F57	488	12.1	11.7++	0.54	42
F88	248	15.9	13.0++	0.85	22
F-O	1285	13.9	12.4++	0.35	
MIDI-PYRENEES					
F09	77	14.1	7.2	0.90	121
F12	134	12.4	7.1+	0.65	123
F31	395	13.1	9.4++	0.49	95
F32	82	11.8	6.5	0.77	130
F46	82	13.9	7.6+	0.90	115
F65	173	19.5	12.2++	0.96	32
F81	177	13.4	8.0++	0.64	113
F82	119	16.6	9.6++	0.93	89
F-P	1239	14.0	8.6++	0.26	
NORD-PAS-DE-CALAIS					
F59	1699	17.3	15.7++	0.39	4
F62	855	15.6	13.7++	0.47	13
F-Q	2554	16.7	15.0++	0.30	
PAYS DE LA LOIRE					
F44	499	13.9	12.1++	0.55	35
F49	304	12.4	10.8++	0.64	61
F53	132	13.0	9.9++	0.88	82
F72	246	12.8	9.9++	0.65	82
F85	235	13.5	10.6++	0.71	66
F-R	1416	13.2	10.9++	0.30	
PICARDIE					
F02	341	16.1	13.4++	0.75	16
F60	366	15.0	14.1++	0.76	8
F80	347	16.4	13.6++	0.75	14
F-S	1054	15.8	13.7++	0.43	
POITOU-CHARENTES					
F16	226	17.1	11.9++	0.83	39
F17	288	14.9	9.9++	0.61	82
F79	136	10.2	7.1+	0.65	123
F86	190	13.5	9.5++	0.73	93
F-T	840	14.0	9.6++	0.35	
PROVENCE-ALPES-COTE D'AZUR					
F04	55	12.3	7.5	1.08	117
F05	45	11.6	7.6	1.18	115
F06	342	11.1	6.4+	0.38	133
F13	822	12.9	9.6++	0.34	89
F83	446	18.1	12.0++	0.59	37
F84	219	14.1	10.1++	0.71	75
F-U	1929	13.5	9.1++	0.22	
RHONE-ALPES					
F01	186	12.3	8.9++	0.68	102
F07	194	19.3	12.8++	0.97	23
F26	223	15.8	11.3++	0.79	50
F38	426	12.5	10.7++	0.53	65
F42	451	15.4	11.9++	0.57	39
F69	622	11.1	9.7++	0.40	87
F73	157	12.9	10.5++	0.86	67
F74	199	11.1	10.0++	0.72	78
F-V	2458	13.0	10.6++	0.22	
F.0	30674	14.9	11.6++	0.07	

UNITED KINGDOM (1976-80)

EAST ANGLIA					
G25	40	2.3	1.6--	0.27	287
G46	45	2.3	1.2--	0.19	325
G55	24	1.4	0.9--	0.18	347
G-A	109	2.0	1.2--	0.12	
EAST MIDLANDS					
G30	64	2.4	1.5--	0.19	296
G44	47	1.9	1.4--	0.21	304
G45	34	2.2	1.4--	0.25	304
G47	24	1.6	1.1--	0.24	337
G50	66	2.3	1.5--	0.19	296
G-B	235	2.1	1.4--	0.10	
NORTHERN					
G14	127	3.7	2.6--	0.23	221
G27	53	3.2	2.5--	0.34	227
G29	37	2.7	1.7--	0.28	281
G33	64	3.6	2.5--	0.32	227
G48	28	3.3	2.2--	0.42	242
G-C	309	3.4	2.4--	0.14	
NORTH-WEST					
G11	197	2.5	1.8--	0.13	268
G12	143	3.2	2.3--	0.19	236
G26	75	2.8	2.1--	0.25	247
G43	111	2.8	1.8--	0.17	268
G-D	526	2.8	1.9--	0.09	

SOUTH-EAST					
G01	502	2.5	1.5--	0.07	296
G22	23	1.5	1.2--	0.25	325
G23	32	1.6	1.2--	0.22	325
G24	35	2.2	1.7--	0.28	281
G34	61	3.4	1.4--	0.19	304
G35	76	1.8	1.2--	0.14	325
G37	110	2.5	1.9--	0.18	257
G39	45	1.6	1.2--	0.18	325
G41	14	4.3	1.9--	0.57	257
G42	104	2.5	1.6--	0.16	287
G51	27	1.6	1.2--	0.25	325
G56	60	2.1	1.3--	0.17	318
G58	56	3.2	1.6--	0.23	287
G-E	1145	2.3	1.5--	0.05	
SOUTH-WEST					
G21	55	2.1	1.3--	0.18	318
G28	28	2.3	1.4--	0.28	304
G31	73	2.6	1.5--	0.19	296
G32	56	3.4	1.7--	0.24	281
G36	37	2.6	1.6--	0.28	287
G53	29	2.4	1.3--	0.25	318
G59	39	2.5	1.9--	0.31	257
G-F	317	2.5	1.5--	0.09	
WEST MIDLANDS					
G15	216	2.7	1.9--	0.13	257
G38	53	3.0	2.0--	0.28	249
G52	18	1.7	1.3--	0.31	318
G54	69	2.3	1.7--	0.21	281
G57	20	1.4	1.1--	0.25	337
G-G	376	2.5	1.7--	0.09	
YORKSHIRE AND HUMBERSIDE					
G13	104	2.7	1.8--	0.18	268
G16	169	2.8	1.9--	0.15	257
G40	85	3.4	2.2--	0.25	242
G49	55	2.8	1.8--	0.25	268
G-H	413	2.9	1.9--	0.10	
WALES					
G61	38	3.4	2.2--	0.38	242
G62	22	2.3	1.3--	0.28	318
G63	37	2.9	2.0--	0.33	249
G64	19	2.9	1.6--	0.39	287
G65	38	2.4	1.7--	0.28	281
G66	7	2.2	1.1--	0.43	337
G67	25	2.2	1.4--	0.29	304
G68	33	3.1	1.9--	0.34	257
G-I	219	2.7	1.7--	0.12	
SCOTLAND(1975-80)					
S01	14	2.5	1.8--	0.50	268
S02	31	2.3	1.5--	0.29	296
S03	24	2.1	1.4--	0.29	304
S04	18	1.8	1.2--	0.30	325
S05	54	2.5	1.9--	0.27	257
S06	4	1.4	0.7--	0.36	351
S07	12	1.5	1.1--	0.32	337
S08	197	2.8	2.1--	0.16	247
S09	10	2.4	1.4--	0.45	304
S10	0	0.0	0.0--	0.00	354
S11	1	1.6	1.6-	1.57	287
S12	3	3.4	1.9--	1.14	257
G-J	368	2.5	1.8--	0.10	
NORTHERN IRELAND					
JE	48	2.9	2.4--	0.36	231
JN	11	1.2	1.2--	0.37	325
JS	16	2.4	1.9--	0.48	257
JW	14	2.3	2.0--	0.56	249
G-K	89	2.3	2.0--	0.22	
G.0	4106	2.5	1.7--	0.03	
ITALIA (1975-79)					
ABRUZZI					
I66	51	7.0	4.1-	0.59	176
I67	38	5.7	4.0-	0.67	182
I68	47	6.8	4.9	0.73	160
I69	62	6.9	4.5	0.58	167
I-A	198	6.6	4.4--	0.32	
BASILICATA					
I76	35	3.4	2.4--	0.42	231
I77	22	4.4	3.5--	0.76	191
I-B	57	3.7	2.7--	0.37	
CALABRIA					
I78	62	3.5	2.9--	0.37	209
I79	88	4.8	4.1--	0.45	176
I80	62	4.2	2.9--	0.39	209
I-C	212	4.2	3.3--	0.24	
CAMPANIA					
I61	95	5.3	5.0	0.52	157
I62	36	5.0	3.2--	0.55	200
I63	574	8.2	8.7++	0.36	104
I64	53	4.9	3.5--	0.50	191
I65	163	6.6	5.5	0.44	147
I-D	921	7.1	6.6++	0.22	
EMILIA-ROMAGNA					
I33	105	15.1	8.7++	0.87	104
I34	86	8.8	5.1	0.57	156
I35	87	8.8	5.4	0.59	150
I36	116	8.2	5.5	0.52	147
I37	151	6.7	4.1--	0.34	176
I38	100	10.7	6.7	0.68	128
I39	55	6.3	4.0--	0.56	182
I40	119	8.2	5.9	0.55	138
I-E	819	8.5	5.4	0.19	
FRIULI-VENEZIA GIULIA					
I30	220	17.1	11.1++	0.76	55
I31	45	12.8	8.2+	1.24	110
I32	95	13.6	7.0	0.75	126
I93	76	11.6	8.9++	1.04	102
I-F	436	14.6	9.3++	0.45	
LAZIO					
I56	54	8.2	5.4	0.74	150
I57	24	6.7	3.9	0.84	184
I58	591	6.6	5.8	0.24	141
I59	83	8.0	7.2+	0.80	121
I60	75	6.7	4.9	0.58	160
I-G	827	6.9	5.6	0.20	
LIGURIA					
I08	57	10.3	5.7	0.79	143
I09	79	10.7	6.2	0.71	135
I10	302	11.7	6.7++	0.40	128
I11	80	13.5	7.5+	0.86	117
I-H	518	11.6	6.6++	0.30	
LOMBARDIA					
I12	227	12.1	10.4++	0.72	68
I13	242	13.2	10.9++	0.71	59
I14	49	11.4	10.1++	1.45	75
I15	1286	13.2	11.2++	0.32	52
I16	300	14.0	13.1++	0.76	19
I17	365	14.9	13.3++	0.70	18
I18	174	13.7	8.2++	0.65	110
I19	141	17.4	12.0++	1.03	37
I20	121	13.1	8.2++	0.77	110
I-I	2905	13.5	11.1++	0.21	
MARCHE					
I41	37	4.6	3.1--	0.52	205
I42	87	8.4	5.4	0.59	150
I43	47	6.6	4.1-	0.61	176
I44	58	6.8	4.7	0.63	164
I-J	229	6.7	4.4--	0.30	
MOLISE					
I70	28	4.9	2.8--	0.55	212
I94	3	1.3	1.1--	0.63	337
I-K	31	3.8	2.3--	0.43	
PIEMONTE					
I01	580	10.0	8.0++	0.34	113
I02	149	15.4	9.0++	0.76	101
I03	137	11.2	7.4++	0.65	119
I04	143	10.5	6.5	0.57	130
I05	59	11.0	5.6	0.79	145
I06	158	13.6	7.1+	0.62	123
I-L	1226	11.1	7.5++	0.22	
PUGLIA					
I71	77	4.6	3.6--	0.43	189
I72	137	3.9	3.2--	0.28	200
I73	45	3.3	3.0--	0.45	206
I74	65	6.8	5.8	0.73	141
I75	97	5.3	4.5-	0.46	167
I-M	421	4.5	3.8--	0.19	
SARDEGNA					
I90	75	7.2	5.6	0.67	145
I91	35	5.1	4.3	0.77	174
I92	90	5.1	4.8	0.51	163
I95	28	7.2	5.0	1.02	157
I-N	228	5.9	4.9-	0.33	
SICILIA					
I81	55	5.3	3.7--	0.52	186
I82	112	3.9	3.2--	0.30	200
I83	75	4.6	3.2--	0.38	200
I84	60	5.0	3.7--	0.49	186
I85	30	4.1	3.4--	0.64	195
I86	23	4.6	3.5--	0.74	191
I87	125	5.1	4.1--	0.38	176
I88	22	3.3	2.3--	0.50	236
I89	51	5.3	4.1-	0.58	176
I-O	553	4.6	3.5--	0.15	
TOSCANA					
I45	65	13.1	8.4++	1.06	109
I46	140	15.0	9.4++	0.82	95
I47	55	8.6	5.2	0.71	154
I48	236	8.2	5.0	0.33	157
I49	112	13.3	8.7++	0.84	104
I50	101	10.8	6.4	0.65	133
I51	57	7.4	4.4-	0.59	170
I52	34	5.4	2.8--	0.50	212
I53	55	10.0	5.7	0.79	143
I-P	855	9.9	6.0	0.21	
TRENTINO-ALTO ADIGE					
I21	88	8.3	7.4+	0.80	119
I22	149	13.9	10.2++	0.86	72
I-Q	237	11.1	9.0++	0.60	
UMBRIA					
I54	135	9.6	6.2	0.54	135
I55	41	7.3	4.4	0.70	170
I-R	176	9.0	5.7	0.43	
VALLE D'AOSTA					
I07	58	20.4	15.0++	1.98	7
VENETO					
I23	250	13.4	10.4++	0.67	68
I24	194	11.2	9.6++	0.69	89
I25	89	16.5	11.5++	1.24	46
I26	211	12.3	10.0++	0.70	78
I27	279	13.6	11.4++	0.69	48
I28	204	10.4	8.7++	0.62	104
I29	82	13.2	9.2++	1.03	99
I-T	1309	12.5	10.1++	0.28	
I.0	12216	8.9	6.7++	0.06	
IRELAND (1976-80)					
CONNAUGHT					
R07	11	2.5	1.8--	0.57	268
R12	2	2.7	1.2--	0.87	325
R16	7	2.4	1.4--	0.53	304
R20	3	2.1	1.4--	0.85	304
R21	7	5.0	2.7-	1.21	217
R-A	30	2.8	1.7--	0.33	
LEINSTER					
R01	5	5.1	4.6	2.14	165
R06	64	2.7	3.0--	0.38	206
R09	9	3.6	4.2	1.42	175
R10	2	1.1	0.9--	0.61	347
R11	3	2.3	1.6--	0.93	287
R14	0	0.0	0.0--	0.00	354
R15	8	3.7	3.5	1.26	191
R17	3	1.3	1.5--	0.87	296
R19	1	0.7	0.4--	0.36	352
R24	3	2.0	1.8--	1.11	268
R25	8	3.3	2.6--	0.95	221
R26	1	0.5	0.4--	0.40	352
R-B	107	2.5	2.4--	0.24	
MUNSTER					
R03	3	1.4	1.0--	0.57	344
R04	39	3.9	3.4--	0.55	195
R08	6	1.9	1.1--	0.44	337
R13	8	2.0	1.8--	0.67	268
R22	13	3.8	2.9--	0.82	209
R23	8	3.6	2.8--	1.00	212
R-C	77	3.1	2.5--	0.29	
ULSTER					
R02	4	2.8	2.0--	1.02	249
R05	9	2.9	1.5--	0.51	296
R18	2	1.5	1.4--	0.98	304
R-D	15	2.6	1.6--	0.43	
R.0	229	2.7	2.2--	0.15	
LUXEMBOURG (1971-80)					
LE	16	8.8	6.2	1.59	135
LN	27	10.2	6.5	1.28	130
LS	117	9.2	6.9+	0.65	127
L.0	160	9.3	6.7+	0.54	
NEDERLAND (1976-80)					
N01	34	2.5	1.8--	0.32	268
N02	28	2.0	1.4--	0.27	304
N03	15	1.4	1.3--	0.33	318
N04	50	2.0	1.5--	0.22	296
N05	69	1.7	1.4--	0.17	304
N06	44	2.0	1.7--	0.27	281
N07	155	2.7	2.0--	0.16	249
N08	203	2.7	2.0--	0.14	249
N09	26	3.1	2.0--	0.42	249
N10	122	2.4	2.3--	0.22	236
N11	70	2.6	2.4--	0.29	231
N.0	816	2.4	1.9--	0.07	
EEC-9					
EEC	56422	7.4	5.6	0.02	

BELGIE-BELGIQUE (1971-78)

BRUSSEL-BRUXELLES					
B21	37	0.8	0.4	0.07	70
VLAANDEREN					
B10	24	0.4	0.2-	0.04	207
B29	15	0.4	0.3	0.07	137
B30	26	0.6	0.3	0.07	137
B40	33	0.6	0.4	0.07	70
B70	9	0.3	0.3	0.09	137
B-V	107	0.5	0.3	0.03	
WALLONIE					
B25	6	0.6	0.3	0.13	137
B50	39	0.7	0.4	0.06	70
B60	26	0.6	0.4	0.08	70
B80	4	0.4	0.4	0.22	70
B90	9	0.6	0.3	0.11	137
B-W	84	0.6	0.4	0.04	
B.0	228	0.6	0.3	0.02	

BR DEUTSCHLAND (1976-80)

BADEN-WURTTEMBERG					
D81	22	0.2	0.1--	0.03	285
D82	19	0.3	0.1--	0.04	285
D83	12	0.2	0.1--	0.03	285
D84	10	0.3	0.1--	0.05	285
D-A	63	0.3	0.1--	0.02	
BAYERN					
D91	42	0.4	0.2--	0.03	207
D92	14	0.5	0.3	0.09	137
D93	6	0.2	0.1--	0.05	285
D94	8	0.3	0.1--	0.05	285
D95	11	0.3	0.1--	0.03	285
D96	8	0.3	0.1--	0.04	285
D97	15	0.4	0.2	0.07	207
D-B	104	0.4	0.2--	0.02	
BERLIN(WEST)					
DB0	39	0.7	0.3	0.06	137
BREMEN					
D40	6	0.3	0.2	0.08	207
HAMBURG					
D20	22	0.5	0.2	0.05	207
HESSEN					
D64	35	0.3	0.2--	0.03	207
D66	5	0.2	0.0--	0.02	346
D-F	40	0.3	0.1--	0.02	
NIEDERSACHSEN					
D31	10	0.2	0.1--	0.04	285
D32	8	0.1	0.1--	0.02	285
D33	9	0.2	0.1--	0.05	285
D34	16	0.3	0.1--	0.04	285
D-G	43	0.2	0.1--	0.02	
NORDRHEIN-WESTFALEN					
D51	55	0.4	0.2--	0.03	207
D53	31	0.3	0.2--	0.03	207
D55	19	0.3	0.2--	0.04	207
D57	7	0.1	0.1--	0.03	285
D59	35	0.4	0.2--	0.03	207
D-H	147	0.3	0.2--	0.02	
RHEINLAND-PFALZ					
D71	14	0.4	0.2-	0.06	207
D72	2	0.2	0.1--	0.05	285
D73	9	0.2	0.1--	0.04	285
D-I	25	0.3	0.1--	0.03	
SAARLAND					
DA0	10	0.4	0.2	0.08	207
SCHLESWIG-HOLSTEIN					
D10	20	0.3	0.2--	0.04	207
D.0	519	0.3	0.2--	0.01	

DANMARK (1971-80)

K15	68	1.0	0.5++	0.06	36
K20	8	0.5	0.4	0.16	70
K25	2	0.2	0.2	0.17	207
K30	7	0.5	0.3	0.12	137
K35	1	0.1	0.1--	0.05	285
K40	0	0.0	0.0--	0.00	346
K42	5	0.2	0.1--	0.05	285
K50	6	0.5	0.3	0.15	137
K55	5	0.5	0.3	0.17	137
K60	4	0.3	0.1-	0.07	285
K65	5	0.4	0.3	0.15	137
K70	3	0.1	0.1--	0.04	285
K76	2	0.2	0.1--	0.07	285
K80	9	0.4	0.3	0.09	137
K.0	125	0.5	0.3	0.03	

FRANCE (1971-78)

ALSACE					
F67	16	0.4	0.3	0.07	137
F68	7	0.3	0.2	0.10	207
F-A	23	0.4	0.2	0.06	
AQUITAINE					
F24	14	0.9	0.4	0.13	70
F33	39	0.9	0.4	0.08	70
F40	6	0.5	0.2	0.11	207
F47	9	0.8	0.4	0.16	70
F64	20	0.9	0.4	0.12	70
F-B	88	0.8	0.4+	0.05	
AUVERGNE					
F03	11	0.7	0.3	0.11	137
F15	4	0.6	0.2	0.15	207
F43	3	0.4	0.2	0.10	207
F63	15	0.6	0.3	0.08	137
F-C	33	0.6	0.3	0.05	
BASSE-NORMANDIE					
F14	11	0.5	0.3	0.10	137
F50	11	0.6	0.3	0.10	137
F61	9	0.7	0.5	0.19	36
F-D	31	0.6	0.3	0.07	
BOURGOGNE					
F21	9	0.5	0.3	0.11	137
F58	7	0.7	0.1--	0.05	285
F71	9	0.4	0.2	0.08	207
F89	13	1.1	0.5	0.16	36
F-E	38	0.6	0.3	0.05	
BRETAGNE					
F22	5	0.2	0.1--	0.05	285
F29	19	0.6	0.3	0.07	137
F35	10	0.3	0.2	0.07	207
F56	9	0.4	0.2	0.08	207
F-F	43	0.4	0.2--	0.04	
CENTRE					
F18	5	0.4	0.3	0.13	137
F28	9	0.7	0.3	0.12	137
F36	7	0.7	0.4	0.17	70
F37	11	0.6	0.4	0.13	70
F41	10	0.9	0.3	0.12	137
F45	11	0.6	0.4	0.13	70
F-G	53	0.6	0.4	0.06	
CHAMPAGNE-ARDENNE					
F08	6	0.5	0.3	0.14	137
F10	7	0.6	0.4	0.16	70
F51	8	0.4	0.3	0.12	137
F52	5	0.6	0.3	0.14	137
F-H	26	0.5	0.3	0.07	
CORSE					
F20	6	0.7	0.4	0.16	70
FRANCHE-COMTE					
F25	7	0.4	0.3	0.13	137
F39	6	0.6	0.3	0.15	137
F70	9	1.0	0.6	0.23	20
F90	2	0.4	0.1-	0.08	285
F-J	24	0.6	0.4	0.08	
HAUTE-NORMANDIE					
F27	11	0.6	0.4	0.13	70
F76	30	0.6	0.4	0.08	·70
F-K	41	0.6	0.4	0.07	
ILE-DE-FRANCE					
F75	125	1.3	0.6++	0.06	20
F77	23	0.8	0.6+	0.13	20
F78	31	0.7	0.6+	0.11	20
F91	17	0.5	0.5	0.12	36
F92	59	1.0	0.6++	0.08	20
F93	46	0.9	0.7++	0.10	9
F94	49	1.0	0.7++	0.10	9
F95	19	0.6	0.5	0.11	36
F-L	369	0.9	0.6++	0.03	
LANGUEDOC-ROUSSILLON					
F11	4	0.4	0.1-	0.07	285
F30	19	0.9	0.5	0.13	36
F34	25	0.9	0.4	0.09	70
F48	2	0.7	0.2	0.18	207
F66	10	0.8	0.4	0.13	70
F-M	60	0.8	0.4	0.06	
LIMOUSIN					
F19	5	0.5	0.2	0.09	207
F23	5	0.8	0.5	0.24	36
F87	8	0.5	0.3	0.13	137
F-N	18	0.6	0.3	0.08	
LORRAINE					
F54	14	0.5	0.3	0.10	137
F55	3	0.4	0.2	0.14	207
F57	23	0.6	0.4	0.09	70
F88	5	0.3	0.2	0.08	207
F-O	45	0.5	0.3	0.05	
MIDI-PYRENEES					
F09	8	1.4	0.7	0.31	9
F12	7	0.6	0.3	0.13	137
F31	26	0.8	0.5	0.10	36
F32	8	1.1	0.6	0.24	20
F46	4	0.7	0.2	0.14	207
F65	7	0.7	0.5	0.19	36
F81	14	1.0	0.4	0.12	70
F82	7	0.9	0.4	0.17	70
F-P	81	0.9	0.4+	0.06	
NORD-PAS-DE-CALAIS					
F59	78	0.8	0.5++	0.07	36
F62	48	0.8	0.5++	0.08	36
F-Q	126	0.8	0.5++	0.05	
PAYS DE LA LOIRE					
F44	18	0.5	0.2	0.07	207
F49	11	0.4	0.2	0.07	207
F53	8	0.7	0.4	0.15	70
F72	16	0.8	0.4	0.11	70
F85	6	0.3	0.1--	0.06	285
F-R	59	0.5	0.3	0.04	
PICARDIE					
F02	15	0.7	0.3	0.09	137
F60	14	0.6	0.4	0.12	70
F80	17	0.8	0.4	0.12	70
F-S	46	0.7	0.4	0.07	
POITOU-CHARENTES					
F16	7	0.5	0.3	0.13	137
F17	12	0.6	0.3	0.12	137
F79	10	0.7	0.4	0.13	70
F86	7	0.5	0.2	0.08	207
F-T	36	0.6	0.3	0.06	
PROVENCE-ALPES-COTE D'AZUR					
F04	2	0.4	0.2	0.13	207
F05	3	0.8	0.6	0.34	20
F06	22	0.6	0.3	0.06	137
F13	50	0.7	0.5+	0.07	36
F83	33	1.3	0.7++	0.13	9
F84	11	0.7	0.5	0.16	36
F-U	121	0.8	0.4++	0.04	
RHONE-ALPES					
F01	8	0.5	0.2	0.08	207
F07	9	0.9	0.4	0.15	70
F26	10	0.7	0.4	0.14	70
F38	10	0.3	0.2	0.06	207
F42	14	0.5	0.2	0.07	207
F69	25	0.4	0.3	0.06	137
F73	5	0.4	0.2	0.09	207
F74	9	0.5	0.4	0.14	70
F-V	90	0.5	0.3	0.03	
F.0	1457	0.7	0.4++	0.01	

UNITED KINGDOM (1976-80)

EAST ANGLIA					
G25	7	0.4	0.2	0.09	207
G46	13	0.6	0.3	0.09	137
G55	9	0.5	0.2	0.10	207
G-A	29	0.5	0.3	0.06	
EAST MIDLANDS					
G30	11	0.4	0.2	0.07	207
G44	14	0.6	0.3	0.10	137
G45	7	0.4	0.2	0.10	207
G47	6	0.4	0.2	0.10	207
G50	14	0.5	0.3	0.08	137
G-B	52	0.5	0.3	0.04	
NORTHERN					
G14	21	0.6	0.3	0.07	137
G27	18	1.0	0.6+	0.16	20
G29	9	0.6	0.4	0.15	70
G33	10	0.5	0.3	0.10	137
G48	4	0.5	0.2	0.11	207
G-C	62	0.6	0.4	0.05	
NORTH-WEST					
G11	69	0.8	0.5++	0.06	36
G12	49	1.0	0.6++	0.10	20
G26	18	0.6	0.4	0.09	70
G43	44	1.0	0.4	0.08	70
G-D	180	0.9	0.5++	0.04	

SOUTH-EAST					
G01	168	0.8	0.4+	0.03	70
G22	5	0.3	0.3	0.12	137
G23	12	0.6	0.3	0.11	137
G24	9	0.6	0.4	0.13	70
G34	27	1.3	0.3	0.07	137
G35	17	0.4	0.2	0.06	207
G37	32	0.7	0.4	0.08	70
G39	18	0.6	0.4	0.10	70
G41	6	1.7	0.6	0.24	20
G42	17	0.4	0.2-	0.05	207
G51	11	0.7	0.3	0.12	137
G56	29	0.9	0.4	0.08	70
G58	8	0.4	0.1--	0.06	285
G-E	359	0.7	0.3	0.02	
SOUTH-WEST					
G21	12	0.4	0.2	0.08	207
G28	10	0.8	0.3	0.09	137
G31	22	0.8	0.4	0.10	70
G32	14	0.8	0.3	0.09	137
G36	6	0.4	0.2	0.09	207
G53	14	1.1	0.5	0.17	36
G59	2	0.1	0.1--	0.04	285
G-F	80	0.6	0.3	0.04	
WEST MIDLANDS					
G15	43	0.5	0.3	0.05	137
G38	10	0.5	0.3	0.11	137
G52	3	0.3	0.1	0.09	285
G54	21	0.7	0.4	0.09	70
G57	3	0.2	0.1--	0.07	285
G-G	80	0.5	0.3	0.04	
YORKSHIRE AND HUMBERSIDE					
G13	24	0.6	0.3	0.07	137
G16	44	0.7	0.4	0.06	70
G40	15	0.6	0.3	0.09	137
G49	14	0.7	0.4	0.11	70
G-H	97	0.6	0.3	0.04	
WALES					
G61	11	0.9	0.4	0.14	70
G62	12	1.2	0.5	0.14	36
G63	7	0.5	0.3	0.13	137
G64	2	0.3	0.1--	0.05	285
G65	20	1.2	0.7+	0.17	9
G66	2	0.6	0.1	0.11	285
G67	5	0.4	0.2	0.10	207
G68	8	0.7	0.3	0.09	137
G-I	67	0.8	0.4	0.05	
SCOTLAND(1975-80)					
S01	4	0.7	0.5	0.24	36
S02	5	0.3	0.2-	0.08	207
S03	8	0.6	0.3	0.11	137
S04	5	0.5	0.3	0.16	137
S05	22	0.9	0.4	0.10	70
S06	2	0.6	0.2	0.17	207
S07	6	0.7	0.4	0.19	70
S08	69	0.9	0.5++	0.07	36
S09	1	0.2	0.2	0.19	207
S10	0	0.0	0.0--	0.00	346
S11	0	0.0	0.0--	0.00	346
S12	1	1.1	0.4	0.35	70
G-J	123	0.8	0.4++	0.04	
NORTHERN IRELAND					
JE	19	1.1	0.8+	0.19	8
JN	6	0.6	0.4	0.18	70
JS	2	0.3	0.1	0.09	285
JW	5	0.8	0.5	0.24	36
G-K	32	0.8	0.5+	0.10	
G.0	1161	0.7	0.4++	0.01	
ITALIA (1975-79)					
ABRUZZI					
I66	3	0.4	0.2	0.14	207
I67	1	0.1	0.1	0.12	285
I68	1	0.1	0.1--	0.07	285
I69	4	0.4	0.3	0.17	137
I-A	9	0.3	0.2	0.07	
BASILICATA					
I76	5	0.5	0.3	0.16	137
I77	3	0.6	0.4	0.23	70
I-B	8	0.5	0.3	0.13	
CALABRIA					
I78	6	0.3	0.3	0.11	137
I79	3	0.2	0.1--	0.07	285
I80	7	0.5	0.3	0.12	137
I-C	16	0.3	0.2	0.06	
CAMPANIA					
I61	8	0.4	0.3	0.12	137
I62	3	0.4	0.2	0.13	207
I63	35	0.5	0.4	0.07	70
I64	3	0.3	0.2	0.09	207
I65	8	0.3	0.2	0.09	207
I-D	57	0.4	0.3	0.05	
EMILIA-ROMAGNA					
I33	2	0.3	0.1--	0.06	285
I34	9	0.9	0.3	0.12	137
I35	6	0.6	0.3	0.14	137
I36	9	0.6	0.4	0.13	70
I37	18	0.7	0.4	0.09	70
I38	10	1.0	0.5	0.16	36
I39	1	0.1	0.1--	0.06	285
I40	9	0.6	0.4	0.13	70
I-E	64	0.6	0.3	0.04	
FRIULI-VENEZIA GIULIA					
I30	16	1.2	0.6	0.17	20
I31	3	0.8	0.4	0.26	70
I32	8	1.0	0.5	0.19	36
I93	4	0.6	0.2	0.09	207
I-F	31	1.0	0.5	0.09	
LAZIO					
I56	1	0.2	0.1--	0.08	285
I57	1	0.3	0.2	0.18	207
I58	46	0.5	0.3	0.05	137
I59	1	0.1	0.1--	0.07	285
I60	1	0.1	0.0--	0.05	346
I-G	50	0.4	0.3	0.04	
LIGURIA					
I08	5	0.8	0.4	0.17	70
I09	6	0.8	0.4	0.18	70
I10	23	0.8	0.4	0.08	70
I11	2	0.3	0.2	0.13	207
I-H	36	0.7	0.4	0.06	
LOMBARDIA					
I12	5	0.3	0.2-	0.07	207
I13	14	0.7	0.5	0.13	36
I14	1	0.2	0.1	0.14	285
I15	74	0.7	0.4+	0.05	70
I16	16	0.7	0.5	0.13	36
I17	27	1.1	0.7++	0.14	9
I18	15	1.1	0.5	0.14	36
I19	13	1.5	0.7	0.22	9
I20	5	0.5	0.2	0.12	207
I-I	170	0.7	0.5++	0.04	
MARCHE					
I41	2	0.2	0.1--	0.07	285
I42	5	0.5	0.2	0.09	207
I43	1	0.1	0.1--	0.07	285
I44	4	0.4	0.2	0.12	207
I-J	12	0.3	0.2--	0.05	
MOLISE					
I70	2	0.3	0.1	0.10	285
I94	1	0.4	0.1	0.13	285
I-K	3	0.4	0.1-	0.08	
PIEMONTE					
I01	51	0.8	0.5++	0.08	36
I02	4	0.4	0.1--	0.06	285
I03	5	0.4	0.3	0.12	137
I04	11	0.8	0.4	0.14	70
I05	1	0.2	0.0--	0.04	346
I06	12	1.0	0.5	0.15	36
I-L	84	0.7	0.4	0.05	
PUGLIA					
I71	6	0.4	0.2	0.10	207
I72	17	0.5	0.3	0.09	137
I73	3	0.2	0.1	0.09	285
I74	2	0.2	0.1	0.10	285
I75	9	0.5	0.4	0.12	70
I-M	37	0.4	0.3	0.05	
SARDEGNA					
I90	3	0.3	0.1--	0.06	285
I91	5	0.7	0.5	0.26	36
I92	5	0.3	0.2	0.09	207
I95	0	0.0	0.0--	0.00	346
I-N	13	0.3	0.2	0.06	
SICILIA					
I81	4	0.4	0.2	0.10	207
I82	8	0.3	0.2	0.07	207
I83	10	0.6	0.4	0.14	70
I84	7	0.6	0.4	0.15	70
I85	6	0.8	0.6	0.27	20
I86	2	0.4	0.2	0.15	207
I87	7	0.3	0.2	0.08	207
I88	5	0.7	0.4	0.21	70
I89	4	0.4	0.3	0.14	137
I-O	53	0.4	0.3	0.04	
TOSCANA					
I45	1	0.2	0.1-	0.10	285
I46	6	0.6	0.2	0.08	207
I47	3	0.4	0.1-	0.08	285
I48	23	0.7	0.4	0.09	70
I49	4	0.5	0.2	0.10	207
I50	3	0.3	0.2	0.10	207
I51	3	0.4	0.2	0.13	207
I52	2	0.3	0.2	0.11	207
I53	3	0.5	0.2	0.12	207
I-P	48	0.5	0.2	0.04	
TRENTINO-ALTO ADIGE					
I21	9	0.8	0.6	0.21	20
I22	4	0.4	0.2	0.10	207
I-Q	13	0.6	0.4	0.11	
UMBRIA					
I54	12	0.8	0.4	0.12	70
I55	4	0.7	0.4	0.21	70
I-R	16	0.8	0.4	0.10	
VALLE D'AOSTA					
I07	3	1.1	0.7	0.43	9
VENETO					
I23	15	0.8	0.5	0.13	36
I24	13	0.7	0.5	0.15	36
I25	8	1.4	0.7	0.25	9
I26	14	0.8	0.6	0.16	20
I27	14	0.7	0.4	0.12	70
I28	14	0.7	0.5	0.13	36
I29	1	0.2	0.1-	0.09	285
I-T	79	0.7	0.5++	0.06	
I.0	802	0.6	0.3++	0.01	
IRELAND (1976-80)					
CONNAUGHT					
R07	6	1.5	0.7	0.31	9
R12	0	0.0	0.0--	0.00	346
R16	5	1.8	0.9	0.40	6
R20	0	0.0	0.0--	0.00	346
R21	1	0.7	0.3	0.31	137
R-A	12	1.2	0.6	0.17	
LEINSTER					
R01	2	2.1	1.5	1.17	2
R06	16	0.6	0.5	0.14	36
R09	1	0.4	0.3	0.27	137
R10	1	0.6	0.2	0.24	207
R11	1	0.8	0.5	0.52	36
R14	1	1.4	1.2	1.17	3
R15	1	0.5	0.5	0.46	36
R17	1	0.5	0.2	0.24	207
R19	1	0.7	0.6	0.60	20
R24	1	0.7	0.5	0.50	36
R25	4	1.7	1.1	0.59	4
R26	2	1.0	0.4	0.31	70
R-B	32	0.7	0.6+	0.10	
MUNSTER					
R03	1	0.5	0.1	0.14	285
R04	12	1.2	0.9+	0.26	6
R08	3	1.0	0.6	0.35	20
R13	1	0.3	0.1	0.12	285
R22	2	0.6	0.3	0.26	137
R23	7	3.2	2.5+	1.02	1
R-C	26	1.1	0.7++	0.15	
ULSTER					
R02	2	1.6	1.0	0.70	5
R05	1	0.3	0.1-	0.10	285
R18	1	0.8	0.7	0.69	9
R-D	4	0.7	0.4	0.24	
R.0	74	0.9	0.6++	0.07	
LUXEMBOURG (1971-80)					
LE	0	0.0	0.0--	0.00	346
LN	2	0.8	0.3	0.19	137
LS	7	0.5	0.3	0.11	137
L.0	9	0.5	0.2	0.09	
NEDERLAND (1976-80)					
N01	2	0.1	0.1--	0.08	285
N02	3	0.2	0.2	0.12	207
N03	2	0.2	0.1-	0.09	285
N04	2	0.1	0.1--	0.06	285
N05	7	0.2	0.1--	0.05	285
N06	4	0.2	0.1-	0.07	285
N07	14	0.2	0.2--	0.04	207
N08	17	0.2	0.1--	0.03	285
N09	3	0.4	0.2	0.12	207
N10	13	0.3	0.2-	0.05	207
N11	3	0.1	0.1--	0.04	285
N.0	70	0.2	0.1--	0.02	
EEC-9					
EEC	4445	0.6	0.3	0.01	

BELGIE-BELGIQUE (1971-78)

BRUSSEL-BRUXELLES					
B21	4296	108.7	67.9++	1.07	56

VLAANDEREN					
B10	6569	106.6	74.2++	0.93	29
B29	3132	87.2	62.0++	1.13	93
B30	3586	84.5	60.3++	1.04	106
B40	5272	100.7	66.5++	0.95	66
B70	2030	72.9	74.2++	1.66	29
B-V	20589	93.5	67.3++	0.48	

WALLONIE					
B25	974	94.9	67.4++	2.20	59
B50	5102	99.5	67.1++	0.96	64
B60	4810	122.1	80.9++	1.19	14
B80	1090	126.2	86.0++	2.67	6
B90	1771	116.8	82.1++	1.99	11
B-W	13747	110.2	74.5++	0.65	
B.0	38632	100.5	69.8++	0.36	

BR DEUTSCHLAND (1976-80)

BADEN-WURTTEMBERG					
D81	3717	44.6	33.1--	0.57	263
D82	3371	59.3	42.8--	0.77	192
D83	2415	54.7	40.4--	0.87	206
D84	1584	44.0	33.9--	0.90	261
D-A	11087	50.4	37.3--	0.37	

BAYERN					
D91	4822	55.4	39.3--	0.59	214
D92	1436	61.3	43.4--	1.19	190
D93	1391	60.2	45.4--	1.26	173
D94	1528	61.9	40.3--	1.08	207
D95	2095	58.3	39.5--	0.90	213
D96	1427	50.0	36.4--	1.00	241
D97	1994	55.1	37.3--	0.87	233
D-B	14693	56.8	39.7--	0.34	

BERLIN (WEST)					
DB0	4601	107.6	62.0++	1.00	93

BREMEN					
D40	1465	89.1	55.6	1.53	124

HAMBURG					
D20	4014	103.6	58.7++	0.99	112

HESSEN					
D64	7121	67.7	46.5--	0.58	167
D66	1802	63.5	38.2--	0.96	221
D-F	8923	66.8	44.6--	0.50	

NIEDERSACHSEN					
D31	2894	74.2	47.4--	0.94	160
D32	3426	70.5	44.2--	0.80	182
D33	2367	67.7	45.1--	0.98	174
D34	3114	61.6	46.8--	0.88	163
D-G	11801	68.2	45.8--	0.45	

NORDRHEIN-WESTFALEN					
D51	11669	94.4	69.2++	0.66	52
D53	7481	79.8	64.3++	0.76	83
D55	4048	69.9	59.1++	0.95	110
D57	2863	66.8	46.8--	0.91	163
D59	7059	79.9	59.8++	0.74	107
D-H	33120	81.5	62.2++	0.35	

RHEINLAND-PFALZ					
D71	2707	83.1	54.5	1.11	127
D72	1018	90.9	61.5++	2.02	99
D73	3322	77.1	53.5	0.97	130
D-I	7047	81.2	54.9+	0.69	

SAARLAND					
DA0	2368	92.4	63.3++	1.36	87

SCHLESWIG-HOLSTEIN					
D10	4456	71.5	47.6--	0.76	158
D.0	103575	70.7	50.2--	0.16	

DANMARK (1971-80)

K15	6860	112.7	70.9++	0.87	44
K20	814	53.8	49.9-	1.76	145
K25	498	53.6	52.8	2.39	133
K30	948	70.0	44.3--	1.49	179
K35	1062	82.4	46.3--	1.47	168
K40	80	33.6	20.5--	2.40	349
K42	1599	72.2	44.3--	1.14	179
K50	696	56.9	38.5--	1.50	218
K55	532	51.1	38.3--	1.69	219
K60	927	58.8	39.6--	1.34	211
K65	583	45.4	34.7--	1.47	253
K70	1769	63.8	45.5--	1.11	171
K76	548	47.9	30.1--	1.33	287
K80	1296	54.9	35.5--	1.01	246
K.0	18212	72.8	48.6--	0.37	

FRANCE (1971-78)

ALSACE					
F67	1908	55.3	44.1--	1.05	184
F68	1359	54.3	45.9--	1.30	170
F-A	3267	54.9	44.9--	0.82	

AQUITAINE					
F24	715	49.1	26.5--	1.05	308
F33	2380	58.3	40.1--	0.85	208
F40	571	51.0	30.7--	1.37	283
F47	557	49.0	28.5--	1.27	298
F64	1095	53.0	34.1--	1.08	258
F-B	5318	53.9	34.0--	0.49	

AUVERGNE					
F03	743	50.2	28.9--	1.13	295
F15	271	40.9	24.7--	1.58	326
F43	312	38.9	23.4--	1.42	338
F63	829	36.4	27.0--	0.96	304
F-C	2155	41.3	26.8--	0.60	

BASSE-NORMANDIE					
F14	910	41.6	36.6--	1.23	240
F50	649	37.3	27.9--	1.12	300
F61	392	34.2	25.8--	1.35	314
F-D	1951	38.5	30.9--	0.71	

BOURGOGNE					
F21	836	46.6	35.5--	1.28	246
F58	544	55.6	30.9--	1.43	281
F71	1173	52.3	34.0--	1.05	260
F89	634	53.4	31.5--	1.36	275
F-E	3187	51.4	33.3--	0.63	

BRETAGNE					
F22	701	34.4	23.6--	0.92	335
F29	1578	50.6	36.0--	0.94	244
F35	700	25.9	21.5--	0.83	345
F56	753	34.2	26.4--	0.98	310
F-F	3732	37.1	27.7--	0.47	

CENTRE					
F18	641	51.2	32.0--	1.34	272
F28	541	40.3	29.3--	1.32	291
F36	416	42.6	23.5--	1.24	337
F37	836	45.0	32.4--	1.17	267
F41	451	40.7	25.4--	1.28	319
F45	843	43.3	31.2--	1.13	277
F-G	3728	43.9	29.4--	0.51	

CHAMPAGNE-ARDENNE					
F08	727	58.5	47.5--	1.82	159
F10	623	55.5	39.1--	1.66	216
F51	960	45.6	39.3--	1.31	214
F52	382	45.0	33.0--	1.75	264
F-H	2692	50.6	40.0--	0.80	

CORSE					
F20	650	67.9	44.3--	1.80	179

FRANCHE-COMTE					
F25	741	39.4	38.0--	1.42	223
F39	447	47.1	32.2--	1.59	270
F70	425	48.7	35.2--	1.81	250
F90	259	50.7	44.2--	2.80	182
F-J	1872	44.4	36.3--	0.86	

HAUTE-NORMANDIE					
F27	756	45.1	37.1--	1.40	235
F76	2298	49.9	42.2--	0.90	197
F-K	3054	48.6	40.8--	0.76	

ILE-DE-FRANCE					
F75	5476	64.4	40.5--	0.57	204
F77	1349	44.8	38.8--	1.09	217
F78	1450	33.6	35.4--	0.95	248
F91	1323	36.0	39.8--	1.12	210
F92	2946	52.4	42.4--	0.79	195
F93	2645	50.0	48.5--	0.96	153
F94	2159	45.5	40.9--	0.89	203
F95	1311	39.2	39.9--	1.12	209
F-L	18659	48.5	41.1--	0.31	

LANGUEDOC-ROUSSILLON					
F11	693	66.5	32.1--	1.31	271
F30	1086	56.4	36.1--	1.14	243
F34	1379	55.4	34.7--	0.98	253
F48	90	30.0	18.2--	2.04	353
F66	837	72.3	37.8--	1.39	227
F-M	4085	59.1	34.5--	0.57	

LIMOUSIN					
F19	467	49.7	26.5--	1.31	308
F23	293	51.1	25.2--	1.63	321
F87	632	46.2	27.0--	1.14	304
F-N	1392	48.3	26.4--	0.76	

LORRAINE					
F54	1745	61.1	52.1	1.28	134
F55	463	57.5	42.0--	2.04	198
F57	2419	59.7	56.3+	1.17	122
F88	771	49.6	37.4--	1.40	231
F-O	5398	58.3	49.8--	0.69	

MIDI-PYRENEES					
F09	286	52.3	24.6--	1.58	329
F12	440	40.6	22.5--	1.14	341
F31	1467	48.8	34.9--	0.94	252
F32	326	46.7	24.7--	1.46	326
F46	276	46.9	24.4--	1.57	330
F65	506	57.0	34.1--	1.58	258
F81	662	50.1	29.2--	1.20	293
F82	335	46.7	27.4--	1.60	302
F-P	4298	48.6	29.2--	0.47	

NORD-PAS-DE-CALAIS					
F59	5619	57.1	49.2--	0.68	150
F62	2973	54.2	44.6--	0.83	177
F-Q	8592	56.1	47.5--	0.53	

PAYS DE LA LOIRE					
F44	1050	29.1	24.8--	0.78	325
F49	748	30.4	24.1--	0.91	333
F53	244	24.1	18.2--	1.19	353
F72	643	33.4	25.1--	1.03	323
F85	481	27.5	19.7--	0.94	350
F-R	3166	29.5	23.2--	0.42	

PICARDIE					
F02	1201	56.6	43.6--	1.32	189
F60	1039	42.6	37.4--	1.20	231
F80	1071	50.7	38.0--	1.21	223
F-S	3311	49.6	39.6--	0.72	

POITOU-CHARENTES					
F16	534	40.5	25.8--	1.18	314
F17	945	48.8	31.1--	1.07	279
F79	469	35.2	23.7--	1.16	334
F86	556	39.6	25.9--	1.16	313
F-T	2504	41.8	27.1--	0.57	

PROVENCE-ALPES-COTE D'AZUR					
F04	200	44.6	25.2--	1.88	321
F05	167	43.1	27.5--	2.21	301
F06	1283	41.7	21.5--	0.65	345
F13	3730	58.4	42.5--	0.71	194
F83	1765	71.7	43.9--	1.08	187
F84	848	54.8	38.3--	1.36	219
F-U	7993	55.8	35.9--	0.42	

RHONE-ALPES					
F01	660	43.6	32.4--	1.31	267
F07	408	40.7	24.7--	1.29	326
F26	620	44.0	30.6--	1.29	284
F38	1553	45.5	38.1--	0.99	222
F42	1486	50.7	37.5--	1.00	230
F69	2589	46.1	39.6--	0.79	211
F73	589	48.4	38.0--	1.60	223
F74	733	40.8	36.2--	1.36	242
F-V	8638	45.7	36.2--	0.40	
F.0	99642	48.4	35.9--	0.12	

UNITED KINGDOM (1976-80)

EAST ANGLIA					
G25	1523	88.5	65.7++	1.72	71
G46	2140	107.4	61.8++	1.38	95
G55	1693	95.4	61.6++	1.54	97
G-A	5356	97.6	62.8++	0.88	

EAST MIDLANDS					
G30	2709	102.8	64.8++	1.27	79
G44	2248	91.3	63.9++	1.37	84
G45	1503	95.5	60.8++	1.60	103
G47	1360	89.0	62.3++	1.73	91
G50	3155	110.1	74.1++	1.34	31
G-B	10975	99.2	66.1++	0.64	

NORTHERN					
G14	5139	151.7	101.3++	1.44	1
G27	2089	124.9	97.4++	2.15	2
G29	1440	104.9	65.6++	1.77	72
G33	1976	110.9	74.8++	1.71	25
G48	1022	119.9	74.8++	2.39	25
G-C	11666	128.7	87.0++	0.82	

NORTH-WEST					
G11	9411	121.4	84.1++	0.88	8
G12	6197	138.5	96.3++	1.25	3
G26	2657	98.7	71.9++	1.42	39
G43	4560	115.9	70.9++	1.08	44
G-D	22825	121.0	82.2++	0.56	

SOUTH-EAST					
G01	25655	128.4	77.5++	0.49	20
G22	1309	88.0	69.0++	1.93	53
G23	1676	83.4	64.7++	1.60	81
G24	1360	86.5	66.4++	1.82	67
G34	2616	146.8	65.2++	1.37	74
G35	4297	102.5	68.7++	1.07	54
G37	4316	98.1	71.7++	1.11	40
G39	2603	94.0	67.7++	1.35	57
G41	426	132.2	60.9+	3.13	102
G42	4534	107.5	67.3++	1.03	61
G51	1356	81.1	65.3++	1.84	73
G56	2822	97.1	61.5++	1.18	99
G58	2176	122.6	62.5++	1.41	89
G-E	55146	112.3	71.2++	0.31	

SOUTH-WEST					
G21	2770	104.0	65.1++	1.27	76
G28	1179	98.7	53.5	1.62	130
G31	2982	108.2	57.9++	1.12	119
G32	2032	122.6	59.3++	1.39	108
G36	1365	94.3	61.0++	1.69	101
G53	1141	94.7	54.3	1.67	128
G59	1354	87.3	63.0++	1.75	88
G-F	12823	102.8	59.6++	0.55	

WEST MIDLANDS					
G15	9326	115.5	80.8++	0.85	15
G38	1618	90.3	60.8++	1.54	103
G52	982	91.6	63.5++	2.07	85
G54	2940	99.8	73.2++	1.37	35
G57	1259	90.9	66.0++	1.89	68
G-G	16125	105.6	74.5++	0.60	

YORKSHIRE AND HUMBERSIDE					
G13	4568	119.2	77.5++	1.17	20
G16	6672	110.8	74.0++	0.92	32
G40	2971	120.3	81.2++	1.52	12
G49	1931	99.4	61.7++	1.45	96
G-H	16142	113.1	74.4++	0.60	

WALES					
G61	1275	115.2	70.6++	2.03	48
G62	846	90.1	51.3	1.80	138
G63	1348	104.9	69.9++	1.93	50
G64	771	117.7	68.5++	2.56	55
G65	1481	94.0	65.0++	1.71	77
G66	258	81.4	44.6--	2.89	177
G67	1220	108.9	72.3++	2.11	38
G68	1168	110.5	67.5++	2.01	58
G-I	8367	103.9	65.5++	0.73	

SCOTLAND(1975-80)					
S01	433	77.8	56.6	2.78	121
S02	1330	99.4	67.3++	1.90	61
S03	1356	117.3	77.9++	2.17	19
S04	1115	111.9	78.5++	2.40	18
S05	2717	126.3	88.3++	1.73	5
S06	295	102.7	58.4	3.51	115
S07	805	100.5	71.1++	2.55	41
S08	9185	129.9	95.3++	1.01	4
S09	433	103.3	67.1++	3.30	64
S10	34	63.9	37.2-	6.65	234
S11	39	62.3	44.9	7.55	176
S12	71	80.9	48.1	6.10	156
G-J	17813	118.9	83.8++	0.64	

NORTHERN IRELAND					
JE	1426	86.9	70.9++	1.93	44
JN	506	55.9	46.8--	2.13	163
JS	242	36.4	29.3--	1.93	291
JW	384	63.9	51.8	2.71	135
G-K	2558	67.1	54.9	1.11	
G.0	179796	110.7	72.9++	0.18	

ITALIA (1975-79)

ABRUZZI					
I66	315	43.0	27.1--	1.57	303
I67	241	36.4	25.7--	1.69	317
I68	312	44.9	32.7--	1.89	266
I69	321	35.8	24.4--	1.38	330
I-A	1189	39.8	27.1--	0.80	

BASILICATA					
I76	254	24.8	18.9--	1.22	352
I77	137	27.2	23.1--	2.01	339
I-B	391	25.6	20.2--	1.05	

CALABRIA					
I78	406	22.9	19.6--	0.99	351
I79	483	26.4	22.9--	1.07	340
I80	475	32.5	24.2--	1.15	332
I-C	1364	26.9	22.2--	0.61	

CAMPANIA					
I61	724	40.5	38.0--	1.43	223
I62	270	37.5	26.1--	1.64	311
I63	3892	55.6	58.6++	0.94	114
I64	384	35.4	25.8--	1.35	314
I65	940	38.1	31.7--	1.05	273
I-D	6210	47.6	44.3--	0.57	

EMILIA-ROMAGNA					
I33	584	83.8	48.3-	2.05	155
I34	828	85.1	49.3-	1.75	148
I35	845	85.1	53.5	1.87	130
I36	1084	76.4	51.6	1.59	136
I37	1756	77.7	48.4--	1.17	154
I38	1051	112.1	69.9++	2.19	50
I39	724	82.3	51.5	1.96	137
I40	896	62.0	44.0--	1.48	186
I-E	7768	80.9	51.2--	0.59	

FRIULI-VENEZIA GIULIA					
I30	1312	102.1	65.2++	1.83	74
I31	400	113.8	75.9++	3.91	23
I32	1011	145.1	74.6++	2.47	28
I93	614	94.0	67.2++	2.76	63
I-F	3337	111.7	69.1++	1.23	

LAZIO					
I56	374	57.1	37.6--	1.98	228
I57	153	42.9	25.1--	2.12	323
I58	5946	66.9	58.0++	0.76	118
I59	510	49.1	45.5--	2.03	171
I60	474	42.4	30.9--	1.45	281
I-G	7457	61.8	51.0--	0.59	

LIGURIA					
I08	430	77.5	42.3--	2.13	196
I09	560	75.8	42.9--	1.86	191
I10	2789	108.1	61.6++	1.19	97
I11	630	106.4	60.6++	2.47	105
I-H	4409	98.8	55.9++	0.86	

LOMBARDIA					
I12	1441	76.9	64.8++	1.74	79
I13	1437	78.3	64.4++	1.73	82
I14	292	68.0	57.3	3.40	120
I15	8473	86.9	73.1++	0.80	36
I16	1603	74.9	70.0++	1.76	49
I17	2027	82.9	73.3++	1.64	33
I18	1420	111.9	66.0++	1.81	68
I19	834	102.8	70.7++	2.49	47
I20	944	101.9	65.0++	2.16	77
I-I	18471	86.0	69.7++	0.52	

MARCHE					
I41	431	53.2	35.6--	1.74	245
I42	653	63.3	41.4--	1.64	202
I43	385	54.3	34.2--	1.78	257
I44	363	42.5	30.1--	1.60	287
I-J	1832	53.8	35.7--	0.85	

MOLISE					
I70	190	32.9	21.7--	1.63	344
I94	83	35.9	21.8--	2.48	343
I-K	273	33.8	21.8--	1.36	

PIEMONTE					
I01	3400	58.4	46.8--	0.81	163
I02	829	85.6	50.8	1.83	141
I03	1008	82.2	55.0	1.78	125
I04	702	51.8	31.0--	1.22	280
I05	365	68.0	37.6--	2.10	228
I06	1107	95.3	48.8--	1.54	152
I-L	7411	66.9	45.4--	0.54	

PUGLIA					
I71	650	38.7	31.2--	1.26	277
I72	1500	42.8	37.1--	0.98	235
I73	677	49.5	47.1--	1.82	161
I74	493	51.9	45.1--	2.05	174
I75	1075	59.3	50.3-	1.55	143
I-M	4395	47.2	40.8--	0.62	

SARDEGNA					
I90	486	46.4	36.8--	1.72	237
I91	202	29.6	26.1--	1.90	311
I92	681	38.7	36.7--	1.42	238
I95	121	31.2	22.1--	2.12	342
I-N	1490	38.4	32.8--	0.87	

SICILIA					
I81	399	38.6	27.0--	1.40	304
I82	1214	42.4	33.8--	0.99	262
I83	652	39.8	28.6--	1.15	297
I84	343	28.8	21.3--	1.19	347
I85	225	31.1	25.3--	1.73	320
I86	118	23.4	16.7--	1.60	355
I87	884	36.4	29.6--	1.02	290
I88	242	36.8	26.6--	1.75	307
I89	348	36.0	28.9--	1.58	295
I-O	4425	36.8	28.3--	0.44	

TOSCANA					
I45	467	94.0	59.1+	2.79	110
I46	878	94.2	58.7+	2.03	112
I47	531	83.2	50.3	2.24	143
I48	2342	81.3	50.4--	1.07	142
I49	768	91.4	56.1	2.06	123
I50	772	82.4	49.9-	1.85	145
I51	452	58.7	36.7--	1.76	238
I52	354	55.9	30.2--	1.65	286
I53	406	73.6	44.1--	2.24	184
I-P	6970	80.3	48.8--	0.60	

TRENTINO-ALTO ADIGE					
I21	524	49.7	42.8--	1.90	192
I22	725	67.5	49.3-	1.88	148
I-Q	1249	58.7	46.3--	1.34	

UMBRIA					
I54	694	49.4	31.6--	1.22	274
I55	295	52.6	32.4--	1.91	267
I-R	989	50.4	31.8--	1.03	

VALLE D'AOSTA					
I07	164	57.5	41.6--	3.27	201

VENETO					
I23	1342	72.1	55.0	1.52	125
I24	1201	69.3	58.2++	1.69	116
I25	568	105.1	71.0++	3.04	43
I26	1265	73.8	59.2++	1.69	109
I27	2113	103.3	83.9++	1.84	9
I28	1748	89.5	74.7++	1.80	27
I29	679	109.4	76.3++	2.98	22
I-T	8916	85.2	67.6++	0.72	
I.0	88710	64.6	48.6--	0.17	

IRELAND (1976-80)

CONNAUGHT					
R07	188	43.5	30.6--	2.34	284
R12	30	40.3	23.6--	4.72	335
R16	129	44.1	25.7--	2.45	317
R20	53	37.2	21.2--	3.14	348
R21	70	50.3	31.3--	3.97	276
R-A	470	43.5	27.2--	1.34	

LEINSTER					
R01	50	50.7	46.2	6.67	169
R06	1633	69.0	75.2++	1.88	24
R09	110	43.4	49.5	4.77	147
R10	96	53.8	40.5--	4.22	204
R11	57	43.5	34.5--	4.69	255
R14	38	47.3	34.4--	5.80	256
R15	122	56.7	54.2	4.96	129
R17	119	51.0	48.1	4.50	156
R19	63	42.3	35.1--	4.51	251
R24	80	52.4	41.8-	4.78	200
R25	137	55.9	43.8-	3.87	188
R26	111	52.9	49.2	4.79	150
R-B	2616	60.7	59.0++	1.17	

MUNSTER					
R03	85	38.7	28.3--	3.18	299
R04	615	61.8	51.0	2.11	140
R08	158	50.8	33.0--	2.74	264
R13	222	56.0	47.1-	3.23	161
R22	194	56.3	42.0--	3.11	198
R23	132	60.1	51.3	4.57	138
R-C	1406	56.5	44.0--	1.20	

ULSTER					
R02	65	45.9	29.7--	3.85	289
R05	137	43.7	29.2--	2.66	293
R18	70	53.3	35.3--	4.35	249
R-D	272	46.4	30.6--	1.95	
R.0	4764	56.3	46.3--	0.69	

LUXEMBOURG (1971-80)

LE	173	95.2	62.5	4.89	89
LN	301	114.0	72.4++	4.32	37
LS	1147	89.9	66.0++	1.98	68
L.0	1621	94.1	66.3++	1.67	

NEDERLAND (1976-80)

N01	1262	92.5	67.4++	1.96	59
N02	1221	85.5	63.4++	1.89	86
N03	836	80.6	62.2++	2.21	92
N04	2158	86.0	71.1++	1.56	41
N05	3658	88.1	73.3++	1.24	33
N06	1987	91.8	79.4++	1.81	17
N07	6126	105.8	79.7++	1.04	16
N08	8211	109.0	81.1++	0.91	13
N09	765	90.1	58.1+	2.20	117
N10	4310	85.2	83.1++	1.28	10
N11	2481	93.3	84.8++	1.72	7
N.0	33015	95.6	76.8++	0.43	

EEC-9

EEC	567967	74.7	53.5	0.07	

BELGIE-BELGIQUE (1971-78)

BRUSSEL-BRUXELLES					
B21	628	14.1	6.6--	0.30	132
VLAANDEREN					
B10	738	11.7	7.0--	0.27	122
B29	260	7.1	4.2--	0.28	210
B30	388	9.0	5.4--	0.29	170
B40	563	10.5	5.9--	0.27	152
B70	132	4.9	4.1--	0.37	215
B-V	2081	9.3	5.6--	0.13	
WALLONIE					
B25	95	8.9	4.9--	0.56	182
B50	470	8.6	4.5--	0.23	194
B60	436	10.3	5.6--	0.30	164
B80	73	8.2	4.5--	0.58	194
B90	120	7.5	4.0--	0.40	228
B-W	1194	9.0	4.8--	0.15	
B.0	3903	9.7	5.5--	0.10	

BR DEUTSCHLAND (1976-80)

BADEN-WURTTEMBERG					
D81	674	7.6	4.0--	0.17	228
D82	565	9.1	4.6--	0.21	186
D83	368	7.6	4.0--	0.23	228
D84	243	6.3	3.4--	0.24	279
D-A	1850	7.8	4.1--	0.10	
BAYERN					
D91	951	10.2	5.1--	0.18	174
D92	189	7.2	3.6--	0.29	262
D93	191	7.6	3.8--	0.30	247
D94	251	9.0	3.8--	0.27	247
D95	392	9.8	4.6--	0.26	186
D96	227	7.3	3.7--	0.27	258
D97	367	9.2	4.5--	0.26	194
D-B	2568	9.1	4.4--	0.10	
BERLIN(WEST)					
DB0	1476	27.8	10.1++	0.32	87
BREMEN					
D40	284	15.3	6.9	0.46	124
HAMBURG					
D20	1024	22.9	9.3++	0.33	97
HESSEN					
D64	1310	11.5	5.7--	0.18	160
D66	321	10.3	4.6--	0.28	186
D-F	1631	11.3	5.4--	0.15	
NIEDERSACHSEN					
D31	506	11.8	5.5--	0.27	167
D32	687	12.6	5.8--	0.25	154
D33	384	10.4	5.0--	0.28	179
D34	426	7.8	4.2--	0.22	210
D-G	2003	10.6	5.1--	0.13	
NORDRHEIN-WESTFALEN					
D51	1877	13.6	7.1--	0.18	119
D53	1216	12.1	6.8--	0.21	125
D55	568	9.1	5.5--	0.24	167
D57	426	9.0	4.5--	0.23	194
D59	1042	10.8	5.7--	0.19	160
D-H	5129	11.5	6.2--	0.09	
RHEINLAND-PFALZ					
D71	325	9.1	4.5--	0.28	194
D72	113	9.1	4.4--	0.45	201
D73	461	9.8	4.8--	0.25	183
D-I	899	9.5	4.6--	0.17	
SAARLAND					
DA0	279	9.8	5.1--	0.33	174
SCHLESWIG-HOLSTEIN					
D10	871	12.9	5.9--	0.23	152
D.0	18014	11.2	5.5--	0.05	

DANMARK (1971-80)

K15	2208	33.2	16.9++	0.39	18
K20	237	15.8	12.7++	0.85	67
K25	100	11.0	9.6	0.99	92
K30	190	14.2	9.4+	0.72	95
K35	225	17.6	9.5+	0.69	94
K40	28	11.9	7.0	1.39	122
K42	364	16.3	9.2++	0.52	100
K50	141	11.5	7.2	0.65	118
K55	137	13.5	9.9+	0.88	89
K60	217	13.6	8.8	0.64	106
K65	154	12.3	9.0	0.75	102
K70	454	16.1	10.8++	0.54	84
K76	128	11.4	7.5	0.71	114
K80	332	14.2	9.0+	0.52	102
K.0	4915	19.3	11.7++	0.18	

FRANCE (1971-78)

ALSACE					
F67	249	6.9	3.8--	0.27	247
F68	159	6.1	3.4--	0.30	279
F-A	408	6.6	3.7--	0.20	
AQUITAINE					
F24	124	8.1	3.5--	0.39	270
F33	384	8.7	4.1--	0.24	215
F40	91	7.8	3.4--	0.43	279
F47	87	7.3	3.4--	0.41	279
F64	171	7.7	4.0--	0.35	228
F-B	857	8.1	3.8--	0.15	
AUVERGNE					
F03	159	10.2	3.9--	0.37	236
F15	50	7.4	3.4--	0.58	279
F43	57	6.8	2.9--	0.45	322
F63	156	6.6	3.8--	0.34	247
F-C	422	7.8	3.7--	0.21	
BASSE-NORMANDIE					
F14	116	5.0	3.0--	0.31	309
F50	98	5.3	2.6--	0.30	344
F61	76	6.3	3.2--	0.42	292
F-D	290	5.4	2.9--	0.19	
BOURGOGNE					
F21	85	4.6	2.5--	0.30	347
F58	75	7.4	2.9--	0.39	322
F71	157	6.8	3.1--	0.29	303
F89	83	6.8	3.0--	0.40	309
F-E	400	6.3	2.9--	0.17	
BRETAGNE					
F22	128	5.9	2.8--	0.28	332
F29	253	7.6	4.0--	0.28	228
F35	150	5.1	2.9--	0.26	322
F56	142	6.2	3.2--	0.29	292
F-F	673	6.3	3.3--	0.14	
CENTRE					
F18	99	7.7	3.2--	0.38	292
F28	61	4.6	2.4--	0.35	350
F36	72	7.2	3.5--	0.50	270
F37	129	6.6	3.3--	0.33	288
F41	79	6.9	2.8--	0.38	332
F45	107	5.4	2.9--	0.32	322
F-G	547	6.3	3.0--	0.15	
CHAMPAGNE-ARDENNE					
F08	59	4.7	3.0--	0.43	309
F10	65	5.6	3.0--	0.43	309
F51	123	5.8	3.6--	0.35	262
F52	29	3.4	2.1--	0.44	354
F-H	276	5.1	3.1--	0.21	
CORSE					
F20	68	7.9	3.6--	0.48	262
FRANCHE-COMTE					
F25	86	4.5	3.4--	0.40	279
F39	57	5.8	3.3--	0.49	288
F70	56	6.3	3.6--	0.55	262
F90	25	4.9	3.1--	0.68	303
F-J	224	5.2	3.4--	0.25	
HAUTE-NORMANDIE					
F27	95	5.5	3.2--	0.37	292
F76	251	5.2	3.0--	0.21	309
F-K	346	5.3	3.0--	0.18	
ILE-DE-FRANCE					
F75	1145	11.6	5.0--	0.17	179
F77	189	6.2	3.8--	0.31	247
F78	252	5.8	4.3--	0.30	204
F91	177	4.8	3.8--	0.31	247
F92	466	7.9	4.6--	0.23	186
F93	345	6.5	4.6--	0.27	186
F94	310	6.2	3.9--	0.25	236
F95	174	5.1	3.7--	0.30	258
F-L	3058	7.5	4.5--	0.09	
LANGUEDOC-ROUSSILLON					
F11	102	9.1	3.7--	0.42	258
F30	125	6.2	2.6--	0.26	344
F34	198	7.4	3.5--	0.29	270
F48	27	9.0	4.2--	0.97	210
F66	79	6.3	3.2--	0.41	292
F-M	531	7.2	3.3--	0.16	
LIMOUSIN					
F19	57	5.8	2.5--	0.40	347
F23	64	10.6	4.3--	0.65	204
F87	98	6.7	2.9--	0.34	322
F-N	219	7.2	3.1--	0.24	
LORRAINE					
F54	160	5.5	3.4--	0.30	279
F55	32	3.9	2.5--	0.48	347
F57	214	5.4	4.1--	0.29	215
F88	98	6.0	3.5--	0.40	270
F-O	504	5.4	3.6--	0.17	
MIDI-PYRENEES					
F09	40	7.1	2.9--	0.53	322
F12	70	6.1	2.2--	0.32	353
F31	204	6.4	3.5--	0.27	270
F32	39	5.6	2.1--	0.38	354
F46	51	8.4	3.6--	0.59	262
F65	67	7.2	3.1--	0.43	303
F81	91	6.6	2.9--	0.35	322
F82	50	6.6	2.7--	0.43	340
F-P	612	6.6	3.0--	0.14	
NORD-PAS-DE-CALAIS					
F59	529	5.2	3.1--	0.15	303
F62	287	5.0	3.0--	0.19	309
F-Q	816	5.1	3.1--	0.12	
PAYS DE LA LOIRE					
F44	190	4.9	3.0--	0.24	309
F49	141	5.4	2.9--	0.28	322
F53	62	5.7	3.0--	0.43	309
F72	133	6.6	3.8--	0.37	247
F85	108	5.9	3.0--	0.34	309
F-R	634	5.6	3.1--	0.14	
PICARDIE					
F02	130	6.1	3.5--	0.34	270
F60	116	4.8	2.8--	0.29	332
F80	131	6.0	3.2--	0.32	292
F-S	377	5.6	3.1--	0.18	
POITOU-CHARENTES					
F16	104	7.5	3.5--	0.39	270
F17	171	8.4	4.1--	0.36	215
F79	76	5.6	2.6--	0.35	344
F86	99	6.8	3.6--	0.42	262
F-T	450	7.2	3.5--	0.19	
PROVENCE-ALPES-COTE D'AZUR					
F04	29	6.5	2.7--	0.58	340
F05	37	9.5	4.3--	0.82	204
F06	237	6.9	3.2--	0.25	292
F13	488	7.3	4.1--	0.20	215
F83	203	8.0	3.8--	0.31	247
F84	84	5.3	2.8--	0.33	332
F-U	1078	7.1	3.6--	0.12	
RHONE-ALPES					
F01	94	6.2	3.2--	0.38	292
F07	75	7.2	3.0--	0.41	309
F26	103	7.0	4.1--	0.45	215
F38	212	6.1	3.5--	0.27	270
F42	211	6.8	3.8--	0.30	247
F69	394	6.7	4.0--	0.22	228
F73	85	6.9	4.0--	0.48	228
F74	107	5.9	3.9--	0.41	236
F-V	1281	6.6	3.7--	0.12	
F.0	14071	6.5	3.5--	0.03	

UNITED KINGDOM (1976-80)

EAST ANGLIA					
G25	423	25.1	15.5++	0.81	32
G46	589	28.4	14.3++	0.64	53
G55	450	25.4	13.2++	0.68	64
G-A	1462	26.4	14.3++	0.41	
EAST MIDLANDS					
G30	582	21.2	11.8++	0.52	75
G44	506	19.9	12.0++	0.57	72
G45	413	25.7	14.7++	0.77	46
G47	393	25.1	14.9++	0.81	44
G50	742	24.9	14.4++	0.56	51
G-B	2636	23.0	13.3++	0.28	
NORTHERN					
G14	1420	39.2	22.4++	0.63	4
G27	576	33.1	23.0++	1.00	3
G29	392	26.8	14.3++	0.79	53
G33	526	28.3	17.1++	0.79	17
G48	257	29.0	16.8++	1.12	19
G-C	3171	33.1	19.7++	0.37	
NORTH-WEST					
G11	2629	31.9	18.2++	0.38	11
G12	2047	42.2	23.8++	0.57	1
G26	655	23.3	14.6++	0.60	48
G43	1200	28.1	14.6++	0.47	48
G-D	6531	32.4	18.3++	0.24	

SOUTH-EAST					
G01	8332	38.3	19.1++	0.23	10
G22	299	20.3	14.2++	0.85	55
G23	511	25.3	15.4++	0.72	36
G24	404	25.9	16.1++	0.85	27
G34	873	40.8	15.2++	0.61	39
G35	1185	26.9	15.1++	0.47	41
G37	1249	28.9	16.6++	0.50	23
G39	754	26.0	15.5++	0.59	32
G41	140	38.7	15.4++	1.49	36
G42	1405	31.4	16.2++	0.47	26
G51	423	27.0	17.2++	0.88	15
G56	951	31.1	16.0++	0.55	30
G58	759	37.6	15.3++	0.64	38
G-E	17285	33.2	17.2++	0.14	
SOUTH-WEST					
G21	720	25.2	12.8++	0.52	66
G28	378	29.3	14.4++	0.81	51
G31	936	32.0	14.0++	0.52	57
G32	655	35.4	14.5++	0.65	50
G36	352	23.2	12.9++	0.73	65
G53	301	23.8	11.2++	0.71	82
G59	400	25.9	15.5++	0.82	32
G-F	3742	28.2	13.6++	0.25	
WEST MIDLANDS					
G15	2112	25.6	15.0++	0.35	42
G38	446	24.1	14.0++	0.71	57
G52	238	21.4	12.5++	0.86	70
G54	657	21.7	13.6++	0.56	60
G57	277	19.5	12.0++	0.76	72
G-G	3730	23.8	14.2++	0.25	
YORKSHIRE AND HUMBERSIDE					
G13	1089	27.2	15.9++	0.51	31
G16	1879	29.4	16.7++	0.42	22
G40	776	29.7	17.2++	0.66	15
G49	547	27.3	14.2++	0.66	55
G-H	4291	28.6	16.2++	0.27	
WALES					
G61	323	27.3	14.7++	0.90	46
G62	198	19.6	9.9++	0.76	89
G63	286	21.3	12.7++	0.79	67
G64	173	24.6	11.4++	0.96	79
G65	364	22.0	13.6++	0.75	60
G66	65	20.5	10.0	1.33	88
G67	333	27.7	15.0++	0.88	42
G68	219	19.1	11.0++	0.78	83
G-I	1961	22.9	12.7++	0.31	
SCOTLAND(1975-80)					
S01	146	25.5	16.1++	1.43	27
S02	411	28.8	16.8++	0.90	19
S03	467	37.3	20.1++	1.02	9
S04	300	28.8	17.5++	1.07	13
S05	855	36.2	21.1++	0.77	6
S06	122	39.1	18.1++	1.82	12
S07	204	24.8	16.1++	1.17	27
S08	2784	36.2	22.1++	0.44	5
S09	128	29.1	16.3++	1.54	25
S10	13	23.8	14.9	4.38	44
S11	5	8.2	3.6-	1.78	262
S12	18	19.9	8.9	2.60	105
G-J	5453	33.8	20.1++	0.29	
NORTHERN IRELAND					
JE	423	25.2	16.5++	0.84	24
JN	126	13.6	9.6+	0.90	92
JS	73	10.8	7.3	0.90	117
JW	116	18.9	12.6++	1.24	69
G-K	738	19.0	12.7++	0.49	
G.0	51000	29.8	16.4++	0.08	
ITALIA (1975-79)					
ABRUZZI					
I66	42	5.5	2.8--	0.45	332
I67	44	6.6	3.5--	0.58	270
I68	49	6.8	4.1--	0.61	215
I69	41	4.4	2.4--	0.39	350
I-A	176	5.7	3.1--	0.25	
BASILICATA					
I76	39	3.7	2.4--	0.41	350
I77	20	4.0	2.9--	0.65	322
I-B	59	3.8	2.5--	0.35	
CALABRIA					
I78	70	3.9	2.8--	0.34	332
I79	71	3.9	2.7--	0.33	340
I80	70	4.7	3.1--	0.40	303
I-C	211	4.1	2.8--	0.20	
CAMPANIA					
I61	106	5.8	4.6--	0.46	186
I62	39	5.3	3.2--	0.54	292
I63	520	7.1	5.8--	0.26	154
I64	50	4.5	3.0--	0.45	309
I65	117	4.6	3.3--	0.32	288
I-D	832	6.2	4.7--	0.17	
EMILIA-ROMAGNA					
I33	89	12.3	6.2-	0.70	147
I34	143	14.0	6.6-	0.58	132
I35	127	12.3	6.3-	0.60	141
I36	162	11.0	6.0--	0.49	149
I37	304	12.5	6.4--	0.39	137
I38	181	18.2	9.4+	0.74	95
I39	132	14.3	7.9	0.73	110
I40	155	10.4	6.3--	0.53	141
I-E	1293	12.8	6.8--	0.20	
FRIULI-VENEZIA GIULIA					
I30	259	19.1	9.3+	0.62	97
I31	66	17.3	7.8	1.03	111
I32	238	29.8	11.6++	0.82	78
I93	90	13.1	6.8	0.78	125
I-F	653	20.2	9.3++	0.39	
LAZIO					
I56	76	11.5	6.8	0.84	125
I57	25	6.9	3.4--	0.74	279
I58	998	10.6	7.5	0.24	114
I59	58	5.6	4.5--	0.60	194
I60	61	5.4	3.1--	0.43	303
I-G	1218	9.6	6.6--	0.19	
LIGURIA					
I08	81	13.5	6.3	0.79	141
I09	85	10.8	5.0--	0.58	179
I10	372	13.1	5.8--	0.32	154
I11	59	9.3	4.3--	0.60	204
I-H	597	12.3	5.5--	0.24	
LOMBARDIA					
I12	203	10.2	6.5--	0.47	135
I13	199	10.2	6.3--	0.46	141
I14	36	8.2	5.1--	0.90	174
I15	1311	12.6	8.3+	0.24	108
I16	228	10.3	7.1	0.48	119
I17	243	9.5	6.4--	0.43	137
I18	165	12.2	5.7--	0.49	160
I19	106	12.3	6.7	0.72	129
I20	117	12.0	6.8	0.67	125
I-I	2608	11.5	7.2--	0.15	
MARCHE					
I41	66	8.0	4.1--	0.53	215
I42	79	7.2	3.9--	0.45	236
I43	61	8.2	4.1--	0.55	215
I44	64	7.2	3.9--	0.51	236
I-J	270	7.6	4.0--	0.25	
MOLISE					
I70	40	6.7	3.9--	0.67	236
I94	14	5.8	3.9--	1.09	236
I-K	54	6.4	3.9--	0.58	
PIEMONTE					
I01	656	10.8	6.6--	0.27	132
I02	128	12.1	5.5--	0.54	167
I03	158	12.0	6.0--	0.51	149
I04	104	7.6	3.4--	0.37	279
I05	71	12.6	4.8--	0.65	183
I06	177	14.3	6.0--	0.51	149
I-L	1294	11.1	5.8--	0.17	
PUGLIA					
I71	90	5.3	3.8--	0.42	247
I72	210	5.8	4.4--	0.32	201
I73	66	4.7	3.9--	0.49	236
I74	39	3.9	3.0--	0.50	309
I75	97	5.0	3.9--	0.40	236
I-M	502	5.2	3.9--	0.18	
SARDEGNA					
I90	67	6.3	4.1--	0.53	215
I91	30	4.3	2.7--	0.53	340
I92	90	5.1	4.1--	0.44	215
I95	23	5.9	4.0--	0.89	228
I-N	210	5.4	3.8--	0.28	
SICILIA					
I81	73	6.8	3.9--	0.49	236
I82	241	8.1	5.6--	0.38	164
I83	107	6.2	3.7--	0.38	258
I84	55	4.6	3.2--	0.45	292
I85	29	3.9	2.9--	0.57	322
I86	20	3.9	2.8--	0.65	332
I87	132	5.3	3.8--	0.34	247
I88	33	4.8	3.0--	0.55	309
I89	55	5.7	4.3--	0.59	204
I-O	745	6.0	4.0--	0.16	
TOSCANA					
I45	49	9.3	4.6--	0.69	186
I46	131	13.0	6.1--	0.59	148
I47	65	9.6	5.1--	0.68	174
I48	395	12.8	6.4--	0.35	137
I49	97	11.0	5.4--	0.59	170
I50	104	10.6	5.2--	0.55	173
I51	53	6.7	3.3--	0.49	288
I52	61	9.3	4.2--	0.60	210
I53	47	8.4	4.4--	0.67	201
I-P	1002	10.9	5.4--	0.18	
TRENTINO-ALTO ADIGE					
I21	96	8.8	5.8--	0.62	154
I22	85	7.6	4.3--	0.49	204
I-Q	181	8.2	4.9--	0.39	
UMBRIA					
I54	96	6.7	3.6--	0.39	262
I55	60	10.4	5.8-	0.78	154
I-R	156	7.7	4.3--	0.36	
VALLE D'AOSTA					
I07	29	10.2	6.5	1.27	135
VENETO					
I23	236	12.1	7.1	0.48	119
I24	181	10.0	6.7-	0.52	129
I25	95	16.3	8.7	0.98	107
I26	184	10.3	6.3--	0.50	141
I27	321	15.0	9.7++	0.56	91
I28	287	14.1	9.2++	0.57	100
I29	82	12.7	7.6	0.88	113
I-T	1386	12.6	7.9	0.22	
I.0	13476	9.4	5.7--	0.05	
IRELAND (1976-80)					
CONNAUGHT					
R07	52	12.8	9.0	1.36	102
R12	4	6.2	3.2--	1.64	292
R16	33	11.9	6.7	1.28	129
R20	17	13.2	8.1	2.02	109
R21	23	17.2	11.3	2.67	80
R-A	129	12.8	8.1	0.77	
LEINSTER					
R01	17	18.0	15.5+	3.91	32
R06	641	25.1	20.8++	0.86	7
R09	51	21.9	23.5++	3.36	2
R10	26	15.5	11.8	2.40	75
R11	22	18.5	15.2+	3.31	39
R14	8	10.9	7.8	2.97	111
R15	55	25.5	20.4++	2.87	8
R17	33	15.0	13.4+	2.43	63
R19	21	15.2	11.8	2.71	75
R24	18	12.3	11.3	2.73	80
R25	56	23.6	17.5++	2.51	13
R26	43	20.5	16.8++	2.74	19
R-B	991	22.5	18.6++	0.62	
MUNSTER					
R03	25	12.2	10.3	2.25	86
R04	188	19.1	13.5++	1.04	62
R08	42	14.4	9.3	1.48	97
R13	56	14.3	10.8+	1.51	84
R22	57	17.6	12.3++	1.73	71
R23	41	18.9	13.9++	2.30	59
R-C	409	17.0	12.1++	0.63	
ULSTER					
R02	24	18.9	12.0	2.70	72
R05	28	9.4	7.4	1.47	116
R18	8	6.6	4.7	1.78	185
R-D	60	11.0	7.8	1.09	
R.0	1589	19.0	14.4++	0.38	
LUXEMBOURG (1971-80)					
LE	18	9.4	5.6	1.41	164
LN	22	8.3	4.1--	0.94	215
LS	139	10.3	5.8--	0.52	154
L.0	179	9.9	5.5--	0.44	
NEDERLAND (1976-80)					
N01	87	6.3	3.9--	0.46	236
N02	67	4.7	2.8--	0.38	332
N03	63	6.1	4.1--	0.54	215
N04	161	6.4	4.5--	0.37	194
N05	294	7.0	5.1--	0.31	174
N06	183	8.2	5.7--	0.45	160
N07	609	10.2	6.4--	0.28	137
N08	788	10.2	6.3--	0.24	141
N09	62	7.3	4.2--	0.59	210
N10	282	5.7	4.6--	0.28	186
N11	192	7.3	5.4--	0.40	170
N.0	2788	8.0	5.4--	0.11	
EEC-9					
EEC	109935	13.7	7.8	0.03	

BELGIE-BELGIQUE (1971-78)

BRUSSEL-BRUXELLES					
B21	79	2.0	1.4+	0.17	54
VLAANDEREN					
B10	80	1.3	1.0	0.11	127
B29	51	1.4	1.1	0.16	103
B30	43	1.0	0.8-	0.12	179
B40	89	1.7	1.2	0.14	85
B70	19	0.7	0.7-	0.16	211
B-V	282	1.3	1.0	0.06	
WALLONIE					
B25	19	1.9	1.6	0.37	31
B50	15	0.3	0.2--	0.06	340
B60	33	0.8	0.6--	0.11	237
B80	9	1.0	0.7	0.24	211
B90	12	0.8	0.5--	0.16	267
B-W	88	0.7	0.5--	0.06	
B.0	449	1.2	0.9--	0.04	

BR DEUTSCHLAND (1976-80)

BADEN-WURTTEMBERG					
D81	156	1.9	1.5++	0.13	40
D82	110	1.9	1.5++	0.15	40
D83	77	1.7	1.4+	0.17	54
D84	56	1.6	1.3	0.18	68
D-A	399	1.8	1.5++	0.08	
BAYERN					
D91	220	2.5	2.0++	0.14	10
D92	46	2.0	1.6+	0.24	31
D93	47	2.0	1.8++	0.27	19
D94	50	2.0	1.5+	0.22	40
D95	90	2.5	1.8++	0.20	19
D96	62	2.2	1.7++	0.23	23
D97	85	2.3	1.8++	0.20	19
D-B	600	2.3	1.8++	0.08	
BERLIN(WEST)					
DB0	141	3.3	2.2++	0.20	7
BREMEN					
D40	38	2.3	1.7+	0.28	23
HAMBURG					
D20	121	3.1	2.1++	0.20	8
HESSEN					
D64	218	2.1	1.6++	0.11	31
D66	50	1.8	1.2	0.18	85
D-F	268	2.0	1.5++	0.10	
NIEDERSACHSEN					
D31	97	2.5	1.9++	0.20	15
D32	98	2.0	1.5++	0.16	40
D33	75	2.1	1.7++	0.20	23
D34	85	1.7	1.4+	0.16	54
D-G	355	2.1	1.6++	0.09	
NORDRHEIN-WESTFALEN					
D51	209	1.7	1.3++	0.09	68
D53	127	1.4	1.2	0.11	85
D55	98	1.7	1.5++	0.16	40
D57	58	1.4	1.1	0.15	103
D59	151	1.7	1.4++	0.12	54
D-H	643	1.6	1.3++	0.05	
RHEINLAND-PFALZ					
D71	66	2.0	1.5+	0.19	40
D72	25	2.2	1.9+	0.38	15
D73	91	2.1	1.7++	0.18	23
D-I	182	2.1	1.6++	0.12	
SAARLAND					
DA0	42	1.6	1.3	0.20	68
SCHLESWIG-HOLSTEIN					
D10	160	2.6	2.0++	0.17	10
D.0	2949	2.0	1.6++	0.03	

DANMARK (1971-80)

K15	209	3.4	2.5++	0.18	4
K20	43	2.8	2.6++	0.39	3
K25	28	3.0	3.0++	0.57	1
K30	41	3.0	2.4++	0.39	5
K35	42	3.3	2.1++	0.35	8
K40	6	2.5	1.7	0.71	23
K42	57	2.6	2.0++	0.27	10
K50	20	1.6	1.3	0.31	68
K55	21	2.0	1.6	0.36	31
K60	31	2.0	1.6	0.29	31
K65	23	1.8	1.4	0.30	54
K70	79	2.8	2.3++	0.27	6
K76	24	2.1	1.6	0.35	31
K80	57	2.4	1.9++	0.26	15
K.0	681	2.7	2.1++	0.08	

FRANCE (1971-78)

ALSACE					
F67	33	1.0	0.8	0.15	179
F68	20	0.8	0.8	0.18	179
F-A	53	0.9	0.8	0.12	
AQUITAINE					
F24	15	1.0	0.7	0.20	211
F33	29	0.7	0.6--	0.11	237
F40	9	0.8	0.5--	0.18	267
F47	7	0.6	0.4--	0.18	307
F64	14	0.7	0.5--	0.14	267
F-B	74	0.8	0.6--	0.07	
AUVERGNE					
F03	17	1.1	0.8	0.20	179
F15	7	1.1	0.9	0.34	152
F43	8	1.0	0.7	0.28	211
F63	10	0.4	0.3--	0.11	325
F-C	42	0.8	0.6--	0.10	
BASSE-NORMANDIE					
F14	13	0.6	0.5--	0.14	267
F50	9	0.5	0.5--	0.18	267
F61	7	0.6	0.5--	0.20	267
F-D	29	0.6	0.5--	0.10	
BOURGOGNE					
F21	13	0.7	0.6-	0.18	237
F58	8	0.8	0.4--	0.13	307
F71	19	0.8	0.6--	0.15	237
F89	9	0.8	0.3--	0.11	325
F-E	49	0.8	0.5--	0.08	
BRETAGNE					
F22	16	0.8	0.6-	0.16	237
F29	44	1.4	1.2	0.18	85
F35	14	0.5	0.4--	0.12	307
F56	24	1.1	0.9	0.18	152
F-F	98	1.0	0.8--	0.08	
CENTRE					
F18	12	1.0	0.8	0.23	179
F28	13	1.0	0.8	0.24	179
F36	11	1.1	0.9	0.28	152
F37	14	0.8	0.6--	0.16	237
F41	5	0.5	0.3--	0.15	325
F45	13	0.7	0.5--	0.16	267
F-G	68	0.8	0.6--	0.08	
CHAMPAGNE-ARDENNE					
F08	11	0.9	0.8	0.26	179
F10	8	0.7	0.4--	0.16	307
F51	16	0.8	0.6-	0.16	237
F52	3	0.4	0.3--	0.17	325
F-H	38	0.7	0.6--	0.10	
CORSE					
F20	2	0.2	0.1--	0.09	345
FRANCHE-COMTE					
F25	9	0.5	0.5--	0.17	267
F39	13	1.4	1.1	0.32	103
F70	8	0.9	0.9	0.31	152
F90	3	0.6	0.5	0.31	267
F-J	33	0.8	0.7-	0.13	
HAUTE-NORMANDIE					
F27	12	0.7	0.6-	0.18	237
F76	42	0.9	0.8	0.12	179
F-K	54	0.9	0.7--	0.10	
ILE-DE-FRANCE					
F75	77	0.9	0.6--	0.08	237
F77	15	0.5	0.5--	0.12	267
F78	40	0.9	0.9	0.15	152
F91	16	0.4	0.5--	0.12	267
F92	34	0.6	0.5--	0.09	267
F93	30	0.6	0.5--	0.10	267
F94	41	0.9	0.8-	0.12	179
F95	18	0.5	0.5--	0.13	267
F-L	271	0.7	0.6--	0.04	
LANGUEDOC-ROUSSILLON					
F11	5	0.5	0.3--	0.14	325
F30	16	0.8	0.6--	0.15	237
F34	18	0.7	0.5--	0.13	267
F48	2	0.7	0.5	0.33	267
F66	11	1.0	0.6	0.21	237
F-M	52	0.8	0.5--	0.07	
LIMOUSIN					
F19	5	0.5	0.3--	0.16	325
F23	9	1.6	1.0	0.40	127
F87	11	0.8	0.5--	0.15	267
F-N	25	0.9	0.5--	0.12	
LORRAINE					
F54	14	0.5	0.4--	0.11	307
F55	7	0.9	0.7	0.27	211
F57	28	0.7	0.7--	0.13	211
F88	10	0.6	0.6--	0.18	237
F-O	59	0.6	0.6--	0.08	
MIDI-PYRENEES					
F09	5	0.9	0.3--	0.12	325
F12	7	0.6	0.4--	0.17	307
F31	13	0.4	0.4--	0.10	307
F32	7	1.0	0.6	0.24	237
F46	5	0.8	0.5-	0.24	267
F65	9	1.0	0.7	0.26	211
F81	3	0.2	0.1--	0.06	345
F82	7	1.0	0.8	0.33	179
F-P	56	0.6	0.4--	0.06	
NORD-PAS-DE-CALAIS					
F59	63	0.6	0.6--	0.08	237
F62	35	0.6	0.5--	0.09	267
F-Q	98	0.6	0.6--	0.06	
PAYS DE LA LOIRE					
F44	25	0.7	0.6--	0.12	237
F49	17	0.7	0.5--	0.14	267
F53	6	0.6	0.5-	0.22	267
F72	12	0.6	0.5--	0.16	267
F85	14	0.8	0.5--	0.15	267
F-R	74	0.7	0.6--	0.07	
PICARDIE					
F02	9	0.4	0.4--	0.13	307
F60	8	0.3	0.3--	0.10	325
F80	10	0.5	0.4--	0.13	307
F-S	27	0.4	0.3--	0.07	
POITOU-CHARENTES					
F16	12	0.9	0.6	0.20	237
F17	19	1.0	0.7	0.18	211
F79	9	0.7	0.6	0.22	237
F86	4	0.3	0.3--	0.15	325
F-T	44	0.7	0.6--	0.09	
PROVENCE-ALPES-COTE D'AZUR					
F04	3	0.7	0.5	0.29	267
F05	1	0.3	0.2--	0.24	340
F06	22	0.7	0.4--	0.10	307
F13	44	0.7	0.5--	0.08	267
F83	17	0.7	0.5--	0.12	267
F84	11	0.7	0.6-	0.18	237
F-U	98	0.7	0.5--	0.05	
RHONE-ALPES					
F01	12	0.8	0.7	0.21	211
F07	10	1.0	0.6-	0.19	237
F26	14	1.0	0.8	0.21	179
F38	22	0.6	0.5--	0.12	267
F42	22	0.8	0.6--	0.13	237
F69	50	0.9	0.8-	0.11	179
F73	5	0.4	0.3--	0.15	325
F74	18	1.0	0.9	0.21	152
F-V	153	0.8	0.7--	0.05	
F.0	1497	0.7	0.6--	0.02	

UNITED KINGDOM (1976-80)

EAST ANGLIA					
G25	20	1.2	1.0	0.23	127
G46	27	1.4	1.1	0.23	103
G55	28	1.6	1.2	0.23	85
G-A	75	1.4	1.1	0.13	
EAST MIDLANDS					
G30	31	1.2	0.9	0.17	152
G44	32	1.3	1.1	0.19	103
G45	16	1.0	0.8	0.21	179
G47	28	1.8	1.5	0.29	40
G50	35	1.2	1.0	0.17	127
G-B	142	1.3	1.0	0.09	
NORTHERN					
G14	31	0.9	0.8	0.14	179
G27	9	0.5	0.4--	0.15	307
G29	18	1.3	1.0	0.25	127
G33	23	1.3	1.0	0.22	127
G48	11	1.3	1.0	0.31	127
G-C	92	1.0	0.8-	0.09	
NORTH-WEST					
G11	65	0.8	0.7--	0.09	211
G12	52	1.2	0.9	0.13	152
G26	34	1.3	1.0	0.17	127
G43	43	1.1	0.8	0.13	179
G-D	194	1.0	0.8--	0.06	

SOUTH-EAST					
G01	313	1.6	1.1	0.07	103
G22	27	1.8	1.5	0.30	40
G23	24	1.2	1.0	0.21	127
G24	20	1.3	1.1	0.25	103
G34	36	2.0	1.2	0.22	85
G35	74	1.8	1.5++	0.18	40
G37	65	1.5	1.2	0.15	85
G39	45	1.6	1.3	0.20	68
G41	10	3.1	2.0	0.67	10
G42	69	1.6	1.3	0.16	68
G51	29	1.7	1.5	0.29	40
G56	53	1.8	1.4+	0.20	54
G58	39	2.2	1.7+	0.29	23
G-E	804	1.6	1.3++	0.05	
SOUTH-WEST					
G21	33	1.2	1.0	0.18	127
G28	28	2.3	1.8+	0.36	19
G31	47	1.7	1.4	0.21	54
G32	27	1.6	1.3	0.27	68
G36	22	1.5	1.3	0.28	68
G53	21	1.7	1.5	0.33	40
G59	21	1.4	1.2	0.26	85
G-F	199	1.6	1.3++	0.10	
WEST MIDLANDS					
G15	97	1.2	0.9	0.09	152
G38	27	1.5	1.2	0.23	85
G52	15	1.4	1.2	0.31	85
G54	26	0.9	0.7	0.15	211
G57	12	0.9	0.7	0.19	211
G-G	177	1.2	0.9	0.07	
YORKSHIRE AND HUMBERSIDE					
G13	47	1.2	1.0	0.15	127
G16	63	1.0	0.8-	0.10	179
G40	38	1.5	1.3	0.21	68
G49	31	1.6	1.2	0.22	85
G-H	179	1.3	1.0	0.08	
WALES					
G61	13	1.2	0.9	0.27	152
G62	17	1.8	1.3	0.34	68
G63	15	1.2	1.0	0.26	127
G64	11	1.7	1.4	0.46	54
G65	19	1.2	0.9	0.22	152
G66	4	1.3	1.0	0.52	127
G67	11	1.0	0.7	0.23	211
G68	15	1.4	1.1	0.30	103
G-I	105	1.3	1.0	0.10	
SCOTLAND(1975-80)					
S01	8	1.4	1.3	0.45	68
S02	23	1.7	1.3	0.29	68
S03	19	1.6	1.4	0.32	54
S04	13	1.3	1.1	0.30	103
S05	28	1.3	1.0	0.19	127
S06	1	0.3	0.1--	0.13	345
S07	7	0.9	0.7	0.25	211
S08	74	1.0	0.9	0.11	152
S09	3	0.7	0.6	0.38	237
S10	2	3.8	2.7	2.10	2
S11	0	0.0	0.0--	0.00	349
S12	0	0.0	0.0--	0.00	349
G-J	178	1.2	1.0	0.08	
NORTHERN IRELAND					
JE	16	1.0	0.9	0.24	152
JN	10	1.1	1.1	0.36	103
JS	4	0.6	0.7	0.35	211
JW	4	0.7	0.8	0.40	179
G-K	34	0.9	0.9	0.16	
G.0	2179	1.3	1.1	0.02	
ITALIA (1975-79)					
ABRUZZI					
I66	9	1.2	0.7	0.23	211
I67	6	0.9	0.7	0.29	211
I68	9	1.3	1.2	0.39	85
I69	8	0.9	0.6	0.23	237
I-A	32	1.1	0.8	0.14	
BASILICATA					
I76	6	0.6	0.5--	0.20	267
I77	5	1.0	0.8	0.39	179
I-B	11	0.7	0.6-	0.18	
CALABRIA					
I78	10	0.6	0.5--	0.16	267
I79	9	0.5	0.5--	0.17	267
I80	5	0.3	0.3--	0.15	325
I-C	24	0.5	0.5--	0.09	

CAMPANIA					
I61	10	0.6	0.6-	0.18	237
I62	4	0.6	0.4--	0.20	307
I63	31	0.4	0.5--	0.08	267
I64	4	0.4	0.3--	0.15	325
I65	13	0.5	0.5--	0.13	267
I-D	62	0.5	0.5--	0.06	
EMILIA-ROMAGNA					
I33	11	1.6	1.0	0.30	127
I34	18	1.9	1.2	0.30	85
I35	9	0.9	0.7	0.22	211
I36	19	1.3	0.9	0.21	152
I37	31	1.4	0.9	0.17	152
I38	10	1.1	0.7	0.23	211
I39	16	1.8	1.1	0.29	103
I40	20	1.4	1.0	0.24	127
I-E	134	1.4	0.9	0.08	
FRIULI-VENEZIA GIULIA					
I30	22	1.7	1.3	0.28	68
I31	9	2.6	2.0	0.69	10
I32	17	2.4	1.6	0.41	31
I93	8	1.2	0.9	0.32	152
I-F	56	1.9	1.4	0.19	
LAZIO					
I56	8	1.2	0.9	0.32	152
I57	4	1.1	1.0	0.50	127
I58	109	1.2	1.1	0.11	103
I59	12	1.2	1.1	0.33	103
I60	9	0.8	0.6-	0.20	237
I-G	142	1.2	1.0	0.09	
LIGURIA					
I08	4	0.7	0.5	0.27	267
I09	10	1.4	0.8	0.27	179
I10	36	1.4	0.9	0.16	152
I11	13	2.2	1.6	0.45	31
I-H	63	1.4	1.0	0.12	
LOMBARDIA					
I12	23	1.2	1.0	0.21	127
I13	24	1.3	1.1	0.22	103
I14	4	0.9	0.9	0.45	152
I15	128	1.3	1.1	0.10	103
I16	15	0.7	0.7-	0.17	211
I17	12	0.5	0.5--	0.15	267
I18	16	1.3	0.9	0.23	152
I19	9	1.1	0.8	0.28	179
I20	13	1.4	1.1	0.31	103
I-I	244	1.1	0.9	0.06	
MARCHE					
I41	8	1.0	0.7	0.27	211
I42	13	1.3	0.9	0.25	152
I43	8	1.1	0.9	0.34	152
I44	6	0.7	0.5-	0.22	267
I-J	35	1.0	0.8	0.13	
MOLISE					
I70	6	1.0	0.6	0.27	237
I94	2	0.9	0.8	0.55	179
I-K	8	1.0	0.7	0.25	
PIEMONTE					
I01	88	1.5	1.2	0.13	85
I02	14	1.4	1.0	0.29	127
I03	21	1.7	1.3	0.28	68
I04	13	1.0	0.7	0.20	211
I05	8	1.5	1.1	0.39	103
I06	25	2.2	1.4	0.29	54
I-L	169	1.5	1.1	0.09	
PUGLIA					
I71	15	0.9	0.8	0.22	179
I72	22	0.6	0.6--	0.13	237
I73	12	0.9	0.8	0.24	179
I74	8	0.8	0.7	0.26	211
I75	9	0.5	0.5--	0.15	267
I-M	66	0.7	0.7--	0.08	
SARDEGNA					
I90	11	1.1	0.8	0.26	179
I91	2	0.3	0.2--	0.15	340
I92	15	0.9	0.8	0.22	179
I95	1	0.3	0.2--	0.16	340
I-N	29	0.7	0.6--	0.12	
SICILIA					
I81	6	0.6	0.5--	0.20	267
I82	20	0.7	0.6--	0.14	237
I83	11	0.7	0.5--	0.15	267
I84	9	0.8	0.7	0.23	211
I85	5	0.7	0.6	0.30	237
I86	2	0.4	0.4-	0.26	307
I87	11	0.5	0.4--	0.13	307
I88	4	0.6	0.4--	0.22	307
I89	12	1.2	1.1	0.31	103
I-O	80	0.7	0.6--	0.06	

TOSCANA					
I45	5	1.0	0.9	0.40	152
I46	8	0.9	0.7	0.24	211
I47	8	1.3	0.8	0.30	179
I48	44	1.5	1.0	0.16	127
I49	6	0.7	0.5-	0.22	267
I50	14	1.5	1.0	0.28	127
I51	9	1.2	0.8	0.28	179
I52	5	0.8	0.3--	0.16	325
I53	11	2.0	1.4	0.43	54
I-P	110	1.3	0.9	0.09	
TRENTINO-ALTO ADIGE					
I21	13	1.2	1.1	0.32	103
I22	15	1.4	1.2	0.31	85
I-Q	28	1.3	1.2	0.22	
UMBRIA					
I54	9	0.6	0.4--	0.13	307
I55	12	2.1	1.3	0.40	68
I-R	21	1.1	0.7-	0.15	
VALLE D'AOSTA					
I07	6	2.1	1.5	0.62	40
VENETO					
I23	19	1.0	0.8	0.19	179
I24	19	1.1	0.9	0.22	152
I25	10	1.9	1.4	0.45	54
I26	22	1.3	1.1	0.24	103
I27	29	1.4	1.2	0.22	85
I28	35	1.8	1.5+	0.26	40
I29	8	1.3	1.0	0.34	127
I-T	142	1.4	1.1	0.10	
I.0	1462	1.1	0.9--	0.02	
IRELAND (1976-80)					
CONNAUGHT					
R07	1	0.2	0.1--	0.09	345
R12	0	0.0	0.0--	0.00	349
R16	3	1.0	0.9	0.52	152
R20	0	0.0	0.0--	0.00	349
R21	2	1.4	1.0	0.69	127
R-A	6	0.6	0.4--	0.17	
LEINSTER					
R01	0	0.0	0.0--	0.00	349
R06	21	0.9	1.0	0.22	127
R09	4	1.6	1.7	0.85	23
R10	1	0.6	0.6	0.62	237
R11	0	0.0	0.0--	0.00	349
R14	2	2.5	1.9	1.36	15
R15	2	0.9	1.1	0.77	103
R17	2	0.9	0.8	0.59	179
R19	0	0.0	0.0--	0.00	349
R24	1	0.7	0.5	0.51	267
R25	2	0.8	0.8	0.59	179
R26	1	0.5	0.4	0.44	307
R-B	36	0.8	0.9	0.14	
MUNSTER					
R03	1	0.5	0.4	0.37	307
R04	7	0.7	0.7	0.27	211
R08	3	1.0	0.6	0.34	237
R13	5	1.3	1.1	0.52	103
R22	1	0.3	0.2--	0.19	340
R23	3	1.4	1.4	0.82	54
R-C	20	0.8	0.7	0.17	
ULSTER					
R02	1	0.7	0.3--	0.28	325
R05	3	1.0	0.8	0.48	179
R18	1	0.8	1.0	0.97	127
R-D	5	0.9	0.7	0.35	
R.0	67	0.8	0.7--	0.09	
LUXEMBOURG (1971-80)					
LE	2	1.1	0.8	0.56	179
LN	2	0.8	0.3--	0.21	325
LS	19	1.5	1.1	0.27	103
L.0	23	1.3	1.0	0.21	
NEDERLAND (1976-80)					
N01	14	1.0	0.9	0.23	152
N02	26	1.8	1.5	0.31	40
N03	11	1.1	0.9	0.27	152
N04	34	1.4	1.2	0.20	85
N05	62	1.5	1.3	0.17	68
N06	32	1.5	1.3	0.24	68
N07	107	1.8	1.6++	0.15	31
N08	150	2.0	1.7++	0.14	23
N09	15	1.8	1.4	0.38	54
N10	64	1.3	1.2	0.16	85
N11	31	1.2	1.1	0.19	103
N.0	546	1.6	1.4++	0.06	
EEC-9					
EEC	9853	1.3	1.0	0.01	

BELGIE-BELGIQUE (1971-78)

BRUSSEL-BRUXELLES

B21	78	1.8	0.9	0.12	119

VLAANDEREN

B10	78	1.2	0.8	0.10	144
B29	42	1.1	0.8	0.13	144
B30	47	1.1	0.7	0.11	170
B40	74	1.4	0.8	0.11	144
B70	16	0.6	0.5-	0.14	242
B-V	257	1.1	0.8-	0.05	

WALLONIE

B25	16	1.5	0.8	0.24	144
B50	29	0.5	0.3--	0.06	308
B60	41	1.0	0.6-	0.11	200
B80	8	0.9	0.5-	0.19	242
B90	11	0.7	0.4--	0.15	279
B-W	105	0.8	0.5--	0.05	
B.0	440	1.1	0.7--	0.04	

BR DEUTSCHLAND (1976-80)

BADEN-WURTTEMBERG

D81	151	1.7	1.0	0.09	99
D82	122	2.0	1.2++	0.12	57
D83	84	1.7	1.1	0.13	78
D84	69	1.8	1.2+	0.15	57
D-A	426	1.8	1.1++	0.06	

BAYERN

D91	201	2.1	1.3++	0.10	43
D92	53	2.0	1.2	0.18	57
D93	44	1.7	1.0	0.16	99
D94	52	1.9	1.1	0.16	78
D95	59	1.5	0.9	0.13	119
D96	51	1.6	1.0	0.14	99
D97	82	2.1	1.3+	0.15	43
D-B	542	1.9	1.1++	0.05	

BERLIN(WEST)

DB0	161	3.0	1.4++	0.14	33

BREMEN

D40	40	2.2	1.2	0.22	57

HAMBURG

D20	128	2.9	1.4++	0.15	33

HESSEN

D64	200	1.8	1.1++	0.09	78
D66	51	1.6	0.8	0.13	144
D-F	251	1.7	1.0+	0.07	

NIEDERSACHSEN

D31	101	2.4	1.3++	0.15	43
D32	131	2.4	1.3++	0.13	43
D33	91	2.5	1.5++	0.18	23
D34	93	1.7	1.1+	0.13	78
D-G	416	2.2	1.3++	0.07	

NORDRHEIN-WESTFALEN

D51	209	1.5	0.9	0.07	119
D53	158	1.6	1.0	0.09	99
D55	84	1.3	0.9	0.10	119
D57	76	1.6	1.0	0.13	99
D59	160	1.7	1.0	0.09	99
D-H	687	1.5	1.0+	0.04	

RHEINLAND-PFALZ

D71	75	2.1	1.3+	0.16	43
D72	21	1.7	1.0	0.24	99
D73	73	1.5	1.0	0.13	99
D-I	169	1.8	1.1+	0.09	

SAAPLAND

DA0	51	1.8	1.1	0.17	78

SCHLESWIG-HOLSTEIN

D10	159	2.4	1.4++	0.13	33
D.0	3030	1.9	1.1++	0.02	

DANMARK (1971-80)

K15	211	3.2	2.0++	0.15	6
K20	31	2.1	1.7++	0.31	11
K25	26	2.9	2.5++	0.52	3
K30	33	2.5	1.7+	0.32	11
K35	33	2.6	1.8++	0.33	8
K40	3	1.3	0.9	0.58	119
K42	58	2.6	1.6++	0.22	18
K50	24	2.0	1.5	0.31	23
K55	16	1.6	1.2	0.31	57
K60	37	2.3	1.7++	0.30	11
K65	26	2.1	1.6+	0.33	18
K70	73	2.6	1.8++	0.23	8
K76	30	2.7	1.8++	0.34	8
K80	58	2.5	1.7++	0.23	11
K.0	659	2.6	1.8++	0.07	

FRANCE (1971-78)

ALSACE

F67	30	0.8	0.5--	0.11	242
F68	16	0.6	0.5--	0.14	242
F-A	46	0.7	0.5--	0.09	

AQUITAINE

F24	6	0.4	0.2--	0.11	332
F33	37	0.8	0.5--	0.09	242
F40	10	0.9	0.5	0.19	242
F47	7	0.6	0.5-	0.19	242
F64	15	0.7	0.5--	0.14	242
F-B	75	0.7	0.5--	0.06	

AUVERGNE

F03	12	0.8	0.5-	0.16	242
F15	11	1.6	0.6	0.21	200
F43	8	1.0	0.6	0.24	200
F63	30	1.3	0.9	0.18	119
F-C	61	1.1	0.7	0.10	

BASSE-NORMANDIE

F14	15	0.7	0.4--	0.12	279
F50	22	1.2	0.9	0.21	119
F61	13	1.1	0.6	0.20	200
F-D	50	0.9	0.6--	0.10	

BOURGOGNE

F21	17	0.9	0.7	0.19	170
F58	6	0.6	0.3--	0.14	308
F71	21	0.9	0.5--	0.11	242
F89	21	1.7	1.1	0.27	78
F-E	65	1.0	0.6--	0.09	

BRETAGNE

F22	20	0.9	0.6	0.15	200
F29	47	1.4	1.0	0.16	99
F35	26	0.9	0.6-	0.13	200
F56	18	0.8	0.6-	0.15	200
F-F	111	1.0	0.7-	0.08	

CENTRE

F18	15	1.2	0.8	0.23	144
F28	8	0.6	0.3--	0.11	308
F36	5	0.5	0.1--	0.04	341
F37	29	1.5	0.9	0.20	119
F41	12	1.0	0.6	0.20	200
F45	17	0.9	0.6	0.16	200
F-G	86	1.0	0.6--	0.07	

CHAMPAGNE-ARDENNE

F08	12	1.0	0.6	0.21	200
F10	8	0.7	0.4--	0.17	279
F51	15	0.7	0.5--	0.13	242
F52	9	1.1	0.7	0.27	170
F-H	44	0.8	0.5--	0.09	

CORSE

F20	5	0.6	0.4--	0.19	279

FRANCHE-COMTE

F25	13	0.7	0.7	0.19	170
F39	7	0.7	0.4--	0.16	279
F70	3	0.3	0.3--	0.18	308
F90	5	1.0	0.7	0.36	170
F-J	28	0.7	0.5--	0.11	

HAUTE-NORMANDIE

F27	14	0.8	0.6	0.18	200
F76	36	0.8	0.6--	0.10	200
F-K	50	0.8	0.6--	0.09	

ILE-DE-FRANCE

F75	82	0.8	0.5--	0.06	242
F77	27	0.9	0.7	0.15	170
F78	38	0.9	0.7	0.12	170
F91	17	0.5	0.3--	0.09	308
F92	58	1.0	0.7-	0.10	170
F93	30	0.6	0.5--	0.09	242
F94	28	0.6	0.4--	0.08	279
F95	23	0.7	0.6-	0.12	200
F-L	303	0.7	0.5--	0.03	

LANGUEDOC-ROUSSILLON

F11	10	0.9	0.4-	0.18	279
F30	14	0.7	0.4--	0.11	279
F34	17	0.6	0.3--	0.09	308
F48	1	0.3	0.1--	0.06	341
F66	12	1.0	0.6	0.19	200
F-M	54	0.7	0.4--	0.06	

LIMOUSIN

F19	8	0.8	0.5-	0.19	242
F23	5	0.8	0.3--	0.17	308
F87	18	1.2	0.7	0.19	170
F-N	31	1.0	0.6--	0.12	

LORRAINE

F54	27	0.9	0.6-	0.12	200
F55	7	0.8	0.7	0.29	170
F57	18	0.5	0.4--	0.09	279
F88	8	0.5	0.3--	0.11	308
F-O	60	0.6	0.4--	0.06	

MIDI-PYRENEES

F09	2	0.4	0.2--	0.15	332
F12	1	0.1	0.0--	0.04	345
F31	20	0.6	0.4--	0.10	279
F32	9	1.3	0.7	0.28	170
F46	4	0.7	0.4-	0.23	279
F65	10	1.1	0.6	0.24	200
F81	15	1.1	0.6	0.18	200
F82	10	1.3	0.7	0.26	170
F-P	71	0.8	0.4--	0.06	

NORD-PAS-DE-CALAIS

F59	71	0.7	0.5--	0.06	242
F62	43	0.7	0.5--	0.08	242
F-Q	114	0.7	0.5--	0.05	

PAYS DE LA LOIRE

F44	41	1.1	0.7	0.12	170
F49	18	0.7	0.4--	0.12	279
F53	4	0.4	0.3--	0.15	308
F72	15	0.7	0.4--	0.13	279
F85	18	1.0	0.7	0.18	170
F-R	96	0.8	0.6--	0.06	

PICARDIE

F02	9	0.4	0.3--	0.10	308
F60	12	0.5	0.3--	0.09	308
F80	18	0.8	0.6	0.17	200
F-S	39	0.6	0.4--	0.07	

POITOU-CHARENTES

F16	21	1.5	1.1	0.26	78
F17	20	1.0	0.5-	0.14	242
F79	11	0.8	0.6	0.20	200
F86	7	0.5	0.4--	0.15	279
F-T	59	0.9	0.6--	0.09	

PROVENCE-ALPES-COTE D'AZUR

F04	1	0.2	0.1--	0.05	341
F05	3	0.8	0.6	0.38	200
F06	20	0.6	0.3--	0.09	308
F13	50	0.7	0.5--	0.08	242
F83	13	0.5	0.3--	0.09	308
F84	17	1.1	0.6	0.18	200
F-U	104	0.7	0.4--	0.05	

RHONE-ALPES

F01	15	1.0	0.7	0.21	170
F07	3	0.3	0.2--	0.15	332
F26	15	1.0	0.5-	0.16	242
F38	19	0.5	0.3--	0.08	308
F42	25	0.8	0.5--	0.11	242
F69	48	0.8	0.5--	0.08	242
F73	12	1.0	0.6	0.19	200
F74	13	0.7	0.6-	0.16	200
F-V	150	0.8	0.5--	0.04	
F.0	1702	0.8	0.5--	0.01	

UNITED KINGDOM (1976-80)

EAST ANGLIA

G25	39	2.3	1.7++	0.29	11
G46	39	1.9	1.2	0.21	57
G55	27	1.5	1.2	0.24	57
G-A	105	1.9	1.3++	0.14	

EAST MIDLANDS

G30	40	1.5	1.1	0.19	78
G44	30	1.2	0.8	0.16	144
G45	24	1.5	1.0	0.22	99
G47	21	1.3	1.0	0.23	99
G50	33	1.1	0.7	0.14	170
G-B	148	1.3	0.9	0.08	

NORTHERN

G14	55	1.5	1.1	0.17	78
G27	13	0.7	0.5-	0.16	242
G29	34	2.3	1.5+	0.30	23
G33	22	1.2	0.9	0.20	119
G48	17	1.9	1.3	0.35	43
G-C	141	1.5	1.1	0.10	

NORTH-WEST

G11	112	1.4	0.9	0.10	119
G12	68	1.4	0.8	0.11	144
G26	47	1.7	1.1	0.17	78
G43	79	1.8	1.3++	0.16	43
G-D	306	1.5	1.0+	0.06	

SOUTH-EAST					
G01	401	1.8	1.2++	0.07	57
G22	23	1.6	1.2	0.27	57
G23	29	1.4	1.1	0.22	78
G24	15	1.0	0.7	0.20	170
G34	48	2.2	1.0	0.19	99
G35	89	2.0	1.4++	0.16	33
G37	90	2.1	1.5++	0.17	23
G39	49	1.7	1.1	0.17	78
G41	10	2.8	1.2	0.46	57
G42	83	1.9	1.3++	0.16	43
G51	23	1.5	1.2	0.26	57
G56	86	2.8	2.0++	0.23	6
G58	42	2.1	1.2	0.23	57
G-E	988	1.9	1.3++	0.04	
SOUTH-WEST					
G21	67	2.3	1.6++	0.21	18
G28	29	2.2	1.4	0.29	33
G31	71	2.4	1.4+	0.20	33
G32	43	2.3	1.3	0.23	43
G36	33	2.2	1.5+	0.28	23
G53	31	2.4	1.7+	0.34	11
G59	33	2.1	1.4+	0.26	33
G-F	307	2.3	1.5++	0.09	
WEST MIDLANDS					
G15	124	1.5	1.1+	0.11	78
G38	15	0.8	0.6	0.16	200
G52	20	1.8	1.4	0.33	33
G54	36	1.2	0.9	0.15	119
G57	22	1.5	1.2	0.27	57
G-G	217	1.4	1.0+	0.07	
YORKSHIRE AND HUMBERSIDE					
G13	64	1.6	1.2	0.16	57
G16	81	1.3	0.9	0.10	119
G40	41	1.6	1.1	0.19	78
G49	26	1.3	0.6-	0.13	200
G-H	212	1.4	1.0	0.07	
WALES					
G61	18	1.5	0.8	0.21	144
G62	35	3.5	2.1++	0.41	5
G63	19	1.4	0.9	0.23	119
G64	18	2.6	1.3	0.36	43
G65	15	0.9	0.6	0.16	200
G66	2	0.6	0.6	0.44	200
G67	20	1.7	1.1	0.26	78
G68	18	1.6	1.1	0.28	78
G-I	145	1.7	1.1	0.10	
SCOTLAND(1975-80)					
S01	9	1.6	1.2	0.43	57
S02	23	1.6	1.0	0.23	99
S03	14	1.1	0.8	0.23	144
S04	21	2.0	1.4	0.33	33
S05	38	1.6	1.2	0.20	57
S06	2	0.6	0.6	0.42	200
S07	19	2.3	1.7+	0.41	11
S08	138	1.8	1.2++	0.11	57
S09	9	2.0	1.5	0.54	23
S10	0	0.0	0.0--	0.00	345
S11	1	1.6	0.9	0.92	119
S12	1	1.1	0.4	0.35	279
G-J	275	1.7	1.2++	0.08	
NORTHERN IRELAND					
JE	29	1.7	1.3	0.26	43
JN	13	1.4	1.1	0.33	78
JS	9	1.3	1.1	0.39	78
JW	9	1.5	1.0	0.37	99
G-K	60	1.5	1.2	0.16	
G.0	2904	1.7	1.2++	0.02	
ITALIA (1975-79)					
ABRUZZI					
I66	9	1.2	0.5-	0.17	242
I67	5	0.7	0.5	0.26	242
I68	9	1.2	0.8	0.28	144
I69	7	0.8	0.6	0.23	200
I-A	30	1.0	0.6-	0.12	
BASILICATA					
I76	10	1.0	0.7	0.23	170
I77	2	0.4	0.3-	0.25	308
I-B	12	0.8	0.6	0.17	
CALABRIA					
I78	12	0.7	0.4--	0.12	279
I79	12	0.7	0.5-	0.15	242
I80	9	0.6	0.6	0.19	200
I-C	33	0.6	0.5--	0.09	
CAMPANIA					
I61	15	0.8	0.6	0.17	200
I62	8	1.1	0.7	0.26	170
I63	22	0.3	0.3--	0.06	308
I64	4	0.4	0.3--	0.14	308
I65	11	0.4	0.3--	0.10	308
I-D	60	0.4	0.4--	0.05	
EMILIA-ROMAGNA					
I33	12	1.7	0.9	0.30	119
I34	13	1.3	0.8	0.25	144
I35	10	1.0	0.6	0.22	200
I36	13	0.9	0.6	0.17	200
I37	23	0.9	0.6-	0.14	200
I38	10	1.0	0.6	0.22	200
I39	12	1.3	0.9	0.25	119
I40	22	1.5	0.9	0.20	119
I-E	115	1.1	0.7-	0.07	
FRIULI-VENEZIA GIULIA					
I30	15	1.1	0.7	0.20	170
I31	6	1.6	0.8	0.34	144
I32	21	2.6	1.3	0.32	43
I93	9	1.3	0.8	0.30	144
I-F	51	1.6	0.9	0.14	
LAZIO					
I56	3	0.5	0.4-	0.21	279
I57	3	0.8	0.5	0.28	242
I58	84	0.9	0.7-	0.08	170
I59	5	0.5	0.3--	0.15	308
I60	6	0.5	0.5-	0.20	242
I-G	101	0.8	0.6--	0.06	
LIGURIA					
I08	15	2.5	1.1	0.33	78
I09	7	0.9	0.4--	0.17	279
I10	39	1.4	0.8	0.14	144
I11	10	1.6	0.7	0.23	170
I-H	71	1.5	0.8	0.10	
LOMBARDIA					
I12	27	1.4	1.0	0.19	99
I13	14	0.7	0.4--	0.12	279
I14	6	1.4	1.0	0.42	99
I15	153	1.5	1.0	0.09	99
I16	16	0.7	0.6	0.15	200
I17	22	0.9	0.7	0.15	170
I18	13	1.0	0.5--	0.15	242
I19	13	1.5	0.9	0.27	119
I20	9	0.9	0.7	0.23	170
I-I	273	1.2	0.8	0.05	
MARCHE					
I41	17	2.0	1.3	0.34	43
I42	8	0.7	0.5-	0.17	242
I43	6	0.8	0.8	0.32	144
I44	7	0.8	0.5-	0.19	242
I-J	38	1.1	0.7	0.12	
MOLISE					
I70	4	0.7	0.5	0.29	242
I94	0	0.0	0.0--	0.00	345
I-K	4	0.5	0.4-	0.20	
PIEMONTE					
I01	85	1.4	0.9	0.11	119
I02	12	1.1	0.6	0.19	200
I03	18	1.4	0.8	0.21	144
I04	10	0.7	0.5-	0.16	242
I05	4	0.7	0.5	0.28	242
I06	18	1.5	0.9	0.26	119
I-L	147	1.3	0.8	0.07	
PUGLIA					
I71	7	0.4	0.4--	0.15	279
I72	26	0.7	0.6--	0.11	200
I73	5	0.4	0.3--	0.12	308
I74	3	0.3	0.2--	0.10	332
I75	5	0.3	0.2--	0.11	332
I-M	46	0.5	0.4--	0.06	
SARDEGNA					
I90	7	0.7	0.4--	0.15	279
I91	8	1.2	0.8	0.28	144
I92	9	0.5	0.4--	0.15	279
I95	2	0.5	0.3-	0.24	308
I-N	26	0.7	0.5--	0.10	
SICILIA					
I81	4	0.4	0.2--	0.11	332
I82	9	0.3	0.2--	0.09	332
I83	12	0.7	0.5--	0.15	242
I84	1	0.1	0.1--	0.10	341
I85	2	0.3	0.2--	0.18	332
I86	1	0.2	0.2--	0.16	332
I87	14	0.6	0.4--	0.12	279
I88	2	0.3	0.3--	0.21	308
I89	7	0.7	0.7	0.25	170
I-O	52	0.4	0.3--	0.05	
TOSCANA					
I45	9	1.7	1.2	0.45	57
I46	11	1.1	0.6	0.19	200
I47	5	0.7	0.4-	0.22	279
I48	42	1.4	0.8	0.14	144
I49	6	0.7	0.6	0.26	200
I50	11	1.1	0.7	0.22	170
I51	5	0.6	0.3--	0.12	308
I52	10	1.5	0.9	0.33	119
I53	7	1.2	0.8	0.32	144
I-P	106	1.2	0.7-	0.08	
TRENTINO-ALTO ADIGE					
I21	18	1.7	1.3	0.32	43
I22	13	1.2	0.7	0.21	170
I-Q	31	1.4	1.0	0.19	
UMBRIA					
I54	14	1.0	0.6	0.17	200
I55	5	0.9	0.4--	0.18	279
I-R	19	0.9	0.5--	0.13	
VALLE D'AOSTA					
I07	4	1.4	0.8	0.44	144
VENETO					
I23	17	0.9	0.5-	0.14	242
I24	19	1.0	0.7	0.17	170
I25	8	1.4	0.7	0.29	170
I26	19	1.1	0.7	0.17	170
I27	20	0.9	0.5--	0.12	242
I28	22	1.1	0.8	0.17	144
I29	9	1.4	0.8	0.28	144
I-T	114	1.0	0.7--	0.07	
I.0	1333	0.9	0.6--	0.02	
IRELAND (1976-80)					
CONNAUGHT					
R07	6	1.5	1.5	0.65	23
R12	0	0.0	0.0--	0.00	345
R16	3	1.1	0.8	0.48	144
R20	0	0.0	0.0--	0.00	345
R21	2	1.5	1.5	1.12	23
R-A	11	1.1	1.0	0.33	
LEINSTER					
R01	0	0.0	0.0--	0.00	345
R06	35	1.4	1.2	0.21	57
R09	0	0.0	0.0--	0.00	345
R10	0	0.0	0.0--	0.00	345
R11	0	0.0	0.0--	0.00	345
R14	1	1.4	0.4	0.42	279
R15	1	0.5	0.3	0.34	308
R17	1	0.5	0.4	0.37	279
R19	0	0.0	0.0--	0.00	345
R24	2	1.4	1.5	1.09	23
R25	7	3.0	2.3	0.94	4
R26	7	3.3	3.4	1.34	1
R-B	54	1.2	1.1	0.15	
MUNSTER					
R03	2	1.0	0.6	0.46	200
R04	9	0.9	0.8	0.28	144
R08	6	2.1	1.6	0.71	18
R13	7	1.8	1.2	0.50	57
R22	5	1.5	1.2	0.57	57
R23	6	2.8	2.7	1.10	2
R-C	35	1.5	1.2	0.21	
ULSTER					
R02	0	0.0	0.0--	0.00	345
R05	2	0.7	0.4	0.30	279
R18	1	0.8	0.9	0.87	119
R-D	3	0.6	0.4	0.26	
R.0	103	1.2	1.0	0.11	
LUXEMBOURG (1971-80)					
LE	1	0.5	0.5	0.54	242
LN	2	0.8	0.4	0.31	279
LS	20	1.5	1.0	0.25	99
L.0	23	1.3	0.9	0.20	
NEDERLAND (1976-80)					
N01	20	1.5	1.0	0.24	99
N02	20	1.4	1.0	0.25	99
N03	13	1.3	0.9	0.26	119
N04	31	1.2	0.9	0.18	119
N05	50	1.2	0.9	0.13	119
N06	35	1.6	1.1	0.20	78
N07	123	2.1	1.5++	0.14	23
N08	144	1.9	1.4++	0.12	33
N09	18	2.1	1.6	0.40	18
N10	49	1.0	0.8	0.12	144
N11	38	1.4	1.1	0.19	78
N.0	541	1.5	1.2++	0.05	
EEC-9					
EEC	10735	1.3	0.9	0.01	

BELGIE-BELGIQUE (1971-78)

BRUSSEL-BRUXELLES					
B21	2176	48.8	25.6++	0.62	97
VLAANDEREN					
B10	2358	37.4	24.5++	0.53	108
B29	1244	33.9	22.5	0.67	133
B30	1781	41.1	26.5++	0.67	70
B40	2092	39.0	24.3++	0.57	110
B70	660	24.4	21.9	0.87	142
B-V	8135	36.4	24.3++	0.29	
WALLONIE					
B25	360	33.6	20.7	1.18	164
B50	2244	41.2	24.0++	0.56	119
B60	1483	35.2	20.2--	0.57	181
B80	302	33.8	21.2	1.32	156
B90	580	36.1	22.2	1.01	136
B-W	4969	37.5	22.1	0.34	
B.0	15280	38.1	23.7++	0.21	

BR DEUTSCHLAND (1976-80)

BADEN-WURTTEMBERG					
D81	2968	33.3	19.8--	0.39	189
D82	2238	36.1	20.3--	0.47	177
D83	1656	34.2	19.9--	0.53	184
D84	1242	32.2	19.4--	0.60	195
D-A	8104	34.0	19.9--	0.24	
BAYERN					
D91	3421	36.6	20.6--	0.39	166
D92	828	31.6	18.2--	0.69	244
D93	768	30.4	17.7--	0.69	259
D94	927	33.2	18.2--	0.66	244
D95	1437	36.1	19.1--	0.55	211
D96	1004	32.4	19.2--	0.66	205
D97	1407	35.4	19.8--	0.58	189
D-B	9792	34.5	19.4--	0.21	
BERLIN(WEST)					
DB0	2865	54.0	23.2+	0.54	126
BREMEN					
D40	776	41.8	21.6	0.87	149
HAMBURG					
D20	2047	45.8	21.8	0.56	147
HESSEN					
D64	4188	36.9	20.8--	0.35	161
D66	1115	35.9	19.2--	0.64	205
D-F	5303	36.7	20.4--	0.31	
NIEDERSACHSEN					
D31	1506	35.1	19.2--	0.55	205
D32	1897	34.9	18.7--	0.48	224
D33	1244	33.7	19.7--	0.61	192
D34	1825	33.6	21.0	0.53	157
D-G	6472	34.3	19.6--	0.27	
NORDRHEIN-WESTFALEN					
D51	5554	40.2	22.9++	0.33	129
D53	3974	39.4	24.2++	0.41	112
D55	2153	34.5	23.1+	0.52	127
D57	1686	35.5	21.0	0.55	157
D59	3602	37.3	22.4	0.40	135
D-H	16969	38.1	22.9++	0.19	
RHEINLAND-PFALZ					
D71	1401	39.4	21.9	0.64	142
D72	470	37.9	22.0	1.10	139
D73	1763	37.4	21.3	0.55	155
D-I	3634	38.2	21.6	0.39	
SAARLAND					
DA0	1017	35.7	20.5	0.69	171
SCHLESWIG-HOLSTEIN					
D10	2447	36.3	20.1--	0.45	182
D.0	59426	37.0	20.8--	0.09	

DANMARK (1971-80)

K15	3418	51.4	27.6++	0.52	43
K20	482	32.0	26.6++	1.25	67
K25	289	31.7	27.9++	1.69	37
K30	561	42.0	26.5++	1.20	70
K35	559	43.8	25.4++	1.17	100
K40	113	48.2	27.9+	2.85	37
K42	905	40.4	23.8+	0.86	121
K50	418	34.2	22.0	1.16	139
K55	385	37.8	26.1++	1.40	84
K60	676	42.4	27.8++	1.14	39
K65	445	35.6	25.9++	1.28	90
K70	1095	38.8	26.8++	0.86	59
K76	448	40.0	25.4++	1.29	100
K80	873	37.2	24.4++	0.87	109
K.0	10667	41.8	26.2++	0.27	

FRANCE (1971-78)

ALSACE					
F67	1152	31.9	21.4	0.69	152
F68	806	31.1	20.6	0.79	166
F-A	1958	31.6	21.1	0.52	
AQUITAINE					
F24	467	30.5	14.7--	0.79	325
F33	1422	32.2	18.8--	0.56	220
F40	366	31.2	18.2--	1.09	244
F47	338	28.3	16.2--	0.99	298
F64	640	29.0	17.5--	0.77	267
F-B	3233	30.7	17.5--	0.35	
AUVERGNE					
F03	593	37.9	19.1--	0.91	211
F15	211	31.3	16.8--	1.35	290
F43	330	39.3	19.2-	1.27	205
F63	668	28.3	17.3--	0.75	275
F-C	1802	33.1	18.1--	0.49	
BASSE-NORMANDIE					
F14	586	25.5	17.5--	0.79	267
F50	519	27.8	16.7--	0.82	293
F61	351	29.0	18.5--	1.10	235
F-D	1456	27.1	17.5--	0.51	
BOURGOGNE					
F21	512	27.8	17.3--	0.85	275
F58	339	33.5	17.3--	1.12	275
F71	699	30.1	17.2--	0.74	280
F89	443	36.3	18.2--	1.04	244
F-E	1993	31.2	17.4--	0.45	
BRETAGNE					
F22	564	26.2	14.7--	0.71	325
F29	845	25.4	15.6--	0.59	311
F35	737	25.3	16.8--	0.68	290
F56	570	24.8	15.0--	0.69	320
F-F	2716	25.4	15.5--	0.33	
CENTRE					
F18	404	31.4	17.6--	1.01	263
F28	393	29.3	19.6-	1.11	194
F36	329	33.0	16.4--	1.09	295
F37	557	28.3	17.5--	0.84	267
F41	366	31.8	17.9--	1.09	255
F45	633	32.0	19.3--	0.87	200
F-G	2682	30.7	18.1--	0.40	
CHAMPAGNE-ARDENNE					
F08	345	27.8	18.5--	1.11	235
F10	295	25.6	14.8--	0.99	321
F51	546	25.6	18.3--	0.85	240
F52	210	24.5	15.8--	1.23	305
F-H	1396	25.9	17.1--	0.51	
CORSE					
F20	196	22.7	11.8--	0.95	345
FRANCHE-COMTE					
F25	390	20.6	15.9--	0.86	302
F39	271	27.8	16.2--	1.12	298
F70	215	24.1	14.3--	1.12	328
F90	128	25.0	17.2--	1.66	280
F-J	1004	23.5	15.8--	0.55	
HAUTE-NORMANDIE					
F27	481	28.1	19.3--	0.97	200
F76	1409	29.4	20.6-	0.59	166
F-K	1890	29.1	20.2--	0.51	
ILE-DE-FRANCE					
F75	4319	43.7	21.6	0.37	149
F77	832	27.4	19.2--	0.74	205
F78	1054	24.3	19.4--	0.64	195
F91	809	21.8	18.8--	0.71	220
F92	1924	32.6	20.4--	0.50	173
F93	1374	26.0	19.3--	0.55	200
F94	1401	28.2	19.9--	0.57	184
F95	852	25.1	20.3-	0.74	177
F-L	12565	31.0	20.3--	0.20	
LANGUEDOC-ROUSSILLON					
F11	358	32.0	14.8--	0.92	321
F30	687	33.9	19.0--	0.81	215
F34	892	33.1	18.7--	0.71	224
F48	107	35.5	17.8	2.09	257
F66	447	35.7	18.7--	0.99	224
F-M	2491	33.7	18.1--	0.41	
LIMOUSIN					
F19	302	30.6	15.9--	1.05	302
F23	212	35.0	15.6--	1.35	311
F87	368	25.3	13.3--	0.81	335
F-N	882	28.9	14.6--	0.58	
LORRAINE					
F54	747	25.7	18.4--	0.72	238
F55	205	24.9	15.4--	1.22	317
F57	912	22.9	17.9--	0.62	255
F88	443	27.2	16.8--	0.90	290
F-O	2307	24.7	17.6--	0.39	
MIDI-PYRENEES					
F09	178	31.7	15.8--	1.39	305
F12	354	31.0	16.1--	1.01	301
F31	901	28.3	18.0--	0.66	250
F32	193	27.5	14.8--	1.24	321
F46	188	30.9	15.8--	1.34	305
F65	293	31.4	17.2--	1.13	280
F81	430	31.1	16.9--	0.93	288
F82	268	35.6	18.8-	1.32	220
F-P	2805	30.3	17.0--	0.36	
NORD-PAS-DE-CALAIS					
F59	3342	32.7	23.1++	0.44	127
F62	1724	30.0	21.0	0.54	157
F-Q	5066	31.7	22.3	0.34	
PAYS DE LA LOIRE					
F44	1068	27.8	19.1--	0.64	211
F49	779	29.8	19.3--	0.78	200
F53	284	26.3	16.5--	1.09	294
F72	564	28.0	17.5--	0.82	267
F85	518	28.1	17.4--	0.87	272
F-R	3213	28.2	18.3--	0.36	
PICARDIE					
F02	624	29.1	18.9--	0.85	217
F60	615	25.4	18.2--	0.81	244
F80	609	27.7	17.4--	0.79	272
F-S	1848	27.3	18.2--	0.47	
POITOU-CHARENTES					
F16	385	27.9	15.7--	0.92	309
F17	619	30.5	17.8--	0.80	257
F79	400	29.5	17.6--	0.99	263
F86	379	26.1	14.8--	0.87	321
F-T	1783	28.7	16.6--	0.45	
PROVENCE-ALPES-COTE D'AZUR					
F04	131	29.4	15.7--	1.55	309
F05	117	30.0	15.6--	1.64	311
F06	757	21.9	9.8--	0.42	353
F13	1864	27.9	17.6--	0.44	263
F83	824	32.4	18.0--	0.70	250
F84	470	29.5	17.7--	0.90	259
F-U	4163	27.6	15.6--	0.27	
RHONE-ALPES					
F01	391	25.9	17.2--	0.96	280
F07	347	33.1	17.7--	1.10	259
F26	421	28.7	16.9--	0.93	288
F38	955	27.5	18.6--	0.65	228
F42	941	30.5	18.3--	0.66	240
F69	1730	29.6	19.9--	0.52	184
F73	371	30.0	19.3-	1.10	200
F74	500	27.7	20.8	0.98	161
F-V	5656	29.0	18.8--	0.27	
F.0	63105	29.4	18.3--	0.08	

UNITED KINGDOM (1976-80)

EAST ANGLIA					
G25	745	44.1	29.5++	1.17	16
G46	981	47.2	26.0++	0.92	88
G55	837	47.3	27.3++	1.04	50
G-A	2563	46.3	27.4++	0.60	
EAST MIDLANDS					
G30	1312	47.8	29.3++	0.87	21
G44	1094	43.1	27.2++	0.89	54
G45	805	50.0	29.8++	1.15	8
G47	707	45.1	29.2++	1.20	23
G50	1397	46.8	29.5++	0.85	16
G-B	5315	46.4	29.0++	0.43	
NORTHERN					
G14	1606	44.3	26.8++	0.73	59
G27	577	33.2	24.1+	1.05	113
G29	665	45.5	26.7++	1.14	62
G33	749	40.4	24.9++	0.98	104
G48	393	44.3	27.3++	1.50	50
G-C	3990	41.7	26.0++	0.44	
NORTH-WEST					
G11	3602	43.7	26.3++	0.48	77
G12	2212	45.6	27.5++	0.64	45
G26	1123	39.9	26.6++	0.85	67
G43	2038	47.6	26.1++	0.65	84
G-D	8975	44.5	26.6++	0.31	

SOUTH-EAST					
G01	10956	50.3	28.5++	0.30	30
G22	550	37.4	26.9++	1.20	57
G23	820	40.5	27.4++	1.01	48
G24	662	42.5	28.4++	1.17	34
G34	1484	69.4	30.5++	0.99	7
G35	2149	48.9	29.8++	0.70	8
G37	1964	45.5	28.8++	0.71	26
G39	1225	42.2	27.5++	0.83	45
G41	216	59.7	25.3	2.03	103
G42	2218	49.6	28.6++	0.67	28
G51	700	44.7	30.8++	1.24	6
G56	1563	51.0	29.3++	0.80	21
G58	1165	57.8	27.7++	0.95	40
G-E	25672	49.3	28.7++	0.20	
SOUTH-WEST					
G21	1325	46.4	26.6++	0.81	67
G28	717	55.5	29.4++	1.23	19
G31	1543	52.8	25.9++	0.77	90
G32	1090	58.9	27.6++	0.99	43
G36	756	49.8	29.8++	1.19	8
G53	682	53.9	29.8++	1.28	8
G59	641	41.6	26.9++	1.14	57
G-F	6754	51.0	27.6++	0.38	
WEST MIDLANDS					
G15	3880	47.0	29.0++	0.50	25
G38	845	45.7	27.7++	1.04	40
G52	511	46.0	28.5++	1.38	30
G54	1321	43.6	28.5++	0.83	30
G57	665	46.8	31.4++	1.29	4
G-G	7222	46.1	28.9++	0.36	
YORKSHIRE AND HUMBERSIDE					
G13	1752	43.8	26.7++	0.69	62
G16	2824	44.1	26.3++	0.54	77
G40	1101	42.1	26.4++	0.87	74
G49	984	49.2	26.7++	0.96	62
G-H	6661	44.4	26.5++	0.36	
WALES					
G61	594	50.2	27.5++	1.28	45
G62	484	47.9	26.7++	1.35	62
G63	575	42.8	27.1++	1.22	56
G64	394	56.0	29.4++	1.72	19
G65	783	47.3	29.1++	1.12	24
G66	150	47.4	25.6	2.36	97
G67	526	43.7	26.4++	1.26	74
G68	553	48.2	28.6++	1.32	28
G-I	4059	47.4	27.7++	0.48	
SCOTLAND(1975-80)					
S01	248	43.4	27.7++	1.91	40
S02	540	37.8	22.5	1.07	133
S03	544	43.4	25.4++	1.20	100
S04	408	39.2	26.0++	1.38	88
S05	1034	43.7	27.3++	0.93	50
S06	149	47.7	26.3	2.44	77
S07	320	38.8	26.8++	1.58	59
S08	3364	43.8	28.4++	0.52	34
S09	220	50.0	29.8++	2.21	8
S10	21	38.5	21.8	5.11	147
S11	27	44.2	26.5	5.83	70
S12	48	53.2	26.7	4.73	62
G-J	6923	42.9	27.2++	0.35	
NORTHERN IRELAND					
JE	709	42.3	29.7++	1.19	14
JN	305	33.0	24.1	1.47	113
JS	175	25.8	19.4	1.55	195
JW	241	39.2	29.5++	2.00	16
G-K	1430	36.7	26.5++	0.74	
G.0	79564	46.4	27.8++	0.11	
ITALIA (1975-79)					
ABRUZZI					
I66	194	25.2	15.8--	1.22	305
I67	130	19.4	12.9--	1.18	337
I68	152	21.0	14.3--	1.20	328
I69	186	20.1	12.4--	0.97	339
I-A	662	21.4	13.7--	0.56	
BASILICATA					
I76	137	13.2	10.0--	0.89	351
I77	52	10.3	8.5--	1.22	355
I-B	189	12.2	9.6--	0.72	
CALABRIA					
I78	262	14.5	11.6--	0.75	346
I79	235	12.8	10.3--	0.70	350
I80	250	16.8	12.3--	0.82	341
I-C	747	14.5	11.4--	0.44	

CAMPANIA					
I61	265	14.5	12.3--	0.77	341
I62	119	16.1	11.0--	1.07	348
I63	1462	20.1	17.5--	0.47	267
I64	145	13.2	10.0--	0.86	351
I65	403	16.0	12.4--	0.64	339
I-D	2394	17.8	14.6--	0.31	
EMILIA-ROMAGNA					
I33	263	36.4	19.8	1.31	189
I34	359	35.0	18.6--	1.07	228
I35	330	32.0	18.6--	1.08	228
I36	476	32.3	20.3	0.97	177
I37	883	36.3	20.7	0.74	164
I38	305	30.6	18.4--	1.10	238
I39	282	30.6	18.1--	1.14	249
I40	393	26.3	17.3--	0.91	275
I-E	3291	32.6	19.2--	0.35	
FRIULI-VENEZIA GIULIA					
I30	487	35.8	19.9-	0.97	184
I31	159	41.6	24.1	2.04	113
I32	407	50.9	23.5	1.31	123
I93	222	32.3	19.2	1.39	205
I-F	1275	39.5	21.2	0.65	
LAZIO					
I56	167	25.2	16.2--	1.31	298
I57	79	21.9	13.0--	1.57	336
I58	2794	29.6	21.9	0.42	142
I59	171	16.5	14.1--	1.09	331
I60	166	14.6	10.6--	0.86	349
I-G	3377	26.7	19.5--	0.34	
LIGURIA					
I08	255	42.5	22.0	1.50	139
I09	308	39.0	20.9	1.27	160
I10	1267	44.7	22.9	0.69	129
I11	243	38.2	20.6	1.43	166
I-H	2073	42.7	22.1	0.52	
LOMBARDIA					
I12	758	37.9	25.8++	0.97	95
I13	683	34.9	23.5	0.94	123
I14	120	27.5	19.4	1.86	195
I15	3662	35.1	24.6++	0.42	106
I16	707	31.9	24.1+	0.93	113
I17	806	31.7	22.1	0.80	138
I18	526	38.8	20.5	0.97	171
I19	382	44.5	25.8++	1.41	95
I20	351	35.9	20.1	1.15	182
I-I	7995	35.1	23.6++	0.27	
MARCHE					
I41	203	24.5	15.3--	1.13	318
I42	321	29.2	17.6--	1.04	263
I43	229	30.9	18.0--	1.25	250
I44	229	25.7	16.3--	1.13	296
I-J	982	27.6	16.8--	0.57	
MOLISE					
I70	113	18.8	11.6--	1.16	346
I94	42	17.5	9.7--	1.60	354
I-K	155	18.4	11.1--	0.95	
PIEMONTE					
I01	2204	36.2	24.1++	0.54	113
I02	432	40.9	20.6	1.10	166
I03	512	39.0	21.9	1.05	142
I04	511	37.2	20.8	0.99	161
I05	213	37.9	19.0	1.45	215
I06	538	43.4	21.6	1.05	149
I-L	4410	37.9	22.4	0.36	
PUGLIA					
I71	283	16.5	13.9--	0.85	333
I72	772	21.3	17.3--	0.65	275
I73	274	19.6	17.2--	1.06	280
I74	228	23.0	18.3--	1.25	240
I75	373	19.4	15.9--	0.84	302
I-M	1930	20.0	16.5--	0.39	
SARDEGNA					
I90	249	23.4	18.6--	1.23	228
I91	156	22.6	18.0-	1.52	250
I92	378	21.3	18.7--	0.99	224
I95	68	17.5	11.9--	1.55	343
I-N	851	21.7	17.7--	0.63	
SICILIA					
I81	239	22.4	15.5--	1.06	314
I82	612	20.5	15.5--	0.65	314
I83	400	23.0	15.3--	0.81	318
I84	218	18.3	13.4--	0.94	334
I85	137	18.6	14.6--	1.29	327
I86	82	15.9	11.9--	1.36	343
I87	651	26.1	20.4	0.83	173
I88	189	27.7	19.7	1.49	192
I89	211	21.8	17.2--	1.21	280
I-O	2739	22.1	16.4--	0.33	

TOSCANA					
I45	164	31.0	18.5-	1.55	235
I46	293	29.1	16.3--	1.03	296
I47	204	30.2	17.2--	1.29	280
I48	1160	37.5	21.4	0.67	152
I49	306	34.6	20.4	1.23	173
I50	312	31.7	18.3--	1.11	240
I51	179	22.7	12.9--	1.03	337
I52	178	27.2	14.3--	1.15	328
I53	132	23.5	14.0--	1.28	332
I-P	2928	31.9	18.2--	0.36	
TRENTINO-ALTO ADIGE					
I21	258	23.8	18.0--	1.16	250
I22	372	33.1	20.4	1.13	173
I-Q	630	28.5	19.4--	0.81	
UMBRIA					
I54	377	26.2	15.5--	0.84	314
I55	168	29.1	17.4--	1.40	272
I-R	545	27.0	16.1--	0.72	
VALLE D'AOSTA					
I07	105	37.0	24.3	2.45	110
VENETO					
I23	600	30.8	19.9-	0.85	184
I24	470	25.9	18.6--	0.89	228
I25	178	30.5	17.0--	1.38	287
I26	507	28.3	18.9--	0.89	217
I27	619	28.9	20.3	0.85	177
I28	532	26.1	18.6--	0.84	228
I29	193	29.9	17.7--	1.37	259
I-T	3099	28.3	19.0--	0.36	
I.0	40377	28.1	18.9--	0.10	
IRELAND (1976-80)					
CONNAUGHT					
R07	126	31.0	24.1	2.32	113
R12	32	49.4	36.4+	7.16	1
R16	96	34.6	23.5	2.73	123
R20	51	39.7	26.3	4.05	77
R21	54	40.3	28.5	4.32	30
R-A	359	35.5	25.6+	1.49	
LEINSTER					
R01	20	21.1	18.9	4.35	217
R06	746	29.2	26.1++	0.99	84
R09	45	19.3	21.4	3.27	152
R10	55	32.9	28.4	4.07	34
R11	41	34.5	28.7	4.71	27
R14	19	25.8	18.6	4.74	228
R15	85	39.5	36.4++	4.11	1
R17	69	31.4	31.0+	3.88	5
R19	39	28.3	25.9	4.35	90
R24	38	25.9	19.4	3.32	195
R25	83	35.0	29.7+	3.50	14
R26	60	28.6	24.9	3.43	104
R-B	1300	29.5	26.3++	0.76	
MUNSTER					
R03	68	33.2	25.6	3.38	97
R04	332	33.7	26.2++	1.52	82
R08	104	35.8	27.2	2.91	54
R13	141	36.1	29.8++	2.67	8
R22	80	24.7	18.8	2.24	220
R23	66	30.5	27.4	3.55	48
R-C	791	32.8	25.9++	0.98	
ULSTER					
R02	41	32.3	25.9	4.30	90
R05	87	29.3	22.2	2.63	136
R18	50	41.4	34.6+	5.26	3
R-D	178	32.7	25.8	2.10	
R.0	2628	31.4	26.0++	0.54	
LUXEMBOURG (1971-80)					
LE	73	38.1	22.6	2.87	132
LN	88	33.3	19.1	2.20	211
LS	460	34.2	21.9	1.06	142
L.0	621	34.5	21.6	0.91	
NEDERLAND (1976-80)					
N01	502	36.6	23.8	1.15	121
N02	514	35.8	24.6+	1.18	106
N03	319	31.1	22.8	1.34	131
N04	887	35.5	26.3++	0.93	77
N05	1462	34.9	25.9++	0.71	90
N06	853	38.1	26.5++	0.97	70
N07	2502	42.0	27.3++	0.59	50
N08	3124	40.2	26.4++	0.51	74
N09	369	43.3	26.1++	1.49	84
N10	1539	30.8	26.2++	0.68	82
N11	809	30.6	24.0+	0.87	119
N.0	12880	36.8	26.1++	0.24	
EEC-9					
EEC	284548	35.5	21.8	0.04	

BELGIE-BELGIQUE (1971-78)

BRUSSEL-BRUXELLES

B21	573	12.9	6.9	0.32	144

VLAANDEREN

B10	742	11.8	7.6++	0.29	123
B29	315	8.6	5.7--	0.34	183
B30	592	13.7	9.0++	0.39	55
B40	607	11.3	7.2	0.32	135
B70	179	6.6	5.9	0.45	174
B-V	2435	10.9	7.3++	0.16	

WALLONIE

B25	119	11.1	6.9	0.67	144
B50	611	11.2	6.6	0.29	153
B60	485	11.5	7.0	0.34	138
B80	125	14.0	8.9+	0.86	61
B90	224	13.9	8.2+	0.60	97
B-W	1564	11.8	7.1	0.19	
B.0	4572	11.4	7.2++	0.11	

BR DEUTSCHLAND (1976-80)

BADEN-WURTTEMBERG

D81	1214	13.6	8.1++	0.25	104
D82	823	13.3	7.6++	0.29	123
D83	659	13.6	7.7++	0.32	119
D84	543	14.1	8.8++	0.41	71
D-A	3239	13.6	8.0++	0.15	

BAYERN

D91	1434	15.3	8.5++	0.24	80
D92	434	16.6	9.8++	0.51	31
D93	343	13.6	8.1++	0.47	104
D94	422	15.1	7.8+	0.42	115
D95	658	16.5	9.2++	0.39	50
D96	464	15.0	8.7++	0.44	73
D97	594	14.9	8.1++	0.36	104
D-B	4349	15.3	8.6++	0.14	

BERLIN(WEST)

DB0	1040	19.6	9.1++	0.34	54

BREMEN

D40	277	14.9	7.9+	0.53	111

HAMBURG

D20	951	21.3	10.3++	0.38	17

HESSEN

D64	1543	13.6	7.8++	0.22	115
D66	427	13.7	7.4	0.40	131
D-F	1970	13.6	7.7++	0.19	

NIEDERSACHSEN

D31	660	15.4	8.2++	0.36	97
D32	747	13.7	7.3	0.30	133
D33	524	14.2	8.2++	0.39	97
D34	689	12.7	7.9++	0.33	111
D-G	2620	13.9	7.9++	0.17	

NORDRHEIN-WESTFALEN

D51	1915	13.9	8.0++	0.20	110
D53	1253	12.4	7.6++	0.23	123
D55	713	11.4	7.6++	0.30	123
D57	637	13.4	7.7++	0.33	119
D59	1230	12.7	7.5++	0.23	129
D-H	5748	12.9	7.7++	0.11	

RHEINLAND-PFALZ

D71	527	14.8	8.1++	0.38	104
D72	176	14.2	7.8	0.64	115
D73	664	14.1	7.9++	0.33	111
D-I	1367	14.4	7.9++	0.23	

SAARLAND

DA0	346	12.2	6.8	0.40	147

SCHLESWIG-HOLSTEIN

D10	1033	15.3	8.4++	0.29	84
D.0	22940	14.3	8.1++	0.06	

DANMARK (1971-80)

K15	1463	22.0	11.7++	0.33	6
K20	199	13.2	11.2++	0.82	7
K25	106	11.6	11.0++	1.09	10
K30	230	17.2	11.1++	0.77	8
K35	243	19.1	11.9++	0.81	5
K40	53	22.6	13.7++	2.02	1
K42	394	17.6	10.8++	0.58	11
K50	184	15.0	9.9++	0.78	28
K55	123	12.1	8.9+	0.83	61
K60	307	19.3	13.0++	0.79	2
K65	159	12.7	9.3++	0.77	45
K70	448	15.9	10.6++	0.53	12
K76	186	16.6	10.5++	0.82	14
K80	402	17.2	11.1++	0.59	8
K.0	4497	17.6	11.2++	0.18	

FRANCE (1971-78)

ALSACE

F67	365	10.1	6.6	0.38	153
F68	249	9.6	6.4	0.45	157
F-A	614	9.9	6.5	0.29	

AQUITAINE

F24	110	7.2	4.0--	0.42	286
F33	304	6.9	4.0--	0.26	286
F40	92	7.8	4.3--	0.51	268
F47	79	6.6	3.5--	0.45	309
F64	142	6.4	4.0--	0.37	286
F-B	727	6.9	4.0--	0.17	

AUVERGNE

F03	155	9.9	5.2--	0.48	208
F15	56	8.3	4.8--	0.72	244
F43	85	10.1	5.9	0.73	174
F63	183	7.7	5.0--	0.40	223
F-C	479	8.8	5.2--	0.26	

BASSE-NORMANDIE

F14	179	7.8	5.8-	0.46	180
F50	148	7.9	5.0--	0.45	223
F61	94	7.8	5.2--	0.58	208
F-D	421	7.8	5.4--	0.28	

BOURGOGNE

F21	186	10.1	6.4	0.52	157
F58	107	10.6	6.3	0.70	159
F71	250	10.8	6.0	0.43	171
F89	99	8.1	4.8--	0.57	244
F-E	642	10.0	5.9--	0.26	

BRETAGNE

F22	179	8.3	5.0--	0.41	223
F29	271	8.2	5.0--	0.33	223
F35	238	8.2	5.8-	0.40	180
F56	193	8.4	5.6--	0.43	186
F-F	881	8.2	5.3--	0.19	

CENTRE

F18	104	8.1	5.0--	0.56	223
F28	110	8.2	5.4-	0.57	200
F36	89	8.9	5.3-	0.64	204
F37	124	6.3	3.8--	0.39	296
F41	79	6.9	3.8--	0.48	296
F45	137	6.9	4.6--	0.43	253
F-G	643	7.4	4.6--	0.20	

CHAMPAGNE-ARDENNE

F08	85	6.8	5.0--	0.59	223
F10	94	8.2	4.7--	0.54	249
F51	159	7.5	5.3--	0.46	204
F52	52	6.1	4.2--	0.64	273
F-H	390	7.2	4.9--	0.27	

CORSE

F20	37	4.3	2.2--	0.40	333

FRANCHE-COMTE

F25	104	5.5	4.5--	0.46	257
F39	83	8.5	5.5-	0.66	190
F70	92	10.3	6.2	0.72	161
F90	38	7.4	5.5	0.97	190
F-J	317	7.4	5.2--	0.32	

HAUTE-NORMANDIE

F27	140	8.2	6.0	0.55	171
F76	360	7.5	5.5--	0.31	190
F-K	500	7.7	5.7--	0.27	

ILE-DE-FRANCE

F75	945	9.6	5.2--	0.19	208
F77	194	6.4	4.9--	0.38	234
F78	244	5.6	4.9--	0.33	234
F91	169	4.6	4.1--	0.34	280
F92	443	7.5	4.9--	0.25	234
F93	303	5.7	4.5--	0.27	257
F94	278	5.6	4.2--	0.27	273
F95	179	5.3	4.5--	0.35	257
F-L	2755	6.8	4.8--	0.10	

LANGUEDOC-ROUSSILLON

F11	94	8.4	4.1--	0.49	280
F30	120	5.9	3.7--	0.37	304
F34	208	7.7	4.4--	0.34	265
F48	27	9.0	5.4	1.25	200
F66	96	7.7	4.4--	0.49	265
F-M	545	7.4	4.2--	0.20	

LIMOUSIN

F19	87	8.8	4.2--	0.52	273
F23	43	7.1	3.3--	0.61	311
F87	121	8.3	4.6--	0.48	253
F-N	251	8.2	4.2--	0.31	

LORRAINE

F54	228	7.8	5.9-	0.42	174
F55	57	6.9	5.1-	0.74	217
F57	326	8.2	6.3	0.37	159
F88	160	9.8	7.0	0.60	138
F-O	771	8.3	6.1--	0.24	

MIDI-PYRENEES

F09	40	7.1	4.0--	0.69	286
F12	86	7.5	4.2--	0.51	273
F31	168	5.3	3.4--	0.29	310
F32	52	7.4	4.5--	0.69	257
F46	56	9.2	4.9-	0.74	234
F65	64	6.9	4.0--	0.54	286
F81	104	7.5	4.7--	0.52	249
F82	49	6.5	4.1--	0.65	280
F-P	619	6.7	4.0--	0.18	

NORD-PAS-DE-CALAIS

F59	853	8.3	6.1--	0.22	166
F62	451	7.8	5.8--	0.29	180
F-Q	1304	8.2	5.9--	0.18	

PAYS DE LA LOIRE

F44	191	5.0	3.8--	0.29	296
F49	158	6.0	4.2--	0.37	273
F53	80	7.4	5.2-	0.63	208
F72	143	7.1	5.1--	0.46	217
F85	115	6.2	4.1--	0.43	280
F-R	687	6.0	4.3--	0.18	

PICARDIE

F02	164	7.6	5.5--	0.47	190
F60	141	5.8	4.7--	0.43	249
F80	159	7.2	5.1--	0.44	217
F-S	464	6.9	5.1--	0.26	

POITOU-CHARENTES

F16	116	8.4	5.2--	0.54	208
F17	171	8.4	4.9--	0.42	234
F79	112	8.3	5.2--	0.54	208
F86	101	7.0	4.9--	0.53	234
F-T	500	8.0	5.0--	0.25	

PROVENCE-ALPES-COTE D'AZUR

F04	35	7.9	4.5-	0.88	257
F05	26	6.7	5.0	1.03	223
F06	159	4.6	2.3--	0.21	326
F13	296	4.4	3.0--	0.19	317
F83	173	6.8	3.8--	0.33	296
F84	91	5.7	3.8--	0.43	296
F-U	780	5.2	3.1--	0.12	

RHONE-ALPES

F01	135	9.0	6.0	0.57	171
F07	121	11.6	6.5	0.68	156
F26	139	9.5	6.1	0.57	166
F38	255	7.3	5.0--	0.34	223
F42	306	9.9	6.1	0.38	166
F69	479	8.2	5.5--	0.27	190
F73	105	8.5	5.1--	0.55	217
F74	126	7.0	5.2--	0.49	208
F-V	1666	8.6	5.6--	0.15	
F.0	15993	7.4	4.9--	0.04	

UNITED KINGDOM (1976-80)

EAST ANGLIA

G25	220	13.0	9.0++	0.65	55
G46	368	17.7	10.3++	0.59	17
G55	277	15.7	9.4++	0.62	40
G-A	865	15.6	9.6++	0.36	

EAST MIDLANDS

G30	411	15.0	9.4++	0.50	40
G44	354	13.9	9.2++	0.53	50
G45	270	16.8	10.1++	0.67	21
G47	204	13.0	8.6++	0.65	76
G50	412	13.8	8.4++	0.44	84
G-B	1651	14.4	9.1++	0.24	

NORTHERN

G14	490	13.5	8.3++	0.40	92
G27	204	11.7	8.4++	0.61	84
G29	212	14.5	8.4++	0.63	84
G33	253	13.6	8.6++	0.57	76
G48	138	15.6	9.9++	0.89	28
G-C	1297	13.6	8.5++	0.25	

NORTH-WEST

G11	1117	13.5	8.2++	0.26	97
G12	681	14.0	8.6++	0.36	76
G26	390	13.9	9.4++	0.50	40
G43	650	15.2	8.5++	0.37	80
G-D	2838	14.1	8.5++	0.17	

SOUTH-EAST

G01	3211	14.7	8.5++	0.16	80
G22	176	12.0	8.7++	0.69	73
G23	236	11.7	8.2+	0.56	97
G24	228	14.6	10.1++	0.70	21
G34	451	21.1	8.9++	0.50	61
G35	678	15.4	9.8++	0.40	31
G37	606	14.0	9.0++	0.39	55
G39	390	13.4	8.9++	0.47	61
G41	96	26.5	12.2++	1.43	4
G42	679	15.2	9.2++	0.39	50
G51	181	11.6	7.5	0.59	129
G56	488	15.9	9.3++	0.45	45
G58	429	21.3	10.0++	0.57	25
G-E	7849	15.1	8.9++	0.11	

SOUTH-WEST

G21	484	16.9	9.7++	0.48	34
G28	222	17.2	10.1++	0.76	21
G31	526	18.0	9.5++	0.47	36
G32	373	20.2	9.3++	0.56	45
G36	237	15.6	8.9++	0.64	61
G53	225	17.8	9.9++	0.72	28
G59	209	13.6	9.2++	0.68	50
G-F	2276	17.2	9.5++	0.22	

WEST MIDLANDS

G15	1082	13.1	8.4++	0.27	84
G38	248	13.4	8.8++	0.60	71
G52	139	12.5	8.4+	0.77	84
G54	422	13.9	9.3++	0.47	45
G57	194	13.6	8.6++	0.66	76
G-G	2085	13.3	8.6++	0.20	

YORKSHIRE AND HUMBERSIDE

G13	560	14.0	8.7++	0.39	73
G16	968	15.1	9.4++	0.33	40
G40	357	13.6	8.9++	0.51	61
G49	339	16.9	9.6++	0.58	35
G-H	2224	14.8	9.2++	0.21	

WALES

G61	163	13.8	8.1	0.70	104
G62	145	14.3	8.3+	0.76	92
G63	146	10.9	6.9	0.61	144
G64	98	13.9	8.2	0.94	97
G65	178	10.7	6.8	0.54	147
G66	61	19.3	10.4+	1.46	16
G67	142	11.8	7.3	0.66	133
G68	131	11.4	7.2	0.67	135
G-I	1064	12.4	7.6++	0.25	

SCOTLAND(1975-80)

S01	69	12.1	8.4	1.07	84
S02	212	14.8	9.0++	0.68	55
S03	132	10.5	5.9	0.56	174
S04	141	13.5	8.3+	0.74	92
S05	316	13.4	8.4++	0.51	84
S06	43	13.8	6.8	1.17	147
S07	122	14.8	10.2++	0.98	19
S08	995	12.9	8.3++	0.28	92
S09	66	15.0	8.9	1.18	61
S10	8	14.7	7.6	3.04	123
S11	8	13.1	7.7	3.21	119
S12	22	24.4	12.6	3.02	3
G-J	2134	13.2	8.3++	0.19	

NORTHERN IRELAND

JE	172	10.3	7.4	0.60	131
JN	87	9.4	6.6	0.74	153
JS	27	4.0	3.2--	0.65	312
JW	49	8.0	5.7	0.86	183
G-K	335	8.6	6.2	0.36	
G.0	24618	14.4	8.7++	0.06	

ITALIA (1975-79)

ABRUZZI

I66	24	3.1	2.3--	0.49	326
I67	38	5.7	3.8--	0.65	296
I68	20	2.8	2.0--	0.46	339
I69	32	3.5	2.3--	0.42	326
I-A	114	3.7	2.5--	0.25	

BASILICATA

I76	23	2.2	1.6--	0.34	347
I77	19	3.8	3.2--	0.74	312
I-B	42	2.7	2.0--	0.33	

CALABRIA

I78	48	2.7	2.2--	0.33	333
I79	41	2.2	1.9--	0.31	341
I80	31	2.1	1.5--	0.29	349
I-C	120	2.3	1.9--	0.18	

CAMPANIA

I61	29	1.6	1.4--	0.27	352
I62	10	1.4	1.0--	0.32	354
I63	187	2.6	2.4--	0.18	324
I64	29	2.6	2.1--	0.39	337
I65	49	1.9	1.5--	0.23	349
I-D	304	2.3	2.0--	0.12	

EMILIA-ROMAGNA

I33	61	8.4	4.5--	0.62	257
I34	90	8.8	4.8--	0.55	244
I35	93	9.0	5.6	0.62	186
I36	145	9.8	6.2	0.53	161
I37	218	9.0	5.3--	0.38	204
I38	101	10.1	5.5-	0.57	190
I39	62	6.7	4.2--	0.57	273
I40	87	5.8	4.1--	0.45	280
I-E	857	8.5	5.1--	0.18	

FRIULI-VENEZIA GIULIA

I30	107	7.9	4.5--	0.47	257
I31	46	12.0	7.7	1.17	119
I32	114	14.3	7.0	0.74	138
I93	46	6.7	4.3--	0.69	268
I-F	313	9.7	5.5--	0.34	

LAZIO

I56	39	5.9	4.0--	0.66	286
I57	6	1.7	1.0--	0.45	354
I58	538	5.7	4.3--	0.19	268
I59	41	4.0	3.7--	0.58	304
I60	34	3.0	2.2--	0.39	333
I-G	658	5.2	3.9--	0.16	

LIGURIA

I08	34	5.7	3.2--	0.60	312
I09	68	8.6	4.8--	0.65	244
I10	272	9.6	5.4--	0.36	200
I11	42	6.6	3.8--	0.63	296
I-H	416	8.6	4.9--	0.26	

LOMBARDIA

I12	154	7.7	5.5--	0.46	190
I13	147	7.5	4.9--	0.42	234
I14	34	7.8	5.2	0.95	208
I15	924	8.9	6.2--	0.21	161
I16	144	6.5	5.0--	0.43	223
I17	178	7.0	5.0--	0.38	223
I18	140	10.3	5.5-	0.50	190
I19	74	8.6	5.0--	0.63	223
I20	83	8.5	4.9--	0.57	234
I-I	1878	8.2	5.6--	0.13	

MARCHE

I41	47	5.7	3.6--	0.55	307
I42	99	9.0	5.3--	0.56	204
I43	34	4.6	2.5--	0.46	322
I44	32	3.6	2.0--	0.38	339
I-J	212	6.0	3.5--	0.25	

MOLISE

I70	22	3.7	2.4--	0.54	324
I94	10	4.2	2.8--	0.91	319
I-K	32	3.8	2.5--	0.47	

PIEMONTE

I01	501	8.2	5.6--	0.26	186
I02	117	11.1	5.9	0.60	174
I03	114	8.7	5.1--	0.51	217
I04	112	8.2	4.4--	0.45	265
I05	45	8.0	4.6--	0.74	253
I06	141	11.4	5.4--	0.50	200
I-L	1030	8.9	5.4--	0.18	

PUGLIA

I71	46	2.7	2.3--	0.35	326
I72	96	2.7	2.3--	0.24	326
I73	49	3.5	3.1--	0.45	315
I74	32	3.2	2.7--	0.49	321
I75	42	2.2	1.9--	0.30	341
I-M	265	2.7	2.4--	0.15	

SARDEGNA

I90	26	2.4	1.9--	0.39	341
I91	17	2.5	2.1--	0.52	337
I92	42	2.4	2.3--	0.35	326
I95	13	3.3	2.9--	0.81	318
I-N	98	2.5	2.2--	0.23	

SICILIA

I81	29	2.7	1.9--	0.37	341
I82	66	2.2	1.7--	0.22	345
I83	40	2.3	1.5--	0.25	349
I84	25	2.1	1.6--	0.33	347
I85	11	1.5	1.2--	0.36	353
I86	14	2.7	2.3--	0.61	326
I87	69	2.8	2.2--	0.28	333
I88	47	6.9	4.9-	0.74	234
I89	21	2.2	1.7--	0.38	345
I-O	322	2.6	2.0--	0.11	

TOSCANA

I45	25	4.7	2.8--	0.59	319
I46	82	8.1	4.5--	0.54	257
I47	49	7.2	4.0--	0.63	286
I48	220	7.1	4.6--	0.33	253
I49	73	8.3	4.9--	0.61	234
I50	70	7.1	3.9--	0.49	295
I51	48	6.1	3.7--	0.58	304
I52	50	7.6	4.0--	0.61	286
I53	61	10.9	6.2	0.84	161
I-P	678	7.4	4.4--	0.18	

TRENTINO-ALTO ADIGE

I21	87	8.0	5.6	0.63	186
I22	99	8.8	5.5-	0.59	190
I-Q	186	8.4	5.5--	0.43	

UMBRIA

I54	57	4.0	2.5--	0.35	322
I55	46	8.0	5.1-	0.79	217
I-R	103	5.1	3.3--	0.34	

VALLE D'AOSTA

I07	26	9.2	6.1	1.24	166

VENETO

I23	126	6.5	4.3--	0.40	268
I24	105	5.8	4.1--	0.41	280
I25	31	5.3	3.1--	0.59	315
I26	97	5.4	3.6--	0.39	307
I27	123	5.7	4.0--	0.38	286
I28	109	5.3	3.8--	0.38	296
I29	42	6.5	4.2--	0.67	273
I-T	633	5.8	3.9--	0.16	
I.0	8287	5.8	4.0--	0.05	

IRELAND (1976-80)

CONNAUGHT

R07	27	6.6	4.7-	0.98	249
R12	11	17.0	10.6	3.62	12
R16	30	10.8	6.8	1.34	147
R20	10	7.8	4.3	1.40	268
R21	16	11.9	10.5	2.80	14
R-A	94	9.3	6.5	0.72	

LEINSTER

R01	5	5.3	6.1	2.77	166
R06	219	8.6	7.8	0.55	115
R09	15	6.4	7.6	1.99	123
R10	11	6.6	4.8	1.54	244
R11	12	10.1	8.9	2.65	61
R14	6	8.1	7.1	2.99	137
R15	15	7.0	7.0	1.86	138
R17	17	7.7	7.0	1.76	138
R19	12	8.7	6.7	2.02	152
R24	10	6.8	5.7	1.91	183
R25	19	8.0	6.8	1.69	147
R26	23	11.0	9.8	2.13	31
R-B	364	8.3	7.5	0.41	

MUNSTER

R03	16	7.8	5.5	1.46	190
R04	87	8.8	7.0	0.79	138
R08	38	13.1	10.0	1.76	25
R13	24	6.1	5.2	1.13	208
R22	30	9.3	6.2	1.20	161
R23	24	11.1	10.0	2.11	25
R-C	219	9.1	7.1	0.51	

ULSTER

R02	10	7.9	5.9	2.01	174
R05	34	11.5	9.5	1.76	36
R18	17	14.1	10.2	2.70	19
R-D	61	11.2	8.8	1.21	
R.0	738	8.8	7.3+	0.28	

LUXEMBOURG (1971-80)

LE	27	14.1	9.5	1.94	36
LN	41	15.5	9.5	1.60	36
LS	174	12.9	8.5+	0.68	80
L.0	242	13.4	8.7++	0.59	

NEDERLAND (1976-80)

N01	187	13.6	9.0++	0.70	55
N02	207	14.4	10.1++	0.75	21
N03	106	10.3	7.9	0.80	111
N04	316	12.6	9.3++	0.55	45
N05	516	12.3	8.9++	0.41	61
N06	263	11.8	8.2++	0.54	97
N07	856	14.4	9.4++	0.34	40
N08	952	12.3	8.1++	0.28	104
N09	121	14.2	8.9+	0.88	61
N10	530	10.6	9.0++	0.40	55
N11	283	10.7	8.3++	0.51	92
N.0	4337	12.4	8.8++	0.14	

EEC-9

EEC	86224	10.8	6.8	0.02	

BELGIE-BELGIQUE (1971-78)

BRUSSEL-BRUXELLES

B21	315	7.1	3.9	0.25	117

VLAANDEREN

B10	217	3.4	2.3--	0.16	206
B29	119	3.2	2.2--	0.21	213
B30	210	4.8	3.1-	0.23	160
B40	259	4.8	3.1-	0.21	160
B70	71	2.6	2.3--	0.28	206
B-V	876	3.9	2.6--	0.09	

WALLONIE

B25	56	5.2	3.2	0.46	153
B50	399	7.3	4.2+	0.23	101
B60	267	6.3	3.6	0.24	133
B80	41	4.6	2.8	0.48	174
B90	93	5.8	3.6	0.41	133
B-W	856	6.5	3.8	0.14	
B.0	2047	5.1	3.2--	0.08	

BR DEUTSCHLAND (1976-80)

BADEN-WURTTEMBERG

D81	535	6.0	3.9	0.18	117
D82	422	6.8	4.1+	0.22	110
D83	286	5.9	3.8	0.24	123
D84	237	6.1	4.2	0.29	101
D-A	1480	6.2	4.0++	0.11	

BAYERN

D91	585	6.3	3.8	0.17	123
D92	201	7.7	4.8++	0.37	69
D93	193	7.6	4.8++	0.37	69
D94	218	7.8	4.6++	0.34	79
D95	340	8.5	4.9++	0.29	66
D96	169	5.4	3.6	0.29	133
D97	272	6.8	4.0	0.27	113
D-B	1978	7.0	4.2++	0.10	

BERLIN(WEST)

DB0	825	15.5	8.4++	0.35	8

BREMEN

D40	154	8.3	4.8++	0.42	69

HAMBURG

D20	460	10.3	5.4++	0.29	50

HESSEN

D64	771	6.8	4.2++	0.16	101
D66	207	6.7	4.0	0.30	113
D-F	978	6.8	4.1++	0.14	

NIEDERSACHSEN

D31	357	8.3	4.9++	0.29	66
D32	527	9.7	5.8++	0.28	39
D33	257	7.0	4.3+	0.29	94
D34	371	6.8	4.6++	0.26	79
D-G	1512	8.0	5.0++	0.14	

NORDRHEIN-WESTFALEN

D51	1269	9.2	5.7++	0.17	41
D53	752	7.5	4.8++	0.19	69
D55	397	6.4	4.3++	0.23	94
D57	342	7.2	4.3++	0.26	94
D59	696	7.2	4.5++	0.18	85
D-H	3456	7.8	4.9++	0.09	

RHEINLAND-PFALZ

D71	207	5.8	3.4	0.26	141
D72	99	8.0	4.7+	0.52	75
D73	328	6.9	4.3++	0.26	94
D-I	634	6.7	4.0+	0.17	

SAARLAND

DA0	209	7.3	4.5+	0.33	85

SCHLESWIG-HOLSTEIN

D10	610	9.1	5.5++	0.24	48
D.0	12296	7.6	4.7++	0.05	

DANMARK (1971-80)

K15	956	14.4	8.7++	0.31	5
K20	117	7.8	6.8++	0.65	22
K25	79	8.7	8.0++	0.92	10
K30	180	13.5	10.5++	0.82	1
K35	145	11.4	7.1++	0.64	14
K40	24	10.2	7.3+	1.57	13
K42	298	13.3	9.3++	0.57	2
K50	137	11.2	8.5++	0.76	6
K55	99	9.7	8.1++	0.84	9
K60	196	12.3	9.1++	0.68	3
K65	96	7.7	6.4++	0.68	30
K70	312	11.1	8.5++	0.51	6
K76	97	8.7	6.7++	0.71	26
K80	288	12.3	9.1++	0.56	3
K.0	3024	11.8	8.5++	0.16	

FRANCE (1971-78)

ALSACE

F67	190	5.3	3.7	0.29	130
F68	109	4.2	3.3	0.34	145
F-A	299	4.8	3.5	0.22	

AQUITAINE

F24	44	2.9	1.7--	0.29	248
F33	171	3.9	2.7--	0.22	183
F40	37	3.2	2.1--	0.38	220
F47	43	3.6	1.9--	0.33	234
F64	50	2.3	1.3--	0.21	271
F-B	345	3.3	2.1--	0.12	

AUVERGNE

F03	51	3.3	2.0--	0.31	227
F15	30	4.4	2.4-	0.50	200
F43	34	4.0	2.8	0.55	174
F63	66	2.8	1.8--	0.24	241
F-C	181	3.3	2.1--	0.17	

BASSE-NORMANDIE

F14	116	5.0	4.1	0.40	110
F50	62	3.3	2.3--	0.32	206
F61	52	4.3	3.2	0.46	153
F-D	230	4.3	3.2	0.23	

BOURGOGNE

F21	108	5.9	4.2	0.44	101
F58	45	4.5	2.8	0.47	174
F71	108	4.7	3.0-	0.32	165
F89	60	4.9	3.2	0.47	153
F-E	321	5.0	3.3	0.21	

BRETAGNE

F22	50	2.3	1.4--	0.23	269
F29	93	2.8	1.7--	0.20	248
F35	78	2.7	1.9--	0.23	234
F56	39	1.7	1.2--	0.21	282
F-F	260	2.4	1.6--	0.11	

CENTRE

F18	47	3.7	2.7-	0.43	183
F28	40	3.0	2.2--	0.38	213
F36	50	5.0	3.2	0.53	153
F37	56	2.8	2.1--	0.31	220
F41	36	3.1	2.0--	0.37	227
F45	66	3.3	2.2--	0.30	213
F-G	295	3.4	2.3--	0.15	

CHAMPAGNE-ARDENNE

F08	43	3.5	2.8	0.45	174
F10	40	3.5	2.6-	0.43	188
F51	69	3.2	2.6--	0.34	188
F52	34	4.0	2.9	0.54	170
F-H	186	3.5	2.7--	0.21	

CORSE

F20	16	1.9	1.1--	0.31	290

FRANCHE-COMTE

F25	61	3.2	2.6--	0.35	188
F39	40	4.1	2.8	0.48	174
F70	34	3.8	2.6-	0.50	188
F90	18	3.5	2.8	0.70	174
F-J	153	3.6	2.6--	0.23	

HAUTE-NORMANDIE

F27	80	4.7	3.6	0.44	133
F76	198	4.1	3.2	0.24	153
F-K	278	4.3	3.3	0.21	

ILE-DE-FRANCE

F75	376	3.8	2.2--	0.13	213
F77	81	2.7	2.1--	0.25	220
F78	145	3.3	3.0-	0.26	165
F91	101	2.7	2.6--	0.27	188
F92	163	2.8	2.0--	0.16	227
F93	180	3.4	2.6--	0.20	188
F94	168	3.4	2.5--	0.21	198
F95	92	2.7	2.3--	0.25	206
F-L	1306	3.2	2.3--	0.07	

LANGUEDOC-ROUSSILLON

F11	39	3.5	2.0--	0.36	227
F30	80	3.9	2.4--	0.29	200
F34	73	2.7	1.6--	0.21	254
F48	5	1.7	0.6--	0.31	337
F66	30	2.4	1.1--	0.23	290
F-M	227	3.1	1.7--	0.13	

LIMOUSIN

F19	23	2.3	1.3--	0.32	271
F23	27	4.5	2.3-	0.54	206
F87	33	2.3	1.4--	0.29	269
F-N	83	2.7	1.6--	0.20	

LORRAINE

F54	124	4.3	3.4	0.32	141
F55	30	3.6	2.5-	0.50	198
F57	217	5.4	4.4+	0.31	90
F88	70	4.3	3.2	0.41	153
F-O	441	4.7	3.6	0.18	

MIDI-PYRENEES

F09	22	3.9	2.1--	0.53	220
F12	29	2.5	1.5--	0.32	260
F31	70	2.2	1.5--	0.20	260
F32	30	4.3	2.4--	0.48	200
F46	42	6.9	4.3	0.75	94
F65	28	3.0	1.9--	0.38	234
F81	39	2.8	1.8--	0.33	241
F82	36	4.8	2.6-	0.49	188
F-P	296	3.2	2.0--	0.13	

NORD-PAS-DE-CALAIS

F59	474	4.6	3.5	0.17	139
F62	240	4.2	3.2-	0.22	153
F-Q	714	4.5	3.3-	0.13	

PAYS DE LA LOIRE

F44	90	2.3	1.8--	0.20	241
F49	62	2.4	1.9--	0.25	234
F53	11	1.0	0.7--	0.24	330
F72	52	2.6	1.7--	0.26	248
F85	37	2.0	1.3--	0.25	271
F-R	252	2.2	1.6--	0.11	

PICARDIE

F02	79	3.7	3.3	0.38	145
F60	63	2.6	2.3--	0.30	206
F80	89	4.0	3.1	0.36	160
F-S	231	3.4	2.9--	0.20	

POITOU-CHARENTES

F16	56	4.1	2.7-	0.39	183
F17	83	4.1	3.0	0.36	165
F79	44	3.2	2.2--	0.36	213
F86	46	3.2	2.6-	0.41	188
F-T	229	3.7	2.7--	0.19	

PROVENCE-ALPES-COTE D'AZUR

F04	9	2.0	1.2--	0.43	282
F05	17	4.4	2.8	0.74	174
F06	66	1.9	1.0--	0.14	302
F13	220	3.3	2.1--	0.16	220
F83	94	3.7	2.3--	0.25	206
F84	47	3.0	2.0--	0.32	227
F-U	453	3.0	1.8--	0.09	

RHONE-ALPES

F01	62	4.1	2.8-	0.39	174
F07	31	3.0	1.8--	0.37	241
F26	49	3.3	2.4--	0.37	200
F38	128	3.7	2.6--	0.25	188
F42	121	3.9	2.4--	0.24	200
F69	257	4.4	3.3	0.22	145
F73	59	4.8	3.3	0.46	145
F74	72	4.0	3.3	0.41	145
F-V	779	4.0	2.8--	0.11	
F.0	7575	3.5	2.5--	0.03	

UNITED KINGDOM (1976-80)

EAST ANGLIA

G25	110	6.5	4.8+	0.49	69
G46	178	8.6	5.2++	0.43	57
G55	114	6.4	4.3	0.43	94
G-A	402	7.3	4.8++	0.26	

EAST MIDLANDS

G30	225	8.2	5.1++	0.37	59
G44	207	8.1	5.6++	0.42	45
G45	126	7.8	5.3++	0.51	54
G47	128	8.2	5.9++	0.55	38
G50	298	10.0	6.3++	0.39	32
G-B	984	8.6	5.7++	0.19	

NORTHERN

G14	368	10.2	6.5++	0.37	28
G27	171	9.8	7.5++	0.60	12
G29	122	8.3	5.0++	0.50	62
G33	188	10.1	7.0++	0.54	19
G48	84	9.5	6.0++	0.71	35
G-C	933	9.8	6.5++	0.23	

NORTH-WEST

G11	837	10.1	6.8++	0.25	22
G12	508	10.5	7.0++	0.33	19
G26	264	9.4	6.5++	0.42	28
G43	472	11.0	6.8++	0.35	22
G-D	2081	10.3	6.8++	0.16	

SOUTH-EAST

G01	1524	7.0	4.2++	0.12	101
G22	88	6.0	4.5	0.50	85
G23	117	5.8	4.2	0.40	101
G24	91	5.8	4.2	0.46	101
G34	187	8.7	4.7+	0.41	75
G35	300	6.8	4.4++	0.27	90
G37	332	7.7	5.3++	0.31	54
G39	169	5.8	3.8	0.31	123
G41	31	8.6	4.6	1.02	79
G42	359	8.0	5.0++	0.29	62
G51	80	5.1	3.6	0.43	133
G56	218	7.1	4.0	0.29	113
G58	163	8.1	3.9	0.37	117
G-E	3659	7.0	4.3++	0.08	

SOUTH-WEST

G21	213	7.5	4.6++	0.34	79
G28	109	8.4	5.5++	0.57	48
G31	270	9.2	5.1++	0.36	59
G32	151	8.2	4.3	0.40	94
G36	138	9.1	6.0++	0.55	35
G53	110	8.7	5.7++	0.60	41
G59	113	7.3	5.0++	0.50	62
G-F	1104	8.3	5.1++	0.17	

WEST MIDLANDS

G15	654	7.9	5.4++	0.22	50
G38	139	7.5	4.9++	0.45	66
G52	79	7.1	4.8+	0.60	69
G54	264	8.7	6.3++	0.40	32
G57	115	8.1	5.7++	0.56	41
G-G	1251	8.0	5.5++	0.16	

YORKSHIRE AND HUMBERSIDE

G13	390	9.8	6.4++	0.35	30
G16	691	10.8	7.1++	0.29	14
G40	272	10.4	7.1++	0.46	14
G49	192	9.6	5.4++	0.43	50
G-H	1545	10.3	6.7++	0.18	

WALES

G61	120	10.1	6.6++	0.66	27
G62	113	11.2	7.1++	0.74	14
G63	107	8.0	5.6++	0.57	45
G64	89	12.6	6.8++	0.82	22
G65	144	8.7	5.6++	0.49	45
G66	26	8.2	5.0	1.04	62
G67	84	7.0	4.7	0.55	75
G68	128	11.2	6.9++	0.66	21
G-I	811	9.5	6.1++	0.23	

SCOTLAND(1975-80)

S01	39	6.8	5.2	0.87	57
S02	98	6.9	4.6	0.49	79
S03	100	8.0	4.7+	0.53	75
S04	97	9.3	7.1++	0.76	14
S05	193	8.2	5.3++	0.41	54
S06	29	9.3	5.8	1.19	39
S07	56	6.8	4.6	0.64	79
S08	627	8.2	5.7++	0.24	41
S09	47	10.7	6.2++	0.99	34
S10	6	11.0	7.7	3.43	11
S11	3	4.9	3.3	1.99	145
S12	5	5.5	2.7	1.38	183
G-J	1300	8.1	5.4++	0.16	

NORTHERN IRELAND

JE	79	4.7	3.4	0.41	141
JN	48	5.2	4.0	0.60	113
JS	17	2.5	2.0--	0.51	227
JW	28	4.6	3.3	0.67	145
G-K	172	4.4	3.3	0.27	
G.0	14242	8.3	5.4++	0.05	

ITALIA (1975-79)

ABRUZZI

I66	15	1.9	1.3--	0.35	271
I67	6	0.9	0.6--	0.24	337
I68	19	2.6	1.9--	0.44	234
I69	11	1.2	0.7--	0.23	330
I-A	51	1.7	1.1--	0.16	

BASILICATA

I76	12	1.2	0.8--	0.24	321
I77	6	1.2	1.0--	0.43	302
I-B	18	1.2	0.9--	0.21	

CALABRIA

I78	19	1.1	0.9--	0.20	312
I79	19	1.0	0.9--	0.21	312
I80	17	1.1	0.8--	0.21	321
I-C	55	1.1	0.9--	0.12	

CAMPANIA

I61	12	0.7	0.6--	0.17	337
I62	2	0.3	0.1--	0.10	355
I63	55	0.8	0.7--	0.09	330
I64	5	0.5	0.3--	0.15	352
I65	28	1.1	0.9--	0.17	312
I-D	102	0.8	0.6--	0.06	

EMILIA-ROMAGNA

I33	6	0.8	0.6--	0.27	337
I34	15	1.5	0.8--	0.23	321
I35	19	1.8	1.0--	0.25	302
I36	13	0.9	0.5--	0.15	347
I37	65	2.7	1.5--	0.19	260
I38	23	2.3	1.2--	0.26	282
I39	17	1.8	1.0--	0.25	302
I40	21	1.4	0.9--	0.20	312
I-E	179	1.8	1.0--	0.08	

FRIULI-VENEZIA GIULIA

I30	48	3.5	2.0--	0.31	227
I31	10	2.6	1.6--	0.54	254
I32	48	6.0	2.9	0.46	170
I93	21	3.1	1.8--	0.42	241
I-F	127	3.9	2.2--	0.21	

LAZIO

I56	8	1.2	0.8--	0.30	321
I57	6	1.7	0.8--	0.36	321
I58	183	1.9	1.5--	0.11	260
I59	3	0.3	0.2--	0.14	353
I60	9	0.8	0.6--	0.19	337
I-G	209	1.7	1.2--	0.09	

LIGURIA

I08	20	3.3	1.9--	0.46	234
I09	19	2.4	1.2--	0.29	282
I10	81	2.9	1.5--	0.18	260
I11	20	3.1	1.7--	0.41	248
I-H	140	2.9	1.5--	0.14	

LOMBARDIA

I12	22	1.1	0.8--	0.17	321
I13	22	1.1	0.7--	0.16	330
I14	8	1.8	1.3--	0.50	271
I15	154	1.5	1.1--	0.09	290
I16	34	1.5	1.2--	0.20	282
I17	40	1.6	1.0--	0.17	302
I18	24	1.8	1.1--	0.24	290
I19	22	2.6	1.3--	0.29	271
I20	20	2.0	1.1--	0.27	290
I-I	346	1.5	1.0--	0.06	

MARCHE

I41	14	1.7	0.9--	0.26	312
I42	18	1.6	0.9--	0.23	312
I43	9	1.2	0.7--	0.23	330
I44	5	0.6	0.4--	0.19	350
I-J	46	1.3	0.7--	0.12	

MOLISE

I70	11	1.8	1.1--	0.34	290
I94	3	1.2	0.7--	0.43	330
I-K	14	1.7	1.0--	0.27	

PIEMONTE

I01	149	2.4	1.7--	0.14	248
I02	29	2.7	1.6--	0.33	254
I03	33	2.5	1.5--	0.28	260
I04	43	3.1	1.9--	0.31	234
I05	14	2.5	1.5--	0.44	260
I06	29	2.3	1.1--	0.22	290
I-L	297	2.6	1.6--	0.10	

PUGLIA

I71	32	1.9	1.5--	0.28	260
I72	60	1.7	1.3--	0.18	271
I73	17	1.2	1.1--	0.26	290
I74	13	1.3	1.0--	0.30	302
I75	15	0.8	0.6--	0.16	337
I-M	137	1.4	1.2--	0.10	

SARDEGNA

I90	6	0.6	0.5--	0.21	347
I91	2	0.3	0.2--	0.16	353
I92	20	1.1	1.0--	0.23	302
I95	7	1.8	1.3--	0.54	271
I-N	35	0.9	0.8--	0.13	

SICILIA

I81	12	1.1	0.9--	0.25	312
I82	21	0.7	0.6--	0.13	337
I83	20	1.2	0.8--	0.19	321
I84	15	1.3	1.0--	0.27	302
I85	8	1.1	0.8--	0.30	321
I86	4	0.8	0.6--	0.30	337
I87	38	1.5	1.2--	0.20	282
I88	11	1.6	1.2--	0.36	282
I89	15	1.5	1.3--	0.33	271
I-O	144	1.2	0.9--	0.08	

TOSCANA

I45	10	1.9	1.3--	0.42	271
I46	10	1.0	0.5--	0.15	347
I47	14	2.1	1.1--	0.33	290
I48	45	1.5	0.9--	0.14	312
I49	14	1.6	1.1--	0.29	290
I50	25	2.5	1.5--	0.32	260
I51	9	1.1	0.6--	0.21	337
I52	7	1.1	0.7--	0.25	330
I53	6	1.1	0.6--	0.26	337
I-P	140	1.5	0.9--	0.08	

TRENTINO-ALTO ADIGE

I21	29	2.7	2.1--	0.40	220
I22	28	2.5	1.6--	0.32	254
I-Q	57	2.6	1.8--	0.25	

UMBRIA

I54	8	0.6	0.4--	0.13	350
I55	8	1.4	0.8--	0.28	321
I-R	16	0.8	0.5--	0.13	

VALLE D'AOSTA

I07	4	1.4	1.2--	0.58	282

VENETO

I23	32	1.6	1.1--	0.19	290
I24	23	1.3	0.9--	0.19	312
I25	15	2.6	1.8--	0.48	241
I26	43	2.4	1.6--	0.25	254
I27	29	1.4	1.0--	0.19	302
I28	36	1.8	1.3--	0.22	271
I29	13	2.0	1.1--	0.33	290
I-T	191	1.7	1.2--	0.09	
I.0	2308	1.6	1.1--	0.02	

IRELAND (1976-80)

CONNAUGHT

R07	12	3.0	2.1-	0.66	220
R12	5	7.7	3.8	1.84	123
R16	10	3.6	3.1	1.09	160
R20	8	6.2	3.9	1.59	117
R21	5	3.7	3.1	1.48	160
R-A	40	4.0	2.9	0.51	

LEINSTER

R01	4	4.2	2.9	1.55	170
R06	76	3.0	2.8-	0.33	174
R09	10	4.3	5.1	1.65	59
R10	5	3.0	2.4	1.14	200
R11	7	5.9	6.0	2.31	35
R14	4	5.4	4.4	2.42	90
R15	6	2.8	2.2	0.93	213
R17	7	3.2	3.0	1.18	165
R19	6	4.4	3.8	1.57	123
R24	7	4.8	4.2	1.62	101
R25	10	4.2	4.2	1.42	101
R26	7	3.3	3.9	1.52	117
R-B	149	3.4	3.2	0.27	

MUNSTER

R03	2	1.0	1.0--	0.73	302
R04	30	3.0	2.2--	0.44	213
R08	10	3.4	3.0	1.00	165
R13	11	2.8	2.9	0.88	170
R22	7	2.2	1.7--	0.68	248
R23	5	2.3	1.6-	0.78	254
R-C	65	2.7	2.2--	0.29	

ULSTER

R02	5	3.9	3.9	1.83	117
R05	5	1.7	1.8-	0.82	241
R18	6	5.0	3.8	1.74	123
R-D	16	2.9	2.7	0.73	
R.0	270	3.2	2.8--	0.18	

LUXEMBOURG (1971-80)

LE	12	6.3	3.6	1.07	133
LN	15	5.7	3.7	1.01	130
LS	104	7.7	5.4++	0.55	50
L.0	131	7.3	5.0++	0.45	

NEDERLAND (1976-80)

N01	66	4.8	3.7	0.48	130
N02	70	4.9	3.8	0.48	123
N03	34	3.3	2.6-	0.46	188
N04	86	3.4	2.7--	0.31	183
N05	193	4.6	3.4	0.26	141
N06	122	5.5	4.1	0.39	110
N07	384	6.4	4.5++	0.25	85
N08	491	6.3	4.5++	0.22	85
N09	54	6.3	4.4	0.65	90
N10	201	4.0	3.5	0.25	139
N11	113	4.3	3.3	0.32	145
N.0	1814	5.2	3.9++	0.10	

EEC-9

EEC	43707	5.5	3.6	0.02	

BELGIE-BELGIQUE (1971-78)

BRUSSEL-BRUXELLES					
B21	825	18.5	9.1	0.36	175
VLAANDEREN					
B10	684	10.8	6.6--	0.27	320
B29	502	13.7	8.4	0.40	227
B30	619	14.3	8.7	0.37	202
B40	729	13.6	8.1--	0.32	252
B70	220	8.1	7.1--	0.49	300
B-V	2754	12.3	7.7--	0.16	
WALLONIE					
B25	147	13.7	7.5-	0.68	280
B50	1120	20.6	11.2++	0.37	45
B60	821	19.5	10.4++	0.39	71
B80	148	16.6	9.3	0.83	157
B90	306	19.0	10.7+	0.67	61
B-W	2542	19.2	10.4++	0.23	
B.0	6121	15.3	8.8-	0.12	

BR DEUTSCHLAND (1976-80)

BADEN-WURTTEMBERG					
D81	1304	14.6	8.4--	0.25	227
D82	998	16.1	8.7	0.30	202
D83	698	14.4	8.3-	0.34	236
D84	527	13.7	8.3-	0.39	236
D-A	3527	14.8	8.4--	0.15	
BAYERN					
D91	1424	15.2	8.0--	0.23	257
D92	459	17.5	10.1	0.51	92
D93	429	17.0	10.0	0.52	99
D94	512	18.3	9.3	0.46	157
D95	742	18.6	9.7	0.39	125
D96	479	15.4	8.9	0.44	191
D97	668	16.8	8.9	0.38	191
D-B	4713	16.6	9.0	0.14	
BERLIN(WEST)					
DB0	1451	27.3	13.1++	0.42	10
BREMEN					
D40	315	17.0	8.6	0.54	209
HAMBURG					
D20	882	19.8	9.4	0.36	148
HESSEN					
D64	1911	16.8	9.2	0.23	167
D66	499	16.1	8.4	0.43	227
D-F	2410	16.7	9.0	0.20	
NIEDERSACHSEN					
D31	739	17.2	9.1	0.38	175
D32	985	18.1	9.5	0.34	142
D33	541	14.6	8.3-	0.39	236
D34	749	13.8	8.5	0.34	218
D-G	3014	16.0	8.9	0.18	
NORDRHEIN-WESTFALEN					
D51	2440	17.7	9.9++	0.22	108
D53	1646	16.3	9.7+	0.25	125
D55	863	13.8	8.8	0.32	197
D57	669	14.1	7.8--	0.33	265
D59	1578	16.3	9.4	0.25	148
D-H	7196	16.2	9.4+	0.12	
RHEINLAND-PFALZ					
D71	564	15.9	8.2-	0.38	241
D72	244	19.7	10.3	0.73	78
D73	864	18.3	9.7	0.36	125
D-I	1672	17.6	9.2	0.25	
SAARLAND					
DA0	492	17.3	9.5	0.46	142
SCHLESWIG-HOLSTEIN					
D10	1220	18.1	9.9+	0.32	108
D.0	26892	16.7	9.2	0.06	

DANMARK (1971-80)

K15	1557	23.4	12.8++	0.36	13
K20	208	13.8	11.3++	0.81	42
K25	134	14.7	13.0++	1.16	11
K30	278	20.8	14.7++	0.94	1
K35	277	21.7	12.2++	0.80	20
K40	44	18.8	12.0	1.92	25
K42	482	21.5	13.5++	0.67	5
K50	238	19.5	13.2++	0.91	7
K55	164	16.1	12.1++	0.99	22
K60	312	19.6	13.2++	0.80	7
K65	167	13.3	10.1	0.82	92
K70	489	17.3	12.1++	0.58	22
K76	165	14.7	9.8	0.82	116
K80	471	20.1	13.6++	0.66	4
K.0	4986	19.5	12.6++	0.19	

FRANCE (1971-78)

ALSACE					
F67	646	17.9	11.0++	0.47	48
F68	471	18.2	11.6++	0.59	33
F-A	1117	18.0	11.3++	0.37	
AQUITAINE					
F24	276	18.0	9.4	0.65	148
F33	773	17.5	10.5++	0.42	67
F40	175	14.9	8.2	0.70	241
F47	229	19.1	10.0	0.75	99
F64	309	14.0	7.7--	0.49	270
F-B	1762	16.7	9.4	0.25	
AUVERGNE					
F03	336	21.5	11.2++	0.70	45
F15	124	18.4	9.8	1.02	116
F43	172	20.5	10.4	0.95	71
F63	428	18.1	10.9++	0.59	51
F-C	1060	19.5	10.8++	0.38	
BASSE-NORMANDIE					
F14	394	17.1	12.1++	0.67	22
F50	255	13.7	8.7	0.60	202
F61	212	17.5	11.1+	0.83	47
F-D	861	16.0	10.6++	0.40	
BOURGOGNE					
F21	278	15.1	9.3	0.62	157
F58	216	21.4	10.9+	0.89	51
F71	338	14.6	8.3	0.51	236
F89	230	18.9	10.9+	0.84	51
F-E	1062	16.6	9.5	0.33	
BRETAGNE					
F22	281	13.0	7.7--	0.51	270
F29	443	13.3	7.7--	0.40	270
F35	350	12.0	7.9--	0.46	260
F56	259	11.2	7.0--	0.47	304
F-F	1333	12.5	7.6--	0.23	
CENTRE					
F18	244	19.0	10.7+	0.78	61
F28	202	15.1	9.7	0.77	125
F36	241	24.2	12.2++	0.95	20
F37	322	16.4	10.1	0.63	92
F41	173	15.0	8.9	0.78	191
F45	299	15.1	9.5	0.61	142
F-G	1481	17.0	10.1++	0.30	
CHAMPAGNE-ARDENNE					
F08	230	18.5	12.6++	0.91	15
F10	177	15.4	9.3	0.79	157
F51	323	15.2	10.8+	0.66	59
F52	132	15.4	10.2	0.99	84
F-H	862	16.0	10.7++	0.41	
CORSE					
F20	82	9.5	4.8--	0.59	351
FRANCHE-COMTE					
F25	277	14.6	11.4++	0.73	39
F39	152	15.6	8.9	0.81	191
F70	172	19.3	11.5+	1.00	36
F90	102	19.9	12.5+	1.39	17
F-J	703	16.5	10.9++	0.45	
HAUTE-NORMANDIE					
F27	286	16.7	11.5++	0.75	36
F76	657	13.7	9.6	0.41	134
F-K	943	14.5	10.1++	0.36	
ILE-DE-FRANCE					
F75	1988	20.1	9.9++	0.25	108
F77	456	15.0	11.0++	0.56	48
F78	495	11.4	9.1	0.44	175
F91	400	10.8	9.2	0.49	167
F92	828	14.0	8.8	0.33	197
F93	723	13.7	10.1++	0.40	92
F94	700	14.1	9.5	0.39	142
F95	422	12.4	9.9	0.51	108
F-L	6012	14.8	9.6++	0.13	
LANGUEDOC-ROUSSILLON					
F11	153	13.7	6.7--	0.63	317
F30	307	15.1	8.2	0.52	241
F34	405	15.0	7.8--	0.44	265
F48	48	15.9	8.2	1.39	241
F66	225	18.0	8.2	0.62	241
F-M	1138	15.4	7.8--	0.26	
LIMOUSIN					
F19	183	18.5	8.7	0.75	202
F23	153	25.3	10.4	1.07	71
F87	236	16.2	8.1	0.62	252
F-N	572	18.8	8.8	0.44	
LORRAINE					
F54	431	14.8	10.7++	0.55	61
F55	137	16.6	10.4	1.00	71
F57	623	15.6	12.0++	0.50	25
F88	271	16.7	10.7+	0.72	61
F-O	1462	15.7	11.1++	0.31	
MIDI-PYRENEES					
F09	98	17.5	8.2	0.97	241
F12	155	13.6	6.8--	0.63	313
F31	449	14.1	8.6	0.45	209
F32	124	17.7	9.2	0.95	167
F46	122	20.0	10.3	1.08	78
F65	163	17.4	10.0	0.86	99
F81	237	17.1	9.3	0.68	157
F82	158	21.0	10.3	0.94	78
F-P	1506	16.3	8.9	0.26	
NORD-PAS-DE-CALAIS					
F59	1601	15.7	10.5++	0.29	67
F62	925	16.1	10.9++	0.39	51
F-Q	2526	15.8	10.7++	0.23	
PAYS DE LA LOIRE					
F44	405	10.5	7.1--	0.39	300
F49	358	13.7	9.3	0.54	157
F53	117	10.8	6.5--	0.66	322
F72	329	16.3	9.9	0.61	108
F85	210	11.4	6.5--	0.52	322
F-R	1419	12.4	7.9--	0.23	
PICARDIE					
F02	374	17.4	11.7++	0.67	30
F60	388	16.0	11.5++	0.65	36
F80	426	19.4	12.9++	0.70	12
F-S	1188	17.5	12.0++	0.39	
POITOU-CHARENTES					
F16	247	17.9	10.4	0.74	71
F17	374	18.4	10.6+	0.62	66
F79	202	14.9	8.2	0.67	241
F86	257	17.7	10.9+	0.77	51
F-T	1080	17.4	10.1++	0.35	
PROVENCE-ALPES-COTE D'AZUR					
F04	51	11.4	6.5--	1.01	322
F05	56	14.3	8.2	1.22	241
F06	336	9.7	4.4--	0.29	353
F13	797	12.0	7.3--	0.28	292
F83	413	16.2	9.1	0.49	175
F84	292	18.4	11.3++	0.73	42
F-U	1945	12.9	7.2--	0.18	
RHONE-ALPES					
F01	215	14.3	8.7	0.66	202
F07	126	12.0	6.5--	0.66	322
F26	203	13.8	8.5	0.66	218
F38	397	11.4	7.2--	0.40	296
F42	475	15.4	8.8	0.45	197
F69	775	13.2	9.0	0.35	182
F73	176	14.2	9.0	0.75	182
F74	198	11.0	8.4	0.63	227
F-V	2565	13.2	8.4--	0.18	
F.0	32679	15.2	9.4++	0.06	

UNITED KINGDOM (1976-80)

EAST ANGLIA					
G25	207	12.3	8.0	0.60	257
G46	336	16.2	8.6	0.52	209
G55	210	11.9	6.9--	0.52	307
G-A	753	13.6	7.9--	0.32	
EAST MIDLANDS					
G30	391	14.3	8.2-	0.45	241
G44	390	15.4	9.4	0.52	148
G45	229	14.2	8.4	0.61	227
G47	235	15.0	9.7	0.68	125
G50	448	15.0	9.0	0.46	182
G-B	1693	14.8	8.9	0.23	
NORTHERN					
G14	550	15.2	9.0	0.42	182
G27	233	13.4	9.6	0.66	134
G29	224	15.3	8.2	0.61	241
G33	286	15.4	9.8	0.62	116
G48	129	14.5	8.5	0.82	218
G-C	1422	14.9	9.1	0.26	
NORTH-WEST					
G11	1312	15.9	9.7	0.29	125
G12	780	16.1	9.8	0.38	116
G26	431	15.3	9.8	0.50	116
G43	717	16.8	9.4	0.40	148
G-D	3240	16.0	9.7++	0.19	

SOUTH-EAST					
G01	2771	12.7	7.0--	0.15	304
G22	159	10.8	7.5--	0.62	280
G23	206	10.2	6.8--	0.50	313
G24	174	11.2	7.4--	0.59	287
G34	361	16.9	7.5--	0.49	280
G35	558	12.7	7.6--	0.35	275
G37	566	13.1	8.1--	0.37	252
G39	324	11.2	6.9--	0.41	307
G41	59	16.3	7.3	1.17	292
G42	644	14.4	7.9--	0.35	260
G51	140	8.9	5.8--	0.52	339
G56	408	13.3	6.9--	0.37	307
G58	284	14.1	6.2--	0.44	335
G-E	6654	12.8	7.2--	0.10	
SOUTH-WEST					
G21	394	13.8	7.5--	0.42	280
G28	219	17.0	9.0	0.69	182
G31	520	17.8	8.5	0.43	218
G32	298	16.1	7.3--	0.49	292
G36	234	15.4	9.1	0.65	175
G53	218	17.2	9.6	0.72	134
G59	199	12.9	7.9-	0.60	260
G-F	2082	15.7	8.2--	0.20	
WEST MIDLANDS					
G15	1151	13.9	8.6	0.27	209
G38	251	13.6	8.4	0.57	227
G52	162	14.6	8.5	0.75	218
G54	458	15.1	10.0	0.49	99
G57	192	13.5	8.9	0.68	191
G-G	2214	14.1	8.9	0.20	
YORKSHIRE AND HUMBERSIDE					
G13	599	15.0	9.3	0.41	157
G16	1033	16.1	9.7	0.33	125
G40	413	15.8	9.8	0.52	116
G49	307	15.3	8.0-	0.51	257
G-H	2352	15.7	9.4	0.21	
WALES					
G61	195	16.5	9.8	0.78	116
G62	198	19.6	10.9+	0.86	51
G63	188	14.0	9.0	0.70	182
G64	150	21.3	10.9	1.01	51
G65	238	14.4	8.9	0.61	191
G66	63	19.9	9.7	1.32	125
G67	153	12.7	7.6-	0.67	275
G68	184	16.1	9.4	0.75	148
G-I	1369	16.0	9.4	0.28	
SCOTLAND(1975-80)					
S01	77	13.5	8.4	1.04	227
S02	168	11.8	7.1--	0.60	300
S03	167	13.3	7.4--	0.64	287
S04	162	15.6	10.2	0.87	84
S05	305	12.9	7.7--	0.48	270
S06	52	16.6	8.8	1.39	197
S07	92	11.2	7.3-	0.80	292
S08	1056	13.7	8.7	0.29	202
S09	82	18.6	9.8	1.20	116
S10	13	23.8	12.5	3.96	17
S11	6	9.8	5.1	2.29	346
S12	9	10.0	3.9--	1.54	355
G-J	2189	13.6	8.3--	0.19	
NORTHERN IRELAND					
JE	162	9.7	6.5--	0.55	322
JN	90	9.7	6.8--	0.76	313
JS	43	6.3	4.3--	0.70	354
JW	69	11.2	7.4	0.95	287
G-K	364	9.3	6.3--	0.35	
G.0	24332	14.2	8.3--	0.06	
ITALIA (1975-79)					
ABRUZZI					
I66	128	16.6	10.0	0.93	99
I67	96	14.3	8.8	0.96	197
I68	112	15.5	10.4	1.02	71
I69	150	16.2	9.6	0.83	134
I-A	486	15.7	9.7	0.46	
BASILICATA					
I76	113	10.9	7.2--	0.71	296
I77	54	10.7	8.3	1.17	236
I-B	167	10.8	7.5-	0.61	
CALABRIA					
I78	214	11.8	9.0	0.64	182
I79	212	11.5	8.6	0.63	209
I80	224	15.0	10.2	0.72	84
I-C	650	12.6	9.3	0.38	
CAMPANIA					
I61	225	12.3	10.3	0.70	78
I62	98	13.3	8.7	0.93	202
I63	1037	14.2	12.3++	0.39	19
I64	144	13.1	8.5	0.74	218
I65	342	13.5	10.2+	0.57	84
I-D	1846	13.7	11.0++	0.26	
EMILIA-ROMAGNA					
I33	130	18.0	9.0	0.85	182
I34	205	20.0	9.2	0.69	167
I35	191	18.5	10.1	0.78	92
I36	234	15.9	9.1	0.62	175
I37	495	20.4	10.5++	0.50	67
I38	148	14.9	7.9	0.68	260
I39	163	17.7	9.2	0.77	167
I40	232	15.5	9.8	0.67	116
I-E	1798	17.8	9.5	0.24	
FRIULI-VENEZIA GIULIA					
I30	246	18.1	9.5	0.65	142
I31	72	18.8	10.2	1.30	84
I32	229	28.6	12.7++	0.93	14
I93	111	16.1	9.0	0.92	182
I-F	658	20.4	10.4++	0.44	
LAZIO					
I56	117	17.6	10.1	0.98	92
I57	44	12.2	5.8--	0.94	339
I58	1334	14.1	10.2++	0.28	84
I59	124	12.0	10.3	0.94	78
I60	163	14.4	9.2	0.76	167
I-G	1782	14.1	9.9++	0.24	
LIGURIA					
I08	145	24.2	11.6+	1.04	33
I09	159	20.1	9.6	0.81	134
I10	563	19.9	9.7	0.44	125
I11	109	17.2	8.6	0.89	209
I-H	976	20.1	9.7	0.34	
LOMBARDIA					
I12	301	15.1	10.0	0.60	99
I13	290	14.8	9.4	0.57	148
I14	54	12.4	8.5	1.20	218
I15	1435	13.8	9.2	0.25	167
I16	303	13.7	9.9	0.59	108
I17	350	13.7	9.3	0.51	157
I18	318	23.5	11.6++	0.71	33
I19	157	18.3	9.3	0.80	157
I20	179	18.3	9.6	0.77	134
I-I	3387	14.9	9.5+	0.17	
MARCHE					
I41	95	11.5	6.4--	0.70	330
I42	161	14.6	7.8	0.66	265
I43	97	13.1	6.7--	0.72	317
I44	117	13.1	7.8	0.75	265
I-J	470	13.2	7.3--	0.35	
MOLISE					
I70	94	15.7	9.3	1.02	157
I94	39	16.2	9.2	1.55	167
I-K	133	15.8	9.3	0.85	
PIEMONTE					
I01	1031	16.9	10.8++	0.35	59
I02	209	19.8	10.3	0.78	78
I03	255	19.4	10.9+	0.73	51
I04	310	22.6	12.0++	0.74	25
I05	109	19.4	9.6	1.03	134
I06	272	22.0	10.1	0.69	92
I-L	2186	18.8	10.7++	0.24	
PUGLIA					
I71	226	13.2	10.4	0.72	71
I72	521	14.4	11.3++	0.51	42
I73	181	13.0	11.0+	0.84	48
I74	168	17.0	13.2++	1.04	7
I75	250	13.0	10.2	0.66	84
I-M	1346	14.0	11.0++	0.31	
SARDEGNA					
I90	94	8.8	6.3--	0.69	333
I91	46	6.7	4.9--	0.76	349
I92	194	10.9	9.4	0.70	148
I95	43	11.1	7.5	1.24	280
I-N	377	9.6	7.5--	0.40	
SICILIA					
I81	177	16.6	10.2	0.83	84
I82	489	16.4	11.8++	0.55	28
I83	372	21.4	13.5++	0.74	5
I84	207	17.4	12.6++	0.91	15
I85	99	13.5	10.0	1.03	99
I86	74	14.4	10.0	1.21	99
I87	471	18.9	14.1++	0.67	3
I88	144	21.1	14.3++	1.25	2
I89	142	14.6	11.4+	0.99	39
I-O	2175	17.6	12.4++	0.28	
TOSCANA					
I45	93	17.6	9.5	1.06	142
I46	186	18.5	9.6	0.77	134
I47	112	16.6	8.4	0.86	227
I48	483	15.6	8.5	0.41	218
I49	157	17.8	9.4	0.80	148
I50	197	20.0	10.5	0.81	67
I51	118	15.0	8.6	0.84	209
I52	109	16.7	8.1	0.83	252
I53	105	18.7	10.7	1.09	61
I-P	1560	17.0	9.1	0.25	
TRENTINO-ALTO ADIGE					
I21	149	13.7	10.0	0.85	99
I22	164	14.6	8.4	0.70	227
I-Q	313	14.2	9.1	0.54	
UMBRIA					
I54	185	12.8	7.2--	0.56	296
I55	99	17.1	9.9	1.04	108
I-R	284	14.1	8.0-	0.50	
VALLE D'AOSTA					
I07	50	17.6	11.8	1.73	28
VENETO					
I23	214	11.0	6.9--	0.49	307
I24	183	10.1	6.7--	0.51	317
I25	87	14.9	8.6	0.98	209
I26	185	10.3	6.5--	0.51	322
I27	265	12.4	8.2	0.53	241
I28	260	12.7	8.5	0.55	218
I29	93	14.4	7.5	0.84	280
I-T	1287	11.7	7.5--	0.22	
I.0	21931	15.3	9.8++	0.07	
IRELAND (1976-80)					
CONNAUGHT					
R07	27	6.6	4.9--	1.02	349
R12	10	15.4	7.4	2.49	287
R16	30	10.8	6.4-	1.37	330
R20	14	10.9	6.4	1.90	330
R21	11	8.2	5.3-	1.86	344
R-A	92	9.1	5.8--	0.68	
LEINSTER					
R01	8	8.5	5.7	2.15	342
R06	174	6.8	5.7--	0.46	342
R09	20	8.6	9.1	2.09	175
R10	12	7.2	5.0--	1.53	348
R11	15	12.6	9.9	2.72	108
R14	11	14.9	11.7	3.71	30
R15	13	6.0	4.7--	1.34	352
R17	14	6.4	5.8-	1.58	339
R19	13	9.4	7.9	2.31	260
R24	13	8.9	7.7	2.26	270
R25	21	8.9	7.6	1.77	275
R26	12	5.7	6.0	1.80	337
R-B	326	7.4	6.3--	0.36	
MUNSTER					
R03	16	7.8	5.3--	1.41	344
R04	73	7.4	5.1--	0.63	346
R08	29	10.0	7.1	1.42	300
R13	36	9.2	7.2	1.27	296
R22	29	8.9	6.6-	1.28	320
R23	19	8.8	6.3	1.55	333
R-C	202	8.4	6.0--	0.45	
ULSTER					
R02	14	11.0	7.6	2.24	275
R05	28	9.4	6.8	1.43	313
R18	12	9.9	7.0	2.25	304
R-D	54	9.9	7.0	1.06	
R.0	674	8.0	6.2--	0.25	
LUXEMBOURG (1971-80)					
LE	32	16.7	8.6	1.61	209
LN	57	21.5	11.4	1.62	39
LS	249	18.5	11.7++	0.77	30
L.0	338	18.8	11.3++	0.65	
NEDERLAND (1976-80)					
N01	144	10.5	6.9--	0.62	307
N02	173	12.1	8.1	0.67	252
N03	86	8.4	6.0--	0.67	337
N04	217	8.7	6.2--	0.44	335
N05	428	10.2	6.9--	0.35	307
N06	239	10.7	7.4--	0.51	287
N07	721	12.1	7.5--	0.30	280
N08	919	11.8	7.6--	0.27	275
N09	106	12.5	7.8	0.83	265
N10	397	8.0	6.5--	0.34	322
N11	234	8.9	6.5--	0.44	322
N.0	3664	10.5	7.1--	0.12	
EEC-9					
EEC	121617	15.2	9.1	0.03	

BELGIE-BELGIQUE (1971-78)

BRUSSEL-BRUXELLES

B21	1162	29.4	16.2++	0.49	41

VLAANDEREN

B10	1382	22.4	14.2+	0.39	134
B29	743	20.7	13.0	0.49	198
B30	1096	25.8	15.5++	0.48	73
B40	1511	28.9	15.8++	0.42	57
B70	347	12.5	12.3	0.67	231
B-V	5079	23.1	14.6++	0.21	

WALLONIE

B25	249	24.3	15.7+	1.02	61
B50	1551	30.2	17.8++	0.47	14
B60	1172	29.8	17.7++	0.53	15
B80	231	26.8	15.8+	1.06	57
B90	445	29.3	17.9++	0.87	11
B-W	3648	29.2	17.5++	0.30	
B.0	9889	25.7	15.7++	0.16	

BR DEUTSCHLAND (1976-80)

BADEN-WURTTEMBERG

D81	1909	22.9	15.6++	0.38	69
D82	1450	25.5	16.8++	0.47	30
D83	1053	23.9	15.9++	0.52	53
D84	849	23.6	16.0++	0.58	49
D-A	5261	23.9	16.0++	0.23	

BAYERN

D91	2181	25.1	15.3++	0.33	85
D92	639	27.3	16.4++	0.66	38
D93	488	21.1	14.0	0.65	143
D94	603	24.4	13.5	0.57	171
D95	901	25.1	14.5+	0.50	122
D96	705	24.7	14.8++	0.57	104
D97	949	26.2	15.0++	0.50	92
D-B	6466	25.0	14.9++	0.19	

BERLIN(WEST)

DB0	1500	35.1	16.2++	0.45	41

BREMEN

D40	577	35.1	19.6++	0.87	4

HAMBURG

D20	1279	33.0	16.3++	0.49	40

HESSEN

D64	2541	24.2	15.1++	0.32	90
D66	796	28.1	15.5++	0.59	73
D-F	3337	25.0	15.2++	0.28	

NIEDERSACHSEN

D31	1043	26.7	15.0++	0.50	92
D32	1402	28.9	15.7++	0.44	61
D33	952	27.2	15.8++	0.54	57
D34	1115	22.1	14.6++	0.46	116
D-G	4512	26.1	15.3++	0.24	

NORDRHEIN-WESTFALEN

D51	3088	25.0	18.3++	0.35	7
D53	2397	25.6	20.8++	0.45	2
D55	1189	20.5	17.9++	0.56	11
D57	1092	25.5	17.1++	0.55	22
D59	1970	22.3	16.5++	0.40	36
D-H	9736	23.9	18.3++	0.20	

RHEINLAND-PFALZ

D71	922	28.3	16.0++	0.56	49
D72	321	28.7	17.3++	1.03	19
D73	1179	27.4	17.2++	0.53	21
D-I	2422	27.9	16.7++	0.36	

SAARLAND

DA0	572	22.3	13.4	0.59	178

SCHLESWIG-HOLSTEIN

D10	1749	28.1	16.0++	0.41	49
D.0	37411	25.5	15.5++	0.08	

DANMARK (1971-80)

K15	1662	27.3	16.2++	0.41	41
K20	271	17.9	15.5+	0.96	73
K25	131	14.1	13.0	1.16	198
K30	355	26.2	13.7	0.75	157
K35	327	25.4	11.6-	0.67	269
K40	67	28.2	13.7	1.74	157
K42	648	29.3	14.8+	0.60	104
K50	285	23.3	13.9	0.85	148
K55	222	21.3	14.0	0.96	143
K60	389	24.7	13.9	0.73	148
K65	231	18.0	11.4-	0.77	272
K70	639	23.0	14.1	0.57	138
K76	281	24.6	12.4	0.77	226
K80	585	24.8	13.5	0.57	171
K.0	6093	24.3	14.2++	0.19	

FRANCE (1971-78)

ALSACE

F67	725	21.0	14.8++	0.57	104
F68	677	27.1	19.8++	0.80	3
F-A	1402	23.6	16.8++	0.47	

AQUITAINE

F24	488	33.5	14.4	0.68	124
F33	1002	24.6	13.3	0.43	184
F40	311	27.8	13.9	0.83	148
F47	341	30.0	13.7	0.77	157
F64	505	24.4	12.3	0.57	231
F-B	2647	26.8	13.4	0.27	

AUVERGNE

F03	608	41.1	18.3++	0.78	7
F15	191	28.8	13.9	1.04	148
F43	276	34.4	15.7+	0.99	61
F63	625	27.4	17.0++	0.71	25
F-C	1700	32.6	16.8++	0.42	

BASSE-NORMANDIE

F14	462	21.1	16.9++	0.81	27
F50	423	24.3	17.1++	0.88	22
F61	303	26.5	17.3++	1.04	19
F-D	1188	23.4	17.1++	0.52	

BOURGOGNE

F21	426	23.7	14.8+	0.74	104
F58	329	33.6	13.7	0.80	157
F71	610	27.2	14.1	0.60	138
F89	394	33.2	14.1	0.75	138
F-E	1759	28.4	14.1+	0.35	

BRETAGNE

F22	493	24.2	14.9+	0.71	98
F29	769	24.6	14.4+	0.54	124
F35	594	22.0	16.9++	0.72	27
F56	553	25.1	17.7++	0.78	15
F-F	2409	23.9	15.8++	0.33	

CENTRE

F18	389	31.0	14.8+	0.79	104
F28	345	25.7	14.6	0.81	116
F36	341	34.9	13.9	0.79	148
F37	521	28.1	15.8++	0.71	57
F41	359	32.4	15.2+	0.84	86
F45	439	22.6	12.8	0.63	209
F-G	2394	28.2	14.5++	0.31	

CHAMPAGNE-ARDENNE

F08	261	21.0	14.8	0.96	104
F10	332	29.6	15.9++	0.93	53
F51	371	17.6	12.3	0.66	231
F52	234	27.6	16.8++	1.13	30
F-H	1198	22.5	14.5++	0.43	

CORSE

F20	115	12.0	6.5--	0.63	347

FRANCHE-COMTE

F25	317	16.9	15.4+	0.90	81
F39	282	29.7	15.5+	0.96	73
F70	233	26.7	14.7	1.00	113
F90	99	19.4	14.4	1.50	124
F-J	931	22.1	15.1++	0.51	

HAUTE-NORMANDIE

F27	350	20.9	14.1	0.78	138
F76	824	17.9	13.6	0.49	167
F-K	1174	18.7	13.7	0.41	

ILE-DE-FRANCE

F75	2151	25.3	13.1	0.29	194
F77	566	18.8	13.4	0.58	178
F78	648	15.0	14.9++	0.60	98
F91	532	14.5	14.8+	0.66	104
F92	1076	19.1	14.6++	0.46	116
F93	837	15.8	15.2++	0.54	86
F94	814	17.1	14.0	0.50	143
F95	531	15.9	15.0++	0.67	92
F-L	7155	18.6	14.1++	0.17	

LANGUEDOC-ROUSSILLON

F11	334	32.0	11.7-	0.67	264
F30	472	24.5	12.9	0.61	203
F34	684	27.5	13.2	0.53	190
F48	85	28.3	11.9	1.34	253
F66	353	30.5	12.3	0.68	231
F-M	1928	27.9	12.6-	0.30	

LIMOUSIN

F19	326	34.7	13.7	0.78	157
F23	344	60.0	19.6++	1.12	4
F87	452	33.1	14.4	0.70	124
F-N	1122	38.9	15.4++	0.48	

LORRAINE

F54	492	17.2	13.0	0.61	198
F55	219	27.2	15.7+	1.11	61
F57	613	15.1	13.7	0.58	157
F88	343	22.1	14.3	0.80	132
F-O	1667	18.0	13.9	0.35	

MIDI-PYRENEES

F09	152	27.8	9.6--	0.82	310
F12	396	36.6	15.6++	0.81	69
F31	597	19.9	12.0--	0.51	245
F32	201	28.8	12.0	0.91	245
F46	214	36.4	15.4	1.11	81
F65	223	25.1	12.4	0.86	226
F81	405	30.6	13.7	0.72	157
F82	242	33.8	15.9+	1.07	53
F-P	2430	27.5	13.2	0.28	

NORD-PAS-DE-CALAIS

F59	1897	19.3	14.5++	0.35	122
F62	1132	20.6	15.4++	0.47	81
F-Q	3029	19.8	14.8++	0.28	

PAYS DE LA LOIRE

F44	766	21.3	15.6++	0.58	69
F49	579	23.5	15.2++	0.65	86
F53	281	27.8	19.2++	1.19	6
F72	420	21.8	13.5	0.68	171
F85	486	27.8	15.9++	0.75	53
F-R	2532	23.6	15.5++	0.32	

PICARDIE

F02	508	23.9	14.7+	0.69	113
F60	501	20.6	15.2++	0.71	86
F80	539	25.5	15.1++	0.67	90
F-S	1548	23.2	15.0++	0.40	

POITOU-CHARENTES

F16	400	30.3	15.4++	0.80	81
F17	613	31.7	15.6++	0.65	69
F79	381	28.6	14.8+	0.79	104
F86	434	30.9	15.5++	0.77	73
F-T	1828	30.5	15.4++	0.37	

PROVENCE-ALPES-COTE D'AZUR

F04	113	25.2	11.1-	1.08	284
F05	105	27.1	13.6	1.36	167
F06	615	20.0	7.3--	0.31	339
F13	1188	18.6	11.6--	0.35	269
F83	643	26.1	13.2	0.54	190
F84	350	22.6	12.5	0.69	222
F-U	3014	21.1	10.8--	0.20	

RHONE-ALPES

F01	376	24.9	14.6	0.77	116
F07	322	32.1	14.9	0.86	98
F26	321	22.8	12.8	0.75	209
F38	664	19.4	14.4	0.57	124
F42	755	25.8	16.6++	0.63	34
F69	1032	18.4	14.4+	0.46	124
F73	290	23.8	16.1++	0.98	45
F74	304	16.9	13.3	0.79	184
F-V	4064	21.5	14.7++	0.24	
F.0	47234	22.9	14.2++	0.07	

UNITED KINGDOM (1976-80)

EAST ANGLIA

G25	330	19.2	13.4	0.76	178
G46	521	26.2	13.6	0.62	167
G55	360	20.3	12.1	0.66	242
G-A	1211	22.1	13.1	0.39	

EAST MIDLANDS

G30	456	17.3	10.5--	0.51	293
G44	398	16.2	10.7--	0.55	290
G45	343	21.8	13.2	0.74	190
G47	276	18.1	12.3	0.77	231
G50	562	19.6	12.8	0.56	209
G-B	2035	18.4	11.8--	0.27	

NORTHERN

G14	528	15.6	10.2--	0.46	300
G27	187	11.2	8.7--	0.65	326
G29	324	23.6	13.5	0.78	171
G33	271	15.2	9.8--	0.61	306
G48	141	16.5	9.7--	0.85	308
G-C	1451	16.0	10.4--	0.28	

NORTH-WEST

G11	1355	17.5	12.1--	0.35	242
G12	756	16.9	11.8--	0.45	258
G26	437	16.2	12.0-	0.60	245
G43	794	20.2	11.3--	0.41	276
G-D	3342	17.7	11.8--	0.21	

SOUTH-EAST					
G01	3915	19.6	11.6--	0.19	269
G22	255	17.1	13.7	0.89	157
G23	347	17.3	13.2	0.73	190
G24	267	17.0	12.8	0.80	209
G34	705	39.6	14.6+	0.58	116
G35	831	19.8	12.8	0.46	209
G37	922	21.0	14.9++	0.51	98
G39	511	18.4	14.2	0.66	134
G41	92	28.5	10.8-	1.18	287
G42	977	23.2	13.6	0.45	167
G51	312	18.7	15.7+	0.98	61
G56	574	19.7	12.6	0.55	219
G58	581	32.7	14.7+	0.64	113
G-E	10289	21.0	12.8--	0.13	
SOUTH-WEST					
G21	600	22.5	13.5	0.57	171
G28	329	27.5	14.0	0.81	143
G31	771	28.0	13.1	0.49	194
G32	545	32.9	13.8	0.61	153
G36	284	19.6	12.0	0.73	245
G53	386	32.0	16.5++	0.86	36
G59	296	19.1	13.3	0.80	184
G-F	3211	25.7	13.6	0.25	
WEST MIDLANDS					
G15	1336	16.6	11.9--	0.34	253
G38	316	17.6	11.3--	0.66	276
G52	208	19.4	12.8	0.93	209
G54	437	14.8	10.8--	0.54	287
G57	223	16.1	12.4	0.88	226
G-G	2520	16.5	11.7--	0.24	
YORKSHIRE AND HUMBERSIDE					
G13	633	16.5	10.5--	0.43	293
G16	1055	17.5	11.1--	0.35	284
G40	468	19.0	12.3	0.59	231
G49	453	23.3	13.3	0.65	184
G-H	2609	18.3	11.5--	0.23	
WALES					
G61	227	20.5	11.7	0.81	264
G62	201	21.4	11.7	0.85	264
G63	231	18.0	11.3--	0.76	276
G64	167	25.5	13.8	1.12	153
G65	220	14.0	9.6--	0.66	310
G66	74	23.3	12.2	1.49	238
G67	227	20.3	13.0	0.89	198
G68	171	16.2	10.0--	0.81	303
G-I	1518	18.8	11.5--	0.30	
SCOTLAND(1975-80)					
S01	114	20.5	12.9	1.24	203
S02	274	20.5	12.5	0.78	222
S03	226	19.5	12.2	0.84	238
S04	189	19.0	12.6	0.95	219
S05	383	17.8	12.7	0.68	215
S06	73	25.4	12.9	1.55	203
S07	109	13.6	9.3--	0.93	317
S08	1003	14.2	10.6--	0.35	292
S09	90	21.5	12.5	1.38	222
S10	9	16.9	8.9	3.05	322
S11	9	14.4	9.4	3.23	316
S12	25	28.5	12.9	2.74	203
G-J	2504	16.7	11.5--	0.24	
NORTHERN IRELAND					
JE	293	17.8	14.3	0.90	132
JN	138	15.3	13.4	1.23	178
JS	81	12.2	10.4-	1.24	297
JW	111	18.5	14.6	1.49	116
G-K	623	16.3	13.5	0.58	
G.0	31313	19.3	12.2--	0.07	

ITALIA (1975-79)

ABRUZZI					
I66	118	16.1	8.5--	0.80	329
I67	106	16.0	9.6--	0.95	310
I68	98	14.1	9.0--	0.93	320
I69	135	15.1	8.7--	0.76	326
I-A	457	15.3	8.9--	0.42	
BASILICATA					
I76	111	10.8	6.7--	0.65	345
I77	65	12.9	9.9--	1.25	304
I-B	176	11.5	7.6--	0.59	
CALABRIA					
I78	144	8.1	6.0--	0.51	353
I79	177	9.7	7.2--	0.56	341
I80	197	13.5	8.0--	0.58	332
I-C	518	10.2	7.1--	0.32	
CAMPANIA					
I61	135	7.6	6.6--	0.58	346
I62	124	17.2	9.9--	0.91	304
I63	597	8.5	8.9--	0.37	322
I64	119	11.0	6.8--	0.64	344
I65	212	8.6	6.4--	0.44	348
I-D	1187	9.1	7.9--	0.23	
EMILIA-ROMAGNA					
I33	177	25.4	12.2	0.94	238
I34	225	23.1	11.7-	0.79	264
I35	259	26.1	16.1++	1.06	45
I36	228	16.1	10.2--	0.70	300
I37	453	20.0	11.8-	0.57	258
I38	185	19.7	11.3-	0.84	276
I39	206	23.4	12.3	0.88	231
I40	259	17.9	12.0	0.76	245
I-E	1992	20.7	12.0--	0.28	
FRIULI-VENEZIA GIULIA					
I30	236	18.4	10.7--	0.71	290
I31	95	27.0	17.6+	1.93	17
I32	217	31.1	14.9	1.07	98
I93	135	20.7	12.7	1.11	215
I-F	683	22.9	12.9	0.50	
LAZIO					
I56	138	21.1	11.9	1.03	253
I57	70	19.6	9.1--	1.13	318
I58	1250	14.1	13.4	0.40	178
I59	84	8.1	7.5--	0.84	337
I60	135	12.1	7.6--	0.67	336
I-G	1677	13.9	11.8--	0.30	
LIGURIA					
I08	162	29.2	13.8	1.13	153
I09	159	21.5	11.2-	0.92	282
I10	689	26.7	13.4	0.52	178
I11	147	24.8	12.5	1.06	222
I-H	1157	25.9	13.0	0.39	
LOMBARDIA					
I12	308	16.4	15.0	0.93	92
I13	315	17.2	14.4	0.87	124
I14	71	16.5	11.8	1.43	258
I15	1523	15.6	14.2+	0.39	134
I16	277	12.9	12.7	0.79	215
I17	343	14.0	12.7	0.71	215
I18	358	28.2	13.3	0.72	184
I19	128	15.8	9.5--	0.87	314
I20	172	18.6	10.3--	0.80	299
I-I	3495	16.3	13.3	0.23	
MARCHE					
I41	150	18.5	10.9-	0.91	286
I42	221	21.4	12.9	0.89	203
I43	136	19.2	10.8--	0.95	287
I44	115	13.5	8.8--	0.84	324
I-J	622	18.3	11.0--	0.45	
MOLISE					
I70	98	17.0	9.5--	0.99	314
I94	34	14.7	7.3--	1.28	339
I-K	132	16.3	8.9--	0.79	
PIEMONTE					
I01	1094	18.8	15.5++	0.50	73
I02	255	26.3	12.6	0.81	219
I03	274	22.3	13.7	0.86	157
I04	349	25.7	13.1	0.73	194
I05	186	34.6	13.7	1.04	157
I06	342	29.4	11.9-	0.69	253
I-L	2500	22.6	13.8	0.29	
PUGLIA					
I71	188	11.2	7.9--	0.59	333
I72	400	11.4	8.7--	0.44	326
I73	122	8.9	7.9--	0.72	333
I74	91	9.6	7.7--	0.82	335
I75	219	12.1	8.8--	0.60	324
I-M	1020	10.9	8.3--	0.26	
SARDEGNA					
I90	151	14.4	9.0--	0.76	320
I91	77	11.3	6.1--	0.74	352
I92	152	8.6	7.2--	0.59	341
I95	43	11.1	5.0--	0.83	355
I-N	423	10.9	7.2--	0.36	
SICILIA					
I81	116	11.2	6.4--	0.61	348
I82	328	11.4	7.5--	0.42	337
I83	196	12.0	7.1--	0.52	343
I84	124	10.4	6.2--	0.58	350
I85	69	9.5	6.2--	0.76	350
I86	46	9.1	5.1--	0.77	354
I87	294	12.1	8.5--	0.50	329
I88	115	17.5	10.5--	1.00	293
I89	114	11.8	8.4--	0.80	331
I-O	1402	11.7	7.4--	0.20	
TOSCANA					
I45	94	18.9	10.5-	1.11	293
I46	174	18.7	9.7--	0.76	308
I47	159	24.9	13.1	1.07	194
I48	644	22.4	11.9--	0.48	253
I49	174	20.7	12.2	0.95	238
I50	213	22.7	11.4-	0.80	272
I51	153	19.9	10.1--	0.84	302
I52	135	21.3	9.6--	0.84	310
I53	100	18.1	9.1--	0.93	318
I-P	1846	21.3	11.1--	0.26	
TRENTINO-ALTO ADIGE					
I21	185	17.6	14.2	1.08	134
I22	188	17.5	11.3-	0.85	276
I-Q	373	17.5	12.5	0.67	
UMBRIA					
I54	298	21.2	11.8-	0.69	258
I55	127	22.7	12.4	1.11	226
I-R	425	21.6	11.9-	0.59	
VALLE D'AOSTA					
I07	58	20.4	14.4	1.95	124
VENETO					
I23	351	18.9	13.5	0.74	171
I24	233	13.4	11.3--	0.76	276
I25	94	17.4	10.4--	1.09	297
I26	274	16.0	12.0	0.75	245
I27	292	14.3	11.4--	0.68	272
I28	238	12.2	9.8--	0.65	306
I29	112	18.1	11.2	1.08	282
I-T	1594	15.2	11.5--	0.30	
I.0	21737	15.8	10.8--	0.07	

IRELAND (1976-80)

CONNAUGHT					
R07	96	22.2	12.4	1.31	226
R12	20	26.9	11.8	2.75	258
R16	100	34.2	15.0	1.56	92
R20	52	36.5	17.9	2.61	11
R21	44	31.6	16.2	2.55	41
R-A	312	28.9	14.4	0.85	
LEINSTER					
R01	20	20.3	16.7	3.89	32
R06	305	12.9	14.0	0.83	143
R09	28	11.1	12.0	2.32	245
R10	31	17.4	11.7	2.15	264
R11	21	16.0	11.8	2.68	258
R14	33	41.1	22.8+	4.06	1
R15	36	16.7	15.5	2.64	73
R17	35	15.0	13.5	2.34	171
R19	37	24.8	16.4	2.77	38
R24	32	20.9	13.8	2.49	153
R25	57	23.3	15.0	2.06	92
R26	39	18.6	16.1	2.67	45
R-B	674	15.6	14.3	0.57	
MUNSTER					
R03	63	28.7	17.6	2.29	17
R04	225	22.6	17.1++	1.18	22
R08	70	22.5	12.0	1.46	245
R13	77	19.4	15.7	1.84	61
R22	74	21.5	14.1	1.69	138
R23	34	15.5	12.1	2.12	242
R-C	543	21.8	15.3++	0.68	
ULSTER					
R02	48	33.9	17.0	2.53	25
R05	74	23.6	11.4	1.36	272
R18	27	20.6	13.3	2.64	184
R-D	149	25.4	13.1	1.10	
R.0	1678	19.8	14.6++	0.37	

LUXEMBOURG (1971-80)

LE	61	33.6	18.3+	2.44	7
LN	73	27.6	14.8	1.83	104
LS	281	22.0	15.7+	0.98	61
L.0	415	24.1	15.9++	0.81	

NEDERLAND (1976-80)

N01	427	31.3	18.0++	0.90	10
N02	421	29.5	16.7++	0.85	32
N03	217	20.9	12.9	0.91	203
N04	548	21.8	15.7++	0.69	61
N05	922	22.2	15.5++	0.52	73
N06	482	22.3	16.9++	0.79	27
N07	1364	23.6	16.0++	0.44	49
N08	1876	24.9	16.6++	0.39	34
N09	271	31.9	16.1++	1.02	45
N10	812	16.0	14.9++	0.54	98
N11	391	14.7	13.0	0.67	198
N.0	7731	22.4	15.8++	0.18	

EEC-9

EEC	163501	21.5	13.3	0.03	

BELGIE-BELGIQUE (1971-78)

BRUSSEL-BRUXELLES					
B21	17	0.4	0.4--	0.09	302
VLAANDEREN					
B10	18	0.3	0.2--	0.06	340
B29	17	0.5	0.4--	0.10	302
B30	14	0.3	0.3--	0.07	329
B40	14	0.3	0.2--	0.06	340
B70	15	0.5	0.5--	0.14	277
B-V	78	0.4	0.3--	0.03	
WALLONIE					
B25	5	0.5	0.4-	0.20	302
B50	30	0.6	0.5--	0.10	277
B60	31	0.8	0.7	0.13	205
B80	10	1.2	1.1	0.36	80
B90	6	0.4	0.4--	0.15	302
B-W	82	0.7	0.6--	0.07	
B.0	177	0.5	0.4--	0.03	

BR DEUTSCHLAND (1976-80)

BADEN-WURTTEMBERG					
D81	81	1.0	0.8	0.10	171
D82	74	1.3	1.1	0.13	80
D83	41	0.9	0.8	0.13	171
D84	39	1.1	0.9	0.15	128
D-A	235	1.1	0.9	0.06	
BAYERN					
D91	99	1.1	0.9	0.09	128
D92	19	0.8	0.7	0.17	205
D93	27	1.2	1.0	0.20	101
D94	40	1.6	1.5+	0.24	25
D95	45	1.3	1.1	0.17	80
D96	35	1.2	1.0	0.18	101
D97	36	1.0	0.9	0.16	128
D-B	301	1.2	1.0+	0.06	
BERLIN(WEST)					
DB0	61	1.4	1.1	0.15	80
BREMEN					
D40	20	1.2	1.0	0.23	101
HAMBURG					
D20	61	1.6	1.3+	0.17	44
HESSEN					
D64	150	1.4	1.2++	0.10	58
D66	36	1.3	1.2	0.20	58
D-F	186	1.4	1.2++	0.09	
NIEDERSACHSEN					
D31	64	1.6	1.3+	0.17	44
D32	67	1.4	1.2	0.15	58
D33	43	1.2	1.2	0.18	58
D34	105	2.1	1.9++	0.19	6
D-G	279	1.6	1.4++	0.09	
NORDRHEIN-WESTFALEN					
D51	199	1.6	1.4++	0.11	33
D53	132	1.4	1.2++	0.11	58
D55	79	1.4	1.3++	0.15	44
D57	81	1.9	1.9++	0.21	6
D59	128	1.4	1.4++	0.13	33
D-H	619	1.5	1.4++	0.06	
RHEINLAND-PFALZ					
D71	44	1.4	1.2	0.18	58
D72	19	1.7	1.6	0.38	17
D73	56	1.3	1.1	0.16	80
D-I	119	1.4	1.2++	0.11	
SAARLAND					
DA0	31	1.2	1.0	0.19	101
SCHLESWIG-HOLSTEIN					
D10	89	1.4	1.2+	0.13	58
D.0	2001	1.4	1.2++	0.03	

DANMARK (1971-80)

K15	132	2.2	1.9++	0.17	6
K20	24	1.6	1.4	0.30	33
K25	13	1.4	1.2	0.34	58
K30	16	1.2	1.1	0.29	80
K35	25	1.9	1.6+	0.34	17
K40	2	0.8	1.0	0.67	101
K42	43	1.9	1.8++	0.28	10
K50	14	1.1	1.1	0.30	80
K55	19	1.8	1.8+	0.41	10
K60	31	2.0	1.8++	0.33	10
K65	26	2.0	1.9++	0.38	6
K70	62	2.2	2.0++	0.25	5
K76	25	2.2	2.1++	0.43	4
K80	39	1.7	1.6++	0.26	17
K.0	471	1.9	1.7++	0.08	

FRANCE (1971-78)

ALSACE					
F67	28	0.8	0.7	0.14	205
F68	24	1.0	0.8	0.17	171
F-A	52	0.9	0.8	0.11	
AQUITAINE					
F24	10	0.7	0.6	0.21	251
F33	38	0.9	0.8	0.14	171
F40	4	0.4	0.3--	0.17	329
F47	12	1.1	1.0	0.30	101
F64	8	0.4	0.4--	0.13	302
F-B	72	0.7	0.7--	0.08	
AUVERGNE					
F03	13	0.9	0.8	0.23	171
F15	11	1.7	1.5	0.46	25
F43	11	1.4	1.3	0.41	44
F63	14	0.6	0.6	0.17	251
F-C	49	0.9	0.9	0.13	
BASSE-NORMANDIE					
F14	35	1.6	1.6+	0.27	17
F50	16	0.9	0.8	0.20	171
F61	13	1.1	1.1	0.30	80
F-D	64	1.3	1.2	0.15	
BOURGOGNE					
F21	18	1.0	0.9	0.21	128
F58	9	0.9	0.9	0.30	128
F71	24	1.1	1.0	0.20	101
F89	17	1.4	1.3	0.32	44
F-E	68	1.1	1.0	0.12	
BRETAGNE					
F22	26	1.3	1.3	0.26	44
F29	49	1.6	1.6++	0.22	17
F35	25	0.9	0.9	0.18	128
F56	21	1.0	0.9	0.20	128
F-F	121	1.2	1.2++	0.11	
CENTRE					
F18	7	0.6	0.4--	0.15	302
F28	8	0.6	0.6	0.20	251
F36	12	1.2	0.9	0.27	128
F37	14	0.8	0.7	0.19	205
F41	11	1.0	0.9	0.28	128
F45	16	0.8	0.8	0.20	171
F-G	68	0.8	0.7-	0.09	
CHAMPAGNE-ARDENNE					
F08	4	0.3	0.3--	0.15	329
F10	11	1.0	0.9	0.27	128
F51	16	0.8	0.7	0.18	205
F52	7	0.8	0.7	0.28	205
F-H	38	0.7	0.7-	0.11	
CORSE					
F20	7	0.7	0.4-	0.18	302
FRANCHE-COMTE					
F25	15	0.8	0.7	0.19	205
F39	9	0.9	0.7	0.24	205
F70	8	0.9	0.9	0.34	128
F90	5	1.0	0.8	0.37	171
F-J	37	0.9	0.8	0.13	
HAUTE-NORMANDIE					
F27	24	1.4	1.3	0.27	44
F76	43	0.9	0.9	0.13	128
F-K	67	1.1	1.0	0.12	
ILE-DE-FRANCE					
F75	112	1.3	1.0	0.10	101
F77	19	0.6	0.5--	0.12	277
F78	43	1.0	0.9	0.15	128
F91	26	0.7	0.7	0.13	205
F92	48	0.9	0.7	0.11	205
F93	51	1.0	0.9	0.14	128
F94	41	0.9	0.8	0.12	171
F95	25	0.7	0.7	0.14	205
F-L	365	0.9	0.8	0.04	
LANGUEDOC-ROUSSILLON					
F11	2	0.2	0.2--	0.17	340
F30	6	0.3	0.3--	0.12	329
F34	14	0.6	0.5--	0.13	277
F48	5	1.7	1.6	0.75	17
F66	6	0.5	0.7	0.29	205
F-M	33	0.5	0.4--	0.08	
LIMOUSIN					
F19	7	0.7	0.6	0.24	251
F23	9	1.6	1.0	0.41	101
F87	13	1.0	0.8	0.22	171
F-N	29	1.0	0.8	0.15	
LORRAINE					
F54	34	1.2	1.1	0.19	80
F55	13	1.6	1.5	0.42	25
F57	29	0.7	0.7	0.13	205
F88	19	1.2	1.2	0.28	58
F-O	95	1.0	0.9	0.10	
MIDI-PYRENEES					
F09	0	0.0	0.0--	0.00	347
F12	10	0.9	1.0	0.32	101
F31	21	0.7	0.6	0.14	251
F32	7	1.0	0.7	0.31	205
F46	5	0.8	0.9	0.40	128
F65	9	1.0	0.8	0.27	171
F81	9	0.7	0.6	0.22	251
F82	10	1.4	1.5	0.50	25
F-P	71	0.8	0.7	0.09	
NORD-PAS-DE-CALAIS					
F59	94	1.0	0.9	0.09	128
F62	39	0.7	0.7-	0.11	205
F-Q	133	0.9	0.8	0.07	
PAYS DE LA LOIRE					
F44	28	0.8	0.7	0.14	205
F49	26	1.1	1.0	0.20	101
F53	9	0.9	0.7	0.24	205
F72	20	1.0	1.1	0.24	80
F85	8	0.5	0.4--	0.15	302
F-R	91	0.8	0.8	0.08	
PICARDIE					
F02	23	1.1	1.0	0.22	101
F60	29	1.2	1.1	0.20	80
F80	17	0.8	0.7	0.17	205
F-S	69	1.0	0.9	0.11	
POITOU-CHARENTES					
F16	13	1.0	0.9	0.25	128
F17	15	0.8	0.7	0.20	205
F79	11	0.8	0.6	0.19	251
F86	15	1.1	0.9	0.25	128
F-T	54	0.9	0.8	0.11	
PROVENCE-ALPES-COTE D'AZUR					
F04	6	1.3	1.0	0.43	101
F05	2	0.5	0.6	0.43	251
F06	14	0.5	0.3--	0.09	329
F13	44	0.7	0.6--	0.09	251
F83	22	0.9	0.8	0.18	171
F84	12	0.8	0.6	0.19	251
F-U	100	0.7	0.6--	0.06	
RHONE-ALPES					
F01	14	0.9	0.8	0.24	171
F07	3	0.3	0.3--	0.15	329
F26	9	0.6	0.5	0.19	277
F38	17	0.5	0.5--	0.11	277
F42	17	0.6	0.5--	0.13	277
F69	43	0.8	0.7-	0.10	205
F73	8	0.7	0.6	0.21	251
F74	24	1.3	1.2	0.24	58
F-V	135	0.7	0.6--	0.06	
F.0	1818	0.9	0.8--	0.02	

UNITED KINGDOM (1976-80)

EAST ANGLIA					
G25	15	0.9	0.8	0.20	171
G46	27	1.4	1.2	0.23	58
G55	25	1.4	1.4	0.28	33
G-A	67	1.2	1.1	0.14	
EAST MIDLANDS					
G30	29	1.1	1.0	0.19	101
G44	25	1.0	1.0	0.19	101
G45	21	1.3	1.2	0.27	58
G47	11	0.7	0.7	0.23	205
G50	28	1.0	0.9	0.18	128
G-B	114	1.0	1.0	0.09	
NORTHERN					
G14	24	0.7	0.7	0.14	205
G27	16	1.0	0.9	0.22	128
G29	12	0.9	0.8	0.25	171
G33	17	1.0	0.9	0.21	128
G48	10	1.2	1.0	0.33	101
G-C	79	0.9	0.8	0.09	
NORTH-WEST					
G11	82	1.1	1.0	0.11	101
G12	40	0.9	0.8	0.13	171
G26	24	0.9	0.9	0.18	128
G43	31	0.8	0.8	0.14	171
G-D	177	0.9	0.9	0.07	

SOUTH-EAST					
G01	179	0.9	0.8	0.06	171
G22	19	1.3	1.2	0.27	58
G23	16	0.8	0.7	0.18	205
G24	18	1.1	1.1	0.25	80
G34	8	0.4	0.4--	0.14	302
G35	43	1.0	1.0	0.15	101
G37	43	1.0	0.9	0.14	128
G39	21	0.8	0.7	0.16	205
G41	1	0.3	0.3	0.34	329
G42	30	0.7	0.7	0.12	205
G51	15	0.9	0.8	0.22	171
G56	29	1.0	0.9	0.17	128
G58	30	1.7	1.5+	0.29	25
G-E	452	0.9	0.8	0.04	
SOUTH-WEST					
G21	25	0.9	0.9	0.19	128
G28	17	1.4	1.3	0.32	44
G31	35	1.3	1.1	0.20	80
G32	22	1.3	1.2	0.26	58
G36	14	1.0	0.8	0.23	171
G53	9	0.7	0.7	0.23	205
G59	15	1.0	0.9	0.24	128
G-F	137	1.1	1.0	0.09	
WEST MIDLANDS					
G15	97	1.2	1.2+	0.12	58
G38	13	0.7	0.7	0.18	205
G52	13	1.2	1.1	0.32	80
G54	22	0.7	0.7	0.15	205
G57	11	0.8	0.7	0.21	205
G-G	156	1.0	1.0	0.08	
YORKSHIRE AND HUMBERSIDE					
G13	44	1.1	1.1	0.16	80
G16	58	1.0	0.9	0.12	128
G40	24	1.0	0.9	0.20	128
G49	21	1.1	1.1	0.24	80
G-H	147	1.0	1.0	0.08	
WALES					
G61	10	0.9	0.9	0.28	128
G62	8	0.9	0.9	0.31	128
G63	10	0.8	0.7	0.24	205
G64	4	0.6	0.7	0.33	205
G65	18	1.1	1.1	0.26	80
G66	3	0.9	1.0	0.59	101
G67	14	1.2	1.2	0.32	58
G68	13	1.2	1.2	0.34	58
G-I	80	1.0	1.0	0.11	
SCOTLAND(1975-80)					
S01	5	0.9	0.8	0.37	171
S02	21	1.6	1.6	0.34	17
S03	18	1.6	1.4	0.34	33
S04	15	1.5	1.4	0.36	33
S05	21	1.0	0.9	0.20	128
S06	3	1.0	0.9	0.53	128
S07	8	1.0	0.9	0.33	128
S08	70	1.0	1.0	0.12	101
S09	6	1.4	1.4	0.60	33
S10	2	3.8	3.9	2.76	1
S11	0	0.0	0.0--	0.00	347
S12	1	1.1	1.3	1.32	44
G-J	170	1.1	1.1+	0.08	
NORTHERN IRELAND					
JE	12	0.7	0.7	0.21	205
JN	6	0.7	0.6	0.25	251
JS	4	0.6	0.7	0.34	205
JW	3	0.5	0.5	0.26	277
G-K	25	0.7	0.7	0.13	
G.0	1604	1.0	0.9	0.02	
ITALIA (1975-79)					
ABRUZZI					
I66	7	1.0	0.7	0.27	205
I67	6	0.9	0.7	0.28	205
I68	8	1.2	1.0	0.38	101
I69	7	0.8	0.7	0.27	205
I-A	28	0.9	0.8	0.15	
BASILICATA					
I76	5	0.5	0.5	0.22	277
I77	3	0.6	0.6	0.33	251
I-B	8	0.5	0.5-	0.18	
CALABRIA					
I78	9	0.5	0.5-	0.16	277
I79	6	0.3	0.3--	0.12	329
I80	8	0.5	0.5-	0.17	277
I-C	23	0.5	0.4--	0.09	
CAMPANIA					
I61	7	0.4	0.4--	0.15	302
I62	6	0.8	0.7	0.29	205
I63	32	0.5	0.5--	0.08	277
I64	6	0.6	0.4-	0.19	302
I65	21	0.9	0.8	0.17	171
I-D	72	0.6	0.5--	0.06	
EMILIA-ROMAGNA					
I33	7	1.0	1.0	0.38	101
I34	9	0.9	0.9	0.32	128
I35	7	0.7	0.5	0.22	277
I36	14	1.0	0.9	0.26	128
I37	21	0.9	0.8	0.18	171
I38	6	0.6	0.5	0.23	277
I39	6	0.7	0.6	0.24	251
I40	16	1.1	0.9	0.23	128
I-E	86	0.9	0.8	0.09	
FRIULI-VENEZIA GIULIA					
I30	13	1.0	0.8	0.23	171
I31	6	1.7	1.2	0.51	58
I32	13	1.9	1.4	0.42	33
I93	10	1.5	1.3	0.43	44
I-F	42	1.4	1.1	0.18	
LAZIO					
I56	6	0.9	0.6	0.29	251
I57	6	1.7	1.0	0.45	101
I58	68	0.8	0.7-	0.09	205
I59	5	0.5	0.5-	0.21	277
I60	10	0.9	0.7	0.24	205
I-G	95	0.8	0.7--	0.07	
LIGURIA					
I08	5	0.9	0.7	0.35	205
I09	3	0.4	0.2--	0.10	340
I10	35	1.4	1.1	0.19	80
I11	5	0.8	0.9	0.42	128
I-H	48	1.1	0.9	0.13	
LOMBARDIA					
I12	8	0.4	0.4--	0.14	302
I13	18	1.0	0.9	0.21	128
I14	3	0.7	0.7	0.44	205
I15	118	1.2	1.0	0.10	101
I16	19	0.9	0.8	0.19	171
I17	31	1.3	1.2	0.22	58
I18	16	1.3	1.0	0.28	101
I19	5	0.6	0.5	0.22	277
I20	9	1.0	0.6	0.21	251
I-I	227	1.1	0.9	0.06	
MARCHE					
I41	13	1.6	1.2	0.35	58
I42	19	1.8	1.6	0.38	17
I43	5	0.7	0.5	0.22	277
I44	3	0.4	0.3--	0.20	329
I-J	40	1.2	1.0	0.16	
MOLISE					
I70	4	0.7	0.5	0.25	277
I94	2	0.9	0.7	0.50	205
I-K	6	0.7	0.5	0.23	
PIEMONTE					
I01	56	1.0	0.9	0.12	128
I02	7	0.7	0.5	0.21	277
I03	9	0.7	0.7	0.23	205
I04	23	1.7	1.4	0.30	33
I05	9	1.7	1.3	0.50	44
I06	19	1.6	1.3	0.31	44
I-L	123	1.1	0.9	0.09	
PUGLIA					
I71	7	0.4	0.4--	0.14	302
I72	24	0.7	0.6	0.13	251
I73	5	0.4	0.4--	0.16	302
I74	4	0.4	0.4-	0.22	302
I75	11	0.6	0.5-	0.16	277
I-M	51	0.5	0.5--	0.07	
SARDEGNA					
I90	6	0.6	0.5-	0.20	277
I91	4	0.6	0.4--	0.19	302
I92	10	0.6	0.5-	0.17	277
I95	2	0.5	0.4	0.31	302
I-N	22	0.6	0.5--	0.10	
SICILIA					
I81	5	0.5	0.3--	0.16	329
I82	13	0.5	0.4--	0.12	302
I83	13	0.8	0.6	0.18	251
I84	8	0.7	0.6	0.22	251
I85	0	0.0	0.0--	0.00	347
I86	2	0.4	0.4	0.28	302
I87	13	0.5	0.5--	0.13	277
I88	1	0.2	0.1--	0.07	345
I89	1	0.1	0.1--	0.10	345
I-O	56	0.5	0.4--	0.05	
TOSCANA					
I45	5	1.0	0.6	0.29	251
I46	19	2.0	1.5	0.36	25
I47	11	1.7	1.4	0.44	33
I48	32	1.1	0.8	0.15	171
I49	11	1.3	1.2	0.36	58
I50	12	1.3	1.1	0.33	80
I51	6	0.8	0.6	0.28	251
I52	4	0.6	0.4-	0.23	302
I53	3	0.5	0.4	0.25	302
I-P	103	1.2	0.9	0.09	
TRENTINO-ALTO ADIGE					
I21	8	0.8	0.7	0.24	205
I22	11	1.0	0.8	0.26	171
I-Q	19	0.9	0.7	0.18	
UMBRIA					
I54	7	0.5	0.4--	0.16	302
I55	4	0.7	0.6	0.29	251
I-R	11	0.6	0.5--	0.14	
VALLE D'AOSTA					
I07	1	0.4	0.3-	0.28	329
VENETO					
I23	25	1.3	1.1	0.23	80
I24	10	0.6	0.5-	0.17	277
I25	9	1.7	1.4	0.49	33
I26	11	0.6	0.6	0.18	251
I27	23	1.1	1.0	0.22	101
I28	19	1.0	0.8	0.19	171
I29	3	0.5	0.4-	0.23	302
I-T	100	1.0	0.8	0.08	
I.0	1161	0.8	0.7--	0.02	
IRELAND (1976-80)					
CONNAUGHT					
R07	1	0.2	0.2--	0.15	340
R12	1	1.3	1.8	1.82	10
R16	1	0.3	0.4	0.42	302
R20	2	1.4	1.8	1.25	10
R21	3	2.2	1.8	1.09	10
R-A	8	0.7	0.7	0.27	
LEINSTER					
R01	0	0.0	0.0--	0.00	347
R06	21	0.9	0.9	0.19	128
R09	1	0.4	0.4	0.40	302
R10	1	0.6	0.4	0.41	302
R11	4	3.1	2.3	1.18	2
R14	0	0.0	0.0--	0.00	347
R15	1	0.5	0.5	0.49	277
R17	3	1.3	1.3	0.76	44
R19	1	0.7	0.9	0.87	128
R24	0	0.0	0.0--	0.00	347
R25	4	1.6	1.7	0.84	16
R26	0	0.0	0.0--	0.00	347
R-B	36	0.8	0.8	0.14	
MUNSTER					
R03	3	1.4	1.2	0.73	58
R04	7	0.7	0.7	0.27	205
R08	3	1.0	0.9	0.55	128
R13	6	1.5	1.5	0.63	25
R22	5	1.5	1.5	0.68	25
R23	2	0.9	0.8	0.59	171
R-C	26	1.0	1.0	0.20	
ULSTER					
R02	2	1.4	1.3	0.90	44
R05	3	1.0	0.7	0.46	205
R18	0	0.0	0.0--	0.00	347
R-D	5	0.9	0.7	0.33	
R.0	75	0.9	0.9	0.10	
LUXEMBOURG (1971-80)					
LE	0	0.0	0.0--	0.00	347
LN	6	2.3	2.3	0.94	2
LS	12	0.9	0.8	0.24	171
L.0	18	1.0	0.9	0.23	
NEDERLAND (1976-80)					
N01	15	1.1	1.0	0.27	101
N02	14	1.0	0.9	0.26	128
N03	8	0.8	0.6	0.23	251
N04	23	0.9	0.8	0.17	171
N05	49	1.2	1.1	0.16	80
N06	20	0.9	0.8	0.18	171
N07	55	1.0	0.8	0.11	171
N08	56	0.7	0.6--	0.09	251
N09	7	0.8	0.8	0.30	171
N10	34	0.7	0.6--	0.10	251
N11	12	0.5	0.4--	0.12	302
N.0	293	0.8	0.8--	0.04	
EEC-9					
EEC	7618	1.0	0.9	0.01	

BELGIE-BELGIQUE (1971-78)

BRUSSEL-BRUXELLES					
B21	607	15.4	9.0++	0.38	30
VLAANDEREN					
B10	812	13.2	8.8++	0.32	34
B29	350	9.7	6.5	0.36	181
B30	399	9.4	6.1--	0.32	214
B40	601	11.5	7.0	0.30	144
B70	230	8.3	8.3+	0.55	56
B-V	2392	10.9	7.3	0.15	
WALLONIE					
B25	111	10.8	7.2	0.69	130
B50	665	13.0	8.4++	0.34	53
B60	578	14.7	9.3++	0.40	23
B80	70	8.1	4.9--	0.60	293
B90	136	9.0	6.1	0.54	214
B-W	1560	12.5	8.1++	0.21	
B.0	4559	11.9	7.8++	0.12	

BR DEUTSCHLAND (1976-80)

BADEN-WURTTEMBERG					
D81	656	7.9	5.6--	0.23	254
D82	504	8.9	6.0--	0.28	225
D83	283	6.4	4.5--	0.28	314
D84	274	7.6	5.4--	0.35	269
D-A	1717	7.8	5.5--	0.14	
BAYERN					
D91	833	9.6	6.3--	0.23	203
D92	194	8.3	5.5--	0.41	264
D93	189	8.2	5.9--	0.45	232
D94	196	7.9	4.8--	0.36	298
D95	326	9.1	5.7--	0.33	246
D96	213	7.5	5.0--	0.36	286
D97	353	9.8	6.1--	0.34	214
D-B	2304	8.9	5.8--	0.13	
BERLIN(WEST)					
DB0	740	17.3	9.2++	0.37	25
BREMEN					
D40	231	14.1	8.2	0.57	67
HAMBURG					
D20	674	17.4	9.3++	0.38	23
HESSEN					
D64	1104	10.5	6.9	0.22	150
D66	291	10.3	5.7--	0.35	246
D-F	1395	10.4	6.6--	0.19	
NIEDERSACHSEN					
D31	474	12.1	7.1	0.35	136
D32	595	12.2	7.1	0.31	136
D33	392	11.2	7.3	0.39	122
D34	534	10.6	7.5	0.34	110
D-G	1995	11.5	7.3	0.17	
NORDRHEIN-WESTFALEN					
D51	1656	13.4	9.8++	0.25	13
D53	1123	12.0	9.6++	0.30	16
D55	591	10.2	9.1++	0.40	28
D57	465	10.8	7.3	0.36	122
D59	1049	11.9	8.8++	0.29	34
D-H	4884	12.0	9.2++	0.14	
RHEINLAND-PFALZ					
D71	426	13.1	7.8	0.40	97
D72	133	11.9	7.5	0.69	110
D73	518	12.0	7.9+	0.37	87
D-I	1077	12.4	7.8++	0.25	
SAARLAND					
DA0	230	9.0	5.8--	0.40	240
SCHLESWIG-HOLSTEIN					
D10	856	13.7	8.2++	0.30	67
D.0	16103	11.0	7.2++	0.06	

DANMARK (1971-80)

K15	1061	17.4	10.8++	0.34	4
K20	147	9.7	8.7+	0.73	39
K25	107	11.5	10.9++	1.06	3
K30	194	14.3	8.4+	0.63	53
K35	234	18.2	9.5++	0.65	19
K40	37	15.6	8.3	1.40	56
K42	356	16.1	9.4++	0.52	20
K50	130	10.6	6.6	0.60	173
K55	121	11.6	8.0	0.75	81
K60	201	12.7	7.8	0.57	97
K65	117	9.1	6.4	0.61	195
K70	319	11.5	7.6	0.44	104
K76	155	13.5	7.4	0.63	115
K80	248	10.5	6.2-	0.41	207
K.0	3427	13.7	8.6++	0.15	

FRANCE (1971-78)

ALSACE					
F67	269	7.8	5.8--	0.37	240
F68	210	8.4	6.7	0.48	166
F-A	479	8.0	6.1--	0.29	
AQUITAINE					
F24	176	12.1	5.5--	0.44	264
F33	434	10.6	6.5	0.33	181
F40	140	12.5	7.0	0.62	144
F47	123	10.8	5.4--	0.52	269
F64	192	9.3	5.1--	0.39	282
F-B	1065	10.8	6.0--	0.19	
AUVERGNE					
F03	184	12.4	6.0-	0.48	225
F15	68	10.3	5.3--	0.66	274
F43	72	9.0	4.7--	0.58	307
F63	198	8.7	5.8--	0.43	240
F-C	522	10.0	5.6--	0.26	
BASSE-NORMANDIE					
F14	123	5.6	4.8--	0.45	298
F50	111	6.4	4.8--	0.48	298
F61	70	6.1	4.3--	0.53	316
F-D	304	6.0	4.7--	0.28	
BOURGOGNE					
F21	152	8.5	6.0-	0.50	225
F58	112	11.4	5.5--	0.56	264
F71	167	7.4	4.1--	0.33	323
F89	143	12.1	5.9-	0.53	232
F-E	574	9.3	5.2--	0.23	
BRETAGNE					
F22	116	5.7	3.7--	0.36	333
F29	187	6.0	3.7--	0.28	333
F35	139	5.1	4.1--	0.35	323
F56	129	5.9	4.3--	0.39	316
F-F	571	5.7	3.9--	0.17	
CENTRE					
F18	140	11.2	6.2	0.56	207
F28	108	8.0	4.9--	0.50	293
F36	89	9.1	4.2--	0.47	321
F37	142	7.6	5.1--	0.45	282
F41	98	8.8	4.8--	0.52	298
F45	151	7.8	4.7--	0.40	307
F-G	728	8.6	5.0--	0.20	
CHAMPAGNE-ARDENNE					
F08	129	10.4	7.9	0.73	87
F10	119	10.6	6.7	0.65	166
F51	161	7.6	6.2	0.50	207
F52	68	8.0	5.4-	0.68	269
F-H	477	9.0	6.6	0.31	
CORSE					
F20	108	11.3	6.9	0.68	150
FRANCHE-COMTE					
F25	135	7.2	6.9	0.61	150
F39	80	8.4	4.7--	0.55	307
F70	72	8.3	5.4-	0.68	269
F90	50	9.8	7.9	1.15	87
F-J	337	8.0	6.0--	0.34	
HAUTE-NORMANDIE					
F27	128	7.6	5.7--	0.52	246
F76	323	7.0	5.5--	0.31	264
F-K	451	7.2	5.5--	0.27	
ILE-DE-FRANCE					
F75	871	10.2	5.9--	0.21	232
F77	245	8.1	6.4	0.42	195
F78	265	6.1	6.6	0.41	173
F91	226	6.1	6.8	0.46	160
F92	492	8.8	6.9	0.32	150
F93	449	8.5	8.0+	0.39	81
F94	405	8.5	7.3	0.37	122
F95	230	6.9	6.9	0.47	150
F-L	3183	8.3	6.7--	0.12	
LANGUEDOC-ROUSSILLON					
F11	193	18.5	7.7	0.60	102
F30	227	11.8	6.6	0.46	173
F34	367	14.7	8.1+	0.45	75
F48	24	8.0	3.2--	0.68	345
F66	192	16.6	7.3	0.56	122
F-M	1003	14.5	7.3	0.24	
LIMOUSIN					
F19	82	8.7	3.7--	0.43	333
F23	57	9.9	3.7--	0.53	333
F87	110	8.0	3.9--	0.40	328
F-N	249	8.6	3.8--	0.26	
LORRAINE					
F54	257	9.0	7.1	0.46	136
F55	81	10.1	6.5	0.76	181
F57	266	6.6	6.2-	0.39	207
F88	147	9.5	6.7	0.57	166
F-O	751	8.1	6.5-	0.25	
MIDI-PYRENEES					
F09	83	15.2	6.2	0.73	207
F12	121	11.2	5.3--	0.51	274
F31	375	12.5	8.1+	0.43	75
F32	84	12.0	5.6-	0.65	254
F46	66	11.2	4.8--	0.62	298
F65	111	12.5	6.7	0.66	166
F81	142	10.7	5.6--	0.49	254
F82	77	10.7	5.3--	0.64	274
F-P	1059	12.0	6.3--	0.20	
NORD-PAS-DE-CALAIS					
F59	840	8.5	7.0	0.25	144
F62	419	7.6	6.0--	0.30	225
F-Q	1259	8.2	6.6-	0.19	
PAYS DE LA LOIRE					
F44	175	4.9	3.8--	0.29	332
F49	118	4.8	3.4--	0.33	340
F53	54	5.3	3.9--	0.55	328
F72	122	6.3	4.0--	0.38	326
F85	91	5.2	3.3--	0.36	342
F-R	560	5.2	3.7--	0.16	
PICARDIE					
F02	193	9.1	6.1-	0.46	214
F60	175	7.2	5.7--	0.44	246
F80	170	8.0	5.0--	0.40	286
F-S	538	8.1	5.6--	0.25	
POITOU-CHARENTES					
F16	110	8.3	4.8--	0.49	298
F17	207	10.7	5.8--	0.42	240
F79	72	5.4	3.0--	0.37	346
F86	89	6.3	3.5--	0.39	339
F-T	478	8.0	4.4--	0.21	
PROVENCE-ALPES-COTE D'AZUR					
F04	53	11.8	6.4	0.94	195
F05	38	9.8	6.1	1.04	214
F06	329	10.7	4.8--	0.29	298
F13	816	12.8	8.5++	0.31	45
F83	412	16.7	9.4++	0.48	20
F84	166	10.7	6.8	0.55	160
F-U	1814	12.7	7.3	0.18	
RHONE-ALPES					
F01	81	5.4	3.6--	0.42	338
F07	97	9.7	5.2--	0.56	281
F26	140	9.9	6.1	0.54	214
F38	231	6.8	5.3--	0.36	274
F42	260	8.9	6.1-	0.39	214
F69	447	8.0	6.6	0.32	173
F73	97	8.0	5.7-	0.60	246
F74	118	6.6	5.6--	0.53	254
F-V	1471	7.8	5.7--	0.15	
F.0	17981	8.7	5.9--	0.05	

UNITED KINGDOM (1976-80)

EAST ANGLIA					
G25	152	8.8	6.5	0.54	181
G46	249	12.5	6.9	0.46	150
G55	187	10.5	6.5	0.49	181
G-A	588	10.7	6.7	0.28	
EAST MIDLANDS					
G30	282	10.7	6.6	0.40	173
G44	232	9.4	6.4	0.43	195
G45	184	11.7	7.3	0.56	122
G47	188	12.3	8.3+	0.62	56
G50	345	12.0	8.3++	0.46	56
G-B	1231	11.1	7.3	0.22	
NORTHERN					
G14	437	12.9	8.5++	0.42	45
G27	226	13.5	10.5++	0.71	6
G29	170	12.4	7.6	0.60	104
G33	221	12.4	8.3+	0.57	56
G48	92	10.8	6.7	0.72	166
G-C	1146	12.6	8.5++	0.26	
NORTH-WEST					
G11	954	12.3	8.5++	0.28	45
G12	624	13.9	9.9++	0.41	11
G26	288	10.7	7.7	0.46	102
G43	572	14.5	8.5++	0.37	45
G-D	2438	12.9	8.7++	0.18	

SOUTH-EAST					
G01	2672	13.4	7.9++	0.16	87
G22	140	9.4	7.4	0.64	115
G23	207	10.3	8.2	0.58	67
G24	131	8.3	6.4	0.57	195
G34	331	18.6	7.6	0.45	104
G35	561	13.4	8.7++	0.38	39
G37	443	10.1	7.1	0.35	136
G39	261	9.4	6.9	0.44	150
G41	63	19.5	8.8	1.18	34
G42	567	13.4	8.5++	0.37	45
G51	131	7.8	6.4	0.60	195
G56	360	12.4	8.0+	0.43	81
G58	259	14.6	7.1	0.47	136
G-E	6126	12.5	7.8++	0.10	
SOUTH-WEST					
G21	333	12.5	7.6	0.43	104
G28	163	13.6	7.1	0.58	136
G31	362	13.1	6.6	0.36	173
G32	267	16.1	7.4	0.48	115
G36	177	12.2	7.6	0.59	104
G53	150	12.4	6.5	0.55	181
G59	180	11.6	8.3	0.64	56
G-F	1632	13.1	7.2	0.19	
WEST MIDLANDS					
G15	846	10.5	7.5	0.26	110
G38	178	9.9	6.5	0.50	181
G52	97	9.0	6.3	0.67	203
G54	293	9.9	7.5	0.45	110
G57	143	10.3	7.8	0.68	97
G-G	1557	10.2	7.3	0.19	
YORKSHIRE AND HUMBERSIDE					
G13	481	12.5	8.1++	0.38	75
G16	776	12.9	8.3++	0.31	56
G40	315	12.8	8.4++	0.48	53
G49	259	13.3	8.0	0.52	81
G-H	1831	12.8	8.2++	0.20	
WALES					
G61	134	12.1	7.4	0.66	115
G62	99	10.5	6.0	0.62	225
G63	162	12.6	8.0	0.64	81
G64	80	12.2	6.8	0.79	160
G65	160	10.2	7.0	0.57	144
G66	36	11.4	6.3	1.09	203
G67	158	14.1	9.2++	0.74	25
G68	100	9.5	5.7-	0.59	246
G-I	929	11.5	7.2	0.24	
SCOTLAND(1975-80)					
S01	50	9.0	5.9	0.85	232
S02	169	12.6	8.1	0.64	75
S03	142	12.3	8.2	0.71	67
S04	114	11.4	8.1	0.78	75
S05	223	10.4	7.4	0.51	115
S06	34	11.8	6.6	1.17	173
S07	86	10.7	7.4	0.82	115
S08	832	11.8	8.7++	0.31	39
S09	41	9.8	5.6	0.90	254
S10	13	24.4	12.6	3.61	1
S11	2	3.2	2.4--	1.75	351
S12	9	10.2	5.0	1.77	286
G-J	1715	11.4	8.0++	0.20	
NORTHERN IRELAND					
JE	128	7.8	6.6	0.62	173
JN	63	7.0	5.6-	0.73	254
JS	28	4.2	3.7--	0.75	333
JW	45	7.5	6.7	1.07	166
G-K	264	6.9	5.9--	0.38	
G.0	19457	12.0	7.8++	0.06	
ITALIA (1975-79)					
ABRUZZI					
I66	79	10.8	6.0	0.69	225
I67	49	7.4	4.9--	0.72	293
I68	54	7.8	5.3-	0.74	274
I69	79	8.8	5.5-	0.63	264
I-A	261	8.7	5.4--	0.34	
BASILICATA					
I76	66	6.4	4.1--	0.52	323
I77	44	8.7	6.9	1.06	150
I-B	110	7.2	4.9--	0.48	
CALABRIA					
I78	107	6.0	4.8--	0.48	298
I79	130	7.1	5.6--	0.51	254
I80	140	9.6	6.5	0.57	181
I-C	377	7.4	5.6--	0.30	
CAMPANIA					
I61	133	7.4	6.5	0.57	181
I62	66	9.2	5.6-	0.70	254
I63	806	11.5	12.1++	0.43	2
I64	94	8.7	5.8-	0.62	240
I65	222	9.0	7.1	0.49	136
I-D	1321	10.1	9.0++	0.25	
EMILIA-ROMAGNA					
I33	93	13.4	7.2	0.77	130
I34	155	15.9	8.3	0.68	56
I35	94	9.5	5.7-	0.60	246
I36	149	10.5	6.9	0.58	150
I37	339	15.0	8.9++	0.50	33
I38	148	15.8	9.6++	0.80	16
I39	132	15.0	8.6+	0.77	42
I40	175	12.1	8.5+	0.65	45
I-E	1285	13.4	8.1++	0.23	
FRIULI-VENEZIA GIULIA					
I30	152	11.8	7.1	0.59	136
I31	61	17.4	10.7++	1.40	5
I32	135	19.4	9.8++	0.89	13
I93	48	7.3	5.0--	0.73	286
I-F	396	13.3	7.8	0.40	
LAZIO					
I56	68	10.4	6.2	0.78	207
I57	32	9.0	4.6--	0.84	311
I58	1015	11.4	10.2++	0.33	8
I59	71	6.8	6.1	0.73	214
I60	87	7.8	5.3--	0.58	274
I-G	1273	10.6	8.7++	0.25	
LIGURIA					
I08	112	20.2	10.1++	1.00	9
I09	122	16.5	8.5	0.80	45
I10	463	18.0	9.6++	0.46	16
I11	111	18.8	10.0++	0.97	10
I-H	808	18.1	9.5++	0.34	
LOMBARDIA					
I12	186	9.9	8.2	0.61	67
I13	208	11.3	9.4++	0.68	20
I14	44	10.2	7.9	1.20	87
I15	1162	11.9	10.3++	0.31	7
I16	158	7.4	6.9	0.55	150
I17	227	9.3	8.3+	0.57	56
I18	202	15.9	8.2	0.60	67
I19	100	12.3	7.9	0.82	87
I20	76	8.2	4.7--	0.55	307
I-I	2363	11.0	8.9++	0.19	
MARCHE					
I41	79	9.7	6.1	0.70	214
I42	141	13.7	8.3	0.71	56
I43	97	13.7	8.1	0.84	75
I44	79	9.2	6.4	0.74	195
I-J	396	11.6	7.3	0.37	
MOLISE					
I70	57	9.9	5.9	0.82	232
I94	18	7.8	3.9--	0.93	328
I-K	75	9.3	5.3--	0.64	
PIEMONTE					
I01	731	12.6	9.9++	0.38	11
I02	166	17.1	9.2++	0.74	25
I03	166	13.5	8.2	0.66	67
I04	178	13.1	7.2	0.56	130
I05	98	18.2	7.9	0.85	87
I06	192	16.5	7.5	0.57	110
I-L	1531	13.8	8.7++	0.23	
PUGLIA					
I71	124	7.4	5.4--	0.50	269
I72	316	9.0	7.3	0.42	122
I73	138	10.1	9.1+	0.78	28
I74	95	10.0	8.3	0.87	56
I75	211	11.6	9.0++	0.63	30
I-M	884	9.5	7.6+	0.26	
SARDEGNA					
I90	94	9.0	6.3	0.67	203
I91	48	7.0	5.0--	0.77	286
I92	141	8.0	7.2	0.61	130
I95	22	5.7	2.9--	0.66	347
I-N	305	7.9	5.9--	0.35	
SICILIA					
I81	106	10.3	6.5	0.66	181
I82	295	10.3	7.4	0.44	115
I83	199	12.1	7.6	0.55	104
I84	90	7.5	5.0--	0.55	286
I85	49	6.8	5.0--	0.73	286
I86	42	8.3	5.9	0.96	232
I87	219	9.0	6.8	0.47	160
I88	63	9.6	6.2	0.80	207
I89	82	8.5	6.4	0.72	195
I-O	1145	9.5	6.6-	0.20	
TOSCANA					
I45	69	13.9	8.5	1.04	45
I46	130	13.9	7.9	0.71	87
I47	78	12.2	6.8	0.79	160
I48	361	12.5	7.3	0.39	122
I49	121	14.4	8.6	0.80	42
I50	134	14.3	7.8	0.70	97
I51	60	7.8	4.2--	0.56	321
I52	68	10.7	4.9--	0.61	293
I53	59	10.7	5.8	0.77	240
I-P	1080	12.4	7.0	0.22	
TRENTINO-ALTO ADIGE					
I21	94	8.9	7.2	0.76	130
I22	131	12.2	8.2	0.74	67
I-Q	225	10.6	7.8	0.53	
UMBRIA					
I54	133	9.5	5.6--	0.49	254
I55	93	16.6	9.8++	1.03	13
I-R	226	11.5	6.8	0.46	
VALLE D'AOSTA					
I07	31	10.9	7.9	1.50	87
VENETO					
I23	176	9.5	6.8	0.52	160
I24	140	8.1	6.5	0.56	181
I25	57	10.5	6.7	0.90	166
I26	163	9.5	7.3	0.59	122
I27	224	11.0	8.8++	0.60	34
I28	219	11.2	8.8++	0.60	34
I29	85	13.7	9.0	1.00	30
I-T	1064	10.2	7.7++	0.24	
I.0	15156	11.0	7.8++	0.06	
IRELAND (1976-80)					
CONNAUGHT					
R07	18	4.2	2.8--	0.70	348
R12	6	8.1	3.3--	1.38	342
R16	16	5.5	2.7--	0.75	349
R20	12	8.4	4.3-	1.27	316
R21	15	10.8	5.6	1.48	254
R-A	67	6.2	3.4--	0.44	
LEINSTER					
R01	2	2.0	1.7--	1.29	354
R06	137	5.8	6.5	0.57	181
R09	11	4.3	5.3	1.65	274
R10	5	2.8	2.4--	1.12	351
R11	4	3.1	2.5--	1.26	350
R14	5	6.2	4.0	1.88	326
R15	13	6.0	5.7	1.62	246
R17	11	4.7	4.3-	1.35	316
R19	6	4.0	3.3--	1.38	342
R24	9	5.9	4.9	1.67	293
R25	13	5.3	3.9--	1.16	328
R26	10	4.8	4.5	1.45	314
R-B	226	5.2	5.1--	0.35	
MUNSTER					
R03	14	6.4	3.4--	0.96	340
R04	62	6.2	5.1--	0.67	282
R08	8	2.6	1.4--	0.51	355
R13	27	6.8	5.9	1.16	232
R22	20	5.8	4.3--	1.00	316
R23	11	5.0	4.8	1.50	298
R-C	142	5.7	4.4--	0.38	
ULSTER					
R02	5	3.5	2.0--	0.95	353
R05	26	8.3	4.6-	0.96	311
R18	12	9.1	5.9	1.76	232
R-D	43	7.3	4.2--	0.66	
R.0	478	5.6	4.5--	0.21	
LUXEMBOURG (1971-80)					
LE	21	11.6	7.0	1.60	144
LN	21	8.0	4.6-	1.06	311
LS	138	10.8	7.8	0.69	97
L.0	180	10.5	7.2	0.55	
NEDERLAND (1976-80)					
N01	149	10.9	7.2	0.61	130
N02	120	8.4	5.1--	0.49	282
N03	89	8.6	6.1	0.67	214
N04	210	8.4	6.5	0.46	181
N05	373	9.0	7.0	0.37	144
N06	165	7.6	6.0-	0.48	225
N07	691	11.9	8.6++	0.33	42
N08	852	11.3	7.9++	0.28	87
N09	95	11.2	6.1	0.66	214
N10	346	6.8	6.5	0.35	181
N11	230	8.6	8.0	0.53	81
N.0	3320	9.6	7.3	0.13	
EEC-9					
EEC	80661	10.6	7.1	0.03	

BELGIE-BELGIQUE (1971-78)

BRUSSEL-BRUXELLES					
B21	248	5.6	2.0+	0.15	60
VLAANDEREN					
B10	250	4.0	2.0+	0.13	60
B29	107	2.9	1.5	0.16	151
B30	144	3.3	1.6	0.14	131
B40	227	4.2	2.0+	0.14	60
B70	50	1.9	1.4	0.20	180
B-V	778	3.5	1.8	0.07	
WALLONIE					
B25	38	3.5	1.4	0.24	180
B50	218	4.0	1.6	0.12	131
B60	190	4.5	1.9	0.15	81
B80	25	2.8	1.2-	0.25	234
B90	40	2.5	1.2-	0.22	234
B-W	511	3.9	1.6	0.08	
B.0	1537	3.8	1.7	0.05	

BR DEUTSCHLAND (1976-80)

BADEN-WURTTEMBERG					
D81	262	2.9	1.3--	0.08	205
D82	214	3.4	1.5	0.11	151
D83	131	2.7	1.2--	0.11	234
D84	125	3.2	1.5	0.15	151
D-A	732	3.1	1.4--	0.05	
BAYERN					
D91	361	3.9	1.5	0.09	151
D92	74	2.8	1.3--	0.16	205
D93	90	3.6	1.5	0.17	151
D94	78	2.8	1.0--	0.13	291
D95	133	3.3	1.3--	0.13	205
D96	99	3.2	1.4-	0.15	180
D97	119	3.0	1.2--	0.12	234
D-B	954	3.4	1.4--	0.05	
BERLIN (WEST)					
DB0	436	8.2	2.5++	0.15	20
BREMEN					
D40	98	5.3	2.2+	0.26	33
HAMBURG					
D20	320	7.2	2.4++	0.15	24
HESSEN					
D64	445	3.9	1.6	0.08	131
D66	109	3.5	1.2--	0.13	234
D-F	554	3.8	1.5--	0.07	
NIEDERSACHSEN					
D31	181	4.2	1.5	0.12	151
D32	261	4.8	1.8	0.12	97
D33	129	3.5	1.3--	0.13	205
D34	180	3.3	1.5	0.12	151
D-G	751	4.0	1.6	0.06	
NORDRHEIN-WESTFALEN					
D51	675	4.9	2.2++	0.09	33
D53	419	4.2	2.0++	0.11	60
D55	242	3.9	2.1++	0.14	50
D57	210	4.4	2.0+	0.15	60
D59	435	4.5	2.1++	0.11	50
D-H	1981	4.4	2.1++	0.05	
RHEINLAND-PFALZ					
D71	124	3.5	1.4-	0.13	180
D72	43	3.5	1.3	0.22	205
D73	170	3.6	1.5	0.13	151
D-I	337	3.5	1.4--	0.08	
SAARLAND					
DA0	86	3.0	1.3--	0.15	205
SCHLESWIG-HOLSTEIN					
D10	326	4.8	1.9+	0.12	81
D.0	6575	4.1	1.7	0.02	

DANMARK (1971-80)

K15	488	7.3	3.1++	0.16	1
K20	62	4.1	2.8++	0.37	6
K25	31	3.4	2.6	0.49	14
K30	79	5.9	2.8++	0.33	6
K35	63	4.9	2.2	0.30	33
K40	20	8.5	3.1	0.73	1
K42	110	4.9	2.5++	0.25	20
K50	39	3.2	1.5	0.27	151
K55	38	3.7	2.0	0.35	60
K60	59	3.7	2.1	0.30	50
K65	35	2.8	1.8	0.33	97
K70	110	3.9	2.2+	0.22	33
K76	44	3.9	2.0	0.32	60
K80	96	4.1	2.1+	0.23	50
K.0	1274	5.0	2.5++	0.08	

FRANCE (1971-78)

ALSACE					
F67	84	2.3	1.1--	0.13	264
F68	73	2.8	1.4	0.18	180
F-A	157	2.5	1.2--	0.11	
AQUITAINE					
F24	72	4.7	1.6	0.23	131
F33	179	4.1	1.6	0.14	131
F40	35	3.0	1.0--	0.20	291
F47	53	4.4	1.6	0.25	131
F64	71	3.2	1.1--	0.16	264
F-B	410	3.9	1.4--	0.08	
AUVERGNE					
F03	61	3.9	1.3	0.21	205
F15	19	2.8	1.4	0.36	180
F43	33	3.9	1.2	0.24	234
F63	73	3.1	1.4	0.19	180
F-C	186	3.4	1.4--	0.12	
BASSE-NORMANDIE					
F14	68	3.0	1.5	0.20	151
F50	38	2.0	0.8--	0.16	327
F61	27	2.2	0.9--	0.21	310
F-D	133	2.5	1.1--	0.11	
BOURGOGNE					
F21	58	3.1	1.2--	0.17	234
F58	31	3.1	1.1-	0.24	264
F71	83	3.6	1.3-	0.16	205
F89	42	3.4	1.1--	0.22	264
F-E	214	3.3	1.2--	0.09	
BRETAGNE					
F22	53	2.5	0.9--	0.16	310
F29	88	2.6	1.2--	0.15	234
F35	54	1.9	0.9--	0.14	310
F56	56	2.4	1.0--	0.14	291
F-F	251	2.3	1.0--	0.07	
CENTRE					
F18	42	3.3	1.1--	0.19	264
F28	26	1.9	0.8--	0.17	327
F36	26	2.6	1.0-	0.26	291
F37	68	3.5	1.3-	0.18	205
F41	39	3.4	1.4	0.27	180
F45	54	2.7	1.1--	0.17	264
F-G	255	2.9	1.1--	0.08	
CHAMPAGNE-ARDENNE					
F08	33	2.7	1.4	0.27	180
F10	41	3.6	1.5	0.27	151
F51	66	3.1	1.5	0.21	151
F52	23	2.7	1.2	0.27	234
F-H	163	3.0	1.4-	0.13	
CORSE					
F20	26	3.0	1.0--	0.24	291
FRANCHE-COMTE					
F25	32	1.7	1.1--	0.21	264
F39	50	5.1	1.8	0.29	97
F70	26	2.9	1.0--	0.23	291
F90	18	3.5	1.3	0.32	205
F-J	126	2.9	1.3--	0.13	
HAUTE-NORMANDIE					
F27	47	2.7	1.2-	0.21	234
F76	118	2.5	1.2--	0.12	234
F-K	165	2.5	1.2--	0.11	
ILE-DE-FRANCE					
F75	458	4.6	1.6	0.08	131
F77	86	2.8	1.3	0.17	205
F78	98	2.3	1.5	0.17	151
F91	73	2.0	1.3-	0.17	205
F92	185	3.1	1.5	0.12	151
F93	165	3.1	1.8	0.15	97
F94	136	2.7	1.3--	0.13	205
F95	100	2.9	1.8	0.21	97
F-L	1301	3.2	1.5--	0.05	
LANGUEDOC-ROUSSILLON					
F11	52	4.6	1.7	0.28	116
F30	80	3.9	1.4	0.18	180
F34	123	4.6	1.7	0.19	116
F48	11	3.6	0.9-	0.31	310
F66	52	4.2	1.4	0.23	180
F-M	318	4.3	1.5	0.10	
LIMOUSIN					
F19	30	3.0	0.8--	0.16	327
F23	26	4.3	1.1-	0.28	264
F87	47	3.2	1.0--	0.17	291
F-N	103	3.4	1.0--	0.11	
LORRAINE					
F54	67	2.3	1.1--	0.15	264
F55	19	2.3	0.8--	0.22	327
F57	84	2.1	1.3-	0.15	205
F88	51	3.1	1.4	0.22	180
F-O	221	2.4	1.2--	0.09	
MIDI-PYRENEES					
F09	21	3.7	1.2	0.34	234
F12	42	3.7	1.0--	0.18	291
F31	109	3.4	1.5	0.16	151
F32	37	5.3	1.5	0.27	151
F46	29	4.8	1.5	0.33	151
F65	29	3.1	1.2-	0.26	234
F81	53	3.8	1.2-	0.19	234
F82	37	4.9	1.8	0.34	97
F-P	357	3.9	1.4--	0.08	
NORD-PAS-DE-CALAIS					
F59	306	3.0	1.5	0.10	151
F62	155	2.7	1.3--	0.11	205
F-Q	461	2.9	1.4--	0.07	
PAYS DE LA LOIRE					
F44	81	2.1	1.1--	0.13	264
F49	61	2.3	1.0--	0.14	291
F53	20	1.9	0.9--	0.23	310
F72	38	1.9	0.7--	0.12	340
F85	43	2.3	1.0--	0.18	291
F-R	243	2.1	1.0--	0.07	
PICARDIE					
F02	61	2.8	1.2-	0.17	234
F60	53	2.2	1.0--	0.16	291
F80	54	2.5	1.1--	0.18	264
F-S	168	2.5	1.1--	0.10	
POITOU-CHARENTES					
F16	44	3.2	1.2-	0.21	234
F17	77	3.8	1.3-	0.17	205
F79	28	2.1	1.0--	0.22	291
F86	41	2.8	1.0--	0.18	291
F-T	190	3.1	1.1--	0.10	
PROVENCE-ALPES-COTE D'AZUR					
F04	16	3.6	1.2	0.32	234
F05	8	2.0	0.8--	0.30	327
F06	111	3.2	0.8--	0.09	327
F13	233	3.5	1.5	0.11	151
F83	101	4.0	1.5	0.16	151
F84	53	3.3	1.6	0.24	131
F-U	522	3.5	1.3--	0.06	
RHONE-ALPES					
F01	42	2.8	1.2-	0.22	234
F07	48	4.6	1.6	0.27	131
F26	43	2.9	1.1--	0.20	264
F38	80	2.3	1.2--	0.15	234
F42	99	3.2	1.3-	0.15	205
F69	173	3.0	1.5	0.13	151
F73	33	2.7	1.2-	0.23	234
F74	38	2.1	1.3	0.22	205
F-V	556	2.9	1.3--	0.06	
F.0	6526	3.0	1.3--	0.02	

UNITED KINGDOM (1976-80)

EAST ANGLIA					
G25	66	3.9	1.7	0.23	116
G46	105	5.1	2.0	0.22	60
G55	82	4.6	1.9	0.24	81
G-A	253	4.6	1.9	0.13	
EAST MIDLANDS					
G30	129	4.7	2.2+	0.21	33
G44	92	3.6	1.7	0.19	116
G45	88	5.5	2.2+	0.26	33
G47	71	4.5	2.2+	0.29	33
G50	133	4.5	2.0	0.19	60
G-B	513	4.5	2.0++	0.10	
NORTHERN					
G14	203	5.6	2.7++	0.21	9
G27	78	4.5	2.6++	0.32	14
G29	88	6.0	2.7++	0.32	9
G33	103	5.5	2.7++	0.28	9
G48	34	3.8	1.7	0.31	116
G-C	506	5.3	2.6++	0.12	
NORTH-WEST					
G11	459	5.6	2.5++	0.13	20
G12	298	6.1	2.8++	0.18	6
G26	124	4.4	2.1+	0.20	50
G43	280	6.5	2.6++	0.18	14
G-D	1161	5.8	2.5++	0.08	

SOUTH-EAST

G01	1244	5.7	2.2++	0.07	33
G22	48	3.3	1.7	0.26	116
G23	89	4.4	2.2+	0.25	33
G24	67	4.3	2.0	0.27	60
G34	172	8.0	2.2++	0.21	33
G35	213	4.8	2.2++	0.17	33
G37	206	4.8	2.2++	0.17	33
G39	114	3.9	2.0	0.19	60
G41	26	7.2	2.6	0.66	14
G42	218	4.9	1.9	0.14	81
G51	68	4.3	2.0	0.26	60
G56	154	5.0	2.0+	0.17	60
G58	134	6.6	2.1	0.22	50
G-E	2753	5.3	2.1++	0.04	

SOUTH-WEST

G21	135	4.7	1.9	0.19	81
G28	58	4.5	1.8	0.26	97
G31	155	5.3	1.8	0.17	97
G32	105	5.7	1.9	0.21	81
G36	61	4.0	1.7	0.24	116
G53	52	4.1	1.6	0.25	131
G59	63	4.1	2.2	0.29	33
G-F	629	4.7	1.8+	0.08	

WEST MIDLANDS

G15	385	4.7	2.2++	0.12	33
G38	75	4.1	1.8	0.22	97
G52	35	3.1	1.7	0.33	116
G54	109	3.6	1.9	0.19	81
G57	56	3.9	2.0	0.29	60
G-G	660	4.2	2.0++	0.08	

YORKSHIRE AND HUMBERSIDE

G13	206	5.2	2.4++	0.18	24
G16	366	5.7	2.6++	0.15	14
G40	139	5.3	2.4++	0.22	24
G49	100	5.0	1.9	0.20	81
G-H	811	5.4	2.4++	0.09	

WALES

G61	70	5.9	2.2	0.28	33
G62	44	4.4	1.7	0.30	116
G63	59	4.4	1.8	0.25	97
G64	40	5.7	2.1	0.38	50
G65	76	4.6	2.3+	0.28	28
G66	12	3.8	1.6	0.48	131
G67	50	4.2	1.7	0.27	116
G68	42	3.7	1.8	0.31	97
G-I	393	4.6	1.9+	0.11	

SCOTLAND(1975-80)

S01	29	5.1	2.3	0.48	28
S02	62	4.3	1.9	0.26	81
S03	75	6.0	2.9++	0.37	5
S04	55	5.3	2.7++	0.40	9
S05	142	6.0	2.7++	0.24	9
S06	13	4.2	1.6	0.53	131
S07	36	4.4	2.5	0.44	20
S08	446	5.8	3.0++	0.15	4
S09	23	5.2	2.3	0.51	28
S10	2	3.7	1.4	1.06	180
S11	3	4.9	1.3	0.73	205
S12	8	8.9	3.1	1.33	1
G-J	894	5.5	2.7++	0.10	

NORTHERN IRELAND

JE	65	3.9	2.2	0.29	33
JN	29	3.1	1.8	0.36	97
JS	12	1.8	1.1	0.33	264
JW	24	3.9	2.0	0.44	60
G-K	130	3.3	1.9	0.18	
G.0	8703	5.1	2.2++	0.03	

ITALIA (1975-79)

ABRUZZI

I66	23	3.0	1.4	0.30	180
I67	14	2.1	0.9--	0.26	310
I68	12	1.7	0.8--	0.23	327
I69	22	2.4	1.1-	0.26	264
I-A	71	2.3	1.1--	0.13	

BASILICATA

I76	22	2.1	1.1-	0.25	264
I77	7	1.4	0.9-	0.35	310
I-B	29	1.9	1.1--	0.21	

CALABRIA

I78	21	1.2	0.7--	0.16	340
I79	31	1.7	1.0--	0.20	291
I80	29	1.9	0.9--	0.19	310
I-C	81	1.6	0.9--	0.10	

CAMPANIA

I61	30	1.6	1.1-	0.21	264
I62	9	1.2	0.6--	0.21	345
I63	142	2.0	1.4-	0.12	180
I64	25	2.3	1.2	0.26	234
I65	37	1.5	0.9--	0.15	310
I-D	243	1.8	1.2--	0.08	

EMILIA-ROMAGNA

I33	22	3.0	1.2	0.26	234
I34	42	4.1	1.7	0.29	116
I35	23	2.2	1.0--	0.21	291
I36	36	2.4	1.1--	0.18	264
I37	70	2.9	1.2--	0.15	234
I38	36	3.6	1.6	0.27	131
I39	29	3.1	1.3	0.26	205
I40	32	2.1	1.2	0.24	234
I-E	290	2.9	1.3--	0.08	

FRIULI-VENEZIA GIULIA

I30	42	3.1	1.4	0.24	180
I31	15	3.9	1.8	0.47	97
I32	59	7.4	2.4+	0.33	24
I93	20	2.9	1.4	0.33	180
I-F	136	4.2	1.7	0.16	

LAZIO

I56	14	2.1	1.0--	0.27	291
I57	6	1.7	0.6--	0.24	345
I58	249	2.6	1.7	0.11	116
I59	16	1.5	1.1-	0.28	264
I60	22	1.9	1.0--	0.22	291
I-G	307	2.4	1.5	0.09	

LIGURIA

I08	38	6.3	2.3	0.40	28
I09	37	4.7	1.8	0.31	97
I10	150	5.3	2.0+	0.18	60
I11	33	5.2	1.6	0.30	131
I-H	258	5.3	2.0+	0.13	

LOMBARDIA

I12	38	1.9	1.1--	0.19	264
I13	52	2.7	1.4	0.20	180
I14	17	3.9	1.9	0.50	81
I15	337	3.2	2.0++	0.11	60
I16	47	2.1	1.3-	0.19	205
I17	64	2.5	1.5	0.20	151
I18	39	2.9	1.1--	0.19	264
I19	18	2.1	1.0--	0.24	291
I20	35	3.6	1.4	0.26	180
I-I	647	2.8	1.6	0.06	

MARCHE

I41	13	1.6	0.8--	0.23	327
I42	33	3.0	1.4	0.26	180
I43	27	3.6	1.6	0.33	131
I44	18	2.0	0.9--	0.23	310
I-J	91	2.6	1.2--	0.13	

MOLISE

I70	9	1.5	0.7--	0.23	340
I94	4	1.7	1.3	0.69	205
I-K	13	1.5	0.9--	0.26	

PIEMONTE

I01	188	3.1	1.8	0.14	97
I02	37	3.5	1.3	0.23	205
I03	63	4.8	2.1	0.28	50
I04	63	4.6	1.9	0.26	81
I05	23	4.1	1.6	0.36	131
I06	53	4.3	1.5	0.23	151
I-L	427	3.7	1.7	0.09	

PUGLIA

I71	32	1.9	1.0--	0.18	291
I72	48	1.3	0.9--	0.14	310
I73	18	1.3	0.9--	0.22	310
I74	25	2.5	1.5	0.31	151
I75	46	2.4	1.4	0.22	180
I-M	169	1.8	1.1--	0.09	

SARDEGNA

I90	20	1.9	1.1	0.27	264
I91	5	0.7	0.4--	0.19	350
I92	31	1.7	1.3	0.24	205
I95	8	2.1	1.1	0.45	264
I-N	64	1.6	1.0--	0.14	

SICILIA

I81	20	1.9	0.8--	0.19	327
I82	69	2.3	1.3-	0.17	205
I83	47	2.7	1.3	0.20	205
I84	14	1.2	0.8--	0.21	327
I85	9	1.2	0.7--	0.25	340
I86	8	1.6	0.9-	0.33	310
I87	52	2.1	1.2--	0.17	234
I88	9	1.3	0.8--	0.26	327
I89	8	0.8	0.5--	0.18	348
I-O	236	1.9	1.0--	0.07	

TOSCANA

I45	12	2.3	0.9-	0.29	310
I46	47	4.7	2.1	0.33	50
I47	23	3.4	1.5	0.34	151
I48	105	3.4	1.4	0.15	180
I49	36	4.1	1.6	0.28	131
I50	32	3.3	1.2	0.24	234
I51	20	2.5	1.1	0.28	264
I52	11	1.7	0.7--	0.21	340
I53	10	1.8	0.8--	0.26	327
I-P	296	3.2	1.4--	0.08	

TRENTINO-ALTO ADIGE

I21	21	1.9	1.3	0.30	205
I22	41	3.7	1.8	0.31	97
I-Q	62	2.8	1.6	0.22	

UMBRIA

I54	46	3.2	1.5	0.24	151
I55	26	4.5	2.2	0.44	33
I-R	72	3.6	1.7	0.21	

VALLE D'AOSTA

I07	7	2.5	1.3	0.51	205

VENETO

I23	61	3.1	1.7	0.24	116
I24	42	2.3	1.4	0.23	180
I25	25	4.3	1.9	0.43	81
I26	40	2.2	1.2-	0.20	234
I27	73	3.4	1.9	0.23	81
I28	49	2.4	1.3	0.20	205
I29	14	2.2	0.9--	0.26	310
I-T	304	2.8	1.5	0.09	
I.0	3803	2.7	1.4--	0.02	

IRELAND (1976-80)

CONNAUGHT

R07	9	2.2	1.4	0.48	180
R12	4	6.2	2.6	1.36	14
R16	9	3.2	1.9	0.73	81
R20	0	0.0	0.0--	0.00	353
R21	3	2.2	1.1	0.68	264
R-A	25	2.5	1.4	0.30	

LEINSTER

R01	0	0.0	0.0--	0.00	353
R06	65	2.5	1.9	0.25	81
R09	2	0.9	0.9	0.64	310
R10	5	3.0	1.7	0.81	116
R11	1	0.8	0.3--	0.32	351
R14	0	0.0	0.0--	0.00	353
R15	5	2.3	1.8	0.81	97
R17	3	1.4	1.1	0.66	264
R19	1	0.7	0.8	0.76	327
R24	6	4.1	2.0	0.87	60
R25	4	1.7	1.2	0.62	234
R26	3	1.4	1.1	0.64	264
R-B	95	2.2	1.6	0.17	

MUNSTER

R03	6	2.9	1.4	0.58	180
R04	18	1.8	1.1-	0.27	264
R08	4	1.4	0.6--	0.31	345
R13	14	3.6	2.0	0.56	60
R22	12	3.7	2.3	0.71	28
R23	3	1.4	0.9	0.56	310
R-C	57	2.4	1.3	0.19	

ULSTER

R02	1	0.8	0.3--	0.28	351
R05	3	1.0	0.5--	0.34	348
R18	4	3.3	1.9	1.02	81
R-D	8	1.5	0.7--	0.28	
R.0	185	2.2	1.4-	0.11	

LUXEMBOURG (1971-80)

LE	8	4.2	1.7	0.63	116
LN	12	4.5	2.0	0.61	60
LS	53	3.9	2.1	0.30	50
L.0	73	4.1	2.0	0.25	

NEDERLAND (1976-80)

N01	35	2.5	1.2	0.24	234
N02	49	3.4	1.6	0.24	131
N03	28	2.7	1.5	0.30	151
N04	63	2.5	1.5	0.19	151
N05	101	2.4	1.2--	0.13	234
N06	75	3.4	1.8	0.22	97
N07	237	4.0	1.8	0.13	97
N08	261	3.4	1.6	0.11	131
N09	37	4.3	2.0	0.37	60
N10	110	2.2	1.6	0.16	131
N11	63	2.4	1.5	0.20	151
N.0	1059	3.0	1.6	0.05	

EEC-9

EEC	29735	3.7	1.7	0.01	

BELGIE-BELGIQUE (1971-78)

BRUSSEL-BRUXELLES					
B21	873	22.1	13.2++	0.46	29
VLAANDEREN					
B10	1138	18.5	12.6++	0.38	47
B29	511	14.2	9.6--	0.44	208
B30	595	14.0	9.6--	0.41	208
B40	886	16.9	10.7	0.37	140
B70	324	11.6	11.8	0.66	76
B-V	3454	15.7	10.9	0.19	
WALLONIE					
B25	186	18.1	12.4	0.93	51
B50	939	18.3	12.0++	0.41	62
B60	827	21.0	13.6++	0.48	24
B80	119	13.8	8.9-	0.85	247
B90	230	15.2	10.4	0.71	158
B-W	2301	18.4	12.1++	0.26	
B.0	6628	17.2	11.6++	0.15	

BR DEUTSCHLAND (1976-80)

BADEN-WURTTEMBERG					
D81	1167	14.0	10.4	0.32	158
D82	925	16.3	11.7+	0.41	80
D83	601	13.6	10.1	0.44	184
D84	528	14.7	11.2	0.51	113
D-A	3221	14.6	10.8	0.20	
BAYERN					
D91	1497	17.2	11.9++	0.32	67
D92	368	15.7	11.4	0.62	97
D93	365	15.8	11.9	0.64	67
D94	418	16.9	11.3	0.58	105
D95	609	16.9	11.2	0.47	113
D96	444	15.6	11.2	0.56	113
D97	615	17.0	11.3	0.48	105
D-B	4316	16.7	11.5++	0.18	
BERLIN(WEST)					
DB0	1137	26.6	15.1++	0.50	4
BREMEN					
D40	349	21.2	12.8++	0.72	36
HAMBURG					
D20	1025	26.4	14.8++	0.50	8
HESSEN					
D64	1890	18.0	12.4++	0.30	51
D66	523	18.4	11.1	0.52	121
D-F	2413	18.1	12.1++	0.26	
NIEDERSACHSEN					
D31	792	20.3	12.7++	0.48	40
D32	934	19.2	11.9+	0.41	67
D33	614	17.6	11.9+	0.52	67
D34	840	16.6	12.3++	0.45	55
D-G	3180	18.4	12.2++	0.23	
NORDRHEIN-WESTFALEN					
D51	2573	20.8	15.5++	0.32	2
D53	1728	18.4	14.9++	0.37	5
D55	933	16.1	14.4++	0.50	12
D57	737	17.2	12.0+	0.46	62
D59	1641	18.6	14.0++	0.36	15
D-H	7612	18.7	14.5++	0.17	
RHEINLAND-PFALZ					
D71	673	20.7	12.8++	0.52	36
D72	214	19.1	12.7+	0.92	40
D73	812	18.9	13.0++	0.48	34
D-I	1699	19.6	12.9++	0.33	
SAARLAND					
DA0	395	15.4	10.5	0.56	150
SCHLESWIG-HOLSTEIN					
D10	1246	20.0	12.7++	0.38	40
D.0	26593	18.2	12.6++	0.08	

DANMARK (1971-80)

K15	1636	26.9	16.9++	0.43	1
K20	247	16.3	14.8++	0.95	8
K25	148	15.9	15.2++	1.26	3
K30	307	22.7	13.8++	0.82	17
K35	351	27.2	14.9++	0.84	5
K40	57	24.0	13.5	1.88	26
K42	543	24.5	14.8++	0.66	8
K50	202	16.5	10.8	0.79	138
K55	177	17.0	12.2	0.94	57
K60	291	18.5	11.6	0.71	85
K65	199	15.5	11.2	0.82	113
K70	506	18.2	12.5++	0.57	48
K76	252	22.0	13.0+	0.87	34
K80	407	17.2	10.7	0.55	140
K.0	5323	21.3	13.8++	0.20	

FRANCE (1971-78)

ALSACE					
F67	498	14.4	11.1	0.52	121
F68	353	14.1	11.7	0.65	80
F-A	851	14.3	11.3	0.41	
AQUITAINE					
F24	263	18.1	8.9--	0.59	247
F33	667	16.3	10.3	0.42	173
F40	199	17.8	10.4	0.80	158
F47	186	16.4	8.8--	0.71	252
F64	307	14.9	8.7--	0.52	257
F-B	1622	16.4	9.6--	0.25	
AUVERGNE					
F03	285	19.3	10.2	0.66	177
F15	116	17.5	10.2	1.01	177
F43	126	15.7	8.7-	0.83	257
F63	345	15.2	10.6	0.59	146
F-C	872	16.7	10.1-	0.36	
BASSE-NORMANDIE					
F14	234	10.7	9.1--	0.61	237
F50	170	9.8	7.5--	0.60	301
F61	119	10.4	7.5--	0.71	301
F-D	523	10.3	8.1--	0.37	
BOURGOGNE					
F21	234	13.0	9.4-	0.64	218
F58	173	17.7	9.4	0.79	218
F71	300	13.4	7.9--	0.49	283
F89	222	18.7	9.8	0.72	199
F-E	929	15.0	9.0--	0.31	
BRETAGNE					
F22	227	11.1	7.3--	0.51	309
F29	335	10.7	7.0--	0.40	316
F35	252	9.3	7.4--	0.48	304
F56	213	9.7	7.2--	0.51	311
F-F	1027	10.2	7.2--	0.23	
CENTRE					
F18	215	17.2	9.9	0.73	193
F28	163	12.1	7.8--	0.65	288
F36	146	15.0	7.6--	0.69	294
F37	225	12.1	8.3--	0.58	275
F41	153	13.8	7.6--	0.67	294
F45	248	12.8	8.2--	0.55	276
F-G	1150	13.6	8.3--	0.26	
CHAMPAGNE-ARDENNE					
F08	192	15.5	11.9	0.90	67
F10	174	15.5	9.9	0.79	193
F51	247	11.7	9.6	0.63	208
F52	116	13.7	9.4	0.90	218
F-H	729	13.7	10.1	0.39	
CORSE					
F20	144	15.0	9.2-	0.79	230
FRANCHE-COMTE					
F25	203	10.8	10.2	0.74	177
F39	131	13.8	8.5--	0.78	266
F70	120	13.8	8.9-	0.87	247
F90	70	13.7	11.1	1.37	121
F-J	524	12.4	9.5--	0.43	
HAUTE-NORMANDIE					
F27	206	12.3	9.3-	0.67	223
F76	507	11.0	8.8--	0.40	252
F-K	713	11.3	8.9--	0.35	
ILE-DE-FRANCE					
F75	1353	15.9	9.4--	0.27	218
F77	394	13.1	10.3	0.54	173
F78	408	9.5	10.1	0.51	184
F91	368	10.0	11.0	0.58	128
F92	737	13.1	10.4	0.39	158
F93	637	12.0	11.4	0.46	97
F94	597	12.6	10.9	0.45	133
F95	347	10.4	10.5	0.57	150
F-L	4841	12.6	10.3--	0.15	
LANGUEDOC-ROUSSILLON					
F11	247	23.7	10.1	0.68	184
F30	324	16.8	9.6-	0.56	208
F34	492	19.8	11.3	0.55	105
F48	42	14.0	6.6--	1.07	326
F66	259	22.4	10.4	0.70	158
F-M	1364	19.7	10.3	0.30	
LIMOUSIN					
F19	122	13.0	6.0--	0.59	336
F23	89	15.5	6.4--	0.76	329
F87	198	14.5	7.4--	0.58	304
F-N	409	14.2	6.7--	0.37	
LORRAINE					
F54	387	13.6	11.1	0.58	121
F55	116	14.4	9.6	0.95	208
F57	438	10.8	10.2	0.50	177
F88	213	13.7	9.9	0.70	193
F-O	1154	12.5	10.3	0.31	
MIDI-PYRENEES					
F09	117	21.4	8.6-	0.86	261
F12	181	16.7	8.4--	0.67	269
F31	486	16.2	10.7	0.50	140
F32	125	17.9	8.9-	0.86	247
F46	94	16.0	7.4--	0.82	304
F65	150	16.9	9.5	0.81	214
F81	209	15.8	8.4--	0.61	269
F82	117	16.3	8.4--	0.82	269
F-P	1479	16.7	9.1--	0.25	
NORD-PAS-DE-CALAIS					
F59	1224	12.4	10.4	0.31	158
F62	618	11.3	9.0--	0.37	239
F-Q	1842	12.0	9.9--	0.24	
PAYS DE LA LOIRE					
F44	284	7.9	6.4--	0.39	329
F49	210	8.5	6.4--	0.46	329
F53	102	10.1	7.8--	0.80	288
F72	203	10.5	7.0--	0.51	316
F85	183	10.5	6.9--	0.54	318
F-R	982	9.1	6.7--	0.22	
PICARDIE					
F02	300	14.1	9.9	0.60	193
F60	271	11.1	9.0--	0.57	239
F80	269	12.7	8.5--	0.55	266
F-S	840	12.6	9.1--	0.33	
POITOU-CHARENTES					
F16	173	13.1	7.8--	0.64	288
F17	338	17.5	10.3	0.60	173
F79	146	10.9	6.4--	0.57	329
F86	173	12.3	7.4--	0.60	304
F-T	830	13.9	8.2--	0.31	
PROVENCE-ALPES-COTE D'AZUR					
F04	72	16.0	9.0	1.13	239
F05	54	13.9	9.3	1.32	223
F06	451	14.6	6.7--	0.35	323
F13	1093	17.1	11.6+	0.36	85
F83	547	22.2	12.8++	0.57	36
F84	246	15.9	10.2	0.67	177
F-U	2463	17.2	10.1--	0.21	
RHONE-ALPES					
F01	155	10.2	7.2--	0.60	311
F07	148	14.8	8.0--	0.69	280
F26	212	15.0	9.6	0.69	208
F38	351	10.3	8.1--	0.45	278
F42	405	13.8	9.8-	0.50	199
F69	667	11.9	9.9-	0.39	193
F73	152	12.5	9.0-	0.75	239
F74	176	9.8	8.6--	0.66	261
F-V	2266	12.0	9.0--	0.20	
F.0	27554	13.4	9.3--	0.06	

UNITED KINGDOM (1976-80)

EAST ANGLIA					
G25	205	11.9	9.0--	0.64	239
G46	339	17.0	9.7-	0.55	203
G55	251	14.1	9.3-	0.61	223
G-A	795	14.5	9.4--	0.35	
EAST MIDLANDS					
G30	397	15.1	9.5--	0.50	214
G44	332	13.5	9.5--	0.53	214
G45	256	16.3	10.4	0.68	158
G47	244	16.0	11.0	0.72	128
G50	477	16.6	11.6	0.55	85
G-B	1706	15.4	10.4	0.26	
NORTHERN					
G14	624	18.4	12.5++	0.51	48
G27	294	17.6	13.9++	0.82	16
G29	224	16.3	10.4	0.72	158
G33	309	17.3	11.6	0.67	85
G48	134	15.7	10.1	0.90	184
G-C	1585	17.5	11.9++	0.31	
NORTH-WEST					
G11	1287	16.6	11.6+	0.33	85
G12	819	18.3	13.1++	0.47	31
G26	401	14.9	10.9	0.56	133
G43	776	19.7	11.9+	0.44	67
G-D	3283	17.4	11.9++	0.21	

SOUTH-EAST					
G01	3645	18.2	11.1	0.19	121
G22	193	13.0	10.2	0.75	177
G23	284	14.1	11.3	0.68	105
G24	186	11.8	9.2-	0.68	230
G34	431	24.2	10.4	0.54	158
G35	731	17.4	11.6	0.44	85
G37	635	14.4	10.5	0.43	150
G39	396	14.3	10.5	0.54	150
G41	80	24.8	11.4	1.38	97
G42	762	18.1	11.6	0.44	85
G51	189	11.3	9.4-	0.73	218
G56	509	17.5	11.5	0.52	93
G58	371	20.9	11.0	0.61	128
G-E	8412	17.1	10.9	0.12	
SOUTH-WEST					
G21	467	17.5	11.2	0.54	113
G28	224	18.7	10.1	0.72	184
G31	538	19.5	10.5	0.48	150
G32	356	21.5	10.0	0.56	191
G36	233	16.1	10.4	0.71	158
G53	214	17.8	9.8	0.70	199
G59	237	15.3	11.2	0.75	113
G-F	2269	18.2	10.5	0.23	
WEST MIDLANDS					
G15	1167	14.5	10.4	0.31	158
G38	246	13.7	9.3-	0.61	223
G52	141	13.2	9.2-	0.81	230
G54	442	15.0	11.4	0.56	97
G57	194	14.0	10.6	0.79	146
G-G	2190	14.3	10.4-	0.23	
YORKSHIRE AND HUMBERSIDE					
G13	662	17.3	11.4	0.46	97
G16	1032	17.1	11.3	0.36	105
G40	433	17.5	11.8	0.58	76
G49	358	18.4	11.4	0.63	97
G-H	2485	17.4	11.4+	0.24	
WALES					
G61	197	17.8	11.3	0.84	105
G62	139	14.8	8.8--	0.77	252
G63	237	18.4	12.2	0.81	57
G64	120	18.3	10.7	1.02	140
G65	233	14.8	10.3	0.69	173
G66	56	17.7	10.9	1.58	133
G67	230	20.5	13.7++	0.92	19
G68	138	13.1	8.0--	0.70	280
G-I	1350	16.8	10.7	0.30	
SCOTLAND(1975-80)					
S01	87	15.6	11.0	1.21	128
S02	246	18.4	12.1	0.80	59
S03	223	19.3	13.3++	0.93	27
S04	160	16.1	11.5	0.93	93
S05	350	16.3	11.5	0.64	93
S06	53	18.5	10.5	1.51	150
S07	127	15.9	11.2	1.02	113
S08	1182	16.7	12.5++	0.38	48
S09	60	14.3	8.5-	1.12	266
S10	15	28.2	14.3	3.81	14
S11	4	6.4	4.5--	2.28	351
S12	18	20.5	11.8	3.02	76
G-J	2525	16.9	12.0++	0.25	
NORTHERN IRELAND					
JE	186	11.3	9.7	0.74	203
JN	85	9.4	7.7--	0.86	292
JS	42	6.3	5.6--	0.91	342
JW	79	13.1	11.7	1.38	80
G-K	392	10.3	8.8--	0.47	
G.0	26992	16.6	11.0+	0.07	
ITALIA (1975-79)					
ABRUZZI					
I66	100	13.7	7.9--	0.81	283
I67	71	10.7	7.4--	0.91	304
I68	75	10.8	7.6--	0.90	294
I69	96	10.7	6.9--	0.72	318
I-A	342	11.5	7.4--	0.41	
BASILICATA					
I76	85	8.3	5.6--	0.64	342
I77	56	11.1	9.0	1.23	239
I-B	141	9.2	6.6--	0.58	
CALABRIA					
I78	130	7.3	6.0--	0.53	336
I79	156	8.5	6.9--	0.57	318
I80	166	11.4	8.0--	0.64	280
I-C	452	8.9	6.9--	0.33	

CAMPANIA					
I61	161	9.0	8.1--	0.64	278
I62	77	10.7	6.7--	0.78	323
I63	964	13.8	14.5++	0.47	11
I64	109	10.1	6.8--	0.68	321
I65	260	10.5	8.6--	0.54	261
I-D	1571	12.0	10.9	0.28	
EMILIA-ROMAGNA					
I33	128	18.4	10.4	0.96	158
I34	215	22.1	11.9	0.83	67
I35	158	15.9	9.7	0.79	203
I36	216	15.2	10.1	0.70	184
I37	507	22.4	13.7++	0.63	19
I38	208	22.2	13.7++	0.96	19
I39	204	23.2	13.7++	0.98	19
I40	252	17.4	12.4+	0.80	51
I-E	1888	19.7	12.1++	0.29	
FRIULI-VENEZIA GIULIA					
I30	229	17.8	11.3	0.76	105
I31	83	23.6	14.9+	1.67	5
I32	179	25.7	13.1+	1.02	31
I93	87	13.3	9.3	1.02	223
I-F	578	19.3	11.7	0.50	
LAZIO					
I56	94	14.3	9.0	0.97	239
I57	43	12.1	6.5--	1.03	328
I58	1365	15.4	13.6++	0.38	24
I59	104	10.0	9.1	0.90	237
I60	118	10.6	7.5--	0.71	301
I-G	1724	14.3	11.8++	0.29	
LIGURIA					
I08	131	23.6	12.1	1.11	59
I09	152	20.6	11.0	0.92	128
I10	602	23.3	12.7++	0.53	40
I11	139	23.5	13.1	1.14	31
I-H	1024	22.9	12.4++	0.40	
LOMBARDIA					
I12	270	14.4	12.1	0.76	59
I13	302	16.5	13.8++	0.83	17
I14	58	13.5	10.5	1.40	150
I15	1621	16.6	14.4++	0.37	12
I16	266	12.4	11.5	0.71	93
I17	327	13.4	12.0	0.68	62
I18	268	21.1	11.4	0.73	97
I19	129	15.9	10.4	0.94	158
I20	132	14.2	8.7--	0.78	257
I-I	3373	15.7	12.7++	0.22	
MARCHE					
I41	114	14.1	9.3	0.89	223
I42	194	18.8	11.9	0.88	67
I43	125	17.6	10.7	0.97	140
I44	95	11.1	7.9--	0.83	283
I-J	528	15.5	10.1	0.45	
MOLISE					
I70	76	13.2	8.2--	0.98	276
I94	23	9.9	5.0--	1.05	347
I-K	99	12.2	7.2--	0.75	
PIEMONTE					
I01	941	16.2	12.8++	0.43	36
I02	220	22.7	12.4	0.88	51
I03	227	18.5	11.8	0.82	76
I04	225	16.6	9.2-	0.64	230
I05	118	22.0	9.7	0.95	203
I06	264	22.7	10.9	0.71	133
I-L	1995	18.0	11.6++	0.27	
PUGLIA					
I71	148	8.8	6.6--	0.56	326
I72	381	10.9	9.0--	0.47	239
I73	170	12.4	11.3	0.88	105
I74	117	12.3	10.4	0.98	158
I75	250	13.8	10.9	0.70	133
I-M	1066	11.4	9.4--	0.29	
SARDEGNA					
I90	131	12.5	8.9-	0.80	247
I91	63	9.2	6.8--	0.91	321
I92	179	10.2	9.2-	0.70	230
I95	30	7.7	4.3--	0.85	352
I-N	403	10.4	8.0--	0.41	
SICILIA					
I81	132	12.8	8.4--	0.76	269
I82	339	11.8	8.7--	0.48	257
I83	230	14.0	9.2--	0.63	230
I84	100	8.4	5.8--	0.60	340
I85	65	9.0	6.7--	0.86	323
I86	51	10.1	7.3--	1.07	309
I87	266	10.9	8.4--	0.53	269
I88	78	11.9	7.9--	0.91	283
I89	99	10.2	7.8--	0.80	288
I-O	1360	11.3	8.1--	0.22	

TOSCANA					
I45	83	16.7	10.4	1.17	158
I46	169	18.1	10.7	0.85	140
I47	100	15.7	8.8-	0.90	252
I48	512	17.8	10.6	0.49	146
I49	176	21.0	12.7	0.98	40
I50	184	19.6	11.1	0.85	121
I51	95	12.3	7.1--	0.74	314
I52	102	16.1	7.6--	0.78	294
I53	89	16.1	9.2	1.01	230
I-P	1510	17.4	10.0--	0.27	
TRENTINO-ALTO ADIGE					
I21	121	11.5	9.5	0.88	214
I22	175	16.3	11.1	0.86	121
I-Q	296	13.9	10.4	0.62	
UMBRIA					
I54	175	12.5	7.6--	0.59	294
I55	112	20.0	12.0	1.18	62
I-R	287	14.6	8.9--	0.54	
VALLE D'AOSTA					
I07	39	13.7	10.1	1.68	184
VENETO					
I23	296	15.9	11.7	0.69	80
I24	206	11.9	9.8	0.69	199
I25	85	15.7	10.2	1.13	177
I26	253	14.8	11.6	0.74	85
I27	334	16.3	13.3++	0.74	27
I28	309	15.8	12.7+	0.73	40
I29	125	20.1	13.7+	1.25	19
I-T	1608	15.4	11.9++	0.30	
I.0	20284	14.8	10.7	0.08	
IRELAND (1976-80)					
CONNAUGHT					
R07	31	7.2	5.3--	1.00	346
R12	10	13.4	6.0-	1.94	336
R16	25	8.5	4.6--	0.99	350
R20	13	9.1	4.8--	1.37	348
R21	19	13.7	7.1-	1.69	314
R-A	98	9.1	5.3--	0.57	
LEINSTER					
R01	2	2.0	1.7--	1.29	355
R06	210	8.9	10.0	0.71	191
R09	16	6.3	7.6	1.96	294
R10	7	3.9	3.3--	1.30	354
R11	10	7.6	6.1-	1.97	335
R14	7	8.7	6.3	2.55	334
R15	20	9.3	8.6	1.96	261
R17	19	8.1	7.6	1.79	294
R19	10	6.7	5.8--	1.85	340
R24	10	6.5	5.4--	1.75	344
R25	24	9.8	7.9	1.72	283
R26	12	5.7	5.4--	1.59	344
R-B	347	8.0	8.0--	0.44	
MUNSTER					
R03	25	11.4	7.2-	1.54	311
R04	102	10.2	8.4--	0.86	269
R08	19	6.1	4.1--	1.00	353
R13	40	10.1	8.8	1.43	252
R22	41	11.9	9.7	1.57	203
R23	19	8.6	8.6	2.01	261
R-C	246	9.9	7.9--	0.52	
ULSTER					
R02	11	7.8	4.7--	1.46	349
R05	34	10.9	6.0--	1.08	336
R18	13	9.9	6.4-	1.83	329
R-D	58	9.9	5.7--	0.78	
R.0	749	8.8	7.3--	0.28	
LUXEMBOURG (1971-80)					
LE	32	17.6	10.6	1.95	146
LN	34	12.9	7.7-	1.40	292
LS	207	16.2	12.0	0.86	62
L.0	273	15.9	11.1	0.69	
NEDERLAND (1976-80)					
N01	231	16.9	11.7	0.80	80
N02	196	13.7	9.3-	0.70	223
N03	153	14.8	10.8	0.90	138
N04	353	14.1	11.4	0.62	97
N05	605	14.6	11.9+	0.50	67
N06	276	12.7	10.5	0.64	150
N07	1032	17.8	13.2++	0.42	29
N08	1279	17.0	12.3++	0.35	55
N09	145	17.1	9.9	0.87	193
N10	588	11.6	11.2	0.47	113
N11	365	13.7	12.7++	0.67	40
N.0	5223	15.1	11.8++	0.17	
EEC-9					
EEC	119619	15.7	10.8	0.03	

BELGIE-BELGIQUE (1971-78)

BRUSSEL-BRUXELLES					
B21	462	10.4	4.2++	0.23	42
VLAANDEREN					
B10	465	7.4	4.0+	0.20	57
B29	233	6.4	3.6	0.26	100
B30	299	6.9	3.6	0.23	100
B40	501	9.3	4.8++	0.24	21
B70	116	4.3	3.4	0.33	131
B-V	1614	7.2	4.0++	0.11	
WALLONIE					
B25	70	6.5	3.0	0.40	199
B50	399	7.3	3.3	0.19	148
B60	366	8.7	4.1+	0.24	50
B80	50	5.6	2.9	0.46	215
B90	103	6.4	3.2	0.35	157
B-W	988	7.5	3.5	0.12	
B.0	3064	7.6	3.9++	0.08	

BR DEUTSCHLAND (1976-80)

BADEN-WURTTEMBERG					
D81	661	7.4	3.7	0.16	88
D82	544	8.8	4.2++	0.21	42
D83	335	6.9	3.3	0.20	148
D84	283	7.3	3.9	0.25	69
D-A	1823	7.7	3.8++	0.10	
BAYERN					
D91	844	9.0	4.2++	0.16	42
D92	198	7.6	3.8	0.30	80
D93	212	8.4	4.3+	0.32	36
D94	265	9.5	4.3+	0.32	36
D95	342	8.6	3.9	0.23	69
D96	251	8.1	4.2+	0.30	42
D97	315	7.9	3.7	0.23	88
D-B	2427	8.6	4.0++	0.09	
BERLIN(WEST)					
DB0	803	15.1	4.9++	0.22	16
BREMEN					
D40	188	10.1	4.5++	0.37	26
HAMBURG					
D20	567	12.7	4.6++	0.22	23
HESSEN					
D64	968	8.5	3.9++	0.14	69
D66	285	9.2	3.9	0.26	69
D-F	1253	8.7	3.9++	0.12	
NIEDERSACHSEN					
D31	398	9.3	3.8	0.21	80
D32	550	10.1	4.4++	0.22	31
D33	302	8.2	3.6	0.23	100
D34	409	7.5	4.0+	0.21	57
D-G	1659	8.8	4.0++	0.11	
NORDRHEIN-WESTFALEN					
D51	1378	10.0	4.9++	0.15	16
D53	838	8.3	4.4++	0.16	31
D55	491	7.9	4.5++	0.22	26
D57	400	8.4	4.0+	0.22	57
D59	855	8.8	4.4++	0.16	31
D-H	3962	8.9	4.5++	0.08	
RHEINLAND-PFALZ					
D71	304	8.6	4.0	0.26	57
D72	87	7.0	3.2	0.38	157
D73	381	8.1	3.7	0.21	88
D-I	772	8.1	3.7	0.15	
SAARLAND					
DA0	204	7.2	3.5	0.27	116
SCHLESWIG-HOLSTEIN					
D10	614	9.1	4.0++	0.19	57
D.0	14272	8.9	4.1++	0.04	

DANMARK (1971-80)

K15	984	14.8	6.8++	0.24	4
K20	137	9.1	6.7++	0.60	5
K25	76	8.3	6.9++	0.82	3
K30	140	10.5	5.5++	0.49	12
K35	182	14.3	7.3++	0.59	2
K40	28	11.9	4.8	0.97	21
K42	244	10.9	5.8++	0.41	9
K50	77	6.3	3.4	0.42	131
K55	96	9.4	5.7++	0.62	11
K60	166	10.4	6.5++	0.54	6
K65	102	8.1	5.5++	0.57	12
K70	283	10.0	6.1++	0.39	8
K76	117	10.4	5.8++	0.58	9
K80	243	10.4	6.2++	0.42	7
K.0	2875	11.3	6.2++	0.13	

FRANCE (1971-78)

ALSACE					
F67	217	6.0	3.4	0.25	131
F68	177	6.8	3.8	0.33	80
F-A	394	6.4	3.6	0.20	
AQUITAINE					
F24	132	8.6	3.1	0.32	179
F33	337	7.6	3.4	0.22	131
F40	81	6.9	2.9	0.38	215
F47	87	7.3	2.7-	0.34	256
F64	144	6.5	2.9	0.31	215
F-B	781	7.4	3.1--	0.13	
AUVERGNE					
F03	122	7.8	2.8-	0.33	239
F15	55	8.2	3.9	0.62	69
F43	65	7.7	3.2	0.48	157
F63	144	6.1	3.1	0.30	179
F-C	386	7.1	3.2	0.19	
BASSE-NORMANDIE					
F14	151	6.6	3.6	0.32	100
F50	106	5.7	2.8-	0.30	239
F61	62	5.1	2.6-	0.37	273
F-D	319	5.9	3.0-	0.19	
BOURGOGNE					
F21	116	6.3	2.9	0.31	215
F58	77	7.6	3.4	0.49	131
F71	174	7.5	3.1	0.28	179
F89	101	8.3	3.4	0.43	131
F-E	468	7.3	3.2-	0.17	
BRETAGNE					
F22	141	6.5	2.9-	0.29	215
F29	179	5.4	2.6--	0.23	273
F35	131	4.5	2.5--	0.24	284
F56	114	5.0	2.4--	0.27	290
F-F	565	5.3	2.6--	0.13	
CENTRE					
F18	92	7.1	2.9	0.36	215
F28	78	5.8	2.9	0.38	215
F36	64	6.4	2.5--	0.38	284
F37	133	6.8	3.1	0.31	179
F41	79	6.9	3.0	0.43	199
F45	121	6.1	2.9	0.31	215
F-G	567	6.5	2.9--	0.14	
CHAMPAGNE-ARDENNE					
F08	76	6.1	3.5	0.46	116
F10	79	6.9	3.1	0.41	179
F51	140	6.6	3.6	0.34	100
F52	42	4.9	2.4--	0.42	290
F-H	337	6.3	3.3	0.20	
CORSE					
F20	52	6.0	2.3--	0.38	299
FRANCHE-COMTE					
F25	76	4.0	2.6--	0.33	273
F39	85	8.7	3.4	0.42	131
F70	68	7.6	4.0	0.56	57
F90	36	7.0	3.3	0.63	148
F-J	265	6.2	3.2	0.22	
HAUTE-NORMANDIE					
F27	100	5.8	3.1	0.36	179
F76	259	5.4	2.9--	0.21	215
F-K	359	5.5	3.0--	0.18	
ILE-DE-FRANCE					
F75	830	8.4	3.3	0.14	148
F77	172	5.7	3.0	0.27	199
F78	206	4.8	3.3	0.25	148
F91	147	4.0	3.0-	0.27	199
F92	343	5.8	3.1-	0.19	179
F93	301	5.7	3.5	0.22	116
F94	270	5.4	3.1	0.22	179
F95	192	5.7	3.9	0.31	69
F-L	2461	6.1	3.3--	0.07	
LANGUEDOC-ROUSSILLON					
F11	95	8.5	3.6	0.45	100
F30	140	6.9	2.7--	0.27	256
F34	196	7.3	3.2	0.29	157
F48	24	8.0	3.0	0.76	199
F66	96	7.7	3.2	0.43	157
F-M	551	7.5	3.1-	0.16	
LIMOUSIN					
F19	71	7.2	2.5--	0.34	284
F23	66	10.9	3.1	0.50	179
F87	104	7.1	2.7-	0.32	256
F-N	241	7.9	2.7--	0.21	
LORRAINE					
F54	147	5.1	3.0-	0.27	199
F55	47	5.7	2.8	0.49	239
F57	201	5.0	3.5	0.27	116
F88	108	6.6	3.2	0.35	157
F-O	503	5.4	3.2-	0.16	
MIDI-PYRENEES					
F09	39	7.0	2.9	0.58	215
F12	94	8.2	3.5	0.47	116
F31	195	6.1	2.9--	0.23	215
F32	65	9.3	3.2	0.47	157
F46	56	9.2	3.4	0.56	131
F65	62	6.6	2.7-	0.40	256
F81	97	7.0	2.9	0.39	215
F82	59	7.8	2.8	0.43	239
F-P	667	7.2	3.0--	0.14	
NORD-PAS-DE-CALAIS					
F59	596	5.8	3.3	0.15	148
F62	296	5.1	2.8--	0.18	239
F-Q	892	5.6	3.1--	0.12	
PAYS DE LA LOIRE					
F44	171	4.4	2.4--	0.21	290
F49	144	5.5	3.0	0.30	199
F53	50	4.6	2.3--	0.38	299
F72	108	5.4	2.6--	0.28	273
F85	108	5.9	2.9	0.32	215
F-R	581	5.1	2.7--	0.13	
PICARDIE					
F02	138	6.4	3.3	0.31	148
F60	116	4.8	2.6--	0.27	273
F80	130	5.9	3.0	0.30	199
F-S	384	5.7	3.0--	0.17	
POITOU-CHARENTES					
F16	88	6.4	2.8-	0.35	239
F17	157	7.7	3.2	0.31	157
F79	70	5.2	2.8	0.38	239
F86	92	6.3	2.7-	0.33	256
F-T	407	6.5	2.9--	0.17	
PROVENCE-ALPES-COTE D'AZUR					
F04	35	7.9	3.6	0.76	100
F05	17	4.4	2.5	0.68	284
F06	198	5.7	1.9--	0.16	318
F13	375	5.6	2.6--	0.15	273
F83	177	6.9	3.0-	0.26	199
F84	82	5.2	2.8-	0.34	239
F-U	884	5.9	2.5--	0.10	
RHONE-ALPES					
F01	104	6.9	3.5	0.40	116
F07	80	7.6	3.1	0.41	179
F26	81	5.5	2.6--	0.33	273
F38	157	4.5	2.6--	0.23	273
F42	209	6.8	3.2	0.26	157
F69	348	5.9	3.2	0.19	157
F73	82	6.6	3.6	0.44	100
F74	82	4.5	3.0	0.35	199
F-V	1143	5.9	3.1--	0.10	
F.0	13207	6.1	3.0--	0.03	

UNITED KINGDOM (1976-80)

EAST ANGLIA					
G25	102	6.0	3.2	0.35	157
G46	168	8.1	3.6	0.32	100
G55	122	6.9	3.1	0.32	179
G-A	392	7.1	3.3	0.19	
EAST MIDLANDS					
G30	182	6.6	3.4	0.28	131
G44	146	5.7	2.8--	0.25	239
G45	123	7.6	3.5	0.35	116
G47	97	6.2	3.2	0.36	157
G50	225	7.5	3.9	0.29	69
G-B	773	6.8	3.4	0.13	
NORTHERN					
G14	317	8.7	4.3++	0.27	36
G27	127	7.3	4.6+	0.44	23
G29	133	9.1	4.3	0.41	36
G33	153	8.2	4.2	0.37	42
G48	64	7.2	3.6	0.49	100
G-C	794	8.3	4.3++	0.17	
NORTH-WEST					
G11	686	8.3	4.1++	0.17	50
G12	444	9.2	4.5++	0.24	26
G26	186	6.6	3.4	0.27	131
G43	424	9.9	4.4++	0.25	31
G-D	1740	8.6	4.2++	0.11	

SOUTH-EAST

G01	1912	8.8	3.7+	0.10	88
G22	69	4.7	2.7-	0.34	256
G23	130	6.4	3.5	0.33	116
G24	112	7.2	4.0	0.40	57
G34	246	11.5	3.8	0.33	80
G35	307	7.0	3.5	0.22	116
G37	303	7.0	3.6	0.23	100
G39	193	6.7	3.6	0.28	100
G41	37	10.2	3.6	0.74	100
G42	345	7.7	3.4	0.21	131
G51	94	6.0	3.2	0.37	157
G56	241	7.9	3.4	0.23	131
G58	205	10.2	3.6	0.33	100
G-E	4194	8.1	3.6	0.06	

SOUTH-WEST

G21	204	7.1	3.1	0.24	179
G28	94	7.3	3.4	0.43	131
G31	235	8.0	3.0-	0.24	199
G32	160	8.7	3.0	0.30	199
G36	103	6.8	3.0	0.34	199
G53	84	6.6	2.7-	0.33	256
G59	108	7.0	4.2	0.44	42
G-F	988	7.5	3.2--	0.12	

WEST MIDLANDS

G15	567	6.9	3.4	0.15	131
G38	118	6.4	3.2	0.32	157
G52	64	5.8	3.1	0.44	179
G54	176	5.8	3.2	0.26	157
G57	84	5.9	3.2	0.37	157
G-G	1009	6.4	3.3-	0.11	

YORKSHIRE AND HUMBERSIDE

G13	313	7.8	3.9	0.24	69
G16	542	8.5	4.0+	0.19	57
G40	215	8.2	4.1	0.30	50
G49	169	8.4	3.7	0.33	88
G-H	1239	8.2	3.9++	0.12	

WALES

G61	97	8.2	3.4	0.40	131
G62	63	6.2	2.8	0.41	239
G63	102	7.6	4.0	0.45	57
G64	66	9.4	3.7	0.53	88
G65	113	6.8	3.7	0.38	88
G66	20	6.3	2.8	0.69	239
G67	79	6.6	2.9	0.37	215
G68	59	5.1	2.7-	0.39	256
G-I	599	7.0	3.3	0.15	

SCOTLAND(1975-80)

S01	45	7.9	4.2	0.72	42
S02	111	7.8	3.9	0.40	69
S03	122	9.7	4.9++	0.50	16
S04	83	8.0	4.4	0.52	31
S05	249	10.5	5.1++	0.36	15
S06	22	7.0	3.1	0.75	179
S07	60	7.3	4.3	0.57	36
S08	712	9.3	4.9++	0.20	16
S09	40	9.1	4.5	0.76	26
S10	6	11.0	5.5	2.47	12
S11	3	4.9	1.3--	0.73	347
S12	16	17.7	8.0	2.50	1
G-J	1469	9.1	4.7++	0.13	

NORTHERN IRELAND

JE	98	5.8	3.5	0.38	116
JN	53	5.7	3.7	0.55	88
JS	22	3.2	2.1--	0.47	311
JW	39	6.4	3.5	0.61	116
G-K	212	5.4	3.3	0.25	
G.0	13409	7.8	3.7++	0.04	

ITALIA (1975-79)

ABRUZZI

I66	31	4.0	2.3-	0.50	299
I67	19	2.8	1.3--	0.32	347
I68	24	3.3	1.8--	0.38	323
I69	27	2.9	1.5--	0.32	338
I-A	101	3.3	1.7--	0.19	

BASILICATA

I76	37	3.6	2.2--	0.38	305
I77	11	2.2	1.6--	0.51	331
I-B	48	3.1	2.0--	0.31	

CALABRIA

I78	39	2.2	1.4--	0.24	343
I79	45	2.4	1.6--	0.26	331
I80	43	2.9	1.7--	0.29	326
I-C	127	2.5	1.6--	0.15	

CAMPANIA

I61	43	2.3	1.7--	0.26	326
I62	11	1.5	0.8--	0.24	352
I63	211	2.9	2.3--	0.16	299
I64	39	3.5	2.2--	0.39	305
I65	57	2.3	1.5--	0.20	338
I-D	361	2.7	1.9--	0.10	

EMILIA-ROMAGNA

I33	40	5.5	2.2--	0.36	305
I34	67	6.5	2.8	0.38	239
I35	48	4.7	2.1--	0.33	311
I36	85	5.8	3.1	0.36	179
I37	150	6.2	2.9--	0.25	215
I38	71	7.1	3.4	0.42	131
I39	60	6.5	3.0	0.43	199
I40	69	4.6	2.7-	0.35	256
I-E	590	5.8	2.8--	0.13	

FRIULI-VENEZIA GIULIA

I30	93	6.8	3.3	0.37	148
I31	30	7.9	3.5	0.68	116
I32	93	11.6	4.0	0.45	57
I93	36	5.2	2.7	0.51	256
I-F	252	7.8	3.5	0.24	

LAZIO

I56	33	5.0	2.9	0.57	215
I57	13	3.6	1.6--	0.48	331
I58	421	4.5	3.1--	0.15	179
I59	31	3.0	2.4--	0.44	290
I60	35	3.1	1.8--	0.34	323
I-G	533	4.2	2.8--	0.13	

LIGURIA

I08	50	8.3	3.2	0.50	157
I09	52	6.6	2.6-	0.38	273
I10	240	8.5	3.5	0.25	116
I11	44	6.9	2.2--	0.36	305
I-H	386	7.9	3.2-	0.18	

LOMBARDIA

I12	98	4.9	3.1	0.32	179
I13	107	5.5	3.2	0.33	157
I14	34	7.8	4.5	0.82	26
I15	585	5.6	3.7	0.16	88
I16	110	5.0	3.2	0.32	157
I17	131	5.1	3.2	0.30	157
I18	84	6.2	2.8-	0.34	239
I19	45	5.2	2.7	0.44	256
I20	60	6.1	2.9	0.42	215
I-I	1254	5.5	3.3-	0.10	

MARCHE

I41	33	4.0	2.2--	0.42	305
I42	53	4.8	2.4--	0.34	290
I43	56	7.6	3.5	0.50	116
I44	27	3.0	1.6--	0.32	331
I-J	169	4.7	2.4--	0.20	

MOLISE

I70	27	4.5	2.5	0.55	284
I94	7	2.9	2.1	0.82	311
I-K	34	4.0	2.4-	0.46	

PIEMONTE

I01	315	5.2	3.1-	0.18	179
I02	72	6.8	3.0	0.46	199
I03	110	8.4	3.8	0.39	80
I04	96	7.0	3.2	0.36	157
I05	33	5.9	2.4-	0.46	290
I06	92	7.4	2.7-	0.32	256
I-L	718	6.2	3.1--	0.13	

PUGLIA

I71	44	2.6	1.6--	0.25	331
I72	74	2.0	1.4--	0.18	343
I73	31	2.2	1.6--	0.30	331
I74	38	3.8	2.4--	0.41	290
I75	67	3.5	2.3--	0.29	299
I-M	254	2.6	1.7--	0.12	

SARDEGNA

I90	41	3.9	2.7	0.45	256
I91	20	2.9	1.9--	0.47	318
I92	56	3.2	2.5--	0.35	284
I95	13	3.3	2.0-	0.61	315
I-N	130	3.3	2.4--	0.22	

SICILIA

I81	41	3.8	2.0--	0.34	315
I82	90	3.0	1.9--	0.21	318
I83	63	3.6	1.9--	0.25	318
I84	24	2.0	1.4--	0.30	343
I85	15	2.0	1.4--	0.39	343
I86	11	2.1	1.5--	0.49	338
I87	67	2.7	1.7--	0.22	326
I88	17	2.5	1.6--	0.42	331
I89	17	1.8	1.3--	0.32	347
I-O	345	2.8	1.7--	0.10	

TOSCANA

I45	28	5.3	2.7	0.53	256
I46	81	8.0	3.8	0.46	80
I47	41	6.1	2.9	0.50	215
I48	192	6.2	2.8--	0.22	239
I49	62	7.0	3.0	0.41	199
I50	62	6.3	3.1	0.45	179
I51	35	4.4	2.2--	0.42	305
I52	32	4.9	1.9--	0.41	318
I53	30	5.3	2.7	0.55	256
I-P	563	6.1	2.8--	0.13	

TRENTINO-ALTO ADIGE

I21	44	4.1	2.9	0.46	215
I22	64	5.7	2.9	0.39	215
I-Q	108	4.9	3.0	0.30	

UMBRIA

I54	75	5.2	2.8-	0.37	239
I55	36	6.2	3.2	0.56	157
I-R	111	5.5	2.9-	0.31	

VALLE D'AOSTA

I07	10	3.5	2.1-	0.68	311

VENETO

I23	123	6.3	3.7	0.35	88
I24	83	4.6	2.9-	0.32	215
I25	36	6.2	3.3	0.61	148
I26	82	4.6	2.7-	0.32	256
I27	129	6.0	3.5	0.33	116
I28	92	4.5	2.6--	0.29	273
I29	24	3.7	2.0--	0.48	315
I-T	569	5.2	3.0--	0.13	
I.0	6663	4.6	2.6--	0.03	

IRELAND (1976-80)

CONNAUGHT

R07	16	3.9	2.8	0.77	239
R12	4	6.2	2.6	1.36	273
R16	14	5.0	2.9	0.88	215
R20	1	0.8	0.5--	0.55	354
R21	3	2.2	1.1--	0.68	351
R-A	38	3.8	2.3--	0.42	

LEINSTER

R01	2	2.1	1.5	1.14	338
R06	119	4.7	3.6	0.34	100
R09	4	1.7	1.7-	0.89	326
R10	5	3.0	1.7-	0.81	326
R11	3	2.5	1.5-	0.87	338
R14	1	1.4	0.8--	0.82	352
R15	7	3.3	2.9	1.15	215
R17	7	3.2	2.8	1.08	239
R19	2	1.5	1.3-	0.93	347
R24	10	6.8	4.6	1.57	23
R25	14	5.9	4.9	1.39	16
R26	7	3.3	2.7	1.11	256
R-B	181	4.1	3.2	0.25	

MUNSTER

R03	11	5.4	2.4	0.76	290
R04	34	3.5	2.4-	0.43	290
R08	14	4.8	3.1	0.95	179
R13	21	5.4	3.6	0.83	100
R22	17	5.2	3.4	0.87	131
R23	7	3.2	2.3	0.93	299
R-C	104	4.3	2.8-	0.29	

ULSTER

R02	1	0.8	0.3--	0.28	355
R05	9	3.0	1.8--	0.65	323
R18	7	5.8	3.7	1.46	88
R-D	17	3.1	1.8--	0.47	
R.0	340	4.1	2.8--	0.16	

LUXEMBOURG (1971-80)

LE	17	8.9	4.1	1.05	50
LN	17	6.4	2.9	0.73	215
LS	94	7.0	3.9	0.42	69
L.0	128	7.1	3.7	0.35	

NEDERLAND (1976-80)

N01	100	7.3	4.0	0.45	57
N02	108	7.5	3.9	0.41	69
N03	66	6.4	4.1	0.54	50
N04	161	6.4	4.1	0.35	50
N05	250	6.0	3.7	0.25	88
N06	154	6.9	4.2	0.37	42
N07	440	7.4	3.8	0.20	80
N08	594	7.7	4.3++	0.20	36
N09	69	8.1	4.1	0.55	50
N10	260	5.2	4.0	0.26	57
N11	151	5.7	3.8	0.32	80
N.0	2353	6.7	4.0++	0.09	

EEC-9

EEC	56311	7.0	3.5	0.02	

BELGIE-BELGIQUE (1971-78)					
BRUSSEL-BRUXELLES					
B21	223	5.6	4.6++	0.33	85
VLAANDEREN					
B10	501	8.1	6.8++	0.31	4
B29	184	5.1	4.2	0.32	120
B30	279	6.6	5.5++	0.34	20
B40	412	7.9	6.4++	0.33	6
B70	138	5.0	4.9++	0.43	59
B-V	1514	6.9	5.8++	0.15	
WALLONIE					
B25	48	4.7	3.9	0.58	153
B50	322	6.3	5.0++	0.29	53
B60	273	6.9	5.5++	0.35	20
B80	28	3.2	2.8	0.55	265
B90	111	7.3	6.0++	0.58	13
B-W	782	6.3	5.0++	0.19	
B.0	2519	6.6	5.4++	0.11	
BR DEUTSCHLAND (1976-80)					
BADEN-WURTTEMBERG					
D81	201	2.4	2.2--	0.16	329
D82	134	2.4	2.1--	0.19	333
D83	133	3.0	2.8--	0.26	265
D84	92	2.6	2.5--	0.27	305
D-A	560	2.5	2.3--	0.10	
BAYERN					
D91	274	3.1	2.7--	0.18	281
D92	67	2.9	2.7--	0.34	281
D93	62	2.7	2.5--	0.33	305
D94	60	2.4	2.1--	0.29	333
D95	102	2.8	2.4--	0.25	317
D96	77	2.7	2.5--	0.30	305
D97	124	3.4	3.0--	0.28	243
D-B	766	3.0	2.6--	0.10	
BERLIN(WEST)					
DB0	192	4.5	3.9	0.31	153
BREMEN					
D40	106	6.4	5.1++	0.54	47
HAMBURG					
D20	146	3.8	2.9--	0.27	256
HESSEN					
D64	342	3.3	2.8--	0.16	265
D66	98	3.5	2.7--	0.29	281
D-F	440	3.3	2.8--	0.14	
NIEDERSACHSEN					
D31	110	2.8	2.5--	0.25	305
D32	150	3.1	2.8--	0.25	265
D33	123	3.5	3.1	0.30	232
D34	163	3.2	3.0--	0.25	243
D-G	546	3.2	2.8--	0.13	
NORDRHEIN-WESTFALEN					
D51	363	2.9	2.6--	0.14	294
D53	275	2.9	2.6--	0.16	294
D55	172	3.0	2.8--	0.22	265
D57	152	3.5	3.1-	0.26	232
D59	246	2.8	2.5--	0.16	305
D-H	1208	3.0	2.7--	0.08	
RHEINLAND-PFALZ					
D71	80	2.5	2.0--	0.24	341
D72	32	2.9	2.4--	0.43	317
D73	115	2.7	2.4--	0.24	317
D-I	227	2.6	2.3--	0.16	
SAARLAND					
DA0	145	5.7	4.7+	0.41	74
SCHLESWIG-HOLSTEIN					
D10	210	3.4	3.1--	0.23	232
D.0	4546	3.1	2.7--	0.04	
DANMARK (1971-80)					
K15	450	7.4	5.7++	0.28	17
K20	75	5.0	4.7	0.55	74
K25	52	5.6	5.7+	0.79	17
K30	84	6.2	5.0+	0.57	53
K35	75	5.8	4.5	0.56	92
K40	10	4.2	3.3	1.15	216
K42	172	7.8	6.1++	0.49	10
K50	75	6.1	5.4++	0.65	24
K55	74	7.1	6.2++	0.73	8
K60	85	5.4	4.7	0.53	74
K65	85	6.6	5.7++	0.64	17
K70	176	6.3	5.5++	0.43	20
K76	100	8.7	7.4++	0.77	1
K80	151	6.4	5.3++	0.45	31
K.0	1664	6.6	5.5++	0.14	
FRANCE (1971-78)					
ALSACE					
F67	84	2.4	2.4--	0.27	317
F68	76	3.0	3.0-	0.35	243
F-A	160	2.7	2.6--	0.22	
AQUITAINE					
F24	63	4.3	3.4	0.47	206
F33	167	4.1	3.5	0.29	194
F40	46	4.1	3.4	0.55	206
F47	41	3.6	2.6-	0.44	294
F64	77	3.7	3.0	0.37	243
F-B	394	4.0	3.3-	0.18	
AUVERGNE					
F03	46	3.1	2.8-	0.46	265
F15	23	3.5	3.2	0.74	225
F43	27	3.4	2.9	0.62	256
F63	65	2.9	2.5--	0.31	305
F-C	161	3.1	2.7--	0.23	
BASSE-NORMANDIE					
F14	47	2.2	1.9--	0.28	345
F50	31	1.8	1.6--	0.29	351
F61	29	2.5	2.3--	0.44	324
F-D	107	2.1	1.9--	0.18	
BOURGOGNE					
F21	46	2.6	2.2--	0.33	329
F58	41	4.2	3.3	0.57	216
F71	82	3.7	3.1	0.36	232
F89	34	2.9	2.1--	0.39	333
F-E	203	3.3	2.6--	0.20	
BRETAGNE					
F22	56	2.7	2.4--	0.34	317
F29	117	3.7	3.3	0.32	216
F35	64	2.4	2.1--	0.27	333
F56	59	2.7	2.5--	0.33	305
F-F	296	2.9	2.6--	0.16	
CENTRE					
F18	41	3.3	2.6--	0.43	294
F28	39	2.9	2.8	0.47	265
F36	29	3.0	2.0--	0.43	341
F37	51	2.7	2.3--	0.34	324
F41	47	4.2	3.5	0.53	194
F45	68	3.5	3.1	0.39	232
F-G	275	3.2	2.7--	0.17	
CHAMPAGNE-ARDENNE					
F08	40	3.2	3.3	0.53	216
F10	36	3.2	2.8	0.49	265
F51	60	2.9	2.7--	0.36	281
F52	22	2.6	2.6-	0.57	294
F-H	158	3.0	2.8--	0.23	
CORSE					
F20	25	2.6	2.1--	0.48	333
FRANCHE-COMTE					
F25	38	2.0	2.1--	0.35	333
F39	33	3.5	2.8	0.50	265
F70	21	2.4	2.0--	0.45	341
F90	13	2.5	2.6	0.74	294
F-J	105	2.5	2.4--	0.24	
HAUTE-NORMANDIE					
F27	35	2.1	2.0--	0.34	341
F76	127	2.8	2.6--	0.24	294
F-K	162	2.6	2.4--	0.20	
ILE-DE-FRANCE					
F75	335	3.9	3.1--	0.19	232
F77	77	2.6	2.5--	0.30	305
F78	133	3.1	3.2	0.28	225
F91	92	2.5	2.7--	0.29	281
F92	178	3.2	2.8--	0.22	265
F93	168	3.2	3.1--	0.24	232
F94	144	3.0	2.9--	0.24	256
F95	114	3.4	3.6	0.34	177
F-L	1241	3.2	3.0--	0.09	
LANGUEDOC-ROUSSILLON					
F11	39	3.7	2.5--	0.43	305
F30	83	4.3	3.5	0.41	194
F34	93	3.7	3.0-	0.33	243
F48	13	4.3	3.6	1.14	177
F66	66	5.7	3.9	0.54	153
F-M	294	4.3	3.2-	0.20	
LIMOUSIN					
F19	43	4.6	3.0	0.50	243
F23	20	3.5	3.0	0.83	243
F87	62	4.5	3.3	0.44	216
F-N	125	4.3	3.1	0.31	
LORRAINE					
F54	57	2.0	1.9--	0.26	345
F55	24	3.0	3.1	0.66	232
F57	85	2.1	2.2--	0.24	329
F88	34	2.2	2.1--	0.37	333
F-O	200	2.2	2.2--	0.16	
MIDI-PYRENEES					
F09	15	2.7	2.4-	0.66	317
F12	33	3.0	2.3--	0.44	324
F31	102	3.4	2.9--	0.30	256
F32	26	3.7	3.0	0.63	243
F46	21	3.6	2.7	0.63	281
F65	38	4.3	3.3	0.59	216
F81	57	4.3	3.3	0.46	216
F82	32	4.5	3.5	0.70	194
F-P	324	3.7	2.9--	0.17	
NORD-PAS-DE-CALAIS					
F59	294	3.0	3.0--	0.18	243
F62	155	2.8	2.7--	0.22	281
F-Q	449	2.9	2.9--	0.14	
PAYS DE LA LOIRE					
F44	93	2.6	2.5--	0.26	305
F49	64	2.6	2.3--	0.30	324
F53	29	2.9	2.6-	0.51	294
F72	41	2.1	1.9--	0.31	345
F85	39	2.2	2.1--	0.35	333
F-R	266	2.5	2.3--	0.14	
PICARDIE					
F02	66	3.1	3.0-	0.38	243
F60	70	2.9	2.8--	0.34	265
F80	61	2.9	2.6--	0.35	294
F-S	197	3.0	2.8--	0.20	
POITOU-CHARENTES					
F16	53	4.0	3.4	0.50	206
F17	66	3.4	2.6--	0.34	294
F79	55	4.1	3.5	0.49	194
F86	45	3.2	2.7-	0.43	281
F-T	219	3.7	3.0--	0.21	
PROVENCE-ALPES-COTE D'AZUR					
F04	21	4.7	4.0	0.97	137
F05	16	4.1	3.3	0.83	216
F06	71	2.3	1.6--	0.20	351
F13	188	2.9	2.5--	0.19	305
F83	87	3.5	2.7--	0.31	281
F84	58	3.7	3.2	0.43	225
F-U	441	3.1	2.5--	0.12	
RHONE-ALPES					
F01	47	3.1	2.9	0.44	256
F07	34	3.4	2.6-	0.47	294
F26	45	3.2	2.7-	0.42	281
F38	121	3.5	3.4	0.32	206
F42	105	3.6	3.0-	0.31	243
F69	201	3.6	3.4	0.25	206
F73	32	2.6	2.2--	0.39	329
F74	54	3.0	2.8-	0.39	265
F-V	639	3.4	3.1--	0.12	
F.0	6441	3.1	2.8--	0.04	
UNITED KINGDOM (1976-80)					
EAST ANGLIA					
G25	72	4.2	3.8	0.47	164
G46	111	5.6	4.4	0.44	102
G55	104	5.9	4.7+	0.48	74
G-A	287	5.2	4.4+	0.27	
EAST MIDLANDS					
G30	127	4.8	3.9	0.36	153
G44	107	4.3	3.7	0.37	169
G45	60	3.8	3.2	0.43	225
G47	96	6.3	5.4++	0.57	24
G50	168	5.9	4.9++	0.39	59
G-B	558	5.0	4.2++	0.18	
NORTHERN					
G14	188	5.5	4.6+	0.35	85
G27	76	4.5	4.1	0.48	130
G29	93	6.8	5.4++	0.60	24
G33	82	4.6	4.0	0.46	137
G48	58	6.8	5.3+	0.72	31
G-C	497	5.5	4.6++	0.21	
NORTH-WEST					
G11	365	4.7	3.9	0.21	153
G12	231	5.2	4.4+	0.30	102
G26	128	4.8	4.2	0.38	120
G43	213	5.4	4.4+	0.31	102
G-D	937	5.0	4.2++	0.14	

SOUTH-EAST					
G01	1198	6.0	4.6++	0.14	85
G22	58	3.9	3.4	0.46	206
G23	105	5.2	4.7+	0.47	74
G24	85	5.4	4.7	0.51	74
G34	147	8.2	6.0++	0.56	13
G35	219	5.2	4.5+	0.31	92
G37	259	5.9	5.2++	0.33	40
G39	147	5.3	4.4	0.37	102
G41	16	5.0	3.6	1.00	177
G42	267	6.3	5.2++	0.34	40
G51	94	5.6	5.2++	0.55	40
G56	187	6.4	5.0++	0.39	53
G58	119	6.7	5.4++	0.53	24
G-E	2901	5.9	4.8++	0.09	
SOUTH-WEST					
G21	156	5.9	4.8++	0.41	66
G28	85	7.1	5.3++	0.62	31
G31	171	6.2	4.7+	0.38	74
G32	115	6.9	4.8+	0.48	66
G36	80	5.5	4.5	0.51	92
G53	85	7.1	5.4++	0.61	24
G59	89	5.7	4.9+	0.53	59
G-F	781	6.3	4.9++	0.18	
WEST MIDLANDS					
G15	385	4.8	4.1	0.22	130
G38	97	5.4	4.6	0.48	85
G52	43	4.0	3.6	0.56	177
G54	178	6.0	5.2++	0.40	40
G57	55	4.0	3.4	0.47	206
G-G	758	5.0	4.2++	0.16	
YORKSHIRE AND HUMBERSIDE					
G13	215	5.6	4.4+	0.31	102
G16	267	4.4	3.7	0.24	169
G40	126	5.1	4.4	0.41	102
G49	101	5.2	4.5	0.47	92
G-H	709	5.0	4.1++	0.16	
WALES					
G61	53	4.8	4.0	0.57	137
G62	51	5.4	4.1	0.61	130
G63	59	4.6	4.1	0.56	130
G64	32	4.9	4.3	0.79	112
G65	91	5.8	5.3++	0.57	31
G66	24	7.6	6.2	1.36	8
G67	66	5.9	4.7	0.62	74
G68	50	4.7	3.6	0.53	177
G-I	426	5.3	4.4++	0.22	
SCOTLAND(1975-80)					
S01	19	3.4	2.8	0.66	265
S02	78	5.8	5.2+	0.60	40
S03	70	6.1	5.2+	0.65	40
S04	52	5.2	5.0	0.72	53
S05	134	6.2	5.3++	0.47	31
S06	10	3.5	2.9	0.96	256
S07	31	3.9	3.5	0.67	194
S08	388	5.5	4.8++	0.25	66
S09	29	6.9	6.1+	1.19	10
S10	0	0.0	0.0--	0.00	355
S11	2	3.2	3.1	2.16	232
S12	7	8.0	7.0	2.75	2
G-J	820	5.5	4.8++	0.17	
NORTHERN IRELAND					
JE	92	5.6	5.3++	0.56	31
JN	47	5.2	5.1	0.76	47
JS	23	3.5	3.5	0.75	194
JW	32	5.3	5.1	0.91	47
G-K	194	5.1	4.9++	0.36	
G.0	8868	5.5	4.5++	0.05	
ITALIA (1975-79)					
ABRUZZI					
I66	39	5.3	4.3	0.73	112
I67	37	5.6	4.8	0.82	66
I68	22	3.2	2.7	0.58	281
I69	31	3.5	2.8	0.53	265
I-A	129	4.3	3.6	0.33	
BASILICATA					
I76	30	2.9	2.5-	0.48	305
I77	19	3.8	3.5	0.83	194
I-B	49	3.2	2.8-	0.41	
CALABRIA					
I78	44	2.5	2.4--	0.37	317
I79	68	3.7	3.6	0.45	177
I80	63	4.3	4.0	0.51	137
I-C	175	3.5	3.3	0.25	

CAMPANIA					
I61	71	4.0	4.0	0.48	137
I62	19	2.6	2.3--	0.54	324
I63	269	3.8	4.0	0.25	137
I64	34	3.1	2.8	0.49	265
I65	115	4.7	4.5+	0.43	92
I-D	508	3.9	3.9	0.17	
EMILIA-ROMAGNA					
I33	34	4.9	3.7	0.73	169
I34	57	5.9	3.9	0.54	153
I35	55	5.5	4.0	0.56	137
I36	84	5.9	4.8+	0.56	66
I37	146	6.5	4.8++	0.42	66
I38	57	6.1	4.6	0.63	85
I39	48	5.5	4.4	0.69	102
I40	58	4.0	3.4	0.46	206
I-E	539	5.6	4.3++	0.20	
FRIULI-VENEZIA GIULIA					
I30	86	6.7	5.3++	0.61	31
I31	21	6.0	4.4	0.99	102
I32	61	8.8	6.9++	1.00	3
I93	39	6.0	5.2	0.85	40
I-F	207	6.9	5.5++	0.41	
LAZIO					
I56	33	5.0	3.6	0.64	177
I57	8	2.2	1.7--	0.61	350
I58	492	5.5	5.0++	0.23	53
I59	44	4.2	4.1	0.62	130
I60	50	4.5	3.7	0.54	169
I-G	627	5.2	4.6++	0.19	
LIGURIA					
I08	32	5.8	3.9	0.77	153
I09	41	5.5	4.0	0.65	137
I10	142	5.5	4.0	0.36	137
I11	38	6.4	4.2	0.72	120
I-H	253	5.7	4.0	0.27	
LOMBARDIA					
I12	83	4.4	4.0	0.45	137
I13	73	4.0	3.6	0.43	177
I14	19	4.4	4.2	0.97	120
I15	437	4.5	3.9	0.19	153
I16	88	4.1	3.9	0.42	153
I17	116	4.7	4.4	0.42	102
I18	80	6.3	4.5	0.55	92
I19	39	4.8	3.7	0.61	169
I20	41	4.4	3.4	0.55	206
I-I	976	4.5	4.0+	0.13	
MARCHE					
I41	47	5.8	4.5	0.67	92
I42	56	5.4	4.2	0.58	120
I43	33	4.7	3.6	0.65	177
I44	40	4.7	3.8	0.62	164
I-J	176	5.2	4.0	0.31	
MOLISE					
I70	30	5.2	4.3	0.79	112
I94	12	5.2	4.2	1.22	120
I-K	42	5.2	4.2	0.67	
PIEMONTE					
I01	266	4.6	4.0	0.25	137
I02	65	6.7	4.9	0.66	59
I03	82	6.7	5.5++	0.63	20
I04	55	4.1	2.9	0.42	256
I05	22	4.1	2.8	0.70	265
I06	94	8.1	5.3++	0.59	31
I-L	584	5.3	4.2++	0.18	
PUGLIA					
I71	62	3.7	3.5	0.45	194
I72	151	4.3	4.2	0.35	120
I73	41	3.0	3.0	0.48	243
I74	40	4.2	3.9	0.63	153
I75	80	4.4	4.2	0.47	120
I-M	374	4.0	3.9	0.20	
SARDEGNA					
I90	47	4.5	4.3	0.63	112
I91	18	2.6	2.7	0.65	281
I92	57	3.2	3.4	0.45	206
I95	12	3.1	2.9	0.86	256
I-N	134	3.5	3.4	0.30	
SICILIA					
I81	30	2.9	2.7-	0.50	281
I82	97	3.4	3.2	0.33	225
I83	67	4.1	3.6	0.46	177
I84	49	4.1	3.7	0.54	169
I85	28	3.9	3.6	0.70	177
I86	19	3.8	3.5	0.82	194
I87	78	3.2	3.0	0.35	243
I88	14	2.1	1.9--	0.53	345
I89	33	3.4	3.2	0.57	225
I-O	415	3.5	3.2--	0.16	

TOSCANA					
I45	28	5.6	4.2	0.86	120
I46	42	4.5	3.5	0.58	194
I47	41	6.4	4.6	0.75	85
I48	156	5.4	4.0	0.34	137
I49	41	4.9	3.3	0.54	216
I50	52	5.6	4.2	0.63	120
I51	40	5.2	3.9	0.66	153
I52	31	4.9	3.5	0.68	194
I53	27	4.9	3.8	0.80	164
I-P	458	5.3	3.9	0.19	
TRENTINO-ALTO ADIGE					
I21	41	3.9	3.6	0.58	177
I22	56	5.2	4.8	0.66	66
I-Q	97	4.6	4.2	0.44	
UMBRIA					
I54	87	6.2	4.8+	0.55	66
I55	26	4.6	3.6	0.76	177
I-R	113	5.8	4.5	0.45	
VALLE D'AOSTA					
I07	13	4.6	3.6	1.04	177
VENETO					
I23	88	4.7	4.1	0.45	130
I24	78	4.5	4.1	0.47	130
I25	23	4.3	3.6	0.77	177
I26	71	4.1	3.8	0.46	164
I27	108	5.3	4.7+	0.45	74
I28	100	5.1	4.6	0.47	85
I29	14	2.3	1.9--	0.55	345
I-T	482	4.6	4.1+	0.19	
I.0	6351	4.6	4.0++	0.05	
IRELAND (1976-80)					
CONNAUGHT					
R07	21	4.9	4.3	0.97	112
R12	3	4.0	3.6	2.21	177
R16	15	5.1	4.3	1.19	112
R20	8	5.6	4.3	1.67	112
R21	8	5.8	5.1	1.83	47
R-A	55	5.1	4.3	0.62	
LEINSTER					
R01	1	1.0	0.6--	0.59	354
R06	132	5.6	6.1++	0.53	10
R09	12	4.7	5.4	1.57	24
R10	13	7.3	6.3	1.77	7
R11	7	5.3	5.1	1.96	47
R14	3	3.7	3.2	1.89	225
R15	6	2.8	2.9	1.17	256
R17	13	5.6	5.4	1.52	24
R19	6	4.0	3.8	1.59	164
R24	5	3.3	3.1	1.40	232
R25	12	4.9	4.5	1.33	92
R26	12	5.7	6.0	1.75	13
R-B	222	5.1	5.3++	0.36	
MUNSTER					
R03	7	3.2	3.1	1.18	232
R04	65	6.5	6.5++	0.82	5
R08	14	4.5	4.0	1.10	137
R13	19	4.8	4.9	1.13	59
R22	13	3.8	4.0	1.12	137
R23	11	5.0	5.1	1.55	47
R-C	129	5.2	5.1++	0.46	
ULSTER					
R02	3	2.1	1.5--	0.86	353
R05	19	6.1	5.8	1.37	16
R18	5	3.8	3.7	1.70	169
R-D	27	4.6	4.2	0.84	
R.0	433	5.1	5.0++	0.24	
LUXEMBOURG (1971-80)					
LE	10	5.5	4.9	1.67	59
LN	16	6.1	5.0	1.32	53
LS	66	5.2	4.3	0.54	112
L.0	92	5.3	4.5	0.48	
NEDERLAND (1976-80)					
N01	57	4.2	3.7	0.51	169
N02	67	4.7	4.4	0.56	102
N03	53	5.1	4.9	0.70	59
N04	121	4.8	4.7+	0.43	74
N05	175	4.2	4.0	0.31	137
N06	80	3.7	3.6	0.41	177
N07	294	5.1	4.5++	0.27	92
N08	398	5.3	4.7++	0.24	74
N09	48	5.7	5.3+	0.77	31
N10	196	3.9	4.0	0.29	137
N11	124	4.7	4.5+	0.41	92
N.0	1613	4.7	4.4++	0.11	
EEC-9					
EEC	32527	4.3	3.7	0.02	

BELGIE-BELGIQUE (1971-78)					
BRUSSEL-BRUXELLES					
B21	227	5.1	3.2++	0.25	80
VLAANDEREN					
B10	564	8.9	6.5++	0.29	1
B29	150	4.1	3.2++	0.28	80
B30	242	5.6	4.4++	0.30	8
B40	333	6.2	4.4++	0.26	8
B70	101	3.7	3.7++	0.38	35
B-V	1390	6.2	4.8++	0.14	
WALLONIE					
B25	37	3.5	2.5	0.43	165
B50	267	4.9	3.7++	0.25	35
B60	205	4.9	3.6++	0.28	44
B80	29	3.2	2.4	0.47	174
B90	82	5.1	3.9++	0.48	25
B-W	620	4.7	3.5++	0.15	
B.0	2237	5.6	4.1++	0.10	
BR DEUTSCHLAND (1976-80)					
BADEN-WURTTEMBERG					
D81	174	2.0	1.5--	0.12	308
D82	115	1.9	1.4--	0.14	325
D83	104	2.1	1.7--	0.18	280
D84	79	2.0	1.8--	0.22	251
D-A	472	2.0	1.5--	0.08	
BAYERN					
D91	235	2.5	1.8--	0.14	251
D92	56	2.1	1.8-	0.28	251
D93	48	1.9	1.3--	0.20	331
D94	54	1.9	1.5--	0.25	308
D95	101	2.5	2.0-	0.23	213
D96	86	2.8	2.2	0.26	190
D97	101	2.5	1.9--	0.21	228
D-B	681	2.4	1.8--	0.08	
BERLIN (WEST)					
DB0	254	4.8	3.6++	0.30	44
BREMEN					
D40	92	5.0	3.5+	0.43	53
HAMBURG					
D20	159	3.6	2.2	0.20	190
HESSEN					
D64	268	2.4	1.8--	0.12	251
D66	81	2.6	1.9-	0.25	228
D-F	349	2.4	1.8--	0.11	
NIEDERSACHSEN					
D31	105	2.4	1.8--	0.19	251
D32	141	2.6	1.9--	0.19	228
D33	100	2.7	1.9-	0.21	228
D34	158	2.9	2.3	0.20	184
D-G	504	2.7	2.0--	0.10	
NORDRHEIN-WESTFALEN					
D51	311	2.3	1.8--	0.11	251
D53	224	2.2	1.8--	0.13	251
D55	121	1.9	1.6--	0.15	295
D57	124	2.6	1.9--	0.19	228
D59	230	2.4	1.8--	0.13	251
D-H	1010	2.3	1.8--	0.06	
RHEINLAND-PFALZ					
D71	69	1.9	1.5--	0.20	308
D72	24	1.9	1.5--	0.35	308
D73	103	2.2	1.7--	0.19	280
D-I	196	2.1	1.6--	0.13	
SAARLAND					
DA0	144	5.1	3.6++	0.35	44
SCHLESWIG-HOLSTEIN					
D10	198	2.9	2.2	0.18	190
D.0	4059	2.5	1.9--	0.03	
DANMARK (1971-80)					
K15	373	5.6	3.8++	0.23	27
K20	63	4.2	3.8++	0.50	27
K25	41	4.5	4.4++	0.70	8
K30	79	5.9	4.6++	0.56	5
K35	60	4.7	3.6+	0.49	44
K40	10	4.3	3.7	1.25	35
K42	133	5.9	4.6++	0.43	5
K50	56	4.6	4.1++	0.58	17
K55	45	4.4	4.2++	0.66	12
K60	79	5.0	4.1++	0.48	17
K65	66	5.3	4.5++	0.57	7
K70	149	5.3	4.2++	0.37	12
K76	55	4.9	4.1++	0.60	17
K80	117	5.0	3.7++	0.37	35
K.0	1326	5.2	4.1++	0.12	
FRANCE (1971-78)					
ALSACE					
F67	64	1.8	1.5--	0.20	308
F68	47	1.8	1.5--	0.23	308
F-A	111	1.8	1.5--	0.15	
AQUITAINE					
F24	36	2.4	2.1	0.42	202
F33	110	2.5	1.8--	0.19	251
F40	30	2.6	1.8	0.36	251
F47	27	2.3	1.6--	0.32	295
F64	58	2.6	1.8--	0.26	251
F-B	261	2.5	1.8--	0.12	
AUVERGNE					
F03	31	2.0	1.8-	0.36	251
F15	15	2.2	2.0	0.59	213
F43	11	1.3	0.9--	0.35	348
F63	49	2.1	1.8-	0.29	251
F-C	106	1.9	1.7--	0.18	
BASSE-NORMANDIE					
F14	39	1.7	1.4--	0.24	325
F50	35	1.9	1.5--	0.28	308
F61	21	1.7	1.3--	0.32	331
F-D	95	1.8	1.4--	0.16	
BOURGOGNE					
F21	31	1.7	1.4--	0.27	325
F58	25	2.5	1.8	0.43	251
F71	51	2.2	1.8-	0.29	251
F89	31	2.5	2.0	0.40	213
F-E	138	2.2	1.7--	0.16	
BRETAGNE					
F22	28	1.3	0.8--	0.17	351
F29	83	2.5	2.0-	0.24	213
F35	46	1.6	1.5--	0.24	308
F56	37	1.6	1.4--	0.26	325
F-F	194	1.8	1.5--	0.12	
CENTRE					
F18	32	2.5	1.9	0.38	228
F28	26	1.9	1.6--	0.32	295
F36	17	1.7	1.4--	0.37	325
F37	32	1.6	1.3--	0.25	331
F41	23	2.0	1.7-	0.38	280
F45	44	2.2	1.9-	0.30	228
F-G	174	2.0	1.6--	0.13	
CHAMPAGNE-ARDENNE					
F08	27	2.2	2.0	0.40	213
F10	27	2.3	1.8	0.37	251
F51	39	1.8	1.6--	0.27	295
F52	15	1.8	1.6	0.44	295
F-H	108	2.0	1.8--	0.18	
CORSE					
F20	11	1.3	1.2--	0.42	340
FRANCHE-COMTE					
F25	33	1.7	1.7-	0.30	280
F39	21	2.2	2.1	0.48	202
F70	15	1.7	1.3--	0.37	331
F90	11	2.1	2.0	0.65	213
F-J	80	1.9	1.7--	0.20	
HAUTE-NORMANDIE					
F27	34	2.0	1.7-	0.31	280
F76	80	1.7	1.5--	0.18	308
F-K	114	1.8	1.6--	0.16	
ILE-DE-FRANCE					
F75	299	3.0	2.0--	0.14	213
F77	53	1.7	1.6--	0.23	295
F78	81	1.9	1.8--	0.20	251
F91	67	1.8	1.7--	0.22	280
F92	153	2.6	1.9--	0.17	228
F93	117	2.2	1.9--	0.19	228
F94	119	2.4	2.0-	0.19	213
F95	60	1.8	1.7--	0.23	280
F-L	949	2.3	1.9--	0.07	
LANGUEDOC-ROUSSILLON					
F11	24	2.1	1.5--	0.33	308
F30	52	2.6	1.9	0.33	228
F34	74	2.7	1.9-	0.26	228
F48	6	2.0	1.6	0.84	295
F66	36	2.9	2.0	0.41	213
F-M	192	2.6	1.9--	0.16	
LIMOUSIN					
F19	18	1.8	1.3--	0.35	331
F23	20	3.3	2.8	0.75	122
F87	54	3.7	2.7	0.39	136
F-N	92	3.0	2.2	0.26	
LORRAINE					
F54	52	1.8	1.7--	0.24	280
F55	12	1.5	1.5-	0.47	308
F57	58	1.5	1.3--	0.18	331
F88	33	2.0	1.8-	0.33	251
F-O	155	1.7	1.5--	0.13	
MIDI-PYRENEES					
F09	12	2.1	1.5-	0.47	308
F12	18	1.6	1.1--	0.29	342
F31	79	2.5	1.9--	0.23	228
F32	22	3.1	2.2	0.51	190
F46	19	3.1	2.2	0.56	190
F65	20	2.1	1.8	0.47	251
F81	32	2.3	1.7-	0.36	280
F82	9	1.2	0.9--	0.31	348
F-P	211	2.3	1.7--	0.13	
NORD-PAS-DE-CALAIS					
F59	180	1.8	1.6--	0.13	295
F62	85	1.5	1.4--	0.16	325
F-Q	265	1.7	1.5--	0.10	
PAYS DE LA LOIRE					
F44	72	1.9	1.6--	0.20	295
F49	35	1.3	1.0--	0.18	343
F53	23	2.1	1.8	0.42	251
F72	54	2.7	2.2	0.31	190
F85	29	1.6	1.5--	0.31	308
F-R	213	1.9	1.6--	0.12	
PICARDIE					
F02	52	2.4	2.0	0.31	213
F60	54	2.2	2.1	0.30	202
F80	42	1.9	1.5--	0.26	308
F-S	148	2.2	1.9--	0.17	
POITOU-CHARENTES					
F16	31	2.2	1.9	0.40	228
F17	59	2.9	2.3	0.33	184
F79	29	2.1	1.7-	0.34	280
F86	29	2.0	1.5--	0.32	308
F-T	148	2.4	1.9--	0.17	
PROVENCE-ALPES-COTE D'AZUR					
F04	7	1.6	1.0--	0.46	343
F05	8	2.0	1.5	0.55	308
F06	48	1.4	1.0--	0.21	343
F13	134	2.0	1.6--	0.15	295
F83	54	2.1	1.9	0.31	228
F84	34	2.1	1.8	0.34	251
F-U	285	1.9	1.5--	0.10	
RHONE-ALPES					
F01	28	1.9	1.6--	0.33	295
F07	37	3.5	2.6	0.50	152
F26	37	2.5	2.2	0.40	190
F38	68	2.0	1.6--	0.21	295
F42	64	2.1	1.5--	0.21	308
F69	158	2.7	2.1	0.18	202
F73	25	2.0	1.7-	0.35	280
F74	36	2.0	1.9	0.33	228
F-V	453	2.3	1.9--	0.10	
F.0	4503	2.1	1.7--	0.03	
UNITED KINGDOM (1976-80)					
EAST ANGLIA					
G25	76	4.5	3.7++	0.45	35
G46	77	3.7	2.9	0.35	110
G55	67	3.8	2.7	0.36	136
G-A	220	4.0	3.0++	0.22	
EAST MIDLANDS					
G30	84	3.1	2.4	0.28	174
G44	71	2.8	2.3	0.29	184
G45	46	2.9	2.4	0.37	174
G47	72	4.6	3.8++	0.48	27
G50	106	3.6	2.8	0.30	122
G-B	379	3.3	2.7	0.15	
NORTHERN					
G14	121	3.3	2.7	0.27	136
G27	70	4.0	3.4+	0.42	63
G29	51	3.5	3.0	0.46	95
G33	59	3.2	2.8	0.39	122
G48	34	3.8	3.3	0.62	72
G-C	335	3.5	2.9++	0.17	
NORTH-WEST					
G11	276	3.3	2.7	0.17	136
G12	167	3.4	2.9	0.24	110
G26	93	3.3	2.8	0.31	122
G43	154	3.6	2.9	0.25	110
G-D	690	3.4	2.8++	0.11	

SOUTH-EAST					
G01	934	4.3	3.2++	0.12	80
G22	51	3.5	3.0	0.43	95
G23	66	3.3	2.8	0.37	122
G24	64	4.1	3.5+	0.46	53
G34	95	4.4	2.9	0.38	110
G35	161	3.7	3.0+	0.25	95
G37	193	4.5	3.5++	0.26	53
G39	94	3.2	2.6	0.29	152
G41	14	3.9	4.0	1.23	20
G42	166	3.7	2.8	0.24	122
G51	89	5.7	4.8++	0.53	3
G56	144	4.7	3.4++	0.31	63
G58	88	4.4	3.0	0.37	95
G-E	2159	4.1	3.2++	0.07	
SOUTH-WEST					
G21	126	4.4	3.0+	0.29	95
G28	53	4.1	3.2	0.47	80
G31	128	4.4	3.0	0.31	95
G32	92	5.0	3.7++	0.45	35
G36	62	4.1	2.9	0.40	110
G53	63	5.0	3.7+	0.51	35
G59	64	4.2	3.3	0.44	72
G-F	588	4.4	3.2++	0.15	
WEST MIDLANDS					
G15	268	3.2	2.7	0.18	136
G38	81	4.4	3.6++	0.42	44
G52	36	3.2	2.8	0.51	122
G54	122	4.0	3.2+	0.31	80
G57	35	2.5	1.9	0.34	228
G-G	542	3.5	2.9++	0.13	
YORKSHIRE AND HUMBERSIDE					
G13	147	3.7	3.1+	0.28	88
G16	226	3.5	2.9+	0.21	110
G40	114	4.4	3.8++	0.39	27
G49	75	3.7	3.1	0.41	88
G-H	562	3.7	3.2++	0.14	
WALES					
G61	50	4.2	3.8+	0.58	27
G62	48	4.7	4.0+	0.64	20
G63	41	3.0	2.6	0.44	152
G64	29	4.1	3.5	0.71	53
G65	34	2.1	1.9	0.35	228
G66	3	0.9	0.7--	0.40	353
G67	47	3.9	2.8	0.45	122
G68	28	2.4	1.8	0.36	251
G-I	280	3.3	2.7	0.18	
SCOTLAND(1975-80)					
S01	25	4.4	4.4+	0.98	8
S02	61	4.3	3.4+	0.46	63
S03	50	4.0	2.8	0.44	122
S04	36	3.5	3.2	0.56	80
S05	117	4.9	3.8++	0.38	27
S06	15	4.8	3.6	1.01	44
S07	30	3.6	2.9	0.55	110
S08	283	3.7	3.0++	0.19	95
S09	13	3.0	2.6	0.81	152
S10	2	3.7	4.2	3.00	12
S11	2	3.3	1.3	0.98	331
S12	2	2.2	0.9--	0.62	348
G-J	636	3.9	3.2++	0.14	
NORTHERN IRELAND					
JE	69	4.1	3.6++	0.46	44
JN	34	3.7	3.3	0.59	72
JS	8	1.2	1.0--	0.38	343
JW	27	4.4	3.7	0.76	35
G-K	138	3.5	3.1+	0.28	
G.0	6529	3.8	3.0++	0.04	
ITALIA (1975-79)					
ABRUZZI					
I66	26	3.4	2.9	0.64	110
I67	25	3.7	3.0	0.62	95
I68	19	2.6	1.8	0.44	251
I69	22	2.4	1.9	0.43	228
I-A	92	3.0	2.3	0.26	
BASILICATA					
I76	17	1.6	1.3--	0.33	331
I77	10	2.0	2.0	0.62	213
I-B	27	1.7	1.5--	0.30	
CALABRIA					
I78	40	2.2	2.1	0.33	202
I79	35	1.9	1.9	0.33	228
I80	38	2.5	2.4	0.40	174
I-C	113	2.2	2.1	0.20	
CAMPANIA					
I61	46	2.5	2.2	0.34	190
I62	20	2.7	2.1	0.48	202
I63	187	2.6	2.4	0.18	174
I64	32	2.9	2.5	0.46	165
I65	56	2.2	2.0	0.28	213
I-D	341	2.5	2.3	0.13	
EMILIA-ROMAGNA					
I33	36	5.0	3.3	0.64	72
I34	50	4.9	3.3	0.54	72
I35	51	5.0	3.3	0.51	72
I36	55	3.7	2.7	0.39	136
I37	106	4.4	3.0	0.31	95
I38	37	3.7	2.8	0.51	122
I39	32	3.5	2.5	0.50	165
I40	63	4.2	3.2	0.43	80
I-E	430	4.3	3.0++	0.16	
FRIULI-VENEZIA GIULIA					
I30	63	4.6	3.5+	0.51	53
I31	17	4.5	2.8	0.80	122
I32	49	6.1	3.4	0.54	63
I93	29	4.2	3.4	0.68	63
I-F	158	4.9	3.4++	0.31	
LAZIO					
I56	20	3.0	2.7	0.66	136
I57	8	2.2	1.7	0.64	280
I58	333	3.5	3.0++	0.17	95
I59	26	2.5	2.5	0.49	165
I60	30	2.6	2.2	0.42	190
I-G	417	3.3	2.8+	0.14	
LIGURIA					
I08	20	3.3	2.4	0.66	174
I09	44	5.6	3.6	0.67	44
I10	126	4.4	2.7	0.27	136
I11	18	2.8	1.8	0.47	251
I-H	208	4.3	2.7	0.22	
LOMBARDIA					
I12	88	4.4	3.3+	0.36	72
I13	47	2.4	1.8-	0.28	251
I14	9	2.1	1.9	0.65	228
I15	375	3.6	2.8+	0.15	122
I16	51	2.3	2.0	0.28	213
I17	88	3.5	3.0	0.33	95
I18	65	4.8	3.5+	0.51	53
I19	36	4.2	2.9	0.55	110
I20	49	5.0	3.3	0.49	72
I-I	808	3.5	2.7++	0.10	
MARCHE					
I41	38	4.6	3.4	0.57	63
I42	41	3.7	2.9	0.48	110
I43	23	3.1	2.3	0.54	184
I44	33	3.7	3.1	0.57	88
I-J	135	3.8	2.9	0.27	
MOLISE					
I70	18	3.0	2.4	0.60	174
I94	6	2.5	2.6	1.15	152
I-K	24	2.9	2.4	0.54	
PIEMONTE					
I01	202	3.3	2.7	0.21	136
I02	36	3.4	2.4	0.51	174
I03	47	3.6	2.5	0.41	165
I04	50	3.6	2.6	0.41	152
I05	21	3.7	2.6	0.63	152
I06	54	4.4	2.7	0.46	136
I-L	410	3.5	2.7	0.15	
PUGLIA					
I71	41	2.4	2.3	0.36	184
I72	118	3.3	3.0	0.28	95
I73	37	2.7	2.4	0.40	174
I74	28	2.8	2.6	0.50	152
I75	62	3.2	2.9	0.38	110
I-M	286	3.0	2.7	0.16	
SARDEGNA					
I90	32	3.0	2.7	0.49	136
I91	9	1.3	1.2--	0.39	340
I92	36	2.0	1.9	0.32	228
I95	10	2.6	2.0	0.69	213
I-N	87	2.2	2.0-	0.22	
SICILIA					
I81	27	2.5	2.2	0.45	190
I82	70	2.3	2.1	0.26	202
I83	38	2.2	1.7--	0.29	280
I84	25	2.1	1.9	0.39	228
I85	9	1.2	1.0--	0.35	343
I86	17	3.3	2.7	0.68	136
I87	58	2.3	2.1	0.28	202
I88	18	2.6	1.8	0.46	251
I89	28	2.9	2.5	0.48	165
I-O	290	2.3	2.0--	0.12	
TOSCANA					
I45	20	3.8	3.5	0.86	53
I46	32	3.2	2.1	0.42	202
I47	31	4.6	3.5	0.73	53
I48	135	4.4	3.1+	0.30	88
I49	26	2.9	1.8	0.39	251
I50	34	3.5	2.8	0.53	122
I51	23	2.9	2.2	0.49	190
I52	21	3.2	2.0	0.52	213
I53	20	3.6	2.1	0.48	202
I-P	342	3.7	2.7	0.16	
TRENTINO-ALTO ADIGE					
I21	24	2.2	1.8	0.38	251
I22	31	2.8	2.1	0.41	202
I-Q	55	2.5	1.9	0.28	
UMBRIA					
I54	53	3.7	2.5	0.40	165
I55	23	4.0	2.6	0.60	152
I-R	76	3.8	2.6	0.34	
VALLE D'AOSTA					
I07	7	2.5	1.8	0.82	251
VENETO					
I23	71	3.6	2.7	0.33	136
I24	63	3.5	3.0	0.41	95
I25	19	3.3	2.6	0.65	152
I26	51	2.8	2.2	0.33	190
I27	94	4.4	3.5++	0.38	53
I28	86	4.2	3.6++	0.41	44
I29	14	2.2	1.7	0.48	280
I-T	398	3.6	2.9++	0.16	
I.0	4704	3.3	2.6++	0.04	
IRELAND (1976-80)					
CONNAUGHT					
R07	16	3.9	3.8	0.96	27
R12	3	4.6	5.0	2.92	2
R16	12	4.3	4.0	1.25	20
R20	4	3.1	2.6	1.30	152
R21	2	1.5	0.7--	0.52	353
R-A	37	3.7	3.3	0.57	
LEINSTER					
R01	1	1.1	0.8-	0.81	351
R06	102	4.0	3.9++	0.39	25
R09	8	3.4	3.7	1.32	35
R10	5	3.0	2.8	1.29	122
R11	1	0.8	0.7-	0.75	353
R14	3	4.1	4.7	2.76	4
R15	3	1.4	1.3	0.76	331
R17	6	2.7	2.7	1.11	136
R19	3	2.2	2.7	1.58	136
R24	3	2.0	1.9	1.09	228
R25	10	4.2	4.0	1.30	20
R26	8	3.8	3.4	1.25	63
R-B	153	3.5	3.3++	0.27	
MUNSTER					
R03	8	3.9	4.2	1.56	12
R04	39	4.0	3.5	0.58	53
R08	5	1.7	1.6	0.75	295
R13	11	2.8	3.0	0.94	95
R22	13	4.0	4.2	1.21	12
R23	8	3.7	3.8	1.37	27
R-C	84	3.5	3.3+	0.38	
ULSTER					
R02	5	3.9	3.1	1.44	88
R05	8	2.7	3.2	1.14	80
R18	3	2.5	2.7	1.59	136
R-D	16	2.9	3.0	0.78	
R.0	290	3.5	3.3++	0.20	
LUXEMBOURG (1971-80)					
LE	5	2.6	1.7	0.83	280
LN	8	3.0	2.6	0.97	152
LS	45	3.3	2.5	0.38	165
L.0	58	3.2	2.4	0.33	
NEDERLAND (1976-80)					
N01	54	3.9	3.4	0.49	63
N02	43	3.0	2.5	0.40	165
N03	49	4.8	4.0++	0.60	20
N04	92	3.7	3.4++	0.37	63
N05	144	3.4	3.1+	0.27	88
N06	58	2.6	2.4	0.34	174
N07	221	3.7	2.9+	0.21	110
N08	298	3.8	3.1++	0.19	88
N09	25	2.9	2.3	0.50	184
N10	157	3.1	3.0+	0.24	95
N11	77	2.9	2.6	0.31	152
N.0	1218	3.5	3.0++	0.09	
EEC-9					
EEC	24924	3.1	2.5	0.02	

BELGIE-BELGIQUE (1971-78)

BRUSSEL-BRUXELLES					
B21	27	0.7	0.4	0.08	153
VLAANDEREN					
B10	33	0.5	0.4	0.07	153
B29	17	0.5	0.3	0.08	226
B30	15	0.4	0.2--	0.06	295
B40	28	0.5	0.4	0.07	153
B70	2	0.1	0.1--	0.05	336
B-V	95	0.4	0.3--	0.03	
WALLONIE					
B25	4	0.4	0.3	0.14	226
B50	31	0.6	0.4	0.08	153
B60	18	0.5	0.3-	0.07	226
B80	6	0.7	0.5	0.23	100
B90	7	0.5	0.3	0.13	226
B-W	66	0.5	0.4-	0.05	
B.0	188	0.5	0.3--	0.03	

BR DEUTSCHLAND (1976-80)

BADEN-WURTTEMBERG					
D81	84	1.0	0.8++	0.09	30
D82	67	1.2	0.9++	0.11	20
D83	76	1.7	1.2++	0.15	12
D84	47	1.3	1.0++	0.15	14
D-A	274	1.2	0.9++	0.06	
BAYERN					
D91	111	1.3	0.9++	0.09	20
D92	44	1.9	1.4++	0.22	6
D93	22	1.0	0.7	0.16	44
D94	33	1.3	0.8+	0.15	30
D95	39	1.1	0.7+	0.12	44
D96	23	0.8	0.6	0.13	62
D97	54	1.5	1.0++	0.15	14
D-B	326	1.3	0.9++	0.05	
BERLIN(WEST)					
DB0	33	0.8	0.4	0.07	153
BREMEN					
D40	13	0.8	0.5	0.16	100
HAMBURG					
D20	34	0.9	0.5	0.09	100
HESSEN					
D64	80	0.8	0.6	0.06	62
D66	26	0.9	0.6	0.12	62
D-F	106	0.8	0.6	0.06	
NIEDERSACHSEN					
D31	27	0.7	0.4	0.09	153
D32	38	0.8	0.5	0.08	100
D33	22	0.6	0.4	0.10	153
D34	28	0.6	0.4	0.08	153
D-G	115	0.7	0.4	0.04	
NORDRHEIN-WESTFALEN					
D51	85	0.7	0.5	0.06	100
D53	58	0.6	0.5	0.07	100
D55	28	0.5	0.4	0.08	153
D57	21	0.5	0.3	0.07	226
D59	57	0.6	0.5	0.07	100
D-H	249	0.6	0.5	0.03	
RHEINLAND-PFALZ					
D71	32	1.0	0.7	0.13	44
D72	9	0.8	0.5	0.18	100
D73	38	0.9	0.6	0.10	62
D-I	79	0.9	0.6+	0.07	
SAARLAND					
DA0	27	1.1	0.7	0.14	44
SCHLESWIG-HOLSTEIN					
D10	34	0.5	0.4	0.07	153
D.0	1290	0.9	0.6++	0.02	

DANMARK (1971-80)

K15	57	0.9	0.6	0.08	62
K20	9	0.6	0.5	0.18	100
K25	4	0.4	0.4	0.22	153
K30	12	0.9	0.6	0.16	62
K35	15	1.2	0.6	0.15	62
K40	2	0.8	0.5	0.33	100
K42	14	0.6	0.4	0.11	153
K50	7	0.6	0.5	0.19	100
K55	5	0.5	0.4	0.18	153
K60	14	0.9	0.6	0.17	62
K65	16	1.2	0.9	0.23	20
K70	14	0.5	0.4	0.10	153
K76	3	0.3	0.1--	0.06	336
K80	20	0.8	0.5	0.13	100
K.0	192	0.8	0.5	0.04	

FRANCE (1971-78)

ALSACE					
F67	43	1.2	1.0++	0.16	14
F68	18	0.7	0.6	0.14	62
F-A	61	1.0	0.8++	0.11	
AQUITAINE					
F24	5	0.3	0.2--	0.08	295
F33	14	0.3	0.3--	0.07	226
F40	3	0.3	0.2-	0.12	295
F47	4	0.4	0.2-	0.11	295
F64	9	0.4	0.3	0.10	226
F-B	35	0.4	0.2--	0.04	
AUVERGNE					
F03	10	0.7	0.4	0.12	153
F15	7	1.1	0.6	0.25	62
F43	3	0.4	0.2-	0.11	295
F63	10	0.4	0.3	0.10	226
F-C	30	0.6	0.4	0.07	
BASSE-NORMANDIE					
F14	13	0.6	0.6	0.17	62
F50	6	0.3	0.2-	0.09	295
F61	5	0.4	0.3	0.13	226
F-D	24	0.5	0.4	0.08	
BOURGOGNE					
F21	17	0.9	0.8	0.20	30
F58	6	0.6	0.4	0.18	153
F71	15	0.7	0.5	0.13	100
F89	8	0.7	0.5	0.20	100
F-E	46	0.7	0.6	0.09	
BRETAGNE					
F22	8	0.4	0.3	0.11	226
F29	16	0.5	0.4	0.09	153
F35	10	0.4	0.3	0.09	226
F56	7	0.3	0.2-	0.10	295
F-F	41	0.4	0.3--	0.05	
CENTRE					
F18	11	0.9	0.7	0.22	44
F28	10	0.7	0.5	0.15	100
F36	4	0.4	0.2--	0.08	295
F37	7	0.4	0.3-	0.10	226
F41	5	0.5	0.4	0.17	153
F45	9	0.5	0.3	0.12	226
F-G	46	0.5	0.4	0.06	
CHAMPAGNE-ARDENNE					
F08	11	0.9	0.6	0.20	62
F10	4	0.4	0.3	0.16	226
F51	8	0.4	0.4	0.13	153
F52	8	0.9	0.9	0.32	20
F-H	31	0.6	0.5	0.09	
CORSE					
F20	5	0.5	0.4	0.18	153
FRANCHE-COMTE					
F25	8	0.4	0.4	0.14	153
F39	4	0.4	0.3	0.14	226
F70	8	0.9	0.7	0.26	44
F90	3	0.6	0.6	0.34	62
F-J	23	0.5	0.5	0.10	
HAUTE-NORMANDIE					
F27	12	0.7	0.5	0.15	100
F76	12	0.3	0.2--	0.06	295
F-K	24	0.4	0.3--	0.06	
ILE-DE-FRANCE					
F75	63	0.7	0.5	0.06	100
F77	15	0.5	0.4	0.12	153
F78	12	0.3	0.3-	0.08	226
F91	8	0.2	0.2--	0.08	295
F92	33	0.6	0.5	0.08	100
F93	21	0.4	0.4	0.08	153
F94	28	0.6	0.5	0.10	100
F95	12	0.4	0.4	0.11	153
F-L	192	0.5	0.4	0.03	
LANGUEDOC-ROUSSILLON					
F11	13	1.2	0.8	0.25	30
F30	10	0.5	0.3	0.11	226
F34	16	0.6	0.4	0.11	153
F48	0	0.0	0.0--	0.00	346
F66	9	0.8	0.4	0.15	153
F-M	48	0.7	0.4	0.07	
LIMOUSIN					
F19	7	0.7	0.3	0.15	226
F23	5	0.9	0.5	0.23	100
F87	13	1.0	0.5	0.14	100
F-N	25	0.9	0.4	0.09	
LORRAINE					
F54	18	0.6	0.6	0.13	62
F55	2	0.2	0.2	0.18	295
F57	29	0.7	0.6	0.12	62
F88	11	0.7	0.5	0.16	100
F-O	60	0.6	0.5	0.07	
MIDI-PYRENEES					
F09	8	1.5	0.8	0.30	30
F12	4	0.4	0.3	0.15	226
F31	20	0.7	0.5	0.11	100
F32	6	0.9	0.6	0.26	62
F46	3	0.5	0.2--	0.10	295
F65	10	1.1	0.7	0.22	44
F81	12	0.9	0.5	0.15	100
F82	5	0.7	0.4	0.17	153
F-P	68	0.8	0.5	0.06	
NORD-PAS-DE-CALAIS					
F59	52	0.5	0.5	0.07	100
F62	22	0.4	0.4	0.08	153
F-Q	74	0.5	0.4	0.05	
PAYS DE LA LOIRE					
F44	12	0.3	0.3	0.09	226
F49	8	0.3	0.2-	0.09	295
F53	8	0.8	0.6	0.23	62
F72	9	0.5	0.4	0.13	153
F85	7	0.4	0.3-	0.10	226
F-R	44	0.4	0.3--	0.05	
PICARDIE					
F02	13	0.6	0.5	0.15	100
F60	7	0.3	0.3	0.10	226
F80	13	0.6	0.5	0.15	100
F-S	33	0.5	0.4	0.08	
POITOU-CHARENTES					
F16	2	0.2	0.1--	0.09	336
F17	7	0.4	0.2-	0.10	295
F79	7	0.5	0.4	0.16	153
F86	9	0.6	0.5	0.16	100
F-T	25	0.4	0.3-	0.06	
PROVENCE-ALPES-COTE D'AZUR					
F04	2	0.4	0.3	0.23	226
F05	1	0.3	0.2	0.17	295
F06	19	0.6	0.3	0.09	226
F13	40	0.6	0.5	0.08	100
F83	24	1.0	0.6	0.13	62
F84	14	0.9	0.6	0.18	62
F-U	100	0.7	0.5	0.05	
RHONE-ALPES					
F01	8	0.5	0.4	0.14	153
F07	10	1.0	0.6	0.22	62
F26	7	0.5	0.3	0.10	226
F38	19	0.6	0.5	0.11	100
F42	17	0.6	0.5	0.11	100
F69	35	0.6	0.5	0.09	100
F73	14	1.2	0.9	0.24	20
F74	16	0.9	0.7	0.19	44
F-V	126	0.7	0.5	0.05	
F.0	1161	0.6	0.4--	0.01	

UNITED KINGDOM (1976-80)

EAST ANGLIA					
G25	5	0.3	0.3	0.11	226
G46	9	0.5	0.3	0.10	226
G55	8	0.5	0.3	0.11	226
G-A	22	0.4	0.3--	0.06	
EAST MIDLANDS					
G30	16	0.6	0.4	0.10	153
G44	11	0.4	0.4	0.12	153
G45	10	0.6	0.4	0.14	153
G47	7	0.5	0.3	0.12	226
G50	11	0.4	0.3-	0.08	226
G-B	55	0.5	0.3-	0.05	
NORTHERN					
G14	19	0.6	0.4	0.09	153
G27	8	0.5	0.4	0.13	153
G29	3	0.2	0.2--	0.10	295
G33	11	0.6	0.4	0.12	153
G48	3	0.4	0.2-	0.11	295
G-C	44	0.5	0.3--	0.05	
NORTH-WEST					
G11	40	0.5	0.4	0.06	153
G12	21	0.5	0.3	0.07	226
G26	13	0.5	0.3	0.10	226
G43	20	0.5	0.3	0.08	226
G-D	94	0.5	0.3--	0.04	

SOUTH-EAST					
G01	84	0.4	0.3--	0.03	226
G22	5	0.3	0.3	0.13	226
G23	6	0.3	0.2-	0.10	295
G24	4	0.3	0.2--	0.09	295
G34	15	0.8	0.4	0.11	153
G35	14	0.3	0.3--	0.07	226
G37	21	0.5	0.4	0.09	153
G39	16	0.6	0.4	0.11	153
G41	1	0.3	0.3	0.27	226
G42	19	0.5	0.3--	0.07	226
G51	4	0.2	0.2--	0.09	295
G56	13	0.4	0.3-	0.08	226
G58	8	0.5	0.3	0.11	226
G-E	210	0.4	0.3--	0.02	
SOUTH-WEST					
G21	7	0.3	0.2--	0.07	295
G28	6	0.5	0.3-	0.11	226
G31	17	0.6	0.4	0.10	153
G32	14	0.8	0.4	0.10	153
G36	7	0.5	0.3	0.12	226
G53	9	0.7	0.5	0.17	100
G59	6	0.4	0.3	0.12	226
G-F	66	0.5	0.3--	0.04	
WEST MIDLANDS					
G15	42	0.5	0.4	0.06	153
G38	9	0.5	0.4	0.12	153
G52	4	0.4	0.2	0.13	295
G54	12	0.4	0.3	0.09	226
G57	3	0.2	0.2--	0.10	295
G-G	70	0.5	0.3--	0.04	
YORKSHIRE AND HUMBERSIDE					
G13	21	0.5	0.4	0.09	153
G16	25	0.4	0.3--	0.06	226
G40	13	0.5	0.4	0.10	153
G49	11	0.6	0.4	0.12	153
G-H	70	0.5	0.3--	0.04	
WALES					
G61	6	0.5	0.3	0.13	226
G62	7	0.7	0.4	0.17	153
G63	3	0.2	0.2-	0.12	295
G64	2	0.3	0.2-	0.13	295
G65	6	0.4	0.3	0.12	226
G66	3	0.9	0.4	0.24	153
G67	2	0.2	0.1--	0.07	336
G68	6	0.6	0.3	0.14	226
G-I	35	0.4	0.3--	0.05	
SCOTLAND(1975-80)					
S01	4	0.7	0.7	0.33	44
S02	7	0.5	0.3	0.11	226
S03	4	0.3	0.3	0.13	226
S04	3	0.3	0.2	0.14	295
S05	5	0.2	0.2--	0.08	295
S06	1	0.3	0.3	0.26	226
S07	3	0.4	0.4	0.21	153
S08	28	0.4	0.3--	0.06	226
S09	1	0.2	0.2-	0.15	295
S10	1	1.9	1.0	1.01	14
S11	0	0.0	0.0--	0.00	346
S12	0	0.0	0.0--	0.00	346
G-J	57	0.4	0.3--	0.04	
NORTHERN IRELAND					
JE	9	0.5	0.5	0.17	100
JN	4	0.4	0.4	0.18	153
JS	3	0.5	0.4	0.23	153
JW	3	0.5	0.4	0.24	153
G-K	19	0.5	0.4	0.10	
G.0	742	0.5	0.3--	0.01	
ITALIA (1975-79)					
ABRUZZI					
I66	7	1.0	0.7	0.28	44
I67	1	0.2	0.1--	0.12	336
I68	2	0.3	0.2	0.15	295
I69	2	0.2	0.1--	0.08	336
I-A	12	0.4	0.3-	0.09	
BASILICATA					
I76	3	0.3	0.2	0.15	295
I77	2	0.4	0.3	0.23	226
I-B	5	0.3	0.3	0.12	
CALABRIA					
I78	9	0.5	0.5	0.15	100
I79	8	0.4	0.4	0.14	153
I80	12	0.8	0.7	0.20	44
I-C	29	0.6	0.5	0.09	

CAMPANIA					
I61	5	0.3	0.3	0.12	226
I62	3	0.4	0.2	0.14	295
I63	37	0.5	0.6	0.09	62
I64	8	0.7	0.6	0.22	62
I65	12	0.5	0.4	0.12	153
I-D	65	0.5	0.5	0.06	
EMILIA-ROMAGNA					
I33	6	0.9	0.5	0.22	100
I34	8	0.8	0.6	0.21	62
I35	10	1.0	0.6	0.19	62
I36	9	0.6	0.4	0.15	153
I37	21	0.9	0.6	0.13	62
I38	5	0.5	0.4	0.16	153
I39	7	0.8	0.5	0.21	100
I40	18	1.2	0.9+	0.22	20
I-E	84	0.9	0.6	0.06	
FRIULI-VENEZIA GIULIA					
I30	20	1.6	1.0+	0.23	14
I31	1	0.3	0.2	0.16	295
I32	2	0.3	0.2	0.14	295
I93	4	0.6	0.5	0.23	100
I-F	27	0.9	0.6	0.12	
LAZIO					
I56	2	0.3	0.2-	0.14	295
I57	3	0.8	0.5	0.28	100
I58	57	0.6	0.6	0.08	62
I59	3	0.3	0.3	0.17	226
I60	2	0.2	0.1--	0.07	336
I-G	67	0.6	0.5	0.06	
LIGURIA					
I08	8	1.4	0.8	0.29	30
I09	10	1.4	0.9	0.31	20
I10	29	1.1	0.6	0.12	62
I11	5	0.8	0.5	0.24	100
I-H	52	1.2	0.7+	0.10	
LOMBARDIA					
I12	15	0.8	0.7	0.20	44
I13	9	0.5	0.4	0.13	153
I14	2	0.5	0.4	0.30	153
I15	95	1.0	0.9++	0.09	20
I16	19	0.9	0.8	0.18	30
I17	22	0.9	0.8	0.17	30
I18	9	0.7	0.4	0.13	153
I19	5	0.6	0.4	0.16	153
I20	12	1.3	0.9	0.26	20
I-I	188	0.9	0.7++	0.05	
MARCHE					
I41	7	0.9	0.6	0.22	62
I42	6	0.6	0.4	0.15	153
I43	6	0.8	0.6	0.24	62
I44	4	0.5	0.3	0.17	226
I-J	23	0.7	0.5	0.10	
MOLISE					
I70	1	0.2	0.1--	0.09	336
I94	1	0.4	0.3	0.34	226
I-K	2	0.2	0.2--	0.11	
PIEMONTE					
I01	54	0.9	0.7++	0.10	44
I02	13	1.3	0.8	0.24	30
I03	16	1.3	0.9+	0.24	20
I04	29	2.1	1.3++	0.25	8
I05	6	1.1	0.7	0.31	44
I06	6	0.5	0.3	0.11	226
I-L	124	1.1	0.8++	0.07	
PUGLIA					
I71	10	0.6	0.5	0.15	100
I72	21	0.6	0.5	0.12	100
I73	9	0.7	0.6	0.21	62
I74	5	0.5	0.5	0.22	100
I75	7	0.4	0.3	0.13	226
I-M	52	0.6	0.5	0.07	
SARDEGNA					
I90	1	0.1	0.1--	0.07	336
I91	6	0.9	0.7	0.31	44
I92	9	0.5	0.5	0.16	100
I95	3	0.8	0.6	0.36	62
I-N	19	0.5	0.4	0.10	
SICILIA					
I81	7	0.7	0.5	0.20	100
I82	13	0.5	0.4	0.11	153
I83	13	0.8	0.6	0.16	62
I84	5	0.4	0.3	0.14	226
I85	6	0.8	0.7	0.29	44
I86	3	0.6	0.4	0.25	153
I87	11	0.5	0.4	0.12	153
I88	3	0.5	0.4	0.24	153
I89	11	1.1	1.0	0.32	14
I-O	72	0.6	0.5	0.06	

TOSCANA					
I45	2	0.4	0.2	0.17	295
I46	10	1.1	0.7	0.23	44
I47	5	0.8	0.5	0.22	100
I48	24	0.8	0.6	0.12	62
I49	3	0.4	0.2-	0.12	295
I50	6	0.6	0.5	0.19	100
I51	5	0.6	0.4	0.20	153
I52	3	0.5	0.2	0.14	295
I53	3	0.5	0.3	0.18	226
I-P	61	0.7	0.5	0.06	
TRENTINO-ALTO ADIGE					
I21	18	1.7	1.4++	0.35	6
I22	23	2.1	1.6++	0.33	3
I-Q	41	1.9	1.5++	0.24	
UMBRIA					
I54	7	0.5	0.3	0.13	226
I55	1	0.2	0.1--	0.13	336
I-R	8	0.4	0.3	0.10	
VALLE D'AOSTA					
I07	6	2.1	1.6	0.65	3
VENETO					
I23	14	0.8	0.6	0.16	62
I24	13	0.7	0.6	0.17	62
I25	5	0.9	0.6	0.27	62
I26	13	0.8	0.6	0.18	62
I27	13	0.6	0.5	0.14	100
I28	12	0.6	0.5	0.15	100
I29	7	1.1	0.8	0.29	30
I-T	77	0.7	0.6	0.07	
I.0	1014	0.7	0.6++	0.02	
IRELAND (1976-80)					
CONNAUGHT					
R07	4	0.9	0.6	0.32	62
R12	1	1.3	1.3	1.32	8
R16	0	0.0	0.0--	0.00	346
R20	1	0.7	0.3	0.34	226
R21	0	0.0	0.0--	0.00	346
R-A	6	0.6	0.4	0.16	
LEINSTER					
R01	1	1.0	0.8	0.79	30
R06	9	0.4	0.5	0.16	100
R09	3	1.2	1.3	0.75	8
R10	1	0.6	0.3	0.31	226
R11	0	0.0	0.0--	0.00	346
R14	2	2.5	1.9	1.36	1
R15	2	0.9	0.8	0.55	30
R17	1	0.4	0.5	0.52	100
R19	0	0.0	0.0--	0.00	346
R24	1	0.7	0.8	0.84	30
R25	5	2.0	1.5	0.69	5
R26	0	0.0	0.0--	0.00	346
R-B	25	0.6	0.6	0.12	
MUNSTER					
R03	1	0.5	0.3	0.27	226
R04	4	0.4	0.3	0.18	226
R08	4	1.3	0.8	0.39	30
R13	1	0.3	0.2	0.17	295
R22	0	0.0	0.0--	0.00	346
R23	1	0.5	0.4	0.38	153
R-C	11	0.4	0.3	0.10	
ULSTER					
R02	2	1.4	1.1	0.77	13
R05	0	0.0	0.0--	0.00	346
R18	1	0.8	0.5	0.51	100
R-D	3	0.5	0.4	0.23	
R.0	45	0.5	0.4	0.07	
LUXEMBOURG (1971-80)					
LE	3	1.7	1.3	0.76	8
LN	7	2.7	1.7	0.66	2
LS	3	0.2	0.2-	0.11	295
L.0	13	0.8	0.6	0.16	
NEDERLAND (1976-80)					
N01	8	0.6	0.4	0.16	153
N02	8	0.6	0.3	0.12	226
N03	8	0.8	0.7	0.24	44
N04	5	0.2	0.2--	0.09	295
N05	15	0.4	0.3	0.08	226
N06	8	0.4	0.3	0.12	226
N07	34	0.6	0.4	0.08	153
N08	41	0.5	0.4	0.06	153
N09	2	0.2	0.2	0.14	295
N10	21	0.4	0.4	0.09	153
N11	13	0.5	0.5	0.13	100
N.0	163	0.5	0.4--	0.03	
EEC-9					
EEC	4808	0.6	0.5	0.01	

BELGIE-BELGIQUE (1971-78)

BRUSSEL-BRUXELLES					
B21	63	1.4	0.7	0.09	135
VLAANDEREN					
B10	79	1.3	0.7	0.09	135
B29	39	1.1	0.6	0.10	187
B30	44	1.0	0.5	0.09	239
B40	58	1.1	0.5-	0.08	239
B70	9	0.3	0.3--	0.09	332
B-V	229	1.0	0.6--	0.04	
WALLONIE					
B25	7	0.7	0.3--	0.14	332
B50	59	1.1	0.5-	0.08	239
B60	36	0.9	0.4--	0.07	294
B80	15	1.7	0.8	0.23	102
B90	36	2.2	1.2+	0.21	23
B-W	153	1.2	0.6--	0.05	
B.0	445	1.1	0.6--	0.03	

BR DEUTSCHLAND (1976-80)

BADEN-WURTTEMBERG					
D81	203	2.3	1.2++	0.09	23
D82	154	2.5	1.2++	0.10	23
D83	140	2.9	1.3++	0.12	17
D84	106	2.8	1.4++	0.15	9
D-A	603	2.5	1.3++	0.06	
BAYERN					
D91	226	2.4	1.1++	0.08	30
D92	88	3.4	1.7++	0.20	5
D93	71	2.8	1.4++	0.18	9
D94	66	2.4	0.9	0.13	64
D95	84	2.1	0.9	0.10	64
D96	79	2.5	1.4++	0.17	9
D97	123	3.1	1.5++	0.14	6
D-B	737	2.6	1.2++	0.05	
BERLIN(WEST)					
DB0	100	1.9	0.6	0.08	187
BREMEN					
D40	34	1.8	0.7	0.13	135
HAMBURG					
D20	78	1.7	0.7	0.09	135
HESSEN					
D64	211	1.9	0.9++	0.07	64
D66	71	2.3	0.9	0.12	64
D-F	282	2.0	0.9++	0.06	
NIEDERSACHSEN					
D31	65	1.5	0.7	0.09	135
D32	85	1.6	0.7	0.09	135
D33	38	1.0	0.5--	0.09	239
D34	57	1.0	0.6	0.09	187
D-G	245	1.3	0.6-	0.04	
NORDRHEIN-WESTFALEN					
D51	202	1.5	0.7	0.05	135
D53	148	1.5	0.7	0.07	135
D55	91	1.5	0.8	0.09	102
D57	61	1.3	0.7	0.10	135
D59	112	1.2	0.6-	0.06	187
D-H	614	1.4	0.7	0.03	
RHEINLAND-PFALZ					
D71	83	2.3	1.0++	0.13	44
D72	27	2.2	1.1	0.23	30
D73	85	1.8	0.9	0.10	64
D-I	195	2.0	1.0++	0.08	
SAARLAND					
DA0	62	2.2	1.1+	0.15	30
SCHLESWIG-HOLSTEIN					
D10	114	1.7	0.8	0.08	102
D.0	3064	1.9	0.9++	0.02	

DANMARK (1971-80)

K15	95	1.4	0.6	0.07	187
K20	12	0.8	0.6	0.18	187
K25	8	0.9	0.7	0.25	135
K30	22	1.6	0.8	0.17	102
K35	20	1.6	0.8	0.19	102
K40	6	2.6	1.0	0.41	44
K42	34	1.5	0.7	0.14	135
K50	23	1.9	0.9	0.20	64
K55	11	1.1	0.5	0.17	239
K60	24	1.5	0.9	0.20	64
K65	13	1.0	0.7	0.20	135
K70	53	1.9	1.0+	0.14	44
K76	18	1.6	0.8	0.20	102
K80	30	1.3	0.6	0.13	187
K.0	369	1.4	0.7	0.04	

FRANCE (1971-78)

ALSACE					
F67	69	1.9	1.2++	0.15	23
F68	52	2.0	1.0+	0.16	44
F-A	121	2.0	1.1++	0.11	
AQUITAINE					
F24	12	0.8	0.2--	0.07	344
F33	47	1.1	0.5-	0.09	239
F40	12	1.0	0.4-	0.13	294
F47	11	0.9	0.5	0.18	239
F64	45	2.0	1.1	0.19	30
F-B	127	1.2	0.6-	0.06	
AUVERGNE					
F03	20	1.3	0.5	0.13	239
F15	14	2.1	1.1	0.34	30
F43	22	2.6	0.9	0.22	64
F63	44	1.9	1.0	0.16	44
F-C	100	1.8	0.9	0.10	
BASSE-NORMANDIE					
F14	35	1.5	0.9	0.16	64
F50	15	0.8	0.3--	0.09	332
F61	11	0.9	0.6	0.21	187
F-D	61	1.1	0.6	0.09	
BOURGOGNE					
F21	25	1.4	0.8	0.17	102
F58	14	1.4	0.6	0.20	187
F71	31	1.3	0.5	0.11	239
F89	21	1.7	0.8	0.21	102
F-E	91	1.4	0.7	0.08	
BRETAGNE					
F22	31	1.4	0.6	0.13	187
F29	42	1.3	0.5	0.09	239
F35	27	0.9	0.5	0.12	239
F56	25	1.1	0.6	0.13	187
F-F	125	1.2	0.6-	0.06	
CENTRE					
F18	8	0.6	0.3--	0.10	332
F28	10	0.7	0.4--	0.12	294
F36	18	1.8	1.0	0.26	44
F37	23	1.2	0.6	0.14	187
F41	14	1.2	0.5	0.15	239
F45	19	1.0	0.5-	0.12	239
F-G	92	1.1	0.5--	0.06	
CHAMPAGNE-ARDENNE					
F08	16	1.3	0.8	0.21	102
F10	15	1.3	0.7	0.21	135
F51	14	0.7	0.4	0.13	294
F52	9	1.1	0.6	0.21	187
F-H	54	1.0	0.6	0.09	
CORSE					
F20	9	1.0	0.6	0.22	187
FRANCHE-COMTE					
F25	24	1.3	0.8	0.19	102
F39	20	2.1	1.0	0.25	44
F70	10	1.1	0.5	0.20	239
F90	9	1.8	0.9	0.32	64
F-J	63	1.5	0.8	0.11	
HAUTE-NORMANDIE					
F27	26	1.5	0.9	0.20	64
F76	45	0.9	0.5	0.09	239
F-K	71	1.1	0.6	0.08	
ILE-DE-FRANCE					
F75	148	1.5	0.6	0.06	187
F77	21	0.7	0.5-	0.11	239
F78	31	0.7	0.4--	0.09	294
F91	19	0.5	0.4--	0.09	294
F92	47	0.8	0.4--	0.06	294
F93	43	0.8	0.5-	0.08	239
F94	53	1.1	0.7	0.10	135
F95	28	0.8	0.6	0.12	187
F-L	390	1.0	0.5--	0.03	
LANGUEDOC-ROUSSILLON					
F11	8	0.7	0.3--	0.14	332
F30	26	1.3	0.6	0.14	187
F34	24	0.9	0.5-	0.11	239
F48	4	1.3	0.4	0.25	294
F66	25	2.0	0.9	0.21	64
F-M	87	1.2	0.6-	0.07	
LIMOUSIN					
F19	26	2.6	1.0	0.24	44
F23	22	3.6	1.1	0.31	30
F87	31	2.1	0.8	0.18	102
F-N	79	2.6	1.0	0.13	
LORRAINE					
F54	39	1.3	0.9	0.15	64
F55	15	1.8	1.1	0.32	30
F57	36	0.9	0.7	0.12	135
F88	36	2.2	1.1	0.22	30
F-O	126	1.3	0.9	0.08	
MIDI-PYRENEES					
F09	6	1.1	0.4	0.22	294
F12	12	1.1	0.4--	0.11	294
F31	23	0.7	0.4--	0.09	294
F32	5	0.7	0.2--	0.09	344
F46	14	2.3	0.7	0.22	135
F65	12	1.3	0.7	0.21	135
F81	11	0.8	0.5	0.17	239
F82	3	0.4	0.2--	0.12	344
F-P	86	0.9	0.4--	0.05	
NORD-PAS-DE-CALAIS					
F59	137	1.3	0.7	0.07	135
F62	61	1.1	0.7	0.09	135
F-Q	198	1.2	0.7	0.06	
PAYS DE LA LOIRE					
F44	32	0.8	0.4--	0.09	294
F49	23	0.9	0.5	0.13	239
F53	9	0.8	0.5	0.18	239
F72	21	1.0	0.5	0.12	239
F85	20	1.1	0.6	0.16	187
F-R	105	0.9	0.5--	0.06	
PICARDIE					
F02	27	1.3	0.6	0.14	187
F60	24	1.0	0.7	0.15	135
F80	21	1.0	0.5	0.13	239
F-S	72	1.1	0.6	0.08	
POITOU-CHARENTES					
F16	16	1.2	0.6	0.16	187
F17	19	0.9	0.5	0.13	239
F79	14	1.0	0.6	0.17	187
F86	24	1.7	0.8	0.19	102
F-T	73	1.2	0.6	0.08	
PROVENCE-ALPES-COTE D'AZUR					
F04	4	0.9	0.3--	0.13	332
F05	10	2.6	1.4	0.50	9
F06	31	0.9	0.4--	0.08	294
F13	77	1.2	0.6	0.07	187
F83	37	1.5	0.7	0.13	135
F84	27	1.7	0.7	0.17	135
F-U	186	1.2	0.6--	0.05	
RHONE-ALPES					
F01	23	1.5	0.9	0.21	64
F07	20	1.9	0.7	0.17	135
F26	21	1.4	0.8	0.20	102
F38	43	1.2	0.7	0.12	135
F42	48	1.6	0.7	0.12	135
F69	75	1.3	0.6	0.08	187
F73	28	2.3	0.9	0.18	64
F74	23	1.3	0.8	0.18	102
F-V	281	1.4	0.7	0.05	
F.0	2597	1.2	0.6--	0.01	

UNITED KINGDOM (1976-80)

EAST ANGLIA					
G25	12	0.7	0.4-	0.13	294
G46	21	1.0	0.5-	0.11	239
G55	24	1.4	0.7	0.16	135
G-A	57	1.0	0.5-	0.08	
EAST MIDLANDS					
G30	35	1.3	0.7	0.12	135
G44	26	1.0	0.5	0.11	239
G45	15	0.9	0.4--	0.10	294
G47	15	1.0	0.5	0.13	239
G50	29	1.0	0.5-	0.09	239
G-B	120	1.0	0.5--	0.05	
NORTHERN					
G14	44	1.2	0.5-	0.08	239
G27	24	1.4	0.9	0.19	64
G29	18	1.2	0.6	0.17	187
G33	15	0.8	0.4--	0.10	294
G48	4	0.5	0.1--	0.07	351
G-C	105	1.1	0.5--	0.06	
NORTH-WEST					
G11	85	1.0	0.5--	0.06	239
G12	62	1.3	0.6	0.09	187
G26	36	1.3	0.7	0.13	135
G43	54	1.3	0.5-	0.08	239
G-D	237	1.2	0.6--	0.04	

SOUTH-EAST					
G01	222	1.0	0.4--	0.03	294
G22	14	1.0	0.6	0.18	187
G23	16	0.8	0.4--	0.11	294
G24	15	1.0	0.6	0.16	187
G34	38	1.8	0.5-	0.09	239
G35	39	0.9	0.5-	0.09	239
G37	51	1.2	0.6	0.09	187
G39	22	0.8	0.4--	0.10	294
G41	9	2.5	0.5	0.18	239
G42	43	1.0	0.5--	0.08	239
G51	17	1.1	0.6	0.16	187
G56	28	0.9	0.4--	0.09	294
G58	31	1.5	0.5	0.11	239
G-E	545	1.0	0.5--	0.02	
SOUTH-WEST					
G21	33	1.2	0.5-	0.10	239
G28	12	0.9	0.4-	0.13	294
G31	39	1.3	0.6	0.10	187
G32	35	1.9	0.7	0.15	135
G36	16	1.1	0.4-	0.11	294
G53	19	1.5	0.6	0.15	187
G59	14	0.9	0.4--	0.11	294
G-F	168	1.3	0.5--	0.05	
WEST MIDLANDS					
G15	92	1.1	0.6	0.07	187
G38	23	1.2	0.6	0.15	187
G52	8	0.7	0.3--	0.11	332
G54	34	1.1	0.6	0.10	187
G57	16	1.1	0.6	0.17	187
G-G	173	1.1	0.6--	0.05	
YORKSHIRE AND HUMBERSIDE					
G13	43	1.1	0.5-	0.08	239
G16	77	1.2	0.5-	0.07	239
G40	29	1.1	0.5	0.10	239
G49	40	2.0	1.0	0.18	44
G-H	189	1.3	0.6-	0.05	
WALES					
G61	20	1.7	0.9	0.23	64
G62	12	1.2	0.6	0.21	187
G63	14	1.0	0.6	0.18	187
G64	9	1.3	0.4--	0.13	294
G65	26	1.6	0.7	0.15	135
G66	4	1.3	0.4	0.22	294
G67	18	1.5	0.9	0.24	64
G68	11	1.0	0.5	0.17	239
G-I	114	1.3	0.7	0.07	
SCOTLAND (1975-80)					
S01	6	1.0	0.4	0.19	294
S02	12	0.8	0.4	0.14	294
S03	15	1.2	0.4-	0.12	294
S04	15	1.4	0.7	0.19	135
S05	40	1.7	0.7	0.12	135
S06	6	1.9	0.6	0.26	187
S07	8	1.0	0.5	0.20	239
S08	87	1.1	0.6-	0.06	187
S09	3	0.7	0.2--	0.11	344
S10	1	1.8	0.5	0.47	239
S11	1	1.6	1.4	1.35	9
S12	3	3.3	1.8	1.13	3
G-J	197	1.2	0.6--	0.04	
NORTHERN IRELAND					
JE	22	1.3	0.7	0.16	135
JN	8	0.9	0.5	0.17	239
JS	6	0.9	0.4	0.20	294
JW	7	1.1	0.8	0.31	102
G-K	43	1.1	0.6	0.10	
G.0	1948	1.1	0.5--	0.01	
ITALIA (1975-79)					
ABRUZZI					
I66	13	1.7	1.0	0.29	44
I67	6	0.9	0.7	0.29	135
I68	9	1.2	0.9	0.30	64
I69	7	0.8	0.4	0.17	294
I-A	35	1.1	0.7	0.13	
BASILICATA					
I76	14	1.3	0.9	0.24	64
I77	7	1.4	1.0	0.38	44
I-B	21	1.4	0.9	0.20	
CALABRIA					
I78	22	1.2	0.9	0.21	64
I79	24	1.3	0.9	0.19	64
I80	22	1.5	0.8	0.18	102
I-C	68	1.3	0.9	0.11	

CAMPANIA					
I61	18	1.0	0.8	0.19	102
I62	8	1.1	0.7	0.27	135
I63	65	0.9	0.7	0.09	135
I64	6	0.5	0.3--	0.10	332
I65	28	1.1	0.8	0.16	102
I-D	125	0.9	0.7	0.07	
EMILIA-ROMAGNA					
I33	9	1.2	0.5	0.17	239
I34	17	1.7	0.9	0.24	64
I35	14	1.4	0.6	0.19	187
I36	23	1.6	0.9	0.20	64
I37	37	1.5	0.7	0.12	135
I38	12	1.2	0.5	0.16	239
I39	16	1.7	0.9	0.23	64
I40	20	1.3	0.9	0.20	64
I-E	148	1.5	0.7	0.07	
FRIULI-VENEZIA GIULIA					
I30	43	3.2	1.5++	0.25	6
I31	6	1.6	0.9	0.39	64
I32	15	1.9	0.7	0.20	135
I93	10	1.5	0.9	0.34	64
I-F	74	2.3	1.1++	0.15	
LAZIO					
I56	11	1.7	0.9	0.29	64
I57	2	0.6	0.3-	0.19	332
I58	121	1.3	0.9+	0.08	64
I59	7	0.7	0.6	0.21	187
I60	17	1.5	1.0	0.25	44
I-G	158	1.3	0.9+	0.07	
LIGURIA					
I08	9	1.5	0.7	0.24	135
I09	11	1.4	0.8	0.25	102
I10	43	1.5	0.6	0.10	187
I11	10	1.6	0.6	0.22	187
I-H	73	1.5	0.6	0.08	
LOMBARDIA					
I12	25	1.3	0.8	0.17	102
I13	26	1.3	0.9	0.18	64
I14	7	1.6	0.9	0.36	64
I15	153	1.5	1.0++	0.08	44
I16	32	1.4	1.0	0.18	44
I17	44	1.7	1.2+	0.18	23
I18	31	2.3	1.1	0.21	30
I19	16	1.9	1.0	0.28	44
I20	12	1.2	0.5	0.17	239
I-I	346	1.5	1.0++	0.05	
MARCHE					
I41	12	1.4	0.8	0.24	102
I42	22	2.0	0.9	0.20	64
I43	10	1.4	0.8	0.27	102
I44	11	1.2	0.8	0.24	102
I-J	55	1.5	0.8	0.12	
MOLISE					
I70	8	1.3	0.8	0.28	102
I94	3	1.2	0.4	0.27	294
I-K	11	1.3	0.7	0.22	
PIEMONTE					
I01	129	2.1	1.3++	0.12	17
I02	27	2.6	1.2+	0.27	23
I03	23	1.8	0.9	0.20	64
I04	33	2.4	1.1+	0.21	30
I05	9	1.6	0.9	0.31	64
I06	19	1.5	0.8	0.21	102
I-L	240	2.1	1.1++	0.08	
PUGLIA					
I71	8	0.5	0.3--	0.12	332
I72	31	0.9	0.7	0.13	135
I73	9	0.6	0.5	0.17	239
I74	6	0.6	0.5	0.20	239
I75	8	0.4	0.3--	0.10	332
I-M	62	0.6	0.5--	0.07	
SARDEGNA					
I90	11	1.0	0.7	0.23	135
I91	11	1.6	1.2	0.37	23
I92	15	0.8	0.7	0.18	135
I95	7	1.8	1.1	0.46	30
I-N	44	1.1	0.8	0.13	
SICILIA					
I81	5	0.5	0.4	0.17	294
I82	31	1.0	0.7	0.13	135
I83	22	1.3	0.6	0.15	187
I84	12	1.0	0.7	0.21	135
I85	14	1.9	1.4	0.39	9
I86	6	1.2	0.8	0.33	102
I87	31	1.2	1.0	0.18	44
I88	4	0.6	0.4	0.19	294
I89	5	0.5	0.4	0.20	294
I-O	130	1.0	0.7	0.07	

TOSCANA					
I45	10	1.9	1.1	0.38	30
I46	17	1.7	0.8	0.20	102
I47	8	1.2	0.6	0.23	187
I48	41	1.3	0.7	0.11	135
I49	7	0.8	0.4-	0.15	294
I50	9	0.9	0.4	0.16	294
I51	11	1.4	0.7	0.22	135
I52	9	1.4	0.6	0.21	187
I53	4	0.7	0.4	0.20	294
I-P	116	1.3	0.6	0.06	
TRENTINO-ALTO ADIGE					
I21	27	2.5	1.8++	0.36	3
I22	31	2.8	1.5++	0.28	6
I-Q	58	2.6	1.6++	0.22	
UMBRIA					
I54	22	1.5	0.9	0.20	64
I55	7	1.2	0.5	0.20	239
I-R	29	1.4	0.8	0.15	
VALLE D'AOSTA					
I07	5	1.8	0.9	0.40	64
VENETO					
I23	21	1.1	0.6	0.15	187
I24	43	2.4	1.4++	0.23	9
I25	7	1.2	0.6	0.24	187
I26	28	1.6	1.0	0.20	44
I27	24	1.1	0.7	0.15	135
I28	27	1.3	0.8	0.16	102
I29	9	1.4	0.9	0.31	64
I-T	159	1.5	0.9+	0.07	
I.0	1957	1.4	0.8++	0.02	
IRELAND (1976-80)					
CONNAUGHT					
R07	6	1.5	0.7	0.30	135
R12	0	0.0	0.0--	0.00	352
R16	2	0.7	0.5	0.37	239
R20	1	0.8	0.2-	0.24	344
R21	3	2.2	1.4	0.84	9
R-A	12	1.2	0.6	0.19	
LEINSTER					
R01	0	0.0	0.0--	0.00	352
R06	27	1.1	0.8	0.16	102
R09	0	0.0	0.0--	0.00	352
R10	1	0.6	0.7	0.70	135
R11	1	0.8	0.5	0.52	239
R14	2	2.7	1.3	0.96	17
R15	2	0.9	0.7	0.47	135
R17	3	1.4	1.0	0.65	44
R19	2	1.5	1.3	0.95	17
R24	1	0.7	0.6	0.57	187
R25	9	3.8	2.3	0.84	1
R26	3	1.4	0.7	0.41	135
R-B	51	1.2	0.8	0.12	
MUNSTER					
R03	2	1.0	0.6	0.48	187
R04	10	1.0	0.5	0.15	239
R08	6	2.1	1.0	0.44	44
R13	1	0.3	0.2-	0.22	344
R22	5	1.5	1.0	0.47	44
R23	2	0.9	0.6	0.43	187
R-C	26	1.1	0.6	0.13	
ULSTER					
R02	2	1.6	1.3	1.06	17
R05	8	2.7	1.9	0.77	2
R18	0	0.0	0.0--	0.00	352
R-D	10	1.8	1.4	0.49	
R.0	99	1.2	0.8	0.08	
LUXEMBOURG (1971-80)					
LE	5	2.6	1.1	0.52	30
LN	5	1.9	1.3	0.60	17
LS	26	1.9	1.1	0.22	30
L.0	36	2.0	1.1+	0.20	
NEDERLAND (1976-80)					
N01	14	1.0	0.6	0.17	187
N02	21	1.5	0.8	0.20	102
N03	3	0.3	0.2--	0.14	344
N04	28	1.1	0.8	0.15	102
N05	46	1.1	0.7	0.12	135
N06	15	0.7	0.5	0.13	239
N07	79	1.3	0.8	0.09	102
N08	113	1.5	0.8	0.08	102
N09	5	0.6	0.3--	0.13	332
N10	28	0.6	0.4--	0.08	294
N11	20	0.8	0.5	0.12	239
N.0	372	1.1	0.7	0.04	
EEC-9					
EEC	10887	1.4	0.7	0.01	

BELGIE-BELGIQUE (1971-78)

BRUSSEL-BRUXELLES					
B21	103	2.6	2.0+	0.20	53
VLAANDEREN					
B10	146	2.4	2.0++	0.17	53
B29	69	1.9	1.6	0.20	119
B30	86	2.0	1.7	0.19	105
B40	105	2.0	1.6	0.16	119
B70	47	1.7	1.6	0.24	119
B-V	453	2.1	1.7++	0.08	
WALLONIE					
B25	15	1.5	1.1	0.30	278
B50	124	2.4	2.0++	0.18	53
B60	104	2.6	2.1++	0.21	44
B80	16	1.9	1.7	0.43	105
B90	42	2.8	2.3+	0.37	28
B-W	301	2.4	2.0++	0.12	
B.0	857	2.2	1.8++	0.06	

BR DEUTSCHLAND (1976-80)

BADEN-WURTTEMBERG					
D81	164	2.0	1.6	0.13	119
D82	115	2.0	1.6	0.15	119
D83	81	1.8	1.6	0.18	119
D84	62	1.7	1.5	0.19	152
D-A	422	1.9	1.6	0.08	
BAYERN					
D91	137	1.6	1.2--	0.11	249
D92	37	1.6	1.3	0.22	217
D93	50	2.2	1.9	0.28	66
D94	49	2.0	1.5	0.23	152
D95	81	2.3	1.8	0.21	84
D96	37	1.3	1.1-	0.19	278
D97	44	1.2	1.0--	0.16	300
D-B	435	1.7	1.4-	0.07	
BERLIN(WEST)					
DB0	87	2.0	1.4	0.16	180
BREMEN					
D40	21	1.3	1.0-	0.23	300
HAMBURG					
D20	81	2.1	1.4	0.16	180
HESSEN					
D64	209	2.0	1.5	0.11	152
D66	45	1.6	1.3	0.20	217
D-F	254	1.9	1.5	0.10	
NIEDERSACHSEN					
D31	85	2.2	1.7	0.20	105
D32	103	2.1	1.6	0.16	119
D33	77	2.2	1.7	0.21	105
D34	92	1.8	1.6	0.17	119
D-G	357	2.1	1.6	0.09	
NORDRHEIN-WESTFALEN					
D51	267	2.2	1.8++	0.11	84
D53	174	1.9	1.6	0.13	119
D55	100	1.7	1.6	0.16	119
D57	69	1.6	1.4	0.17	180
D59	167	1.9	1.6	0.13	119
D-H	777	1.9	1.6+	0.06	
RHEINLAND-PFALZ					
D71	64	2.0	1.6	0.21	119
D72	19	1.7	1.2	0.30	249
D73	77	1.8	1.4	0.17	180
D-I	160	1.8	1.5	0.12	
SAARLAND					
DA0	51	2.0	1.6	0.23	119
SCHLESWIG-HOLSTEIN					
D10	111	1.8	1.4	0.14	180
D.0	2756	1.9	1.5	0.03	

DANMARK (1971-80)

K15	105	1.7	1.4	0.14	180
K20	26	1.7	1.6	0.31	119
K25	19	2.0	1.9	0.44	66
K30	28	2.1	1.6	0.31	119
K35	30	2.3	1.9	0.36	66
K40	2	0.8	0.5--	0.34	351
K42	32	1.4	1.0--	0.18	300
K50	20	1.6	1.3	0.29	217
K55	12	1.2	0.9-	0.26	323
K60	18	1.1	1.0-	0.24	300
K65	13	1.0	0.9-	0.27	323
K70	31	1.1	0.9--	0.17	323
K76	17	1.5	1.2	0.31	249
K80	35	1.5	1.2	0.21	249
K.0	388	1.6	1.3--	0.07	

FRANCE (1971-78)

ALSACE					
F67	55	1.6	1.4	0.19	180
F68	24	1.0	0.9--	0.18	323
F-A	79	1.3	1.2-	0.13	
AQUITAINE					
F24	28	1.9	1.4	0.30	180
F33	73	1.8	1.4	0.17	180
F40	19	1.7	1.4	0.34	180
F47	17	1.5	1.2	0.31	249
F64	41	2.0	1.6	0.26	119
F-B	178	1.8	1.4	0.11	
AUVERGNE					
F03	26	1.8	1.5	0.30	152
F15	8	1.2	0.9-	0.32	323
F43	16	2.0	1.6	0.43	119
F63	47	2.1	1.7	0.25	105
F-C	97	1.9	1.5	0.16	
BASSE-NORMANDIE					
F14	27	1.2	1.2	0.23	249
F50	27	1.6	1.4	0.27	180
F61	14	1.2	1.1	0.30	278
F-D	68	1.3	1.2	0.15	
BOURGOGNE					
F21	25	1.4	1.4	0.28	180
F58	15	1.5	0.8-	0.25	338
F71	37	1.6	1.2	0.21	249
F89	17	1.4	1.1	0.28	278
F-E	94	1.5	1.2--	0.13	
BRETAGNE					
F22	40	2.0	1.5	0.26	152
F29	42	1.3	1.2	0.19	249
F35	31	1.1	1.0--	0.18	300
F56	26	1.2	1.0-	0.20	300
F-F	139	1.4	1.2--	0.10	
CENTRE					
F18	29	2.3	1.9	0.37	66
F28	22	1.6	1.4	0.30	180
F36	14	1.4	1.3	0.37	217
F37	35	1.9	1.5	0.26	152
F41	24	2.2	1.8	0.38	84
F45	25	1.3	1.1	0.22	278
F-G	149	1.8	1.5	0.12	
CHAMPAGNE-ARDENNE					
F08	14	1.1	1.1	0.30	278
F10	16	1.4	1.1	0.30	278
F51	35	1.7	1.5	0.26	152
F52	12	1.4	1.0	0.31	300
F-H	77	1.4	1.3	0.15	
CORSE					
F20	10	1.0	0.7--	0.23	345
FRANCHE-COMTE					
F25	25	1.3	1.3	0.26	217
F39	12	1.3	1.0	0.31	300
F70	14	1.6	1.2	0.34	249
F90	9	1.8	1.6	0.54	119
F-J	60	1.4	1.3	0.17	
HAUTE-NORMANDIE					
F27	26	1.6	1.4	0.28	180
F76	59	1.3	1.2-	0.16	249
F-K	85	1.4	1.2	0.14	
ILE-DE-FRANCE					
F75	159	1.9	1.4	0.12	180
F77	41	1.4	1.3	0.20	217
F78	46	1.1	1.0--	0.16	300
F91	43	1.2	1.2	0.19	249
F92	90	1.6	1.3	0.14	217
F93	83	1.6	1.5	0.16	152
F94	82	1.7	1.5	0.17	152
F95	45	1.3	1.2	0.18	249
F-L	589	1.5	1.3--	0.06	
LANGUEDOC-ROUSSILLON					
F11	20	1.9	1.1	0.28	278
F30	24	1.2	1.0-	0.21	300
F34	49	2.0	1.7	0.24	105
F48	5	1.7	1.6	0.71	119
F66	27	2.3	1.8	0.36	84
F-M	125	1.8	1.4	0.13	
LIMOUSIN					
F19	17	1.8	1.2	0.30	249
F23	8	1.4	0.9	0.38	323
F87	24	1.8	1.2	0.26	249
F-N	49	1.7	1.1-	0.17	
LORRAINE					
F54	57	2.0	1.8	0.24	84
F55	17	2.1	1.9	0.47	66
F57	60	1.5	1.4	0.19	180
F88	19	1.2	1.1	0.27	278
F-O	153	1.7	1.5	0.13	
MIDI-PYRENEES					
F09	17	3.1	2.6	0.68	13
F12	18	1.7	1.4	0.34	180
F31	58	1.9	1.5	0.21	152
F32	14	2.0	1.6	0.47	119
F46	15	2.5	1.8	0.51	84
F65	11	1.2	1.0	0.31	300
F81	22	1.7	1.3	0.30	217
F82	13	1.8	1.4	0.41	180
F-P	168	1.9	1.5	0.12	
NORD-PAS-DE-CALAIS					
F59	166	1.7	1.6	0.12	119
F62	82	1.5	1.3	0.15	217
F-Q	248	1.6	1.5	0.10	
PAYS DE LA LOIRE					
F44	52	1.4	1.3	0.18	217
F49	29	1.2	1.1	0.21	278
F53	24	2.4	1.9	0.39	66
F72	23	1.2	1.1-	0.22	278
F85	32	1.8	1.4	0.27	180
F-R	160	1.5	1.3-	0.10	
PICARDIE					
F02	33	1.6	1.4	0.26	180
F60	32	1.3	1.2	0.21	249
F80	24	1.1	1.0-	0.21	300
F-S	89	1.3	1.2-	0.13	
POITOU-CHARENTES					
F16	19	1.4	1.1	0.26	278
F17	43	2.2	1.7	0.27	105
F79	27	2.0	1.7	0.34	105
F86	24	1.7	1.4	0.29	180
F-T	113	1.9	1.5	0.15	
PROVENCE-ALPES-COTE D'AZUR					
F04	5	1.1	0.8-	0.37	338
F05	5	1.3	1.1	0.48	278
F06	27	0.9	0.5--	0.12	351
F13	99	1.5	1.3	0.13	217
F83	46	1.9	1.4	0.22	180
F84	17	1.1	0.9--	0.23	323
F-U	199	1.4	1.1--	0.08	
RHONE-ALPES					
F01	25	1.7	1.3	0.27	217
F07	17	1.7	1.4	0.35	180
F26	34	2.4	2.0	0.35	53
F38	51	1.5	1.3	0.19	217
F42	51	1.7	1.4	0.21	180
F69	62	1.1	1.0--	0.13	300
F73	21	1.7	1.5	0.32	152
F74	27	1.5	1.3	0.25	217
F-V	288	1.5	1.3--	0.08	
F.0	3217	1.6	1.3--	0.02	

UNITED KINGDOM (1976-80)

EAST ANGLIA					
G25	29	1.7	1.5	0.27	152
G46	34	1.7	1.4	0.26	180
G55	24	1.4	1.1-	0.22	278
G-A	87	1.6	1.3	0.15	
EAST MIDLANDS					
G30	52	2.0	1.6	0.23	119
G44	42	1.7	1.4	0.23	180
G45	37	2.4	1.9	0.32	66
G47	22	1.4	1.3	0.28	217
G50	45	1.6	1.3	0.19	217
G-B	198	1.8	1.5	0.11	
NORTHERN					
G14	47	1.4	1.2	0.18	249
G27	31	1.9	1.7	0.30	105
G29	24	1.7	1.4	0.29	180
G33	39	2.2	1.8	0.29	84
G48	23	2.7	2.1	0.46	44
G-C	164	1.8	1.5	0.12	
NORTH-WEST					
G11	131	1.7	1.4	0.12	180
G12	71	1.6	1.3	0.16	217
G26	47	1.7	1.5	0.22	152
G43	74	1.9	1.5	0.18	152
G-D	323	1.7	1.4	0.08	

SOUTH-EAST					
G01	297	1.5	1.2--	0.07	249
G22	21	1.4	1.2	0.27	249
G23	24	1.2	1.0-	0.21	300
G24	34	2.2	1.8	0.32	84
G34	35	2.0	1.5	0.29	152
G35	69	1.6	1.4	0.17	180
G37	56	1.3	1.1--	0.14	278
G39	46	1.7	1.4	0.20	180
G41	6	1.9	1.4	0.64	180
G42	63	1.5	1.1-	0.15	278
G51	18	1.1	0.9-	0.22	323
G56	47	1.6	1.3	0.20	217
G58	26	1.5	1.2	0.25	249
G-E	742	1.5	1.2--	0.05	
SOUTH-WEST					
G21	33	1.2	1.0--	0.18	300
G28	17	1.4	1.0-	0.24	300
G31	36	1.3	1.1-	0.18	278
G32	25	1.5	1.0-	0.22	300
G36	19	1.3	1.2	0.27	249
G53	23	1.9	1.5	0.32	152
G59	14	0.9	0.8--	0.21	338
G-F	167	1.3	1.0--	0.08	
WEST MIDLANDS					
G15	127	1.6	1.3	0.12	217
G38	32	1.8	1.3	0.24	217
G52	9	0.8	0.7--	0.23	345
G54	44	1.5	1.3	0.20	217
G57	35	2.5	2.2	0.38	34
G-G	247	1.6	1.4	0.09	
YORKSHIRE AND HUMBERSIDE					
G13	89	2.3	1.8	0.20	84
G16	96	1.6	1.3	0.14	217
G40	42	1.7	1.5	0.24	152
G49	36	1.9	1.6	0.27	119
G-H	263	1.8	1.5	0.10	
WALES					
G61	16	1.4	1.2	0.32	249
G62	18	1.9	1.3	0.32	217
G63	28	2.2	1.8	0.34	84
G64	16	2.4	1.9	0.49	66
G65	24	1.5	1.3	0.27	217
G66	6	1.9	1.2	0.52	249
G67	10	0.9	0.8--	0.24	338
G68	18	1.7	1.2	0.30	249
G-I	136	1.7	1.3	0.12	
SCOTLAND(1975-80)					
S01	6	1.1	1.0	0.41	300
S02	14	1.0	0.9-	0.25	323
S03	12	1.0	0.9-	0.26	323
S04	14	1.4	1.1	0.30	278
S05	22	1.0	0.9--	0.19	323
S06	9	3.1	2.3	0.80	28
S07	11	1.4	1.1	0.34	278
S08	95	1.3	1.2--	0.12	249
S09	4	1.0	0.7-	0.36	345
S10	2	3.8	3.4	2.46	2
S11	1	1.6	0.9	0.93	323
S12	1	1.1	0.9	0.89	323
G-J	191	1.3	1.1--	0.08	
NORTHERN IRELAND					
JE	16	1.0	0.9-	0.23	323
JN	11	1.2	1.1	0.35	278
JS	11	1.7	1.6	0.49	119
JW	20	3.3	3.1+	0.70	4
G-K	58	1.5	1.4	0.19	
G.0	2576	1.6	1.3--	0.03	
ITALIA (1975-79)					
ABRUZZI					
I66	15	2.0	1.4	0.37	180
I67	15	2.3	1.7	0.44	105
I68	13	1.9	1.5	0.42	152
I69	18	2.0	1.6	0.39	119
I-A	61	2.0	1.5	0.20	
BASILICATA					
I76	22	2.1	1.9	0.41	66
I77	3	0.6	0.5--	0.28	351
I-B	25	1.6	1.4	0.29	
CALABRIA					
I78	26	1.5	1.3	0.27	217
I79	35	1.9	1.8	0.31	84
I80	24	1.6	1.5	0.31	152
I-C	85	1.7	1.6	0.17	
CAMPANIA					
I61	30	1.7	1.6	0.30	119
I62	19	2.6	2.3	0.55	28
I63	127	1.8	1.9+	0.17	66
I64	18	1.7	1.4	0.34	180
I65	49	2.0	1.9	0.27	66
I-D	243	1.9	1.8++	0.12	
EMILIA-ROMAGNA					
I33	26	3.7	2.5	0.53	20
I34	38	3.9	2.7++	0.46	10
I35	33	3.3	2.3	0.42	28
I36	46	3.2	2.3+	0.35	28
I37	53	2.3	1.7	0.24	105
I38	27	2.9	2.0	0.39	53
I39	18	2.0	1.3	0.32	217
I40	32	2.2	1.8	0.33	84
I-E	273	2.8	2.0++	0.13	
FRIULI-VENEZIA GIULIA					
I30	28	2.2	1.7	0.33	105
I31	6	1.7	1.3	0.59	217
I32	24	3.4	2.0	0.45	53
I93	21	3.2	2.6	0.58	13
I-F	79	2.6	1.9	0.23	
LAZIO					
I56	12	1.8	1.4	0.42	180
I57	12	3.4	2.5	0.77	20
I58	188	2.1	1.9++	0.14	66
I59	25	2.4	2.2	0.45	34
I60	25	2.2	1.8	0.38	84
I-G	262	2.2	1.9++	0.12	
LIGURIA					
I08	18	3.2	2.7	0.65	10
I09	24	3.2	2.0	0.44	53
I10	89	3.5	2.5++	0.28	20
I11	14	2.4	1.6	0.47	119
I-H	145	3.2	2.3++	0.20	
LOMBARDIA					
I12	70	3.7	3.2++	0.40	3
I13	45	2.5	2.0	0.31	53
I14	7	1.6	1.4	0.55	180
I15	236	2.4	2.1++	0.14	44
I16	69	3.2	3.0++	0.36	7
I17	58	2.4	2.1+	0.28	44
I18	53	4.2	2.6++	0.39	13
I19	26	3.2	2.5+	0.51	20
I20	44	4.7	3.6++	0.57	1
I-I	608	2.8	2.4++	0.10	
MARCHE					
I41	13	1.6	1.3	0.39	217
I42	35	3.4	2.6+	0.45	13
I43	12	1.7	1.2	0.35	249
I44	23	2.7	2.2	0.46	34
I-J	83	2.4	1.9	0.21	
MOLISE					
I70	15	2.6	2.0	0.54	53
I94	8	3.5	3.0	1.10	7
I-K	23	2.8	2.3	0.50	
PIEMONTE					
I01	164	2.8	2.4++	0.19	26
I02	25	2.6	1.9	0.39	66
I03	29	2.4	1.9	0.38	66
I04	35	2.6	2.0	0.36	53
I05	6	1.1	0.7-	0.32	345
I06	37	3.2	2.2	0.39	34
I-L	296	2.7	2.2++	0.13	
PUGLIA					
I71	37	2.2	2.0	0.34	53
I72	73	2.1	1.9	0.23	66
I73	29	2.1	2.1	0.40	44
I74	17	1.8	1.7	0.42	105
I75	39	2.1	2.0	0.32	53
I-M	195	2.1	2.0++	0.14	
SARDEGNA					
I90	22	2.1	1.8	0.40	84
I91	16	2.3	2.2	0.55	34
I92	17	1.0	1.0-	0.23	300
I95	5	1.3	1.2	0.55	249
I-N	60	1.5	1.4	0.19	
SICILIA					
I81	28	2.7	2.3	0.44	28
I82	58	2.0	1.8	0.24	84
I83	31	1.9	1.6	0.30	119
I84	24	2.0	1.8	0.37	84
I85	13	1.8	1.7	0.48	105
I86	12	2.4	1.9	0.58	66
I87	53	2.2	2.1+	0.29	44
I88	11	1.7	1.3	0.40	217
I89	16	1.7	1.5	0.38	152
I-O	246	2.0	1.8++	0.12	
TOSCANA					
I45	12	2.4	1.8	0.55	84
I46	33	3.5	3.1++	0.56	4
I47	16	2.5	2.2	0.58	34
I48	63	2.2	1.6	0.21	119
I49	27	3.2	2.7+	0.55	10
I50	29	3.1	2.2	0.42	34
I51	19	2.5	1.5	0.34	152
I52	24	3.8	2.9+	0.67	9
I53	13	2.4	1.5	0.45	152
I-P	236	2.7	2.1++	0.14	
TRENTINO-ALTO ADIGE					
I21	16	1.5	1.5	0.38	152
I22	16	1.5	1.2	0.30	249
I-Q	32	1.5	1.3	0.24	
UMBRIA					
I54	34	2.4	1.8	0.33	84
I55	15	2.7	1.9	0.51	66
I-R	49	2.5	1.9	0.28	
VALLE D'AOSTA					
I07	6	2.1	1.5	0.64	152
VENETO					
I23	55	3.0	2.5++	0.34	20
I24	47	2.7	2.5++	0.36	20
I25	16	3.0	2.2	0.58	34
I26	28	1.6	1.4	0.27	180
I27	45	2.2	1.9	0.29	66
I28	58	3.0	2.6++	0.35	13
I29	16	2.6	2.1	0.53	44
I-T	265	2.5	2.2++	0.14	
I.0	3272	2.4	2.0++	0.04	
IRELAND (1976-80)					
CONNAUGHT					
R07	10	2.3	2.1	0.69	44
R12	2	2.7	3.1	2.19	4
R16	4	1.4	1.1	0.66	278
R20	1	0.7	0.5-	0.49	351
R21	3	2.2	2.2	1.30	34
R-A	20	1.9	1.7	0.40	
LEINSTER					
R01	3	3.0	2.4	1.42	26
R06	39	1.6	1.8	0.29	84
R09	4	1.6	1.8	0.92	84
R10	5	2.8	2.6	1.17	13
R11	2	1.5	1.2	0.88	249
R14	1	1.2	1.6	1.62	119
R15	3	1.4	1.2	0.71	249
R17	2	0.9	0.9	0.62	323
R19	3	2.0	1.6	0.95	119
R24	4	2.6	2.6	1.31	13
R25	5	2.0	1.6	0.74	119
R26	2	1.0	1.0	0.73	300
R-B	73	1.7	1.7	0.20	
MUNSTER					
R03	4	1.8	1.8	0.94	84
R04	17	1.7	1.5	0.37	152
R08	5	1.6	1.0	0.45	300
R13	3	0.8	0.8	0.47	338
R22	5	1.5	1.1	0.55	278
R23	4	1.8	2.2	1.08	34
R-C	38	1.5	1.4	0.23	
ULSTER					
R02	4	2.8	2.0	1.05	53
R05	2	0.6	0.5--	0.37	351
R18	1	0.8	0.7	0.65	345
R-D	7	1.2	0.9	0.35	
R.0	138	1.6	1.5	0.13	
LUXEMBOURG (1971-80)					
LE	1	0.6	0.6	0.58	350
LN	3	1.1	0.8	0.50	338
LS	20	1.6	1.3	0.29	217
L.0	24	1.4	1.1	0.23	
NEDERLAND (1976-80)					
N01	32	2.3	2.1	0.37	44
N02	26	1.8	1.5	0.30	152
N03	16	1.5	1.5	0.37	152
N04	36	1.4	1.3	0.22	217
N05	62	1.5	1.3	0.17	217
N06	35	1.6	1.4	0.24	180
N07	105	1.8	1.5	0.15	152
N08	89	1.2	1.0--	0.10	300
N09	15	1.8	1.6	0.42	119
N10	54	1.1	1.0--	0.14	300
N11	24	0.9	0.8--	0.17	338
N.0	494	1.4	1.2--	0.06	
EEC-9					
EEC	13722	1.8	1.5	0.01	

BELGIE-BELGIQUE (1971-78)

BRUSSEL-BRUXELLES					
B21	58	1.3	0.8	0.13	165
VLAANDEREN					
B10	89	1.4	1.1	0.12	63
B29	55	1.5	1.2+	0.17	51
B30	43	1.0	0.8	0.13	165
B40	73	1.4	1.1+	0.14	63
B70	26	1.0	0.9	0.17	127
B-V	286	1.3	1.0++	0.06	
WALLONIE					
B25	9	0.8	0.7	0.23	204
B50	61	1.1	0.8	0.12	165
B60	50	1.2	0.8	0.12	165
B80	9	1.0	0.6	0.23	254
B90	25	1.6	1.2	0.27	51
B-W	154	1.2	0.8	0.07	
B.0	498	1.2	0.9+	0.05	

BR DEUTSCHLAND (1976-80)

BADEN-WURTTEMBERG					
D81	122	1.4	0.9	0.09	127
D82	87	1.4	0.9	0.11	127
D83	65	1.3	0.9	0.13	127
D84	48	1.2	0.8	0.13	165
D-A	322	1.4	0.9	0.05	
BAYERN					
D91	121	1.3	0.8	0.08	165
D92	24	0.9	0.5--	0.11	297
D93	41	1.6	1.0	0.18	88
D94	36	1.3	0.9	0.16	127
D95	63	1.6	0.9	0.13	127
D96	26	0.8	0.6-	0.12	254
D97	37	0.9	0.6--	0.10	254
D-B	348	1.2	0.8	0.05	
BERLIN (WEST)					
DB0	103	1.9	1.0	0.13	88
BREMEN					
D40	24	1.3	0.9	0.21	127
HAMBURG					
D20	73	1.6	0.7	0.11	204
HESSEN					
D64	158	1.4	0.9	0.08	127
D66	42	1.4	0.7	0.13	204
D-F	200	1.4	0.9	0.07	
NIEDERSACHSEN					
D31	86	2.0	1.3++	0.16	40
D32	95	1.7	1.0	0.12	88
D33	36	1.0	0.5--	0.10	297
D34	63	1.2	0.8	0.11	165
D-G	280	1.5	0.9	0.06	
NORDRHEIN-WESTFALEN					
D51	174	1.3	0.8	0.07	165
D53	130	1.3	0.9	0.09	127
D55	66	1.1	0.8	0.11	165
D57	62	1.3	0.8	0.12	165
D59	113	1.2	0.8	0.08	165
D-H	545	1.2	0.8	0.04	
RHEINLAND-PFALZ					
D71	64	1.8	1.1	0.15	63
D72	24	1.9	1.2	0.27	51
D73	69	1.5	1.0	0.14	88
D-I	157	1.7	1.1+	0.10	
SAARLAND					
DA0	29	1.0	0.7	0.14	204
SCHLESWIG-HOLSTEIN					
D10	84	1.2	0.8	0.10	165
D.0	2165	1.3	0.9	0.02	

DANMARK (1971-80)

K15	103	1.5	1.0	0.11	88
K20	18	1.2	0.9	0.22	127
K25	8	0.9	0.7	0.26	204
K30	17	1.3	0.9	0.24	127
K35	16	1.3	1.0	0.27	88
K40	3	1.3	0.8	0.50	165
K42	24	1.1	0.6	0.14	254
K50	4	0.3	0.2--	0.13	351
K55	11	1.1	0.7	0.23	204
K60	10	0.6	0.4--	0.14	333
K65	7	0.6	0.5-	0.18	297
K70	21	0.7	0.6-	0.13	254
K76	15	1.3	0.9	0.25	127
K80	19	0.8	0.6	0.15	254
K.0	276	1.1	0.8	0.05	

FRANCE (1971-78)

ALSACE					
F67	32	0.9	0.7	0.13	204
F68	31	1.2	1.0	0.18	88
F-A	63	1.0	0.8	0.11	
AQUITAINE					
F24	12	0.8	0.5-	0.16	297
F33	44	1.0	0.7	0.12	204
F40	17	1.4	0.9	0.26	127
F47	15	1.3	1.0	0.28	88
F64	19	0.9	0.5-	0.14	297
F-B	107	1.0	0.7-	0.08	
AUVERGNE					
F03	16	1.0	0.8	0.23	165
F15	9	1.3	0.7	0.26	204
F43	10	1.2	0.6	0.25	254
F63	27	1.1	0.9	0.19	127
F-C	62	1.1	0.8	0.12	
BASSE-NORMANDIE					
F14	22	1.0	0.7	0.17	204
F50	12	0.6	0.5	0.17	297
F61	18	1.5	1.0	0.25	88
F-D	52	1.0	0.7	0.11	
BOURGOGNE					
F21	17	0.9	0.7	0.18	204
F58	15	1.5	1.0	0.30	88
F71	26	1.1	0.8	0.17	165
F89	15	1.2	0.8	0.26	165
F-E	73	1.1	0.8	0.11	
BRETAGNE					
F22	15	0.7	0.6	0.18	254
F29	26	0.8	0.5--	0.11	297
F35	31	1.1	0.8	0.16	165
F56	15	0.7	0.4--	0.12	333
F-F	87	0.8	0.6--	0.07	
CENTRE					
F18	17	1.3	1.0	0.27	88
F28	13	1.0	0.9	0.26	127
F36	13	1.3	1.0	0.33	88
F37	28	1.4	1.1	0.22	63
F41	13	1.1	0.9	0.27	127
F45	12	0.6	0.5-	0.15	297
F-G	96	1.1	0.9	0.10	
CHAMPAGNE-ARDENNE					
F08	12	1.0	0.8	0.24	165
F10	13	1.1	0.9	0.28	127
F51	19	0.9	0.7	0.18	204
F52	6	0.7	0.6	0.26	254
F-H	50	0.9	0.8	0.12	
CORSE					
F20	5	0.6	0.3--	0.15	346
FRANCHE-COMTE					
F25	11	0.6	0.5-	0.15	297
F39	8	0.8	0.7	0.27	204
F70	13	1.5	0.9	0.30	127
F90	3	0.6	0.4	0.27	333
F-J	35	0.8	0.6	0.11	
HAUTE-NORMANDIE					
F27	15	0.9	0.8	0.21	165
F76	42	0.9	0.7	0.12	204
F-K	57	0.9	0.7	0.10	
ILE-DE-FRANCE					
F75	121	1.2	0.8	0.08	165
F77	23	0.8	0.6	0.14	254
F78	30	0.7	0.6-	0.11	254
F91	27	0.7	0.6-	0.12	254
F92	59	1.0	0.7	0.10	204
F93	47	0.9	0.8	0.11	165
F94	39	0.8	0.7	0.11	204
F95	26	0.8	0.7	0.14	204
F-L	372	0.9	0.7--	0.04	
LANGUEDOC-ROUSSILLON					
F11	17	1.5	1.1	0.30	63
F30	14	0.7	0.5-	0.15	297
F34	25	0.9	0.7	0.14	204
F48	3	1.0	0.4	0.26	333
F66	19	1.5	0.7	0.18	204
F-M	78	1.1	0.7	0.09	
LIMOUSIN					
F19	10	1.0	0.5	0.18	297
F23	4	0.7	0.7	0.39	204
F87	12	0.8	0.5-	0.18	297
F-N	26	0.9	0.5--	0.12	
LORRAINE					
F54	36	1.2	0.9	0.17	127
F55	8	1.0	0.6	0.28	254
F57	32	0.8	0.7	0.13	204
F88	17	1.0	0.7	0.19	204
F-O	93	1.0	0.8	0.09	
MIDI-PYRENEES					
F09	4	0.7	0.6	0.35	254
F12	9	0.8	0.6	0.23	254
F31	37	1.2	1.0	0.17	88
F32	10	1.4	0.9	0.37	127
F46	8	1.3	1.1	0.43	63
F65	6	0.6	0.6	0.26	254
F81	14	1.0	0.6	0.19	254
F82	11	1.5	1.0	0.35	88
F-P	99	1.1	0.8	0.09	
NORD-PAS-DE-CALAIS					
F59	90	0.9	0.7	0.08	204
F62	43	0.7	0.6--	0.10	254
F-Q	133	0.8	0.7--	0.06	
PAYS DE LA LOIRE					
F44	32	0.8	0.6	0.12	254
F49	39	1.5	1.2	0.21	51
F53	8	0.7	0.5-	0.18	297
F72	25	1.2	1.0	0.22	88
F85	24	1.3	0.7	0.18	204
F-R	128	1.1	0.8	0.08	
PICARDIE					
F02	24	1.1	0.8	0.19	165
F60	16	0.7	0.6	0.16	254
F80	24	1.1	0.9	0.19	127
F-S	64	0.9	0.8	0.10	
POITOU-CHARENTES					
F16	23	1.7	1.0	0.25	88
F17	30	1.5	1.1	0.23	63
F79	18	1.3	0.9	0.24	127
F86	15	1.0	0.8	0.24	165
F-T	86	1.4	1.0	0.12	
PROVENCE-ALPES-COTE D'AZUR					
F04	3	0.7	0.5	0.31	297
F05	4	1.0	1.1	0.56	63
F06	14	0.4	0.3--	0.09	346
F13	54	0.8	0.6--	0.09	254
F83	31	1.2	0.8	0.17	165
F84	20	1.3	1.1	0.26	63
F-U	126	0.8	0.6--	0.06	
RHONE-ALPES					
F01	12	0.8	0.7	0.21	204
F07	5	0.5	0.5	0.23	297
F26	4	0.3	0.2--	0.09	351
F38	28	0.8	0.7	0.13	204
F42	29	0.9	0.7	0.14	204
F69	41	0.7	0.5--	0.09	297
F73	11	0.9	0.5-	0.16	297
F74	20	1.1	0.9	0.21	127
F-V	150	0.8	0.6--	0.05	
F.0	2042	1.0	0.7--	0.02	

UNITED KINGDOM (1976-80)

EAST ANGLIA					
G25	14	0.8	0.7	0.20	204
G46	16	0.8	0.5-	0.14	297
G55	24	1.4	1.0	0.23	88
G-A	54	1.0	0.7	0.11	
EAST MIDLANDS					
G30	24	0.9	0.6	0.14	254
G44	25	1.0	0.9	0.18	127
G45	19	1.2	0.9	0.23	127
G47	20	1.3	0.9	0.22	127
G50	24	0.8	0.5-	0.12	297
G-B	112	1.0	0.7	0.07	
NORTHERN					
G14	32	0.9	0.6-	0.11	254
G27	19	1.1	0.8	0.19	165
G29	16	1.1	0.8	0.22	165
G33	18	1.0	0.6	0.17	254
G48	13	1.5	1.0	0.30	88
G-C	98	1.0	0.7	0.08	
NORTH-WEST					
G11	92	1.1	0.8	0.09	165
G12	46	0.9	0.6--	0.09	254
G26	18	0.6	0.4--	0.11	333
G43	44	1.0	0.6	0.11	254
G-D	200	1.0	0.6--	0.05	

SOUTH-EAST					
G01	199	0.9	0.6--	0.05	254
G22	14	1.0	0.8	0.21	165
G23	10	0.5	0.4--	0.12	333
G24	18	1.2	1.0	0.24	88
G34	31	1.4	0.8	0.18	165
G35	36	0.8	0.5--	0.10	297
G37	35	0.8	0.7	0.12	204
G39	12	0.4	0.3--	0.10	346
G41	3	0.8	0.7	0.44	204
G42	60	1.3	0.9	0.13	127
G51	19	1.2	1.0	0.23	88
G56	31	1.0	0.7	0.14	204
G58	21	1.0	0.5-	0.14	297
G-E	489	0.9	0.6--	0.03	
SOUTH-WEST					
G21	23	0.8	0.5-	0.12	297
G28	10	0.8	0.6	0.22	254
G31	33	1.1	0.6-	0.12	254
G32	30	1.6	0.9	0.20	127
G36	12	0.8	0.5	0.17	297
G53	16	1.3	0.7	0.21	204
G59	11	0.7	0.6	0.18	254
G-F	135	1.0	0.6--	0.06	
WEST MIDLANDS					
G15	103	1.2	1.0	0.11	88
G38	10	0.5	0.3--	0.11	346
G52	7	0.6	0.6	0.25	254
G54	39	1.3	1.0	0.16	88
G57	9	0.6	0.5-	0.17	297
G-G	168	1.1	0.8	0.07	
YORKSHIRE AND HUMBERSIDE					
G13	50	1.3	0.9	0.14	127
G16	51	0.8	0.5--	0.08	297
G40	36	1.4	1.0	0.19	88
G49	25	1.2	0.8	0.17	165
G-H	162	1.1	0.8	0.07	
WALES					
G61	16	1.4	1.0	0.27	88
G62	15	1.5	1.0	0.29	88
G63	20	1.5	1.1	0.27	63
G64	11	1.6	1.1	0.38	63
G65	16	1.0	0.6	0.17	254
G66	4	1.3	0.6	0.42	254
G67	13	1.1	0.7	0.20	204
G68	16	1.4	0.8	0.21	165
G-I	111	1.3	0.9	0.09	
SCOTLAND(1975-80)					
S01	4	0.7	0.5	0.29	297
S02	9	0.6	0.4-	0.16	333
S03	15	1.2	0.9	0.25	127
S04	8	0.8	0.5	0.20	297
S05	23	1.0	0.6	0.15	254
S06	1	0.3	0.3-	0.27	346
S07	13	1.6	1.3	0.37	40
S08	105	1.4	1.0	0.11	88
S09	3	0.7	0.6	0.35	254
S10	0	0.0	0.0--	0.00	353
S11	3	4.9	3.7	2.30	1
S12	1	1.1	0.5	0.51	297
G-J	185	1.1	0.8	0.07	
NORTHERN IRELAND					
JE	13	0.8	0.6	0.16	254
JN	10	1.1	0.8	0.27	165
JS	4	0.6	0.5	0.27	297
JW	9	1.5	1.4	0.47	28
G-K	36	0.9	0.8	0.13	
G.0	1750	1.0	0.7--	0.02	
ITALIA (1975-79)					
ABRUZZI					
I66	13	1.7	1.1	0.35	63
I67	14	2.1	1.6	0.45	15
I68	9	1.2	1.0	0.36	88
I69	15	1.6	1.3	0.34	40
I-A	51	1.7	1.2+	0.19	
BASILICATA					
I76	17	1.6	1.5	0.38	19
I77	4	0.8	0.7	0.36	204
I-B	21	1.4	1.2	0.28	
CALABRIA					
I78	18	1.0	0.6	0.16	254
I79	17	0.9	0.7	0.17	204
I80	18	1.2	1.0	0.26	88
I-C	53	1.0	0.8	0.11	
CAMPANIA					
I61	15	0.8	0.7	0.19	204
I62	9	1.2	0.9	0.31	127
I63	80	1.1	1.0	0.11	88
I64	6	0.5	0.5	0.23	297
I65	20	0.8	0.8	0.17	165
I-D	130	1.0	0.9	0.08	
EMILIA-ROMAGNA					
I33	13	1.8	1.1	0.35	63
I34	27	2.6	1.5+	0.32	19
I35	24	2.3	1.6+	0.35	15
I36	35	2.4	1.7++	0.31	12
I37	39	1.6	1.1	0.20	63
I38	16	1.6	1.1	0.30	63
I39	15	1.6	1.1	0.33	63
I40	18	1.2	0.8	0.21	165
I-E	187	1.9	1.3++	0.10	
FRIULI-VENEZIA GIULIA					
I30	23	1.7	1.4	0.30	28
I31	5	1.3	0.7	0.33	204
I32	9	1.1	0.5	0.20	297
I93	17	2.5	1.8+	0.46	7
I-F	54	1.7	1.2	0.17	
LAZIO					
I56	12	1.8	1.4	0.42	28
I57	7	1.9	1.7	0.68	12
I58	141	1.5	1.2++	0.11	51
I59	13	1.3	1.1	0.32	63
I60	13	1.1	0.9	0.28	127
I-G	186	1.5	1.2++	0.09	
LIGURIA					
I08	11	1.8	1.3	0.44	40
I09	14	1.8	1.2	0.35	51
I10	62	2.2	1.4++	0.19	28
I11	9	1.4	1.0	0.36	88
I-H	96	2.0	1.3++	0.14	
LOMBARDIA					
I12	31	1.6	1.3	0.24	40
I13	30	1.5	1.1	0.20	63
I14	4	0.9	0.6	0.34	254
I15	176	1.7	1.3++	0.10	40
I16	40	1.8	1.6++	0.25	15
I17	46	1.8	1.5++	0.23	19
I18	37	2.7	1.9++	0.35	6
I19	15	1.7	1.4	0.39	28
I20	28	2.9	1.8++	0.38	7
I-I	407	1.8	1.4++	0.07	
MARCHE					
I41	16	1.9	1.4	0.41	28
I42	19	1.7	1.0	0.26	88
I43	4	0.5	0.5	0.26	297
I44	5	0.6	0.4-	0.20	333
I-J	44	1.2	0.9	0.15	
MOLISE					
I70	9	1.5	1.1	0.39	63
I94	2	0.8	0.6	0.46	254
I-K	11	1.3	0.9	0.30	
PIEMONTE					
I01	110	1.8	1.3++	0.13	40
I02	19	1.8	1.2	0.31	51
I03	27	2.1	1.5+	0.31	19
I04	25	1.8	1.4	0.31	28
I05	19	3.4	2.3+	0.63	4
I06	29	2.3	1.2	0.27	51
I-L	229	2.0	1.3++	0.10	
PUGLIA					
I71	19	1.1	0.8	0.20	165
I72	32	0.9	0.7	0.13	204
I73	12	0.9	0.7	0.21	204
I74	16	1.6	1.3	0.34	40
I75	27	1.4	1.2	0.24	51
I-M	106	1.1	0.9	0.09	
SARDEGNA					
I90	19	1.8	1.5	0.35	19
I91	8	1.2	1.0	0.37	88
I92	19	1.1	1.0	0.24	88
I95	6	1.5	1.5	0.64	19
I-N	52	1.3	1.2+	0.17	
SICILIA					
I81	12	1.1	0.9	0.27	127
I82	36	1.2	1.1	0.18	63
I83	17	1.0	0.7	0.19	204
I84	20	1.7	1.3	0.30	40
I85	7	1.0	0.8	0.32	165
I86	6	1.2	0.8	0.34	165
I87	31	1.2	1.1	0.20	63
I88	11	1.6	1.3	0.40	40
I89	10	1.0	1.0	0.30	88
I-O	150	1.2	1.0	0.08	
TOSCANA					
I45	5	0.9	0.9	0.43	127
I46	27	2.7	1.5+	0.33	19
I47	10	1.5	0.9	0.30	127
I48	57	1.8	1.1	0.17	63
I49	14	1.6	1.0	0.29	88
I50	15	1.5	0.9	0.26	127
I51	6	0.8	0.7	0.31	204
I52	11	1.7	1.1	0.40	63
I53	8	1.4	0.9	0.35	127
I-P	153	1.7	1.1+	0.10	
TRENTINO-ALTO ADIGE					
I21	14	1.3	1.1	0.30	63
I22	24	2.1	1.6+	0.35	15
I-Q	38	1.7	1.3+	0.23	
UMBRIA					
I54	19	1.3	0.9	0.21	127
I55	10	1.7	1.2	0.43	51
I-R	29	1.4	1.0	0.20	
VALLE D'AOSTA					
I07	7	2.5	1.8	0.72	7
VENETO					
I23	31	1.6	1.2	0.23	51
I24	41	2.3	2.1++	0.34	5
I25	18	3.1	1.8+	0.47	7
I26	33	1.8	1.4+	0.26	28
I27	41	1.9	1.4+	0.22	28
I28	35	1.7	1.4+	0.24	28
I29	11	1.7	1.5	0.46	19
I-T	210	1.9	1.5++	0.11	
I.0	2214	1.5	1.2++	0.03	
IRELAND (1976-80)					
CONNAUGHT					
R07	3	0.7	0.4	0.24	333
R12	1	1.5	0.8	0.78	165
R16	2	0.7	0.7	0.55	204
R20	3	2.3	1.2	0.80	51
R21	2	1.5	0.7	0.47	204
R-A	11	1.1	0.7	0.22	
LEINSTER					
R01	1	1.1	1.5	1.45	19
R06	30	1.2	1.0	0.19	88
R09	1	0.4	0.6	0.56	254
R10	1	0.6	0.4	0.44	333
R11	2	1.7	1.4	1.02	28
R14	3	4.1	3.2	1.88	2
R15	3	1.4	1.0	0.60	88
R17	1	0.5	0.6	0.56	254
R19	2	1.5	1.3	1.04	40
R24	1	0.7	0.7	0.69	204
R25	3	1.3	1.0	0.66	88
R26	3	1.4	1.4	0.82	28
R-B	51	1.2	1.0	0.15	
MUNSTER					
R03	2	1.0	1.1	0.81	63
R04	6	0.6	0.7	0.29	204
R08	2	0.7	0.4	0.30	333
R13	0	0.0	0.0--	0.00	353
R22	6	1.9	1.8	0.74	7
R23	2	0.9	0.7	0.53	204
R-C	18	0.7	0.7	0.18	
ULSTER					
R02	2	1.6	1.0	0.74	88
R05	8	2.7	2.6	0.98	3
R18	0	0.0	0.0--	0.00	353
R-D	10	1.8	1.7	0.55	
R.0	90	1.1	1.0	0.10	
LUXEMBOURG (1971-80)					
LE	3	1.6	1.7	1.00	12
LN	1	0.4	0.4	0.39	333
LS	12	0.9	0.7	0.20	204
L.0	16	0.9	0.7	0.19	
NEDERLAND (1976-80)					
N01	11	0.8	0.5	0.17	297
N02	9	0.6	0.4--	0.14	333
N03	7	0.7	0.5	0.19	297
N04	19	0.8	0.5-	0.13	297
N05	42	1.0	0.8	0.13	165
N06	17	0.8	0.6	0.15	254
N07	65	1.1	0.7	0.10	204
N08	70	0.9	0.7	0.09	204
N09	10	1.2	0.6	0.23	254
N10	31	0.6	0.5--	0.10	297
N11	21	0.8	0.7	0.15	204
N.0	302	0.9	0.6--	0.04	
EEC-9					
EEC	9353	1.2	0.8	0.01	

BELGIE-BELGIQUE (1971-78)

BRUSSEL-BRUXELLES					
B21	196	5.0	3.7++	0.28	26
VLAANDEREN					
B10	189	3.1	2.4	0.18	182
B29	137	3.8	3.0	0.27	87
B30	94	2.2	1.8--	0.19	298
B40	170	3.2	2.4	0.20	182
B70	81	2.9	2.9	0.32	104
B-V	671	3.0	2.4-	0.10	
WALLONIE					
B25	32	3.1	2.6	0.48	144
B50	199	3.9	2.8	0.20	112
B60	160	4.1	3.0	0.25	87
B80	28	3.2	2.5	0.49	160
B90	38	2.5	2.1	0.35	248
B-W	457	3.7	2.7	0.13	
B.0	1324	3.4	2.7	0.08	

BR DEUTSCHLAND (1976-80)

BADEN-WURTTEMBERG					
D81	187	2.2	1.7--	0.13	315
D82	169	3.0	2.3	0.19	202
D83	113	2.6	2.1--	0.20	248
D84	79	2.2	1.8--	0.21	298
D-A	548	2.5	2.0--	0.09	
BAYERN					
D91	249	2.9	2.1--	0.14	248
D92	68	2.9	2.2	0.28	224
D93	50	2.2	1.8--	0.27	298
D94	73	3.0	2.1	0.27	248
D95	82	2.3	1.6--	0.19	323
D96	90	3.2	2.5	0.27	160
D97	103	2.8	2.3	0.24	202
D-B	715	2.8	2.1--	0.08	
BERLIN(WEST)					
DB0	161	3.8	2.5	0.23	160
BREMEN					
D40	45	2.7	1.8--	0.28	298
HAMBURG					
D20	157	4.1	2.6	0.22	144
HESSEN					
D64	329	3.1	2.3-	0.13	202
D66	105	3.7	2.5	0.26	160
D-F	434	3.3	2.4-	0.12	
NIEDERSACHSEN					
D31	76	1.9	1.5--	0.19	334
D32	114	2.3	1.6--	0.16	323
D33	87	2.5	1.9--	0.21	288
D34	103	2.0	1.7--	0.17	315
D-G	380	2.2	1.7--	0.09	
NORDRHEIN-WESTFALEN					
D51	350	2.8	2.3-	0.13	202
D53	290	3.1	2.7	0.16	126
D55	147	2.5	2.3	0.20	202
D57	123	2.9	2.3	0.21	202
D59	249	2.8	2.2-	0.15	224
D-H	1159	2.9	2.4--	0.07	
RHEINLAND-PFALZ					
D71	92	2.8	2.0--	0.22	273
D72	39	3.5	2.8	0.47	112
D73	127	2.9	2.3	0.21	202
D-I	258	3.0	2.2--	0.15	
SAARLAND					
DA0	91	3.6	2.6	0.30	144
SCHLESWIG-HOLSTEIN					
D10	175	2.8	2.1--	0.17	248
D.0	4123	2.8	2.2--	0.04	

DANMARK (1971-80)

K15	322	5.3	3.7++	0.21	26
K20	70	4.6	4.4++	0.53	3
K25	36	3.9	3.8	0.65	21
K30	54	4.0	2.6	0.37	144
K35	75	5.8	3.9++	0.49	14
K40	8	3.4	2.2	0.85	224
K42	99	4.5	3.2	0.34	60
K50	48	3.9	3.1	0.46	78
K55	46	4.4	3.3	0.51	54
K60	79	5.0	3.6+	0.42	31
K65	61	4.8	3.8+	0.50	21
K70	130	4.7	3.6++	0.33	31
K76	67	5.9	4.0++	0.52	10
K80	105	4.4	3.2	0.33	60
K.0	1200	4.8	3.5++	0.11	

FRANCE (1971-78)

ALSACE					
F67	114	3.3	2.9	0.29	104
F68	67	2.7	2.4	0.30	182
F-A	181	3.0	2.7	0.21	
AQUITAINE					
F24	55	3.8	2.6	0.39	144
F33	126	3.1	2.2	0.21	224
F40	36	3.2	2.4	0.41	182
F47	47	4.1	3.2	0.52	60
F64	61	3.0	2.1	0.28	248
F-B	325	3.3	2.4	0.14	
AUVERGNE					
F03	40	2.7	1.8-	0.32	298
F15	14	2.1	1.7	0.51	315
F43	24	3.0	1.8-	0.40	298
F63	61	2.7	2.2	0.29	224
F-C	139	2.7	2.0--	0.18	
BASSE-NORMANDIE					
F14	49	2.2	2.1	0.31	248
F50	42	2.4	2.0-	0.31	273
F61	23	2.0	1.6--	0.35	323
F-D	114	2.2	2.0--	0.19	
BOURGOGNE					
F21	57	3.2	2.5	0.34	160
F58	42	4.3	2.6	0.44	144
F71	73	3.3	2.3	0.29	202
F89	48	4.0	2.7	0.42	126
F-E	220	3.5	2.5	0.18	
BRETAGNE					
F22	46	2.3	1.8--	0.27	298
F29	82	2.6	2.1-	0.24	248
F35	73	2.7	2.4	0.29	182
F56	48	2.2	1.9--	0.28	288
F-F	249	2.5	2.0--	0.13	
CENTRE					
F18	40	3.2	2.2	0.37	224
F28	43	3.2	2.4	0.38	182
F36	41	4.2	3.3	0.55	54
F37	63	3.4	2.5	0.33	160
F41	38	3.4	2.5	0.44	160
F45	62	3.2	2.4	0.33	182
F-G	287	3.4	2.5	0.16	
CHAMPAGNE-ARDENNE					
F08	38	3.1	2.6	0.43	144
F10	35	3.1	2.4	0.43	182
F51	51	2.4	2.2	0.31	224
F52	21	2.5	2.1	0.49	248
F-H	145	2.7	2.3	0.20	
CORSE					
F20	19	2.0	1.8-	0.43	298
FRANCHE-COMTE					
F25	36	1.9	1.9-	0.33	288
F39	29	3.1	2.5	0.50	160
F70	18	2.1	1.6--	0.39	323
F90	10	2.0	1.6-	0.51	323
F-J	93	2.2	1.9--	0.20	
HAUTE-NORMANDIE					
F27	40	2.4	2.1	0.34	248
F76	145	3.1	2.8	0.24	112
F-K	185	2.9	2.6	0.20	
ILE-DE-FRANCE					
F75	350	4.1	3.2++	0.19	60
F77	74	2.5	2.2	0.27	224
F78	95	2.2	2.3	0.24	202
F91	89	2.4	2.6	0.28	144
F92	162	2.9	2.4	0.19	182
F93	144	2.7	2.7	0.23	126
F94	126	2.7	2.6	0.23	144
F95	89	2.7	2.7	0.29	126
F-L	1129	2.9	2.6	0.08	
LANGUEDOC-ROUSSILLON					
F11	35	3.4	2.5	0.46	160
F30	60	3.1	2.1	0.29	248
F34	91	3.7	3.0	0.35	87
F48	5	1.7	1.4-	0.63	337
F66	37	3.2	2.2	0.40	224
F-M	228	3.3	2.4	0.18	
LIMOUSIN					
F19	25	2.7	1.6--	0.35	323
F23	25	4.4	2.0	0.44	273
F87	43	3.1	2.1	0.35	248
F-N	93	3.2	2.0--	0.22	
LORRAINE					
F54	71	2.5	2.4	0.29	182
F55	21	2.6	2.3	0.54	202
F57	89	2.2	2.2	0.24	224
F88	26	1.7	1.6--	0.32	323
F-O	207	2.2	2.1--	0.15	
MIDI-PYRENEES					
F09	11	2.0	1.6	0.61	323
F12	31	2.9	2.0	0.41	273
F31	75	2.5	2.1-	0.26	248
F32	22	3.2	2.0	0.45	273
F46	18	3.1	2.3	0.65	202
F65	29	3.3	2.5	0.49	160
F81	40	3.0	2.0	0.35	273
F82	27	3.8	2.5	0.52	160
F-P	253	2.9	2.1--	0.15	
NORD-PAS-DE-CALAIS					
F59	238	2.4	2.2--	0.15	224
F62	129	2.4	2.1--	0.19	248
F-Q	367	2.4	2.2--	0.12	
PAYS DE LA LOIRE					
F44	75	2.1	1.8--	0.21	298
F49	70	2.8	2.5	0.30	160
F53	32	3.2	2.7	0.49	126
F72	50	2.6	2.2	0.33	224
F85	50	2.9	2.1	0.32	248
F-R	277	2.6	2.2--	0.13	
PICARDIE					
F02	51	2.4	2.1	0.31	248
F60	62	2.5	2.3	0.31	202
F80	53	2.5	2.1	0.30	248
F-S	166	2.5	2.2-	0.18	
POITOU-CHARENTES					
F16	53	4.0	2.8	0.40	112
F17	62	3.2	2.3	0.32	202
F79	54	4.0	3.2	0.48	60
F86	43	3.1	2.2	0.36	224
F-T	212	3.5	2.6	0.19	
PROVENCE-ALPES-COTE D'AZUR					
F04	18	4.0	2.8	0.72	112
F05	9	2.3	1.7	0.68	315
F06	60	1.9	1.2--	0.18	350
F13	200	3.1	2.5	0.19	160
F83	93	3.8	2.7	0.29	126
F84	42	2.7	2.0	0.32	273
F-U	422	2.9	2.2--	0.11	
RHONE-ALPES					
F01	42	2.8	2.1	0.33	248
F07	30	3.0	2.0	0.38	273
F26	45	3.2	2.3	0.37	202
F38	101	3.0	2.6	0.26	144
F42	101	3.4	2.7	0.29	126
F69	197	3.5	3.2+	0.23	60
F73	47	3.9	3.1	0.48	78
F74	36	2.0	1.9-	0.32	288
F-V	599	3.2	2.7	0.11	
F.0	5910	2.9	2.3--	0.03	

UNITED KINGDOM (1976-80)

EAST ANGLIA					
G25	64	3.7	3.2	0.41	60
G46	91	4.6	3.0	0.33	87
G55	80	4.5	3.2	0.37	60
G-A	235	4.3	3.1+	0.21	
EAST MIDLANDS					
G30	98	3.7	2.6	0.27	144
G44	107	4.3	3.5+	0.34	37
G45	79	5.0	3.5+	0.42	37
G47	82	5.4	4.2++	0.48	6
G50	150	5.2	3.9++	0.33	14
G-B	516	4.7	3.5++	0.16	
NORTHERN					
G14	164	4.8	3.6++	0.29	31
G27	51	3.0	2.5	0.36	160
G29	54	3.9	2.7	0.39	126
G33	68	3.8	2.8	0.35	112
G48	42	4.9	3.5	0.57	37
G-C	379	4.2	3.1++	0.17	
NORTH-WEST					
G11	268	3.5	2.6	0.17	144
G12	162	3.6	2.8	0.23	112
G26	98	3.6	2.9	0.30	104
G43	136	3.5	2.4	0.22	182
G-D	664	3.5	2.7	0.11	

SOUTH-EAST					
G01	981	4.9	3.4++	0.11	45
G22	54	3.6	2.9	0.40	104
G23	86	4.3	3.7++	0.41	26
G24	73	4.6	3.9++	0.46	14
G34	102	5.7	3.0	0.33	87
G35	199	4.7	3.4++	0.25	45
G37	225	5.1	4.0++	0.28	10
G39	112	4.0	3.2	0.30	60
G41	17	5.3	3.2	0.86	60
G42	203	4.8	3.5++	0.26	37
G51	60	3.6	3.0	0.39	87
G56	172	5.9	4.2++	0.34	6
G58	99	5.6	3.2	0.36	60
G-E	2383	4.9	3.5++	0.07	
SOUTH-WEST					
G21	126	4.7	3.2+	0.30	60
G28	73	6.1	3.9++	0.49	14
G31	149	5.4	3.5++	0.31	37
G32	92	5.5	3.2	0.36	60
G36	63	4.4	3.1	0.41	78
G53	64	5.3	3.5	0.45	37
G59	72	4.6	3.7+	0.44	26
G-F	639	5.1	3.4++	0.14	
WEST MIDLANDS					
C15	350	4.3	3.3++	0.18	54
G38	91	5.1	3.8++	0.41	21
G52	40	3.7	2.7	0.43	126
G54	118	4.0	3.1	0.29	78
G57	50	3.6	2.9	0.41	104
G-G	649	4.3	3.3++	0.13	
YORKSHIRE AND HUMBERSIDE					
G13	148	3.9	2.8	0.24	112
G16	241	4.0	3.0	0.20	87
G40	89	3.6	2.7	0.30	126
G49	79	4.1	2.7	0.32	126
G-H	557	3.9	2.8	0.12	
WALES					
G61	58	5.2	4.0+	0.55	10
G62	41	4.4	3.0	0.50	87
G63	51	4.0	3.1	0.46	78
G64	29	4.4	3.0	0.60	87
G65	51	3.2	2.4	0.34	182
G66	14	4.4	2.5	0.73	160
G67	52	4.6	3.2	0.45	60
G68	45	4.3	3.0	0.48	87
G-I	341	4.2	3.0+	0.17	
SCOTLAND(1975-80)					
S01	18	3.2	2.6	0.62	144
S02	72	5.4	3.9++	0.48	14
S03	47	4.1	2.9	0.43	104
S04	50	5.0	3.8+	0.55	21
S05	120	5.6	4.2++	0.40	6
S06	16	5.6	3.2	0.84	60
S07	32	4.0	3.0	0.55	87
S08	333	4.7	3.7++	0.21	26
S09	17	4.1	3.1	0.78	78
S10	2	3.8	2.5	1.82	160
S11	6	9.6	8.2	3.43	1
S12	7	8.0	4.4	1.74	3
G-J	720	4.8	3.6++	0.14	
NORTHERN IRELAND					
JE	64	3.9	3.4	0.44	45
JN	28	3.1	2.7	0.53	126
JS	17	2.6	2.1	0.54	248
JW	29	4.8	4.7+	0.90	2
G-K	138	3.6	3.2+	0.28	
G.0	7221	4.4	3.3++	0.04	
ITALIA (1975-79)					
ABRUZZI					
I66	20	2.7	2.0	0.47	273
I67	12	1.8	1.6-	0.49	323
I68	18	2.6	2.0	0.49	273
I69	20	2.2	1.8-	0.42	298
I-A	70	2.3	1.9--	0.23	
BASILICATA					
I76	23	2.2	1.9	0.41	288
I77	4	0.8	0.7--	0.36	353
I-B	27	1.8	1.5--	0.30	
CALABRIA					
I78	26	1.5	1.3--	0.27	345
I79	29	1.6	1.4--	0.26	337
I80	31	2.1	1.8--	0.33	298
I-C	86	1.7	1.5--	0.16	
CAMPANIA					
I61	24	1.3	1.3--	0.27	345
I62	20	2.8	2.4	0.55	182
I63	132	1.9	1.9--	0.17	288
I64	17	1.6	1.3--	0.33	345
I65	38	1.5	1.4--	0.23	337
I-D	231	1.8	1.7--	0.11	
EMILIA-ROMAGNA					
I33	21	3.0	2.2	0.53	224
I34	37	3.8	2.7	0.50	126
I35	35	3.5	2.3	0.41	202
I36	61	4.3	3.4	0.45	45
I37	94	4.2	3.0	0.33	87
I38	50	5.3	3.4	0.49	45
I39	35	4.0	2.5	0.44	160
I40	64	4.4	3.3	0.42	54
I-E	397	4.1	2.9	0.15	
FRIULI-VENEZIA GIULIA					
I30	39	3.0	2.2	0.37	224
I31	19	5.4	3.9	0.92	14
I32	42	6.0	3.4	0.56	45
I93	18	2.8	2.0	0.50	273
I-F	118	3.9	2.7	0.26	
LAZIO					
I56	22	3.4	2.2	0.49	224
I57	14	3.9	2.8	0.77	112
I58	270	3.0	2.8	0.17	112
I59	35	3.4	3.2	0.54	60
I60	28	2.5	2.0	0.40	273
I-G	369	3.1	2.7	0.14	
LIGURIA					
I08	28	5.0	2.9	0.57	104
I09	26	3.5	2.2	0.46	224
I10	107	4.1	2.7	0.27	126
I11	28	4.7	3.0	0.60	87
I-H	189	4.2	2.7	0.21	
LOMBARDIA					
I12	56	3.0	2.7	0.38	126
I13	58	3.2	2.8	0.38	112
I14	8	1.9	1.7	0.59	315
I15	304	3.1	2.7	0.16	126
I16	48	2.2	2.1	0.30	248
I17	88	3.6	3.2	0.34	60
I18	65	5.1	3.4	0.46	45
I19	34	4.2	3.0	0.54	87
I20	33	3.6	2.4	0.44	182
I-I	694	3.2	2.7	0.11	
MARCHE					
I41	28	3.5	2.4	0.48	182
I42	28	2.7	1.8-	0.35	298
I43	22	3.1	2.3	0.53	202
I44	25	2.9	2.5	0.52	160
I-J	103	3.0	2.2	0.23	
MOLISE					
I70	9	1.6	1.3--	0.42	345
I94	5	2.2	2.2	0.99	224
I-K	14	1.7	1.5--	0.41	
PIEMONTE					
I01	139	2.4	2.0--	0.17	273
I02	31	3.2	2.2	0.42	224
I03	40	3.3	2.4	0.39	182
I04	39	2.9	1.9-	0.32	288
I05	21	3.9	2.6	0.60	144
I06	39	3.4	2.1	0.37	248
I-L	309	2.8	2.1--	0.12	
PUGLIA					
I71	37	2.2	1.9-	0.33	288
I72	62	1.8	1.6--	0.21	323
I73	20	1.5	1.4--	0.32	337
I74	14	1.5	1.4--	0.37	337
I75	44	2.4	2.2	0.33	224
I-M	177	1.9	1.7--	0.13	
SARDEGNA					
I90	25	2.4	1.9	0.40	288
I91	15	2.2	1.8	0.48	298
I92	37	2.1	2.1	0.35	248
I95	7	1.8	1.4-	0.55	337
I-N	84	2.2	1.9--	0.22	
SICILIA					
I81	31	3.0	2.3	0.43	202
I82	79	2.8	2.4	0.28	182
I83	31	1.9	1.4--	0.25	337
I84	25	2.1	1.6--	0.34	323
I85	18	2.5	2.4	0.58	182
I86	15	3.0	2.1	0.58	248
I87	49	2.0	1.8--	0.26	298
I88	10	1.5	1.2--	0.39	350
I89	25	2.6	2.4	0.48	182
I-O	283	2.4	2.0--	0.12	
TOSCANA					
I45	17	3.4	2.5	0.64	160
I46	36	3.9	2.5	0.44	160
I47	21	3.3	2.0	0.46	273
I48	102	3.5	2.6	0.27	144
I49	37	4.4	3.2	0.55	60
I50	28	3.0	2.1	0.42	248
I51	32	4.2	2.5	0.46	160
I52	21	3.3	1.8-	0.41	298
I53	30	5.4	3.5	0.67	37
I-P	324	3.7	2.5	0.15	
TRENTINO-ALTO ADIGE					
I21	17	1.6	1.5--	0.38	334
I22	30	2.8	2.0	0.38	273
I-Q	47	2.2	1.8--	0.27	
UMBRIA					
I54	47	3.3	2.3	0.35	202
I55	21	3.7	2.8	0.64	112
I-R	68	3.5	2.4	0.31	
VALLE D'AOSTA					
I07	5	1.8	1.5	0.69	334
VENETO					
I23	64	3.4	2.8	0.36	112
I24	50	2.9	2.6	0.37	144
I25	18	3.3	2.3	0.55	202
I26	62	3.6	2.9	0.38	104
I27	71	3.5	3.0	0.36	87
I28	51	2.6	2.3	0.33	202
I29	18	2.9	2.2	0.54	224
I-T	334	3.2	2.7	0.15	
I.0	3929	2.9	2.3--	0.04	
IRELAND (1976-80)					
CONNAUGHT					
R07	19	4.4	3.1	0.74	78
R12	6	8.1	3.4	1.39	45
R16	10	3.4	2.2	0.78	224
R20	5	3.5	3.0	1.44	87
R21	3	2.2	1.7	1.03	315
R-A	43	4.0	2.6	0.44	
LEINSTER					
R01	4	4.1	4.1	2.06	9
R06	69	2.9	3.1	0.38	78
R09	5	2.0	2.3	1.05	202
R10	4	2.2	1.8	0.92	298
R11	2	1.5	1.3	0.97	345
R14	2	2.5	1.7	1.22	315
R15	4	1.9	1.9	0.97	288
R17	5	2.1	2.4	1.09	182
R19	5	3.4	2.5	1.18	160
R24	4	2.6	2.3	1.15	202
R25	7	2.9	2.1	0.81	248
R26	8	3.8	3.9	1.41	14
R-B	119	2.8	2.8	0.26	
MUNSTER					
R03	7	3.2	2.7	1.07	126
R04	39	3.9	3.5	0.58	37
R08	8	2.6	1.7	0.66	315
R13	9	2.3	2.2	0.75	224
R22	13	3.8	3.1	0.88	78
R23	0	0.0	0.0--	0.00	355
R-C	76	3.1	2.6	0.31	
ULSTER					
R02	1	0.7	0.5--	0.53	354
R05	8	2.6	1.8	0.65	298
R18	4	3.0	2.7	1.37	126
R-D	13	2.2	1.7	0.49	
R.0	251	3.0	2.6	0.17	
LUXEMBOURG (1971-80)					
LE	3	1.7	1.4	0.83	337
LN	4	1.5	0.9--	0.45	352
LS	35	2.7	2.2	0.37	224
L.0	42	2.4	1.9--	0.29	
NEDERLAND (1976-80)					
N01	53	3.9	2.8	0.40	112
N02	69	4.8	3.6+	0.46	31
N03	43	4.1	3.4	0.53	45
N04	104	4.1	3.6++	0.36	31
N05	200	4.8	4.0++	0.29	10
N06	93	4.3	3.6++	0.38	31
N07	310	5.4	4.4++	0.26	3
N08	360	4.8	3.8++	0.21	21
N09	36	4.2	3.0	0.52	87
N10	167	3.3	3.3+	0.26	54
N11	97	3.6	3.3+	0.34	54
N.0	1532	4.4	3.7++	0.10	
EEC-9					
EEC	25532	3.4	2.6	0.02	

BELGIE-BELGIQUE (1971-78)

BRUSSEL-BRUXELLES					
B21	145	3.3	1.6	0.15	118
VLAANDEREN					
B10	128	2.0	1.4	0.14	160
B29	87	2.4	1.5	0.17	136
B30	50	1.2	0.7--	0.11	333
B40	100	1.9	1.2-	0.14	217
B70	49	1.8	1.6	0.23	118
B-V	414	1.9	1.3--	0.07	
WALLONIE					
B25	20	1.9	1.1	0.27	255
B50	142	2.6	1.5	0.14	136
B60	111	2.6	1.6	0.17	118
B80	17	1.9	1.3	0.37	183
B90	55	3.4	2.1	0.32	49
B-W	345	2.6	1.5	0.09	
B.0	904	2.3	1.4--	0.05	

BR DEUTSCHLAND (1976-80)

BADEN-WURTTEMBERG					
D81	174	2.0	1.2--	0.10	217
D82	159	2.6	1.4	0.12	160
D83	86	1.8	1.0--	0.12	279
D84	65	1.7	0.8--	0.11	323
D-A	484	2.0	1.1--	0.06	
BAYERN					
D91	237	2.5	1.3	0.10	183
D92	57	2.2	1.2-	0.17	217
D93	43	1.7	0.9--	0.16	309
D94	69	2.5	1.2-	0.16	217
D95	93	2.3	1.2-	0.15	217
D96	66	2.1	1.2	0.18	217
D97	83	2.1	1.3	0.16	183
D-B	648	2.3	1.2--	0.06	
BERLIN (WEST)					
DB0	228	4.3	1.6	0.15	118
BREMEN					
D40	58	3.1	1.5	0.23	136
HAMBURG					
D20	133	3.0	1.4	0.16	160
HESSEN					
D64	298	2.6	1.4	0.09	160
D66	76	2.4	1.3	0.19	183
D-F	374	2.6	1.4	0.08	
NIEDERSACHSEN					
D31	100	2.3	1.2-	0.15	217
D32	109	2.0	1.0--	0.11	279
D33	101	2.7	1.4	0.16	160
D34	115	2.1	1.2--	0.13	217
D-G	425	2.3	1.2--	0.07	
NORDRHEIN-WESTFALEN					
D51	380	2.8	1.5	0.09	136
D53	249	2.5	1.6	0.11	118
D55	123	2.0	1.3-	0.12	183
D57	103	2.2	1.2-	0.14	217
D59	212	2.2	1.3--	0.10	183
D-H	1067	2.4	1.4-	0.05	
RHEINLAND-PFALZ					
D71	90	2.5	1.3	0.16	183
D72	29	2.3	1.3	0.26	183
D73	113	2.4	1.3	0.14	183
D-I	232	2.4	1.3-	0.10	
SAARLAND					
DA0	57	2.0	1.1--	0.16	255
SCHLESWIG-HOLSTEIN					
D10	151	2.2	1.2--	0.12	217
D.0	3857	2.4	1.3--	0.02	

DANMARK (1971-80)

K15	308	4.6	2.3++	0.15	31
K20	33	2.2	1.9	0.34	73
K25	19	2.1	1.8	0.43	83
K30	74	5.5	3.2++	0.41	3
K35	65	5.1	2.5++	0.36	21
K40	6	2.6	1.3	0.55	183
K42	71	3.2	1.7	0.23	105
K50	29	2.4	1.9	0.39	73
K55	43	4.2	3.0++	0.48	6
K60	49	3.1	1.8	0.27	83
K65	33	2.6	1.8	0.34	83
K70	100	3.5	2.1+	0.22	49
K76	48	4.3	2.6+	0.41	13
K80	82	3.5	2.1+	0.25	49
K.0	960	3.8	2.2++	0.08	

FRANCE (1971-78)

ALSACE					
F67	90	2.5	1.6	0.19	118
F68	38	1.5	1.0--	0.18	279
F-A	128	2.1	1.3	0.13	
AQUITAINE					
F24	27	1.8	1.0-	0.24	279
F33	114	2.6	1.6	0.18	118
F40	26	2.2	1.5	0.36	136
F47	25	2.1	1.2	0.29	217
F64	50	2.3	1.3	0.22	183
F-B	242	2.3	1.4	0.11	
AUVERGNE					
F03	20	1.3	0.6--	0.17	338
F15	19	2.8	1.6	0.44	118
F43	19	2.3	0.8--	0.26	323
F63	31	1.3	0.8--	0.17	323
F-C	89	1.6	0.9--	0.11	
BASSE-NORMANDIE					
F14	32	1.4	1.0--	0.20	279
F50	39	2.1	1.1-	0.20	255
F61	22	1.8	1.1	0.27	255
F-D	93	1.7	1.1--	0.13	
BOURGOGNE					
F21	36	2.0	1.1-	0.22	255
F58	25	2.5	1.5	0.39	136
F71	59	2.5	1.2	0.19	217
F89	32	2.6	1.0-	0.22	279
F-E	152	2.4	1.2--	0.12	
BRETAGNE					
F22	41	1.9	1.2	0.22	217
F29	71	2.1	1.2-	0.16	217
F35	57	2.0	1.1-	0.17	255
F56	34	1.5	0.9--	0.19	309
F-F	203	1.9	1.1--	0.09	
CENTRE					
F18	20	1.6	1.0-	0.25	279
F28	23	1.7	1.1	0.25	255
F36	23	2.3	1.3	0.32	183
F37	40	2.0	1.3	0.25	183
F41	28	2.4	1.0-	0.22	279
F45	45	2.3	1.4	0.24	160
F-G	179	2.1	1.2--	0.10	
CHAMPAGNE-ARDENNE					
F08	14	1.1	0.9--	0.25	309
F10	29	2.5	1.7	0.35	105
F51	45	2.1	1.4	0.23	160
F52	18	2.1	1.4	0.35	160
F-H	106	2.0	1.3	0.14	
CORSE					
F20	20	2.3	1.0	0.27	279
FRANCHE-COMTE					
F25	27	1.4	1.1-	0.22	255
F39	12	1.2	1.0	0.35	279
F70	18	2.0	1.0	0.28	279
F90	8	1.6	1.2	0.44	217
F-J	65	1.5	1.0--	0.14	
HAUTE-NORMANDIE					
F27	30	1.8	1.0-	0.21	279
F76	101	2.1	1.6	0.17	118
F-K	131	2.0	1.4	0.14	
ILE-DE-FRANCE					
F75	312	3.2	1.7	0.12	105
F77	55	1.8	1.2	0.18	217
F78	80	1.8	1.5	0.18	136
F91	51	1.4	1.2	0.19	217
F92	124	2.1	1.4	0.14	160
F93	94	1.8	1.3	0.14	183
F94	93	1.9	1.3	0.15	183
F95	53	1.6	1.3	0.19	183
F-L	862	2.1	1.4-	0.05	
LANGUEDOC-ROUSSILLON					
F11	22	2.0	0.9--	0.24	309
F30	41	2.0	1.3	0.22	183
F34	63	2.3	1.4	0.22	160
F48	3	1.0	0.6-	0.40	338
F66	33	2.6	2.0	0.44	61
F-M	162	2.2	1.3	0.13	
LIMOUSIN					
F19	17	1.7	0.9-	0.28	309
F23	12	2.0	1.1	0.40	255
F87	27	1.9	1.1	0.24	255
F-N	56	1.8	1.0--	0.16	
LORRAINE					
F54	44	1.5	0.9--	0.15	309
F55	10	1.2	0.6--	0.23	338
F57	59	1.5	1.2	0.17	217
F88	17	1.0	0.5--	0.16	344
F-O	130	1.4	0.9--	0.09	
MIDI-PYRENEES					
F09	13	2.3	1.3	0.57	183
F12	19	1.7	0.6--	0.16	338
F31	46	1.4	1.0--	0.18	279
F32	13	1.9	1.1	0.39	255
F46	15	2.5	1.2	0.40	217
F65	9	1.0	0.8-	0.30	323
F81	24	1.7	1.2	0.28	217
F82	15	2.0	1.2	0.35	217
F-P	154	1.7	1.0--	0.10	
NORD-PAS-DE-CALAIS					
F59	176	1.7	1.2--	0.10	217
F62	96	1.7	1.2--	0.13	217
F-Q	272	1.7	1.2--	0.08	
PAYS DE LA LOIRE					
F44	66	1.7	1.1--	0.16	255
F49	55	2.1	1.3	0.20	183
F53	11	1.0	0.6--	0.20	338
F72	28	1.4	0.9--	0.19	309
F85	38	2.1	1.1-	0.21	255
F-R	198	1.7	1.1--	0.09	
PICARDIE					
F02	51	2.4	1.4	0.23	160
F60	42	1.7	1.4	0.23	160
F80	38	1.7	1.2	0.21	217
F-S	131	1.9	1.4	0.13	
POITOU-CHARENTES					
F16	29	2.1	1.1	0.25	255
F17	40	2.0	1.0--	0.19	279
F79	31	2.3	1.4	0.29	160
F86	36	2.5	1.8	0.33	83
F-T	136	2.2	1.3-	0.13	
PROVENCE-ALPES-COTE D'AZUR					
F04	7	1.6	1.0	0.46	279
F05	7	1.8	1.0	0.48	279
F06	77	2.2	1.1-	0.20	255
F13	162	2.4	1.5	0.13	136
F83	59	2.3	1.1--	0.16	255
F84	44	2.8	1.7	0.29	105
F-U	356	2.4	1.3--	0.08	
RHONE-ALPES					
F01	31	2.1	1.1	0.25	255
F07	21	2.0	0.9--	0.24	309
F26	26	1.8	1.1-	0.23	255
F38	71	2.0	1.3	0.18	183
F42	59	1.9	1.4	0.20	160
F69	138	2.4	1.6	0.16	118
F73	29	2.3	1.6	0.32	118
F74	32	1.8	1.3	0.25	183
F-V	407	2.1	1.4-	0.08	
F.0	4272	2.0	1.2--	0.02	

UNITED KINGDOM (1976-80)

EAST ANGLIA					
G25	59	3.5	2.1	0.30	49
G46	78	3.8	2.0	0.26	61
G55	62	3.5	1.9	0.28	73
G-A	199	3.6	2.0++	0.16	
EAST MIDLANDS					
G30	105	3.8	2.2++	0.25	39
G44	84	3.3	2.1+	0.24	49
G45	61	3.8	2.3+	0.33	31
G47	71	4.5	2.6++	0.34	13
G50	113	3.8	2.2++	0.22	39
G-B	434	3.8	2.2++	0.12	
NORTHERN					
G14	137	3.8	2.0+	0.19	61
G27	42	2.4	1.4	0.24	160
G29	40	2.7	1.5	0.26	136
G33	61	3.3	1.9	0.28	73
G48	21	2.4	1.5	0.35	136
G-C	301	3.1	1.8	0.11	
NORTH-WEST					
G11	246	3.0	1.7	0.12	105
G12	125	2.6	1.5	0.14	136
G26	81	2.9	1.8	0.21	83
G43	128	3.0	1.6	0.16	118
G-D	580	2.9	1.6	0.08	

SOUTH-EAST					
G01	948	4.4	2.3++	0.09	31
G22	41	2.8	2.0	0.32	61
G23	72	3.6	2.2+	0.28	39
G24	62	4.0	2.6++	0.37	13
G34	132	6.2	2.1+	0.25	49
G35	194	4.4	2.5++	0.20	21
G37	183	4.2	2.4++	0.20	26
G39	102	3.5	2.2++	0.23	39
G41	23	6.4	3.1	0.81	4
G42	183	4.1	2.1++	0.18	49
G51	46	2.9	1.9	0.32	73
G56	145	4.7	2.6++	0.24	13
G58	109	5.4	2.3++	0.27	31
G-E	2240	4.3	2.3++	0.06	
SOUTH-WEST					
G21	122	4.3	2.3++	0.24	31
G28	45	3.5	1.6	0.28	118
G31	155	5.3	2.4++	0.23	26
G32	99	5.4	2.1+	0.28	49
G36	56	3.7	2.2	0.32	39
G53	64	5.1	2.7++	0.38	9
G59	55	3.6	2.2+	0.32	39
G-F	596	4.5	2.3++	0.11	
WEST MIDLANDS					
G15	280	3.4	2.0++	0.13	61
G38	62	3.4	1.8	0.26	83
G52	33	3.0	1.8	0.37	83
G54	101	3.3	2.3++	0.24	31
G57	40	2.8	1.8	0.30	83
G-G	516	3.3	2.0++	0.10	
YORKSHIRE AND HUMBERSIDE					
G13	133	3.3	1.9	0.18	73
G16	195	3.0	1.6	0.13	118
G40	90	3.4	2.0+	0.24	61
G49	81	4.0	1.9	0.25	73
G-H	499	3.3	1.8++	0.09	
WALES					
G61	40	3.4	1.8	0.34	83
G62	49	4.8	2.5+	0.39	21
G63	38	2.8	1.9	0.34	73
G64	33	4.7	2.6	0.58	13
G65	47	2.8	1.8	0.29	83
G66	7	2.2	1.3	0.54	183
G67	53	4.4	2.2	0.34	39
G68	36	3.1	1.7	0.31	105
G-I	303	3.5	2.0++	0.13	
SCOTLAND (1975-80)					
S01	21	3.7	2.3	0.56	31
S02	63	4.4	2.1+	0.30	49
S03	54	4.3	2.3+	0.35	31
S04	46	4.4	2.6+	0.41	13
S05	120	5.1	2.7++	0.28	9
S06	12	3.8	3.1	1.09	4
S07	28	3.4	2.0	0.40	61
S08	326	4.2	2.5++	0.15	21
S09	16	3.6	1.7	0.47	105
S10	1	1.8	1.0	0.95	279
S11	3	4.9	3.9	2.43	2
S12	3	3.3	1.5	1.06	136
G-J	693	4.3	2.4++	0.10	
NORTHERN IRELAND					
JE	64	3.8	2.6++	0.35	13
JN	33	3.6	2.7+	0.50	9
JS	8	1.2	0.7--	0.27	333
JW	22	3.6	2.5	0.56	21
G-K	127	3.3	2.3++	0.22	
G.0	6488	3.8	2.1++	0.03	
ITALIA (1975-79)					
ABRUZZI					
I66	17	2.2	1.2	0.34	217
I67	13	1.9	1.4	0.44	160
I68	16	2.2	1.5	0.40	136
I69	13	1.4	1.0-	0.29	279
I-A	59	1.9	1.2	0.18	
BASILICATA					
I76	5	0.5	0.3--	0.16	349
I77	2	0.4	0.3--	0.23	349
I-B	7	0.5	0.3--	0.13	
CALABRIA					
I78	15	0.8	0.6--	0.16	338
I79	24	1.3	1.0--	0.21	279
I80	18	1.2	1.0-	0.25	279
I-C	57	1.1	0.8--	0.12	
CAMPANIA					
I61	15	0.8	0.7--	0.20	333
I62	10	1.4	0.9-	0.29	309
I63	98	1.3	1.2--	0.12	217
I64	15	1.4	1.0-	0.27	279
I65	38	1.5	1.2	0.20	217
I-D	176	1.3	1.1--	0.08	
EMILIA-ROMAGNA					
I33	17	2.3	1.4	0.37	160
I34	27	2.6	1.6	0.36	118
I35	20	1.9	1.2	0.30	217
I36	30	2.0	1.3	0.27	183
I37	90	3.7	2.0+	0.24	61
I38	34	3.4	1.8	0.34	83
I39	29	3.1	1.7	0.34	105
I40	31	2.1	1.4	0.26	160
I-E	278	2.8	1.6	0.11	
FRIULI-VENEZIA GIULIA					
I30	30	2.2	1.3	0.26	183
I31	12	3.1	1.7	0.51	105
I32	29	3.6	1.3	0.25	183
I93	21	3.1	2.1	0.50	49
I-F	92	2.8	1.5	0.18	
LAZIO					
I56	18	2.7	1.5	0.38	136
I57	4	1.1	0.5--	0.24	344
I58	232	2.5	1.8+	0.12	83
I59	18	1.7	1.4	0.33	160
I60	18	1.6	1.1	0.28	255
I-G	290	2.3	1.7	0.10	
LIGURIA					
I08	8	1.3	0.9	0.37	309
I09	21	2.7	1.3	0.34	183
I10	95	3.4	1.8	0.20	83
I11	18	2.8	1.6	0.40	118
I-H	142	2.9	1.6	0.15	
LOMBARDIA					
I12	43	2.2	1.4	0.23	160
I13	43	2.2	1.5	0.24	136
I14	10	2.3	1.2	0.42	217
I15	217	2.1	1.5	0.11	136
I16	39	1.8	1.3	0.21	183
I17	45	1.8	1.2	0.19	217
I18	32	2.4	1.3	0.26	183
I19	16	1.9	0.8--	0.21	323
I20	23	2.4	1.2	0.29	217
I-I	468	2.1	1.4-	0.07	
MARCHE					
I41	24	2.9	1.7	0.38	105
I42	21	1.9	1.0-	0.23	279
I43	15	2.0	1.3	0.38	183
I44	13	1.5	1.0-	0.29	279
I-J	73	2.0	1.2-	0.16	
MOLISE					
I70	7	1.2	0.9	0.36	309
I94	3	1.2	0.9	0.56	309
I-K	10	1.2	0.9-	0.30	
PIEMONTE					
I01	78	1.3	0.8--	0.10	323
I02	34	3.2	1.5	0.30	136
I03	31	2.4	1.5	0.30	136
I04	28	2.0	1.2	0.25	217
I05	11	2.0	1.0	0.32	279
I06	30	2.4	1.2	0.27	217
I-L	212	1.8	1.1--	0.08	
PUGLIA					
I71	22	1.3	1.2	0.26	217
I72	33	0.9	0.7--	0.13	333
I73	20	1.4	1.3	0.30	183
I74	10	1.0	0.9-	0.29	309
I75	18	0.9	0.7--	0.18	333
I-M	103	1.1	0.9--	0.09	
SARDEGNA					
I90	27	2.5	1.8	0.38	83
I91	7	1.0	0.8-	0.33	323
I92	38	2.1	1.8	0.30	83
I95	3	0.8	0.5--	0.32	344
I-N	75	1.9	1.5	0.18	
SICILIA					
I81	18	1.7	1.2	0.31	217
I82	47	1.6	1.3	0.20	183
I83	25	1.4	1.0-	0.22	279
I84	17	1.4	1.1	0.29	255
I85	9	1.2	1.0	0.33	279
I86	1	0.2	0.1--	0.10	352
I87	29	1.2	1.0-	0.20	279
I88	12	1.8	1.5	0.45	136
I89	15	1.5	1.3	0.34	183
I-O	173	1.4	1.1--	0.09	
TOSCANA					
I45	13	2.5	1.5	0.45	136
I46	21	2.1	1.1	0.28	255
I47	22	3.3	2.1	0.51	49
I48	55	1.8	1.1--	0.15	255
I49	21	2.4	1.2	0.29	217
I50	28	2.8	1.5	0.30	136
I51	17	2.2	1.3	0.33	183
I52	13	2.0	1.2	0.36	217
I53	13	2.3	1.4	0.45	160
I-P	203	2.2	1.3--	0.10	
TRENTINO-ALTO ADIGE					
I21	17	1.6	1.1	0.27	255
I22	21	1.9	1.1	0.26	255
I-Q	38	1.7	1.1-	0.19	
UMBRIA					
I54	24	1.7	1.0-	0.22	279
I55	15	2.6	1.8	0.49	83
I-R	39	1.9	1.2	0.21	
VALLE D'AOSTA					
I07	5	1.8	1.3	0.60	183
VENETO					
I23	30	1.5	0.9--	0.18	309
I24	51	2.8	2.0	0.30	61
I25	23	3.9	2.4	0.57	26
I26	42	2.3	1.5	0.24	136
I27	49	2.3	1.7	0.26	105
I28	47	2.3	1.6	0.25	118
I29	18	2.8	1.4	0.35	160
I-T	260	2.4	1.6	0.11	
I.0	2760	1.9	1.3--	0.03	
IRELAND (1976-80)					
CONNAUGHT					
R07	12	3.0	2.0	0.61	61
R12	2	3.1	0.8	0.54	323
R16	9	3.2	2.2	0.76	39
R20	0	0.0	0.0--	0.00	353
R21	6	4.5	2.4	1.11	26
R-A	29	2.9	1.8	0.36	
LEINSTER					
R01	5	5.3	4.8	2.17	1
R06	58	2.3	1.8	0.25	83
R09	5	2.1	2.2	1.00	39
R10	3	1.8	1.7	0.99	105
R11	1	0.8	0.5	0.52	344
R14	1	1.4	0.8	0.82	323
R15	3	1.4	1.4	0.80	160
R17	0	0.0	0.0--	0.00	353
R19	3	2.2	1.7	1.07	105
R24	5	3.4	1.8	0.84	83
R25	4	1.7	1.8	0.88	83
R26	3	1.4	1.0	0.60	279
R-B	91	2.1	1.7	0.18	
MUNSTER					
R03	6	2.9	2.2	1.00	39
R04	24	2.4	1.8	0.39	83
R08	9	3.1	2.0	0.75	61
R13	6	1.5	1.5	0.63	136
R22	11	3.4	2.1	0.65	49
R23	5	2.3	2.4	1.08	26
R-C	61	2.5	1.9	0.26	
ULSTER					
R02	1	0.8	0.2--	0.23	351
R05	4	1.3	1.2	0.63	217
R18	0	0.0	0.0--	0.00	353
R-D	5	0.9	0.7-	0.34	
R.0	186	2.2	1.7	0.13	
LUXEMBOURG (1971-80)					
LE	2	1.0	0.8	0.59	323
LN	2	0.8	0.5--	0.39	344
LS	20	1.5	1.0-	0.26	279
L.0	24	1.3	0.9--	0.20	
NEDERLAND (1976-80)					
N01	37	2.7	1.5	0.27	136
N02	39	2.7	1.6	0.28	118
N03	29	2.8	1.8	0.35	83
N04	73	2.9	2.0	0.26	61
N05	164	3.9	2.7++	0.23	9
N06	99	4.4	2.9++	0.32	7
N07	278	4.7	2.8++	0.18	8
N08	327	4.2	2.6++	0.16	13
N09	29	3.4	1.9	0.38	73
N10	112	2.2	1.8	0.18	83
N11	69	2.6	1.9	0.23	73
N.0	1256	3.6	2.4++	0.07	
EEC-9					
EEC	20707	2.6	1.5	0.01	

BELGIE-BELGIQUE (1971-78)

BRUSSEL-BRUXELLES					
B21	116	2.9	1.8	0.17	130
VLAANDEREN					
B10	129	2.1	1.4-	0.13	239
B29	93	2.6	1.8	0.19	130
B30	120	2.8	1.9	0.18	111
B40	134	2.6	1.6	0.15	183
B70	57	2.0	2.0	0.27	87
B-V	533	2.4	1.7	0.07	
WALLONIE					
B25	38	3.7	2.6+	0.43	26
B50	116	2.3	1.4-	0.14	239
B60	103	2.6	1.8	0.18	130
B80	14	1.6	1.2	0.32	294
B90	56	3.7	2.5+	0.34	35
B-W	327	2.6	1.7	0.10	
B.0	976	2.5	1.7	0.06	

BR DEUTSCHLAND (1976-80)

BADEN-WURTTEMBERG					
D81	139	1.7	1.3--	0.11	269
D82	84	1.5	1.1--	0.12	313
D83	57	1.3	1.0--	0.13	325
D84	60	1.7	1.2--	0.17	294
D-A	340	1.5	1.1--	0.07	
BAYERN					
D91	226	2.6	1.8	0.13	130
D92	42	1.8	1.4	0.22	239
D93	54	2.3	1.7	0.23	160
D94	62	2.5	1.6	0.22	183
D95	81	2.3	1.5	0.18	212
D96	74	2.6	1.8	0.22	130
D97	92	2.5	1.6	0.18	183
D-B	631	2.4	1.7	0.07	
BERLIN(WEST)					
DB0	144	3.4	2.0	0.18	87
BREMEN					
D40	67	4.1	2.5+	0.32	35
HAMBURG					
D20	132	3.4	2.0	0.20	87
HESSEN					
D64	217	2.1	1.5-	0.10	212
D66	68	2.4	1.5	0.19	212
D-F	285	2.1	1.5--	0.09	
NIEDERSACHSEN					
D31	86	2.2	1.4-	0.16	239
D32	107	2.2	1.3--	0.14	269
D33	63	1.8	1.3-	0.17	269
D34	91	1.8	1.3--	0.14	269
D-G	347	2.0	1.3--	0.07	
NORDRHEIN-WESTFALEN					
D51	321	2.6	1.9	0.11	111
D53	192	2.0	1.7	0.13	160
D55	94	1.6	1.4-	0.15	239
D57	92	2.1	1.5	0.17	212
D59	178	2.0	1.5-	0.11	212
D-H	877	2.2	1.6	0.06	
RHEINLAND-PFALZ					
D71	92	2.8	1.8	0.20	130
D72	28	2.5	1.7	0.34	160
D73	116	2.7	1.8	0.18	130
D-I	236	2.7	1.8	0.12	
SAARLAND					
DA0	43	1.7	1.1--	0.17	313
SCHLESWIG-HOLSTEIN					
D10	234	3.8	2.5++	0.17	35
D.0	3336	2.3	1.6--	0.03	

DANMARK (1971-80)

K15	194	3.2	2.0	0.15	87
K20	44	2.9	2.8+	0.43	18
K25	18	1.9	1.8	0.43	130
K30	49	3.6	2.2	0.33	59
K35	51	4.0	2.1	0.30	70
K40	10	4.2	2.9	0.96	13
K42	82	3.7	2.2	0.25	59
K50	29	2.4	1.6	0.29	183
K55	30	2.9	2.1	0.39	70
K60	53	3.4	2.1	0.31	70
K65	47	3.7	2.6+	0.40	26
K70	101	3.6	2.5++	0.26	35
K76	59	5.2	3.0++	0.40	9
K80	87	3.7	2.3+	0.26	50
K.0	854	3.4	2.2++	0.08	

FRANCE (1971-78)

ALSACE					
F67	71	2.1	1.5	0.19	212
F68	44	1.8	1.5	0.23	212
F-A	115	1.9	1.5	0.15	
AQUITAINE					
F24	47	3.2	1.6	0.24	183
F33	104	2.5	1.6	0.16	183
F40	24	2.1	1.2	0.27	294
F47	25	2.2	1.2-	0.24	294
F64	42	2.0	1.2--	0.19	294
F-B	242	2.5	1.4--	0.10	
AUVERGNE					
F03	45	3.0	1.6	0.25	183
F15	18	2.7	1.6	0.40	183
F43	15	1.9	1.1-	0.30	313
F63	40	1.8	1.3-	0.21	269
F-C	118	2.3	1.4--	0.13	
BASSE-NORMANDIE					
F14	36	1.6	1.4	0.24	239
F50	33	1.9	1.4	0.26	239
F61	22	1.9	1.3	0.29	269
F-D	91	1.8	1.4-	0.15	
BOURGOGNE					
F21	41	2.3	1.7	0.28	160
F58	28	2.9	1.4	0.27	239
F71	68	3.0	1.8	0.23	130
F89	22	1.9	1.0--	0.25	325
F-E	159	2.6	1.5	0.13	
BRETAGNE					
F22	39	1.9	1.2-	0.20	294
F29	91	2.9	2.0	0.22	87
F35	54	2.0	1.6	0.22	183
F56	39	1.8	1.3-	0.21	269
F-F	223	2.2	1.6	0.11	
CENTRE					
F18	38	3.0	1.9	0.33	111
F28	30	2.2	1.5	0.28	212
F36	18	1.8	1.0--	0.25	325
F37	43	2.3	1.6	0.25	183
F41	25	2.3	1.5	0.31	212
F45	50	2.6	1.7	0.26	160
F-G	204	2.4	1.5	0.11	
CHAMPAGNE-ARDENNE					
F08	15	1.2	0.9--	0.24	335
F10	32	2.9	1.8	0.33	130
F51	47	2.2	1.9	0.28	111
F52	24	2.8	2.1	0.45	70
F-H	118	2.2	1.7	0.16	
CORSE					
F20	17	1.8	1.2	0.30	294
FRANCHE-COMTE					
F25	25	1.3	1.2	0.25	294
F39	22	2.3	1.4	0.31	239
F70	19	2.2	1.6	0.38	183
F90	9	1.8	1.6	0.53	183
F-J	75	1.8	1.4	0.17	
HAUTE-NORMANDIE					
F27	44	2.6	2.0	0.30	87
F76	72	1.6	1.3--	0.16	269
F-K	116	1.8	1.5	0.14	
ILE-DE-FRANCE					
F75	224	2.6	1.5-	0.11	212
F77	52	1.7	1.3-	0.18	269
F78	61	1.4	1.5	0.19	212
F91	51	1.4	1.5	0.21	212
F92	98	1.7	1.4-	0.14	239
F93	60	1.1	1.1--	0.14	313
F94	100	2.1	1.8	0.18	130
F95	61	1.8	1.8	0.23	130
F-L	707	1.8	1.5--	0.06	
LANGUEDOC-ROUSSILLON					
F11	30	2.9	1.4	0.27	239
F30	26	1.4	0.9--	0.18	335
F34	63	2.5	1.5	0.20	212
F48	6	2.0	0.8-	0.35	345
F66	29	2.5	1.2-	0.23	294
F-M	154	2.2	1.3--	0.11	
LIMOUSIN					
F19	33	3.5	1.6	0.31	183
F23	13	2.3	0.9--	0.28	335
F87	42	3.1	1.6	0.27	183
F-N	88	3.1	1.5	0.17	
LORRAINE					
F54	54	1.9	1.6	0.23	183
F55	14	1.7	1.1-	0.31	313
F57	96	2.4	2.2+	0.23	59
F88	27	1.7	1.3	0.26	269
F-O	191	2.1	1.8	0.13	
MIDI-PYRENEES					
F09	17	3.1	1.3	0.32	269
F12	30	2.8	1.6	0.30	183
F31	81	2.7	1.8	0.21	130
F32	21	3.0	1.7	0.39	160
F46	20	3.4	1.6	0.37	183
F65	24	2.7	1.6	0.34	183
F81	29	2.2	1.2-	0.24	294
F82	14	2.0	1.2	0.35	294
F-P	236	2.7	1.5	0.11	
NORD-PAS-DE-CALAIS					
F59	166	1.7	1.4--	0.11	239
F62	105	1.9	1.5	0.15	212
F-Q	271	1.8	1.4--	0.09	
PAYS DE LA LOIRE					
F44	81	2.2	1.8	0.20	130
F49	53	2.2	1.7	0.24	160
F53	15	1.5	1.0--	0.25	325
F72	38	2.0	1.3	0.22	269
F85	44	2.5	1.7	0.28	160
F-R	231	2.1	1.6	0.11	
PICARDIE					
F02	51	2.4	1.8	0.26	130
F60	38	1.6	1.4	0.23	239
F80	34	1.6	1.2-	0.22	294
F-S	123	1.8	1.5-	0.14	
POITOU-CHARENTES					
F16	39	3.0	1.7	0.28	160
F17	49	2.5	1.6	0.24	183
F79	39	2.9	1.8	0.30	130
F86	34	2.4	1.4	0.24	239
F-T	161	2.7	1.6	0.13	
PROVENCE-ALPES-COTE D'AZUR					
F04	12	2.7	1.5	0.45	212
F05	7	1.8	1.3	0.53	269
F06	83	2.7	1.2--	0.14	294
F13	122	1.9	1.4--	0.13	239
F83	68	2.8	1.6	0.21	183
F84	30	1.9	1.2-	0.22	294
F-U	322	2.2	1.3--	0.08	
RHONE-ALPES					
F01	45	3.0	2.1	0.33	70
F07	19	1.9	1.1-	0.28	313
F26	35	2.5	1.7	0.29	160
F38	60	1.8	1.4	0.19	239
F42	73	2.5	1.7	0.20	160
F69	113	2.0	1.7	0.17	160
F73	21	1.7	1.4	0.30	239
F74	29	1.6	1.4	0.26	239
F-V	395	2.1	1.6	0.08	
F.0	4357	2.1	1.5--	0.02	

UNITED KINGDOM (1976-80)

EAST ANGLIA					
G25	56	3.3	2.5+	0.34	35
G46	53	2.7	1.6	0.23	183
G55	50	2.8	1.9	0.28	111
G-A	159	2.9	1.9	0.16	
EAST MIDLANDS					
G30	77	2.9	1.9	0.22	111
G44	52	2.1	1.6	0.23	183
G45	42	2.7	1.7	0.27	160
G47	36	2.4	1.7	0.30	160
G50	75	2.6	1.8	0.21	130
G-B	282	2.5	1.7	0.11	
NORTHERN					
G14	81	2.4	1.6	0.18	183
G27	28	1.7	1.3	0.25	269
G29	56	4.1	2.7++	0.37	24
G33	43	2.4	1.7	0.26	160
G48	30	3.5	2.2	0.42	59
G-C	238	2.6	1.8	0.12	
NORTH-WEST					
G11	190	2.5	1.7	0.13	160
G12	120	2.7	1.9	0.18	111
G26	73	2.7	2.0	0.24	87
G43	110	2.8	1.8	0.17	130
G-D	493	2.6	1.8	0.08	

SOUTH-EAST					
G01	702	3.5	2.2++	0.08	59
G22	35	2.4	1.9	0.33	111
G23	50	2.5	2.1	0.30	70
G24	46	2.9	2.4	0.36	44
G34	81	4.5	2.1	0.25	70
G35	120	2.9	2.0	0.18	87
G37	113	2.6	1.9	0.18	111
G39	79	2.9	2.2	0.25	59
G41	12	3.7	2.0	0.65	87
G42	126	3.0	2.0	0.18	87
G51	56	3.3	2.8++	0.39	18
G56	126	4.3	2.8++	0.25	18
G58	83	4.7	2.5++	0.29	35
G-E	1629	3.3	2.2++	0.06	
SOUTH-WEST					
G21	89	3.3	2.2	0.24	59
G28	42	3.5	2.0	0.32	87
G31	125	4.5	2.6++	0.24	26
G32	71	4.3	2.1	0.26	70
G36	53	3.7	2.4+	0.34	44
G53	40	3.3	1.9	0.31	111
G59	62	4.0	2.8++	0.36	18
G-F	482	3.9	2.3++	0.11	
WEST MIDLANDS					
G15	199	2.5	1.8	0.13	130
G38	49	2.7	1.9	0.28	111
G52	28	2.6	1.7	0.33	160
G54	69	2.3	1.7	0.21	160
G57	41	3.0	2.2	0.36	59
G-G	386	2.5	1.8	0.09	
YORKSHIRE AND HUMBERSIDE					
G13	117	3.1	2.0	0.19	87
G16	157	2.6	1.8	0.14	130
G40	62	2.5	1.7	0.22	160
G49	71	3.7	2.4+	0.29	44
G-H	407	2.9	1.9	0.10	
WALES					
G61	39	3.5	2.2	0.37	59
G62	21	2.2	1.4	0.31	239
G63	35	2.7	1.9	0.32	111
G64	12	1.8	1.1-	0.32	313
G65	43	2.7	2.0	0.31	87
G66	9	2.8	1.8	0.63	130
G67	41	3.7	2.6+	0.41	26
G68	40	3.8	2.5	0.40	35
G-I	240	3.0	2.0+	0.13	
SCOTLAND(1975-80)					
S01	21	3.8	2.9	0.65	13
S02	46	3.4	2.4	0.36	44
S03	43	3.7	2.5+	0.39	35
S04	29	2.9	2.0	0.38	87
S05	60	2.8	1.9	0.26	111
S06	12	4.2	2.4	0.72	44
S07	24	3.0	2.3	0.48	50
S08	196	2.8	2.1+	0.15	70
S09	7	1.7	1.1	0.44	313
S10	2	3.8	1.8	1.27	130
S11	1	1.6	1.6	1.56	183
S12	5	5.7	2.0	0.88	87
G-J	446	3.0	2.1++	0.10	
NORTHERN IRELAND					
JE	39	2.4	2.0	0.34	87
JN	29	3.2	2.7	0.52	24
JS	17	2.6	2.1	0.53	70
JW	19	3.2	2.6	0.61	26
G-K	104	2.7	2.3+	0.23	
G.0	4866	3.0	2.0++	0.03	

ITALIA (1975-79)

ABRUZZI					
I66	14	1.9	1.2	0.33	294
I67	12	1.8	1.4	0.40	239
I68	20	2.9	2.0	0.46	87
I69	9	1.0	0.6--	0.21	351
I-A	55	1.8	1.2--	0.17	
BASILICATA					
I76	12	1.2	0.9--	0.26	335
I77	5	1.0	0.8-	0.38	345
I-B	17	1.1	0.9--	0.21	
CALABRIA					
I78	26	1.5	1.2-	0.23	294
I79	21	1.1	0.9--	0.21	335
I80	19	1.3	1.0--	0.24	325
I-C	66	1.3	1.0--	0.13	
CAMPANIA					
I61	16	0.9	0.9--	0.22	335
I62	10	1.4	0.9--	0.30	335
I63	89	1.3	1.3--	0.14	269
I64	14	1.3	1.0-	0.28	325
I65	37	1.5	1.3-	0.21	269
I-D	166	1.3	1.2--	0.09	
EMILIA-ROMAGNA					
I33	26	3.7	2.0	0.39	87
I34	28	2.9	1.6	0.31	183
I35	17	1.7	1.0--	0.24	325
I36	35	2.5	1.7	0.30	160
I37	55	2.4	1.5	0.21	212
I38	28	3.0	2.0	0.38	87
I39	20	2.3	1.3	0.29	269
I40	44	3.0	2.3	0.35	50
I-E	253	2.6	1.7	0.11	
FRIULI-VENEZIA GIULIA					
I30	44	3.4	2.1	0.32	70
I31	12	3.4	2.4	0.73	44
I32	18	2.6	1.4	0.34	239
I93	19	2.9	2.0	0.47	87
I-F	93	3.1	1.9	0.20	
LAZIO					
I56	16	2.4	1.5	0.38	212
I57	8	2.2	1.3	0.46	269
I58	158	1.8	1.6	0.13	183
I59	16	1.5	1.5	0.37	212
I60	17	1.5	1.1-	0.27	313
I-G	215	1.8	1.5-	0.10	
LIGURIA					
I08	15	2.7	1.3	0.37	269
I09	27	3.7	2.0	0.40	87
I10	92	3.6	2.0	0.22	87
I11	18	3.0	1.7	0.41	160
I-H	152	3.4	1.9	0.16	
LOMBARDIA					
I12	40	2.1	2.1	0.37	70
I13	42	2.3	1.9	0.31	111
I14	5	1.2	0.8--	0.35	345
I15	199	2.0	1.8	0.13	130
I16	35	1.6	1.6	0.27	183
I17	52	2.1	1.9	0.27	111
I18	54	4.3	2.3	0.32	50
I19	30	3.7	2.3	0.43	50
I20	34	3.7	2.2	0.39	59
I-I	491	2.3	1.9	0.09	
MARCHE					
I41	21	2.6	1.6	0.35	183
I42	20	1.9	1.3	0.29	269
I43	17	2.4	1.5	0.36	212
I44	17	2.0	1.3	0.32	269
I-J	75	2.2	1.4-	0.16	
MOLISE					
I70	6	1.0	0.6--	0.25	351
I94	5	2.2	1.7	0.78	160
I-K	11	1.4	0.9--	0.29	
PIEMONTE					
I01	132	2.3	1.8	0.16	130
I02	21	2.2	1.1--	0.24	313
I03	28	2.3	1.6	0.31	183
I04	46	3.4	1.8	0.27	130
I05	15	2.8	1.4	0.38	239
I06	22	1.9	0.9--	0.20	335
I-L	264	2.4	1.5-	0.10	
PUGLIA					
I71	30	1.8	1.5	0.28	212
I72	49	1.4	1.2--	0.18	294
I73	19	1.4	1.3	0.31	269
I74	18	1.9	1.7	0.41	160
I75	21	1.2	1.0--	0.21	325
I-M	137	1.5	1.3--	0.11	
SARDEGNA					
I90	13	1.2	1.0--	0.28	325
I91	12	1.8	1.4	0.42	239
I92	23	1.3	1.3	0.26	269
I95	2	0.5	0.5--	0.35	355
I-N	50	1.3	1.1--	0.16	
SICILIA					
I81	15	1.5	1.1-	0.28	313
I82	44	1.5	1.2--	0.19	294
I83	20	1.2	0.8--	0.20	345
I84	10	0.8	0.6--	0.19	351
I85	11	1.5	1.3	0.39	269
I86	5	1.0	0.9	0.42	335
I87	23	0.9	0.8--	0.17	345
I88	12	1.8	1.4	0.40	239
I89	10	1.0	0.8--	0.26	345
I-O	150	1.2	1.0--	0.08	
TOSCANA					
I45	12	2.4	1.5	0.43	212
I46	34	3.6	2.1	0.37	70
I47	15	2.3	1.5	0.41	212
I48	87	3.0	1.8	0.20	130
I49	25	3.0	1.9	0.38	111
I50	28	3.0	1.8	0.35	130
I51	24	3.1	1.8	0.37	130
I52	24	3.8	1.9	0.40	111
I53	15	2.7	1.5	0.40	212
I-P	264	3.0	1.8	0.11	
TRENTINO-ALTO ADIGE					
I21	17	1.6	1.3	0.33	269
I22	23	2.1	1.5	0.32	212
I-Q	40	1.9	1.4	0.23	
UMBRIA					
I54	30	2.1	1.4	0.27	239
I55	14	2.5	1.5	0.40	212
I-R	44	2.2	1.4	0.22	
VALLE D'AOSTA					
I07	4	1.4	1.1	0.54	313
VENETO					
I23	54	2.9	2.1	0.28	70
I24	48	2.8	2.3	0.34	50
I25	15	2.8	1.8	0.48	130
I26	47	2.7	2.2	0.33	59
I27	66	3.2	2.5+	0.32	35
I28	62	3.2	2.6+	0.33	26
I29	14	2.3	1.5	0.41	212
I-T	306	2.9	2.2++	0.13	
I.0	2853	2.1	1.5--	0.03	

IRELAND (1976-80)

CONNAUGHT					
R07	19	4.4	2.9	0.70	13
R12	6	8.1	4.2	1.76	1
R16	13	4.4	2.0	0.58	87
R20	4	2.8	1.9	1.08	111
R21	5	3.6	2.9	1.45	13
R-A	47	4.3	2.6+	0.41	
LEINSTER					
R01	3	3.0	3.0	1.78	9
R06	68	2.9	3.2++	0.39	5
R09	7	2.8	3.5	1.36	3
R10	1	0.6	0.6	0.60	351
R11	2	1.5	1.4	1.00	239
R14	2	2.5	2.1	1.51	70
R15	5	2.3	1.9	0.87	111
R17	5	2.1	2.6	1.16	26
R19	6	4.0	2.6	1.12	26
R24	7	4.6	3.1	1.18	6
R25	10	4.1	3.0	0.96	9
R26	9	4.3	3.9	1.33	2
R-B	125	2.9	2.9++	0.26	
MUNSTER					
R03	6	2.7	1.8	0.78	130
R04	18	1.8	1.4	0.34	239
R08	7	2.3	1.2	0.46	294
R13	15	3.8	3.1	0.82	6
R22	13	3.8	2.8	0.82	18
R23	2	0.9	0.9	0.62	335
R-C	61	2.5	1.8	0.24	
ULSTER					
R02	4	2.8	1.4	0.69	239
R05	7	2.2	1.5	0.60	212
R18	3	2.3	1.4	0.83	239
R-D	14	2.4	1.4	0.39	
R.0	247	2.9	2.4++	0.16	

LUXEMBOURG (1971-80)

LE	5	2.8	2.1	0.97	70
LN	5	1.9	1.0	0.48	325
LS	25	2.0	1.4	0.30	239
L.0	35	2.0	1.4	0.25	

NEDERLAND (1976-80)

N01	59	4.3	3.1++	0.42	6
N02	74	5.2	3.3++	0.41	4
N03	38	3.7	2.6+	0.44	26
N04	68	2.7	2.1	0.26	70
N05	155	3.7	2.9++	0.24	13
N06	72	3.3	2.8++	0.33	18
N07	176	3.0	2.3++	0.17	50
N08	318	4.2	3.0++	0.17	9
N09	29	3.4	2.0	0.40	87
N10	121	2.4	2.3++	0.21	50
N11	67	2.5	2.3+	0.29	50
N.0	1177	3.4	2.6++	0.08	

EEC-9

EEC	18701	2.5	1.7	0.01

BELGIE-BELGIQUE (1971-78)

BRUSSEL-BRUXELLES					
B21	136	3.1	1.2	0.11	175
VLAANDEREN					
B10	102	1.6	0.9--	0.10	293
B29	93	2.5	1.5	0.16	66
B30	95	2.2	1.2	0.13	175
B40	109	2.0	1.0-	0.11	261
B70	49	1.8	1.5	0.22	66
B-V	448	2.0	1.1	0.06	
WALLONIE					
B25	29	2.7	1.5	0.30	66
B50	121	2.2	1.1	0.11	219
B60	92	2.2	1.1	0.13	219
B80	21	2.3	1.4	0.32	96
B90	45	2.8	1.3	0.21	136
B-W	308	2.3	1.1	0.07	
B.0	892	2.2	1.1-	0.04	

BR DEUTSCHLAND (1976-80)

BADEN-WURTTEMBERG					
D81	146	1.6	0.8--	0.07	312
D82	111	1.8	0.9--	0.10	293
D83	83	1.7	0.8--	0.10	312
D84	62	1.6	0.9--	0.13	293
D-A	402	1.7	0.9--	0.05	
BAYERN					
D91	236	2.5	1.2	0.09	175
D92	73	2.8	1.3	0.17	136
D93	62	2.5	1.2	0.16	175
D94	81	2.9	1.2	0.15	175
D95	95	2.4	1.1	0.13	219
D96	70	2.3	1.1	0.14	219
D97	117	2.9	1.3	0.13	136
D-B	734	2.6	1.2	0.05	
BERLIN (WEST)					
DB0	245	4.6	1.5+	0.12	66
BREMEN					
D40	46	2.5	0.9-	0.15	293
HAMBURG					
D20	145	3.2	1.2	0.11	175
HESSEN					
D64	235	2.1	1.0--	0.07	261
D66	74	2.4	1.2	0.17	175
D-F	309	2.1	1.0--	0.07	
NIEDERSACHSEN					
D31	95	2.2	1.0-	0.11	261
D32	121	2.2	1.0--	0.10	261
D33	68	1.8	0.8--	0.11	312
D34	78	1.4	0.7--	0.09	330
D-G	362	1.9	0.9--	0.05	
NORDRHEIN-WESTFALEN					
D51	341	2.5	1.2	0.07	175
D53	225	2.2	1.1	0.08	219
D55	103	1.7	1.0--	0.10	261
D57	97	2.0	0.9--	0.10	293
D59	210	2.2	1.1-	0.08	219
D-H	976	2.2	1.1--	0.04	
RHEINLAND-PFALZ					
D71	109	3.1	1.4	0.15	96
D72	25	2.0	0.9	0.20	293
D73	140	3.0	1.3	0.12	136
D-I	274	2.9	1.3	0.09	
SAARLAND					
DA0	50	1.8	0.9--	0.13	293
SCHLESWIG-HOLSTEIN					
D10	211	3.1	1.4	0.11	96
D.0	3754	2.3	1.1--	0.02	

DANMARK (1971-80)

K15	232	3.5	1.5++	0.11	66
K20	26	1.7	1.3	0.26	136
K25	16	1.8	1.4	0.35	96
K30	34	2.5	1.2	0.21	175
K35	50	3.9	1.9+	0.29	17
K40	8	3.4	1.3	0.48	136
K42	75	3.4	1.7+	0.20	31
K50	30	2.5	1.4	0.27	96
K55	16	1.6	1.0	0.26	261
K60	51	3.2	1.7	0.25	31
K65	29	2.3	1.5	0.29	66
K70	85	3.0	1.8++	0.20	18
K76	32	2.9	1.4	0.26	96
K80	56	2.4	1.4	0.19	96
K.0	740	2.9	1.5++	0.06	

FRANCE (1971-78)

ALSACE					
F67	95	2.6	1.4	0.16	96
F68	72	2.8	1.3	0.17	136
F-A	167	2.7	1.4	0.11	
AQUITAINE					
F24	39	2.5	1.1	0.20	219
F33	105	2.4	1.1	0.13	219
F40	15	1.3	0.4--	0.13	346
F47	25	2.1	1.1	0.24	219
F64	48	2.2	1.0	0.17	261
F-B	232	2.2	1.0--	0.08	
AUVERGNE					
F03	57	3.6	1.3	0.21	136
F15	19	2.8	1.1	0.31	219
F43	19	2.3	1.1	0.30	219
F63	43	1.8	0.9	0.16	293
F-C	138	2.5	1.1	0.11	
BASSE-NORMANDIE					
F14	45	2.0	1.2	0.20	175
F50	39	2.1	1.1	0.20	219
F61	27	2.2	1.2	0.25	175
F-D	111	2.1	1.2	0.12	
BOURGOGNE					
F21	41	2.2	1.1	0.19	219
F58	31	3.1	1.2	0.25	175
F71	66	2.8	1.3	0.19	136
F89	34	2.8	1.2	0.25	175
F-E	172	2.7	1.2	0.11	
BRETAGNE					
F22	56	2.6	1.3	0.19	136
F29	82	2.5	1.1	0.14	219
F35	43	1.5	0.9-	0.15	293
F56	50	2.2	1.2	0.18	175
F-F	231	2.2	1.1	0.08	
CENTRE					
F18	36	2.8	1.3	0.27	136
F28	35	2.6	1.1	0.22	219
F36	25	2.5	1.2	0.28	175
F37	50	2.5	1.4	0.22	96
F41	37	3.2	1.3	0.25	136
F45	56	2.8	1.4	0.21	96
F-G	239	2.7	1.3	0.10	
CHAMPAGNE-ARDENNE					
F08	28	2.3	1.3	0.28	136
F10	39	3.4	1.6	0.29	47
F51	56	2.6	1.4	0.21	96
F52	27	3.2	1.6	0.35	47
F-H	150	2.8	1.5	0.14	
CORSE					
F20	15	1.7	0.7--	0.20	330
FRANCHE-COMTE					
F25	29	1.5	1.0	0.20	261
F39	19	1.9	1.0	0.27	261
F70	23	2.6	1.2	0.30	175
F90	13	2.5	1.0	0.29	261
F-J	84	2.0	1.0	0.13	
HAUTE-NORMANDIE					
F27	37	2.2	1.4	0.25	96
F76	91	1.9	1.1	0.13	219
F-K	128	2.0	1.2	0.11	
ILE-DE-FRANCE					
F75	313	3.2	1.2	0.08	175
F77	73	2.4	1.2	0.17	175
F78	70	1.6	1.1	0.15	219
F91	65	1.8	1.3	0.18	136
F92	130	2.2	1.1	0.10	219
F93	81	1.5	1.0	0.12	261
F94	119	2.4	1.4	0.14	96
F95	62	1.8	1.4	0.19	96
F-L	913	2.3	1.2	0.04	
LANGUEDOC-ROUSSILLON					
F11	25	2.2	0.7--	0.16	330
F30	40	2.0	1.0	0.17	261
F34	74	2.7	1.2	0.16	175
F48	8	2.7	0.8	0.33	312
F66	36	2.9	1.1	0.20	219
F-M	183	2.5	1.0--	0.09	
LIMOUSIN					
F19	27	2.7	1.1	0.23	219
F23	30	5.0	1.6	0.34	47
F87	33	2.3	0.9	0.19	293
F-N	90	3.0	1.1	0.14	
LORRAINE					
F54	78	2.7	1.6	0.20	47
F55	13	1.6	0.7-	0.22	330
F57	85	2.1	1.4	0.16	96
F88	39	2.4	1.5	0.26	66
F-O	215	2.3	1.4	0.10	
MIDI-PYRENEES					
F09	12	2.1	0.8-	0.24	312
F12	41	3.6	1.1	0.21	219
F31	57	1.8	1.0	0.14	261
F32	22	3.1	1.3	0.31	136
F46	16	2.6	1.0	0.29	261
F65	30	3.2	1.5	0.30	66
F81	42	3.0	1.4	0.24	96
F82	23	3.1	1.3	0.30	136
F-P	243	2.6	1.1	0.08	
NORD-PAS-DE-CALAIS					
F59	223	2.2	1.3	0.10	136
F62	114	2.0	1.1	0.11	219
F-Q	337	2.1	1.3	0.08	
PAYS DE LA LOIRE					
F44	86	2.2	1.1	0.13	219
F49	48	1.8	1.0	0.16	261
F53	21	1.9	1.1	0.27	219
F72	47	2.3	1.1	0.19	219
F85	30	1.6	0.9	0.18	293
F-R	232	2.0	1.0-	0.08	
PICARDIE					
F02	48	2.2	1.2	0.19	175
F60	47	1.9	1.0	0.17	261
F80	50	2.3	1.4	0.22	96
F-S	145	2.1	1.2	0.11	
POITOU-CHARENTES					
F16	33	2.4	1.3	0.25	136
F17	58	2.9	1.2	0.18	175
F79	32	2.4	1.2	0.24	175
F86	39	2.7	1.5	0.28	66
F-T	162	2.6	1.3	0.12	
PROVENCE-ALPES-COTE D'AZUR					
F04	8	1.8	1.0	0.39	261
F05	12	3.1	1.7	0.54	31
F06	70	2.0	0.8--	0.11	312
F13	121	1.8	1.0--	0.10	261
F83	62	2.4	1.1	0.16	219
F84	25	1.6	0.7--	0.15	330
F-U	298	2.0	0.9--	0.06	
RHONE-ALPES					
F01	49	3.2	1.7	0.26	31
F07	30	2.9	1.4	0.30	96
F26	34	2.3	1.1	0.21	219
F38	74	2.1	1.3	0.16	136
F42	87	2.8	1.3	0.16	136
F69	165	2.8	1.5+	0.13	66
F73	28	2.3	1.2	0.25	175
F74	33	1.8	1.2	0.22	175
F-V	500	2.6	1.4	0.07	
F.0	4985	2.3	1.2--	0.02	

UNITED KINGDOM (1976-80)

EAST ANGLIA					
G25	57	3.4	1.8+	0.26	18
G46	54	2.6	1.2	0.18	175
G55	62	3.5	1.5	0.22	66
G-A	173	3.1	1.5+	0.12	
EAST MIDLANDS					
G30	87	3.2	1.5	0.18	66
G44	50	2.0	1.0	0.15	261
G45	61	3.8	1.8+	0.25	18
G47	30	1.9	0.8-	0.16	312
G50	90	3.0	1.5	0.17	66
G-B	318	2.8	1.4	0.08	
NORTHERN					
G14	94	2.6	1.3	0.15	136
G27	39	2.2	1.2	0.21	175
G29	37	2.5	1.3	0.23	136
G33	45	2.4	1.3	0.20	136
G48	24	2.7	1.2	0.25	175
G-C	239	2.5	1.3	0.09	
NORTH-WEST					
G11	209	2.5	1.2	0.09	175
G12	135	2.8	1.4	0.13	96
G26	74	2.6	1.5	0.19	66
G43	101	2.4	1.0	0.12	261
G-D	519	2.6	1.3	0.06	

SOUTH-EAST					
G01	693	3.2	1.5++	0.06	66
G22	33	2.2	1.4	0.25	96
G23	58	2.9	1.7+	0.24	31
G24	43	2.8	1.5	0.25	66
G34	100	4.7	1.5	0.19	66
G35	137	3.1	1.6+	0.15	47
G37	132	3.1	1.5	0.14	66
G39	67	2.3	1.2	0.16	175
G41	10	2.8	1.4	0.53	96
G42	106	2.4	1.0	0.11	261
G51	39	2.5	1.4	0.24	96
G56	113	3.7	1.7++	0.17	31
G58	98	4.9	1.6+	0.20	47
G-E	1629	3.1	1.5++	0.04	
SOUTH-WEST					
G21	97	3.4	1.7+	0.19	31
G28	36	2.8	1.2	0.22	175
G31	131	4.5	1.8++	0.18	18
G32	72	3.9	1.5	0.22	66
G36	47	3.1	1.4	0.22	96
G53	57	4.5	1.8+	0.26	18
G59	38	2.5	1.2	0.21	175
G-F	478	3.6	1.6++	0.08	
WEST MIDLANDS					
G15	217	2.6	1.4	0.10	96
G38	49	2.7	1.3	0.21	136
G52	28	2.5	1.3	0.26	136
G54	69	2.3	1.4	0.17	96
G57	43	3.0	1.7	0.28	31
G-G	406	2.6	1.4+	0.07	
YORKSHIRE AND HUMBERSIDE					
G13	100	2.5	1.3	0.13	136
G16	156	2.4	1.1	0.10	219
G40	70	2.7	1.5	0.19	66
G49	75	3.7	1.6	0.20	47
G-H	401	2.7	1.3	0.07	
WALES					
G61	44	3.7	1.8	0.30	18
G62	34	3.4	1.5	0.28	66
G63	41	3.0	1.6	0.28	47
G64	27	3.8	1.5	0.32	66
G65	49	3.0	1.5	0.23	66
G66	15	4.7	2.2	0.66	9
G67	30	2.5	1.4	0.28	96
G68	29	2.5	1.3	0.25	136
G-I	269	3.1	1.5++	0.10	
SCOTLAND(1975-80)					
S01	15	2.6	1.3	0.36	136
S02	43	3.0	1.3	0.22	136
S03	48	3.8	1.7	0.28	31
S04	30	2.9	1.6	0.32	47
S05	72	3.0	1.4	0.18	96
S06	9	2.9	1.5	0.51	66
S07	19	2.3	1.3	0.32	136
S08	157	2.0	1.1	0.09	219
S09	20	4.5	1.7	0.39	31
S10	1	1.8	0.5	0.47	341
S11	2	3.3	2.0	1.50	12
S12	4	4.4	1.7	0.94	31
G-J	420	2.6	1.3	0.07	
NORTHERN IRELAND					
JE	43	2.6	1.4	0.23	96
JN	19	2.1	1.2	0.29	175
JS	13	1.9	1.2	0.36	175
JW	12	2.0	1.1	0.35	219
G-K	87	2.2	1.3	0.15	
G.0	4939	2.9	1.4++	0.02	
ITALIA (1975-79)					
ABRUZZI					
I66	21	2.7	1.4	0.32	96
I67	2	0.3	0.2--	0.14	352
I68	10	1.4	0.7-	0.23	330
I69	18	1.9	1.1	0.27	219
I-A	51	1.7	0.9-	0.13	
BASILICATA					
I76	16	1.5	1.0	0.26	261
I77	5	1.0	0.7	0.34	330
I-B	21	1.4	0.9	0.21	
CALABRIA					
I78	10	0.6	0.4--	0.12	346
I79	27	1.5	1.0	0.20	261
I80	9	0.6	0.4--	0.12	346
I-C	46	0.9	0.6--	0.09	

CAMPANIA					
I61	16	0.9	0.8-	0.20	312
I62	10	1.4	0.9	0.30	293
I63	99	1.4	1.1	0.12	219
I64	8	0.7	0.5--	0.16	341
I65	17	0.7	0.5--	0.12	341
I-D	150	1.1	0.9--	0.07	
EMILIA-ROMAGNA					
I33	27	3.7	1.6	0.34	47
I34	29	2.8	1.4	0.31	96
I35	34	3.3	1.6	0.29	47
I36	37	2.5	1.3	0.22	136
I37	56	2.3	1.1	0.15	219
I38	26	2.6	1.3	0.26	136
I39	21	2.3	1.1	0.26	219
I40	38	2.5	1.5	0.25	66
I-E	268	2.7	1.3	0.08	
FRIULI-VENEZIA GIULIA					
I30	38	2.8	1.2	0.22	175
I31	11	2.9	1.4	0.46	96
I32	42	5.3	2.0+	0.33	12
I93	21	3.1	1.7	0.40	31
I-F	112	3.5	1.6+	0.16	
LAZIO					
I56	14	2.1	1.1	0.30	219
I57	6	1.7	0.8	0.37	312
I58	156	1.7	1.1	0.09	219
I59	13	1.3	1.0	0.29	261
I60	10	0.9	0.5--	0.17	341
I-G	199	1.6	1.0--	0.07	
LIGURIA					
I08	23	3.8	1.7	0.39	31
I09	24	3.0	1.3	0.29	136
I10	90	3.2	1.5	0.18	66
I11	17	2.7	1.2	0.33	175
I-H	154	3.2	1.4	0.13	
LOMBARDIA					
I12	63	3.2	1.8+	0.23	18
I13	45	2.3	1.4	0.22	96
I14	10	2.3	1.3	0.45	136
I15	195	1.9	1.2	0.09	175
I16	39	1.8	1.1	0.19	219
I17	65	2.6	1.6	0.21	47
I18	34	2.5	1.0	0.18	261
I19	31	3.6	1.6	0.31	47
I20	18	1.8	0.8-	0.19	312
I-I	500	2.2	1.3	0.06	
MARCHE					
I41	20	2.4	1.2	0.28	175
I42	28	2.5	1.2	0.25	175
I43	10	1.4	0.6--	0.19	340
I44	13	1.5	0.9	0.25	293
I-J	71	2.0	1.0-	0.12	
MOLISE					
I70	3	0.5	0.2--	0.11	352
I94	2	0.8	0.4--	0.28	346
I-K	5	0.6	0.2--	0.11	
PIEMONTE					
I01	118	1.9	1.2	0.11	175
I02	28	2.6	1.2	0.27	175
I03	39	3.0	1.6	0.27	47
I04	30	2.2	1.0	0.20	261
I05	17	3.0	1.2	0.32	175
I06	34	2.7	1.1	0.21	219
I-L	266	2.3	1.2	0.08	
PUGLIA					
I71	27	1.6	1.0	0.21	261
I72	43	1.2	0.9--	0.14	293
I73	19	1.4	1.1	0.25	219
I74	12	1.2	0.9	0.27	293
I75	20	1.0	0.8-	0.18	312
I-M	121	1.3	0.9--	0.09	
SARDEGNA					
I90	18	1.7	1.0	0.26	261
I91	15	2.2	1.4	0.39	96
I92	25	1.4	1.1	0.23	219
I95	5	1.3	0.8	0.41	312
I-N	63	1.6	1.1	0.15	
SICILIA					
I81	12	1.1	0.8	0.24	312
I82	31	1.0	0.8--	0.15	312
I83	16	0.9	0.7--	0.18	330
I84	13	1.1	0.8	0.24	312
I85	4	0.5	0.5--	0.23	341
I86	5	1.0	0.7	0.31	330
I87	31	1.2	0.9	0.17	293
I88	8	1.2	0.7-	0.26	330
I89	16	1.6	1.3	0.33	136
I-O	136	1.1	0.8--	0.07	

TOSCANA					
I45	14	2.6	1.4	0.41	96
I46	42	4.2	1.6	0.27	47
I47	23	3.4	1.4	0.32	96
I48	73	2.4	1.2	0.15	175
I49	23	2.6	1.2	0.26	175
I50	29	2.9	1.3	0.26	136
I51	14	1.8	0.9	0.25	293
I52	25	3.8	1.6	0.35	47
I53	10	1.8	0.8	0.27	312
I-P	253	2.8	1.3	0.09	
TRENTINO-ALTO ADIGE					
I21	13	1.2	0.8-	0.23	312
I22	26	2.3	1.1	0.23	219
I-Q	39	1.8	1.0	0.17	
UMBRIA					
I54	27	1.9	1.0	0.19	261
I55	11	1.9	1.1	0.33	219
I-R	38	1.9	1.0	0.17	
VALLE D'AOSTA					
I07	4	1.4	0.8	0.39	312
VENETO					
I23	51	2.6	1.4	0.21	96
I24	49	2.7	1.7	0.25	31
I25	12	2.1	1.0	0.32	261
I26	47	2.6	1.6	0.25	47
I27	47	2.2	1.4	0.20	96
I28	63	3.1	1.8+	0.23	18
I29	19	2.9	1.8	0.46	18
I-T	288	2.6	1.5++	0.10	
I.0	2785	1.9	1.1--	0.02	
IRELAND (1976-80)					
CONNAUGHT					
R07	9	2.2	1.4	0.50	96
R12	5	7.7	3.8	1.81	2
R16	13	4.7	2.2	0.71	9
R20	4	3.1	1.8	0.89	18
R21	3	2.2	1.0	0.58	261
R-A	34	3.4	1.8	0.34	
LEINSTER					
R01	2	2.1	2.0	1.48	12
R06	47	1.8	1.4	0.22	96
R09	3	1.3	1.3	0.75	136
R10	4	2.4	1.8	0.91	18
R11	4	3.4	2.5	1.33	5
R14	1	1.4	1.3	1.33	136
R15	10	4.6	3.9+	1.29	1
R17	7	3.2	2.5	0.99	5
R19	4	2.9	2.5	1.29	5
R24	2	1.4	0.9	0.73	293
R25	1	0.4	0.2--	0.24	352
R26	6	2.9	2.6	1.11	4
R-B	91	2.1	1.6+	0.18	
MUNSTER					
R03	1	0.5	0.3--	0.30	350
R04	21	2.1	1.5	0.36	66
R08	2	0.7	0.3--	0.21	350
R13	7	1.8	1.2	0.49	175
R22	6	1.9	1.5	0.66	66
R23	5	2.3	1.5	0.67	66
R-C	42	1.7	1.2	0.20	
ULSTER					
R02	3	2.4	1.6	0.93	47
R05	5	1.7	1.0	0.47	261
R18	0	0.0	0.0--	0.00	355
R-D	8	1.5	0.9	0.35	
R.0	175	2.1	1.5+	0.12	
LUXEMBOURG (1971-80)					
LE	7	3.7	1.5	0.58	66
LN	5	1.9	0.9	0.43	293
LS	33	2.5	1.3	0.23	136
L.0	45	2.5	1.3	0.20	
NEDERLAND (1976-80)					
N01	50	3.6	1.8+	0.28	18
N02	54	3.8	2.1++	0.31	11
N03	34	3.3	2.3++	0.41	8
N04	65	2.6	1.7+	0.22	31
N05	127	3.0	2.0++	0.19	12
N06	53	2.4	1.4	0.21	96
N07	181	3.0	1.6++	0.13	47
N08	289	3.7	2.0++	0.13	12
N09	44	5.2	2.8++	0.46	3
N10	115	2.3	1.7++	0.16	31
N11	67	2.5	1.8+	0.22	18
N.0	1079	3.1	1.8++	0.06	
EEC-9					
EEC	19394	2.4	1.2	0.01	

BELGIE-BELGIQUE (1971-78)

BRUSSEL-BRUXELLES					
B21	418	10.6	7.5++	0.40	53
VLAANDEREN					
B10	443	7.2	5.7-	0.29	254
B29	298	8.3	6.6	0.41	132
B30	347	8.2	6.5	0.37	142
B40	400	7.6	5.5--	0.29	279
B70	128	4.6	4.6--	0.42	337
B-V	1616	7.3	5.9--	0.15	
WALLONIE					
B25	98	9.5	7.2	0.75	68
B50	473	9.2	6.7	0.33	117
B60	332	8.4	6.3	0.37	180
B80	73	8.5	6.3	0.78	180
B90	128	8.4	6.3	0.59	180
B-W	1104	8.9	6.5	0.21	
B.0	3138	8.2	6.3	0.12	

BR DEUTSCHLAND (1976-80)

BADEN-WURTTEMBERG					
D81	634	7.6	5.9	0.25	235
D82	450	7.9	6.1	0.32	215
D83	366	8.3	6.4	0.36	163
D84	282	7.8	6.4	0.40	163
D-A	1732	7.9	6.1	0.16	
BAYERN					
D91	638	7.3	5.6--	0.24	268
D92	161	6.9	5.3-	0.45	297
D93	183	7.9	6.4	0.49	163
D94	201	8.1	6.0	0.46	223
D95	316	8.8	6.9	0.42	95
D96	237	8.3	6.3	0.43	180
D97	300	8.3	6.2	0.38	198
D-B	2036	7.9	6.0--	0.14	
BERLIN(WEST)					
DB0	476	11.1	6.9	0.37	95
BREMEN					
D40	139	8.5	5.4	0.50	290
HAMBURG					
D20	361	9.3	6.0	0.36	223
HESSEN					
D64	873	8.3	6.1	0.22	215
D66	272	9.6	6.3	0.42	180
D-F	1145	8.6	6.1	0.20	
NIEDERSACHSEN					
D31	363	9.3	6.5	0.38	142
D32	519	10.7	7.9++	0.38	31
D33	312	8.9	6.4	0.39	163
D34	430	8.5	7.1	0.36	79
D-G	1624	9.4	7.0++	0.19	
NORDRHEIN-WESTFALEN					
D51	1059	8.6	6.9+	0.22	95
D53	706	7.5	6.6	0.26	132
D55	396	6.8	6.0	0.31	223
D57	344	8.0	6.2	0.36	198
D59	651	7.4	6.2	0.26	198
D-H	3156	7.8	6.5	0.12	
RHEINLAND-PFALZ					
D71	312	9.6	7.0	0.44	88
D72	100	8.9	6.5	0.71	142
D73	364	8.5	6.5	0.37	142
D-I	776	8.9	6.7	0.26	
SAARLAND					
DA0	210	8.2	6.4	0.50	163
SCHLESWIG-HOLSTEIN					
D10	548	8.8	6.4	0.30	163
D.0	12203	8.3	6.4	0.06	

DANMARK (1971-80)

K15	583	9.6	6.9	0.31	95
K20	111	7.3	6.9	0.66	95
K25	72	7.7	7.2	0.86	68
K30	160	11.8	8.2+	0.70	19
K35	167	13.0	8.1+	0.69	24
K40	33	13.9	9.2	1.75	5
K42	236	10.7	6.8	0.47	108
K50	90	7.4	5.5	0.61	279
K55	86	8.3	6.5	0.74	142
K60	150	9.5	7.6	0.66	47
K65	106	8.3	6.5	0.67	142
K70	261	9.4	7.3	0.48	64
K76	121	10.6	7.2	0.71	68
K80	243	10.3	7.9++	0.55	31
K.0	2419	9.7	7.2++	0.15	

FRANCE (1971-78)

ALSACE					
F67	281	8.1	6.9	0.43	95
F68	199	8.0	6.7	0.50	117
F-A	480	8.1	6.8	0.33	
AQUITAINE					
F24	157	10.8	6.5	0.61	142
F33	375	9.2	6.7	0.38	117
F40	125	11.2	8.0+	0.79	28
F47	123	10.8	7.3	0.72	64
F64	188	9.1	6.4	0.51	163
F-B	968	9.8	6.8	0.24	
AUVERGNE					
F03	149	10.1	6.6	0.63	132
F15	60	9.1	5.5	0.77	279
F43	91	11.3	7.8	0.91	36
F63	237	10.4	8.4++	0.58	16
F-C	537	10.3	7.4++	0.35	
BASSE-NORMANDIE					
F14	160	7.3	6.3	0.51	180
F50	116	6.7	5.7	0.56	254
F61	99	8.6	7.2	0.75	68
F-D	375	7.4	6.2	0.33	
BOURGOGNE					
F21	173	9.6	7.7+	0.63	42
F58	114	11.6	6.4	0.67	163
F71	250	11.1	7.8++	0.54	36
F89	142	12.0	7.2	0.68	68
F-E	679	10.9	7.5++	0.31	
BRETAGNE					
F22	197	9.7	7.0	0.53	88
F29	253	8.1	6.2	0.41	198
F35	228	8.4	7.2	0.49	68
F56	184	8.4	6.7	0.52	117
F-F	862	8.6	6.7	0.24	
CENTRE					
F18	132	10.5	6.8	0.66	108
F28	121	9.0	7.0	0.67	88
F36	85	8.7	5.2	0.65	307
F37	157	8.5	6.5	0.55	142
F41	108	9.7	6.6	0.69	132
F45	203	10.4	7.8+	0.59	36
F-G	806	9.5	6.8	0.26	
CHAMPAGNE-ARDENNE					
F08	115	9.3	7.4	0.72	58
F10	104	9.3	6.9	0.72	95
F51	169	8.0	6.9	0.55	95
F52	64	7.5	5.6	0.74	268
F-H	452	8.5	6.8	0.33	
CORSE					
F20	72	7.5	5.8	0.76	246
FRANCHE-COMTE					
F25	119	6.3	6.0	0.56	223
F39	107	11.3	8.6+	0.92	10
F70	83	9.5	7.0	0.83	88
F90	50	9.8	8.5	1.23	12
F-J	359	8.5	7.1	0.39	
HAUTE-NORMANDIE					
F27	118	7.0	5.7	0.55	254
F76	355	7.7	6.8	0.37	108
F-K	473	7.5	6.5	0.31	
ILE-DE-FRANCE					
F75	983	11.6	8.2++	0.30	19
F77	237	7.9	6.8	0.46	108
F78	288	6.7	6.9	0.41	95
F91	208	5.7	6.0	0.43	223
F92	507	9.0	7.7++	0.36	42
F93	374	7.1	7.0	0.37	88
F94	384	8.1	7.3+	0.39	64
F95	243	7.3	7.4+	0.48	58
F-L	3224	8.4	7.3++	0.13	
LANGUEDOC-ROUSSILLON					
F11	120	11.5	6.2	0.66	198
F30	171	8.9	6.3	0.54	180
F34	251	10.1	6.5	0.46	142
F48	29	9.7	5.3	1.06	297
F66	133	11.5	7.5	0.75	53
F-M	704	10.2	6.5	0.28	
LIMOUSIN					
F19	82	8.7	5.8	0.76	246
F23	68	11.9	6.0	0.85	223
F87	138	10.1	6.6	0.63	132
F-N	288	10.0	6.2	0.43	
LORRAINE					
F54	225	7.9	6.7	0.46	117
F55	58	7.2	5.5	0.77	279
F57	239	5.9	5.6-	0.38	268
F88	111	7.1	5.6	0.56	268
F-O	633	6.8	6.0	0.25	
MIDI-PYRENEES					
F09	54	9.9	5.7	0.92	254
F12	118	10.9	6.3	0.66	180
F31	255	8.5	6.4	0.43	163
F32	76	10.9	6.5	0.90	142
F46	62	10.5	5.8	0.85	246
F65	82	9.2	7.0	0.84	88
F81	160	12.1	7.6	0.67	47
F82	80	11.2	7.9	1.03	31
F-P	887	10.0	6.6	0.25	
NORD-PAS-DE-CALAIS					
F59	819	8.3	7.4++	0.27	58
F62	407	7.4	6.6	0.34	132
F-Q	1226	8.0	7.1++	0.21	
PAYS DE LA LOIRE					
F44	315	8.7	7.6++	0.44	47
F49	230	9.4	7.4	0.51	58
F53	98	9.7	7.8	0.81	36
F72	173	9.0	7.3	0.58	64
F85	191	10.9	8.2++	0.63	19
F-R	1007	9.4	7.6++	0.25	
PICARDIE					
F02	192	9.0	6.9	0.52	95
F60	178	7.3	6.7	0.52	117
F80	211	10.0	7.9+	0.57	31
F-S	581	8.7	7.1+	0.31	
POITOU-CHARENTES					
F16	127	9.6	6.5	0.63	142
F17	187	9.7	6.2	0.49	198
F79	150	11.2	7.6	0.67	47
F86	140	10.0	6.5	0.59	142
F-T	604	10.1	6.6	0.29	
PROVENCE-ALPES-COTE D'AZUR					
F04	39	8.7	6.6	1.24	132
F05	45	11.6	7.7	1.26	42
F06	259	8.4	4.7--	0.37	333
F13	510	8.0	6.3	0.30	180
F83	234	9.5	6.8	0.49	108
F84	133	8.6	6.5	0.59	142
F-U	1220	8.5	6.1	0.19	
RHONE-ALPES					
F01	121	8.0	6.7	0.65	117
F07	111	11.1	8.1	0.85	24
F26	110	7.8	5.4	0.55	290
F38	268	7.9	6.9	0.43	95
F42	244	8.3	6.5	0.44	142
F69	446	7.9	7.1	0.35	79
F73	90	7.4	6.0	0.65	223
F74	142	7.9	7.2	0.63	68
F-V	1532	8.1	6.8+	0.18	
F.0	17969	8.7	6.8++	0.05	

UNITED KINGDOM (1976-80)

EAST ANGLIA					
G25	126	7.3	6.2	0.57	198
G46	160	8.0	5.7	0.49	254
G55	121	6.8	4.9--	0.48	319
G-A	407	7.4	5.5--	0.29	
EAST MIDLANDS					
G30	199	7.5	5.7	0.42	254
G44	154	6.3	5.1--	0.43	310
G45	108	6.9	5.2-	0.53	307
G47	116	7.6	6.2	0.60	198
G50	208	7.3	6.0	0.45	223
G-B	785	7.1	5.6--	0.21	
NORTHERN					
G14	229	6.8	5.3--	0.37	297
G27	99	5.9	5.1-	0.53	310
G29	95	6.9	4.8--	0.52	325
G33	111	6.2	4.8--	0.49	325
G48	59	6.9	4.9-	0.68	319
G-C	593	6.5	5.1--	0.22	
NORTH-WEST					
G11	487	6.3	5.1--	0.24	310
G12	315	7.0	5.5--	0.32	279
G26	187	6.9	5.7	0.43	254
G43	309	7.9	5.7-	0.35	254
G-D	1298	6.9	5.4--	0.16	

SOUTH-EAST					
G01	1493	7.5	5.5--	0.15	279
G22	97	6.5	5.6	0.58	268
G23	129	6.4	5.5	0.50	279
G24	110	7.0	5.9	0.58	235
G34	181	10.2	5.4-	0.47	290
G35	314	7.5	5.7-	0.34	254
G37	315	7.2	5.9	0.35	235
G39	178	6.4	5.4-	0.42	290
G41	22	6.8	4.3-	1.01	340
G42	349	8.3	6.3	0.36	180
G51	104	6.2	5.7	0.60	254
G56	255	8.8	6.8	0.45	108
G58	169	9.5	6.1	0.54	215
G-E	3716	7.6	5.7--	0.10	
SOUTH-WEST					
G21	203	7.6	5.9	0.44	235
G28	109	9.1	6.7	0.71	117
G31	253	9.2	5.5-	0.38	279
G32	153	9.2	5.3-	0.48	297
G36	84	5.8	4.5--	0.52	339
G53	110	9.1	6.8	0.71	108
G59	115	7.4	6.2	0.60	198
G-F	1027	8.2	5.8--	0.20	
WEST MIDLANDS					
G15	530	6.6	5.5--	0.25	279
G38	144	8.0	6.3	0.56	180
G52	81	7.6	5.8	0.68	246
G54	210	7.1	6.1	0.44	215
G57	91	6.6	5.8	0.63	246
G-G	1056	6.9	5.8--	0.19	
YORKSHIRE AND HUMBERSIDE					
G13	270	7.0	5.5--	0.35	279
G16	415	6.9	5.4--	0.28	290
G40	192	7.8	6.3	0.48	180
G49	141	7.3	5.0--	0.45	316
G-H	1018	7.1	5.5--	0.18	
WALES					
G61	98	8.9	5.8	0.61	246
G62	65	6.9	5.3	0.72	297
G63	81	6.3	4.7--	0.56	333
G64	57	8.7	6.0	0.87	223
G65	97	6.2	4.9--	0.51	319
G66	17	5.4	4.3	1.18	340
G67	85	7.6	5.5	0.62	279
G68	86	8.1	6.0	0.68	223
G-I	586	7.3	5.3--	0.23	
SCOTLAND(1975-80)					
S01	38	6.8	5.7	0.98	254
S02	93	7.0	5.0-	0.55	316
S03	89	7.7	6.2	0.69	198
S04	74	7.4	6.2	0.76	198
S05	148	6.9	5.4-	0.47	290
S06	29	10.1	6.1	1.20	215
S07	46	5.7	4.8-	0.74	325
S08	430	6.1	5.1--	0.26	310
S09	20	4.8	3.2--	0.76	353
S10	6	11.3	5.9	2.50	235
S11	5	8.0	6.5	3.02	142
S12	15	17.1	11.0	3.15	1
G-J	993	6.6	5.3--	0.18	
NORTHERN IRELAND					
JE	120	7.3	6.5	0.62	142
JN	72	8.0	7.2	0.88	68
JS	31	4.7	4.1--	0.75	346
JW	48	8.0	7.1	1.08	79
G-K	271	7.1	6.4	0.40	
G.0	11750	7.2	5.6--	0.05	
ITALIA (1975-79)					
ABRUZZI					
I66	58	7.9	6.1	0.85	215
I67	60	9.1	6.6	0.90	132
I68	50	7.2	5.6	0.83	268
I69	77	8.6	6.3	0.76	180
I-A	245	8.2	6.1	0.41	
BASILICATA					
I76	80	7.8	6.2	0.72	198
I77	29	5.8	5.2	0.98	307
I-B	109	7.1	5.9	0.59	
CALABRIA					
I78	108	6.1	5.6	0.55	268
I79	102	5.6	4.8--	0.48	325
I80	128	8.8	7.4	0.67	58
I-C	338	6.7	5.8	0.32	
CAMPANIA					
I61	99	5.5	5.3-	0.53	297
I62	52	7.2	5.9	0.85	235
I63	411	5.9	6.0	0.30	223
I64	65	6.0	4.8-	0.63	325
I65	180	7.3	6.4	0.49	163
I-D	807	6.2	5.9-	0.21	
EMILIA-ROMAGNA					
I33	84	12.1	8.1	0.95	24
I34	86	8.8	6.4	0.76	163
I35	104	10.5	7.6	0.79	47
I36	150	10.6	8.5++	0.73	12
I37	284	12.6	9.0++	0.57	8
I38	113	12.1	8.4+	0.84	16
I39	114	13.0	9.2++	0.95	5
I40	149	10.3	8.0+	0.69	28
I-E	1084	11.3	8.2++	0.27	
FRIULI-VENEZIA GIULIA					
I30	116	9.0	6.5	0.64	142
I31	29	8.3	5.8	1.15	246
I32	68	9.8	6.8	0.97	108
I93	58	8.9	6.7	0.93	117
I-F	271	9.1	6.4	0.42	
LAZIO					
I56	81	12.4	8.5+	1.00	12
I57	29	8.1	5.3	1.12	297
I58	729	8.2	7.7++	0.29	42
I59	79	7.6	7.2	0.82	68
I60	88	7.9	6.4	0.71	163
I-G	1006	8.3	7.5++	0.24	
LIGURIA					
I08	46	8.3	4.7-	0.76	333
I09	70	9.5	6.6	0.91	132
I10	293	11.4	7.5+	0.48	53
I11	74	12.5	8.4	1.08	16
I-H	483	10.8	7.1	0.36	
LOMBARDIA					
I12	184	9.8	9.3++	0.72	3
I13	144	7.8	6.9	0.60	95
I14	37	8.6	7.4	1.25	58
I15	904	9.3	8.6++	0.29	10
I16	138	6.4	6.3	0.54	180
I17	170	7.0	6.5	0.51	142
I18	166	13.1	9.2++	0.82	5
I19	94	11.6	9.6++	1.08	2
I20	82	8.9	6.4	0.75	163
I-I	1919	8.9	7.9++	0.19	
MARCHE					
I41	76	9.4	6.4	0.78	163
I42	85	8.2	6.2	0.71	198
I43	80	11.3	8.0	0.97	28
I44	66	7.7	5.9	0.75	235
I-J	307	9.0	6.6	0.40	
MOLISE					
I70	49	8.5	6.1	0.92	215
I94	22	9.5	6.7	1.56	117
I-K	71	8.8	6.3	0.79	
PIEMONTE					
I01	465	8.0	7.1+	0.34	79
I02	92	9.5	6.2	0.72	198
I03	129	10.5	7.8	0.74	36
I04	134	9.9	6.7	0.65	117
I05	49	9.1	5.6	0.95	268
I06	164	14.1	8.1+	0.75	24
I-L	1033	9.3	7.1++	0.24	
PUGLIA					
I71	134	8.0	6.9	0.61	95
I72	262	7.5	6.7	0.42	117
I73	66	4.8	4.6--	0.57	337
I74	66	6.9	6.2	0.78	198
I75	137	7.6	6.7	0.58	117
I-M	665	7.1	6.4	0.25	
SARDEGNA					
I90	80	7.6	6.4	0.74	163
I91	44	6.5	4.9	0.79	319
I92	130	7.4	7.1	0.63	79
I95	30	7.7	6.4	1.27	163
I-N	284	7.3	6.4	0.39	
SICILIA					
I81	81	7.8	6.0	0.70	223
I82	167	5.8	5.0--	0.40	316
I83	122	7.4	6.3	0.60	180
I84	76	6.4	5.4	0.65	290
I85	35	4.8	4.2--	0.72	343
I86	33	6.5	5.6	1.01	268
I87	165	6.8	5.9	0.47	235
I88	41	6.2	4.7-	0.77	333
I89	51	5.3	4.8-	0.68	325
I-O	771	6.4	5.4--	0.20	
TOSCANA					
I45	27	5.4	4.2-	0.87	343
I46	101	10.8	7.6	0.82	47
I47	60	9.4	7.2	1.03	68
I48	275	9.5	6.5	0.42	142
I49	104	12.4	8.7+	0.92	9
I50	90	9.6	6.3	0.73	180
I51	71	9.2	6.5	0.85	142
I52	75	11.8	7.5	1.01	53
I53	67	12.1	8.2	1.11	19
I-P	870	10.0	6.9+	0.26	
TRENTINO-ALTO ADIGE					
I21	45	4.3	3.8--	0.59	349
I22	87	8.1	6.7	0.76	117
I-Q	132	6.2	5.3-	0.48	
UMBRIA					
I54	125	8.9	5.9	0.55	235
I55	64	11.4	8.5	1.15	12
I-R	189	9.6	6.6	0.51	
VALLE D'AOSTA					
I07	20	7.0	5.3	1.26	297
VENETO					
I23	184	9.9	8.2++	0.62	19
I24	129	7.4	6.7	0.60	117
I25	51	9.4	7.1	1.06	79
I26	127	7.4	6.3	0.58	180
I27	175	8.6	7.7+	0.60	42
I28	159	8.1	7.1	0.58	79
I29	51	8.2	5.9	0.88	235
I-T	876	8.4	7.2++	0.25	
I.0	11480	8.4	6.9++	0.07	
IRELAND (1976-80)					
CONNAUGHT					
R07	27	6.2	4.3-	0.91	340
R12	8	10.8	7.0	2.84	88
R16	19	6.5	3.7--	0.93	350
R20	7	4.9	2.7--	1.08	355
R21	9	6.5	4.2	1.46	343
R-A	70	6.5	4.1--	0.54	
LEINSTER					
R01	7	7.1	5.8	2.25	246
R06	110	4.7	4.8--	0.47	325
R09	15	5.9	5.9	1.53	235
R10	11	6.2	5.1	1.57	310
R11	11	8.4	6.5	2.07	142
R14	6	7.5	5.7	2.40	254
R15	10	4.6	4.8	1.56	325
R17	23	9.8	9.3	1.99	3
R19	7	4.7	3.9	1.47	348
R24	10	6.5	5.3	1.71	297
R25	14	5.7	4.9	1.33	319
R26	18	8.6	7.9	1.92	31
R-B	242	5.6	5.4--	0.35	
MUNSTER					
R03	22	10.0	7.8	1.73	36
R04	78	7.8	7.2	0.84	68
R08	22	7.1	4.9	1.11	319
R13	23	5.8	5.3	1.12	297
R22	28	8.1	6.8	1.34	108
R23	8	3.6	2.8--	1.02	354
R-C	181	7.3	6.2	0.47	
ULSTER					
R02	10	7.1	5.6	1.89	268
R05	16	5.1	3.5--	0.92	351
R18	6	4.6	3.5	1.50	351
R-D	32	5.5	3.9--	0.73	
R.0	525	6.2	5.3--	0.24	
LUXEMBOURG (1971-80)					
LE	10	5.5	4.0	1.35	347
LN	22	8.3	5.7	1.30	254
LS	89	7.0	5.6	0.61	268
L.0	121	7.0	5.4	0.52	
NEDERLAND (1976-80)					
N01	135	9.9	7.1	0.64	79
N02	115	8.1	6.1	0.60	215
N03	66	6.4	5.1	0.66	310
N04	168	6.7	5.7	0.46	254
N05	327	7.9	6.6	0.38	132
N06	185	8.5	7.5	0.56	53
N07	437	7.5	6.2	0.31	198
N08	690	9.2	7.1++	0.28	79
N09	77	9.1	6.3	0.78	180
N10	323	6.4	6.2	0.35	198
N11	178	6.7	6.4	0.49	163
N.0	2701	7.8	6.5	0.13	
EEC-9					
EEC	62306	8.2	6.4	0.03	

BELGIE-BELGIQUE (1971-78)

BRUSSEL-BRUXELLES					
B21	373	8.4	4.2	0.28	164
VLAANDEREN					
B10	331	5.2	3.7-	0.23	252
B29	230	6.3	4.4	0.32	124
B30	250	5.8	3.7	0.26	252
B40	322	6.0	3.6-	0.23	269
B70	123	4.6	4.1	0.38	192
B-V	1256	5.6	3.8--	0.12	
WALLONIE					
B25	76	7.1	4.4	0.57	124
B50	387	7.1	4.0	0.24	212
B60	308	7.3	4.3	0.29	146
B80	39	4.4	3.0-	0.56	326
B90	110	6.8	4.0	0.46	212
B-W	920	7.0	4.1	0.16	
B.0	2549	6.4	4.0-	0.09	

BR DEUTSCHLAND (1976-80)

BADEN-WURTTEMBERG					
D81	592	6.6	4.1	0.19	192
D82	458	7.4	4.6	0.27	91
D83	373	7.7	4.6	0.29	91
D84	266	6.9	4.6	0.33	91
D-A	1689	7.1	4.4	0.13	
BAYERN					
D91	593	6.3	3.6--	0.18	269
D92	169	6.4	3.8	0.36	237
D93	161	6.4	4.0	0.37	212
D94	206	7.4	3.9	0.32	228
D95	256	6.4	3.9	0.29	228
D96	202	6.5	3.8	0.31	237
D97	266	6.7	4.0	0.30	212
D-B	1853	6.5	3.8--	0.11	
BERLIN(WEST)					
DB0	600	11.3	4.6	0.29	91
BREMEN					
D40	144	7.8	4.5	0.48	110
HAMBURG					
D20	417	9.3	4.5	0.31	110
HESSEN					
D64	784	6.9	3.9	0.17	228
D66	234	7.5	3.8	0.30	237
D-F	1018	7.0	3.9	0.15	
NIEDERSACHSEN					
D31	330	7.7	4.7	0.35	76
D32	454	8.4	4.5	0.27	110
D33	271	7.3	4.3	0.32	146
D34	337	6.2	4.0	0.25	212
D-G	1392	7.4	4.4	0.14	
NORDRHEIN-WESTFALEN					
D51	1012	7.3	4.5	0.17	110
D53	706	7.0	4.4	0.19	124
D55	366	5.9	4.1	0.24	192
D57	327	6.9	4.1	0.26	192
D59	688	7.1	4.2	0.19	164
D-H	3099	7.0	4.3	0.09	
RHEINLAND-PFALZ					
D71	268	7.5	4.6	0.37	91
D72	101	8.1	4.7	0.57	76
D73	341	7.2	4.2	0.28	164
D-I	710	7.5	4.4	0.21	
SAARLAND					
DA0	182	6.4	4.0	0.38	212
SCHLESWIG-HOLSTEIN					
D10	502	7.5	4.0	0.21	212
D.0	11606	7.2	4.2	0.05	

DANMARK (1971-80)

K15	525	7.9	4.5	0.23	110
K20	92	6.1	5.2	0.56	38
K25	61	6.7	5.7	0.77	14
K30	103	7.7	4.8	0.54	60
K35	102	8.0	4.8	0.53	60
K40	17	7.3	5.0	1.41	45
K42	181	8.1	4.9	0.40	51
K50	75	6.1	4.3	0.57	146
K55	67	6.6	5.0	0.67	45
K60	109	6.8	4.7	0.50	76
K65	90	7.2	5.7+	0.65	14
K70	167	5.9	4.2	0.36	164
K76	80	7.1	4.6	0.57	91
K80	149	6.4	4.6	0.42	91
K.0	1818	7.1	4.7++	0.12	

FRANCE (1971-78)

ALSACE					
F67	253	7.0	4.7	0.34	76
F68	163	6.3	3.7	0.33	252
F-A	416	6.7	4.3	0.24	
AQUITAINE					
F24	112	7.3	3.8	0.46	237
F33	290	6.6	3.8	0.28	237
F40	88	7.5	4.1	0.56	192
F47	101	8.4	4.4	0.56	124
F64	166	7.5	4.2	0.39	164
F-B	757	7.2	4.0	0.18	
AUVERGNE					
F03	155	9.9	5.3+	0.55	31
F15	52	7.7	4.5	0.76	110
F43	83	9.9	5.7	0.79	14
F63	181	7.7	5.3+	0.45	31
F-C	471	8.7	5.3++	0.30	
BASSE-NORMANDIE					
F14	130	5.6	4.0	0.40	212
F50	122	6.5	4.3	0.45	146
F61	87	7.2	4.2	0.53	164
F-D	339	6.3	4.2	0.26	
BOURGOGNE					
F21	122	6.6	4.7	0.49	76
F58	76	7.5	4.1	0.58	192
F71	171	7.4	3.9	0.37	228
F89	106	8.7	4.0	0.49	212
F-E	475	7.4	4.2	0.24	
BRETAGNE					
F22	137	6.4	3.9	0.39	228
F29	218	6.6	4.3	0.35	146
F35	174	6.0	4.2	0.36	164
F56	139	6.0	3.6	0.36	269
F-F	668	6.2	4.0	0.18	
CENTRE					
F18	93	7.2	3.6	0.48	269
F28	101	7.5	4.9	0.57	51
F36	102	10.2	5.8+	0.76	11
F37	102	5.2	3.3-	0.39	303
F41	96	8.3	4.7	0.59	76
F45	126	6.4	4.1	0.43	192
F-G	620	7.1	4.3	0.21	
CHAMPAGNE-ARDENNE					
F08	78	6.3	4.2	0.55	164
F10	96	8.3	4.7	0.58	76
F51	138	6.5	4.4	0.43	124
F52	67	7.8	5.9+	0.83	9
F-H	379	7.0	4.7	0.28	
CORSE					
F20	55	6.4	3.6	0.62	269
FRANCHE-COMTE					
F25	80	4.2	3.2-	0.39	314
F39	71	7.3	4.2	0.60	164
F70	45	5.0	2.7--	0.48	341
F90	38	7.4	4.8	0.91	60
F-J	234	5.5	3.6-	0.27	
HAUTE-NORMANDIE					
F27	109	6.4	3.9	0.44	228
F76	284	5.9	4.2	0.28	164
F-K	393	6.0	4.1	0.24	
ILE-DE-FRANCE					
F75	1005	10.2	5.4++	0.24	27
F77	191	6.3	4.5	0.36	110
F78	251	5.8	4.5	0.30	110
F91	199	5.4	4.1	0.31	192
F92	421	7.1	4.4	0.26	124
F93	327	6.2	4.7	0.28	76
F94	366	7.4	5.4++	0.33	27
F95	214	6.3	4.8	0.36	60
F-L	2974	7.3	4.8++	0.10	
LANGUEDOC-ROUSSILLON					
F11	83	7.4	3.7	0.56	252
F30	133	6.6	4.1	0.44	192
F34	192	7.1	4.0	0.37	212
F48	24	8.0	5.7	1.43	14
F66	83	6.6	3.9	0.54	228
F-M	515	7.0	4.0	0.23	
LIMOUSIN					
F19	93	9.4	5.3	0.70	31
F23	65	10.7	6.0	1.04	8
F87	108	7.4	4.3	0.54	146
F-N	266	8.7	4.9	0.40	
LORRAINE					
F54	186	6.4	4.5	0.36	110
F55	43	5.2	2.9-	0.55	330
F57	233	5.9	4.6	0.33	91
F88	107	6.6	4.4	0.49	124
F-O	569	6.1	4.4	0.20	
MIDI-PYRENEES					
F09	40	7.1	5.2	1.10	38
F12	72	6.3	3.5	0.56	283
F31	218	6.8	4.7	0.37	76
F32	60	8.5	4.6	0.75	91
F46	38	6.2	3.2	0.63	314
F65	70	7.5	4.7	0.77	76
F81	120	8.7	5.3	0.60	31
F82	54	7.2	3.5	0.58	283
F-P	672	7.3	4.4	0.21	
NORD-PAS-DE-CALAIS					
F59	671	6.6	4.7+	0.20	76
F62	354	6.2	4.5	0.27	110
F-Q	1025	6.4	4.6++	0.16	
PAYS DE LA LOIRE					
F44	244	6.3	4.5	0.33	110
F49	193	7.4	4.8	0.39	60
F53	76	7.0	4.3	0.56	146
F72	145	7.2	4.8	0.47	60
F85	143	7.8	5.0	0.49	45
F-R	801	7.0	4.7+	0.19	
PICARDIE					
F02	164	7.6	4.8	0.44	60
F60	137	5.6	3.7	0.37	252
F80	173	7.9	5.4+	0.48	27
F-S	474	7.0	4.6	0.25	
POITOU-CHARENTES					
F16	102	7.4	4.6	0.55	91
F17	153	7.5	4.2	0.43	164
F79	107	7.9	4.9	0.57	51
F86	129	8.9	5.7+	0.62	14
F-T	491	7.9	4.8+	0.27	
PROVENCE-ALPES-COTE D'AZUR					
F04	32	7.2	4.3	1.00	146
F05	29	7.4	4.2	0.95	164
F06	183	5.3	2.8--	0.29	334
F13	423	6.3	4.2	0.24	164
F83	179	7.0	4.1	0.39	192
F84	113	7.1	4.6	0.50	91
F-U	959	6.4	3.9-	0.15	
RHONE-ALPES					
F01	97	6.4	4.5	0.52	110
F07	83	7.9	4.8	0.66	60
F26	117	8.0	5.3	0.59	31
F38	238	6.9	4.7	0.34	76
F42	224	7.3	4.6	0.36	91
F69	363	6.2	4.1	0.24	192
F73	73	5.9	3.6	0.47	269
F74	88	4.9	3.4	0.40	292
F-V	1283	6.6	4.3	0.14	
F.0	14836	6.9	4.4++	0.04	

UNITED KINGDOM (1976-80)

EAST ANGLIA					
G25	90	5.3	3.7	0.43	252
G46	135	6.5	3.5	0.36	283
G55	100	5.7	3.5	0.42	283
G-A	325	5.9	3.6-	0.23	
EAST MIDLANDS					
G30	144	5.2	3.7	0.36	252
G44	153	6.0	4.2	0.39	164
G45	107	6.7	4.5	0.51	110
G47	88	5.6	3.4	0.42	292
G50	167	5.6	3.3--	0.29	303
G-B	659	5.8	3.8-	0.17	
NORTHERN					
G14	175	4.8	3.1--	0.27	321
G27	91	5.2	4.4	0.50	124
G29	86	5.9	3.1--	0.39	321
G33	75	4.0	2.6--	0.33	346
G48	45	5.1	2.6--	0.45	346
G-C	472	4.9	3.2--	0.17	
NORTH-WEST					
G11	450	5.5	3.4--	0.19	292
G12	294	6.1	4.0	0.27	212
G26	150	5.3	3.3--	0.29	303
G43	288	6.7	3.7	0.27	252
G-D	1182	5.9	3.6--	0.12	

SOUTH-EAST					
G01	1380	6.3	3.6--	0.12	269
G22	76	5.2	3.4	0.42	292
G23	85	4.2	2.9--	0.35	330
G24	96	6.2	4.6	0.52	91
G34	181	8.5	3.6	0.40	269
G35	249	5.7	3.4--	0.24	292
G37	254	5.9	3.8	0.27	237
G39	161	5.5	3.7	0.32	252
G41	22	6.1	3.1	0.87	321
G42	307	6.9	3.8	0.26	237
G51	93	5.9	4.1	0.47	192
G56	189	6.2	3.8	0.33	237
G58	156	7.7	3.7	0.40	252
G-E	3249	6.2	3.6--	0.08	
SOUTH-WEST					
G21	142	5.0	2.8--	0.27	334
G28	84	6.5	3.3-	0.43	303
G31	196	6.7	3.7	0.34	252
G32	137	7.4	3.2--	0.37	314
G36	90	5.9	3.5	0.43	283
G53	86	6.8	3.8	0.51	237
G59	80	5.2	3.3-	0.42	303
G-F	815	6.2	3.3--	0.14	
WEST MIDLANDS					
G15	420	5.1	3.4--	0.19	292
G38	94	5.1	3.3-	0.38	303
G52	64	5.8	3.4	0.47	292
G54	176	5.8	3.8	0.32	237
G57	84	5.9	4.2	0.53	164
G-G	838	5.3	3.5--	0.14	
YORKSHIRE AND HUMBERSIDE					
G13	224	5.6	3.7	0.28	252
G16	342	5.3	3.2--	0.20	314
G40	151	5.8	3.8	0.36	237
G49	144	7.2	4.4	0.44	124
G-H	861	5.7	3.6--	0.14	
WALES					
G61	99	8.4	4.8	0.57	60
G62	76	7.5	4.4	0.62	124
G63	74	5.5	3.2-	0.45	314
G64	42	6.0	3.4	0.65	292
G65	73	4.4	3.0--	0.39	326
G66	17	5.4	2.8	0.79	334
G67	78	6.5	3.3-	0.43	303
G68	70	6.1	3.7	0.50	252
G-I	529	6.2	3.6--	0.18	
SCOTLAND(1975-80)					
S01	31	5.4	3.2	0.64	314
S02	93	6.5	4.3	0.52	146
S03	78	6.2	3.8	0.51	237
S04	50	4.8	2.8--	0.44	334
S05	147	6.2	3.5-	0.35	283
S06	27	8.6	6.3	1.57	4
S07	34	4.1	3.0-	0.57	326
S08	382	5.0	3.3--	0.19	303
S09	32	7.3	3.8	0.78	237
S10	4	7.3	6.1	3.26	7
S11	3	4.9	3.1	1.94	321
S12	4	4.4	1.9-	1.12	352
G-J	885	5.5	3.5--	0.14	
NORTHERN IRELAND					
JE	99	5.9	4.0	0.44	212
JN	37	4.0	2.9-	0.53	330
JS	28	4.1	3.3	0.66	303
JW	22	3.6	2.8-	0.65	334
G-K	186	4.8	3.4--	0.27	
G.0	10001	5.8	3.6--	0.04	
ITALIA (1975-79)					
ABRUZZI					
I66	48	6.2	4.1	0.67	192
I67	37	5.5	3.6	0.64	269
I68	31	4.3	3.5	0.67	283
I69	62	6.7	4.6	0.66	91
I-A	178	5.8	4.0	0.33	
BASILICATA					
I76	51	4.9	4.1	0.61	192
I77	21	4.2	3.5	0.79	283
I-B	72	4.7	3.9	0.48	
CALABRIA					
I78	81	4.5	3.7	0.43	252
I79	100	5.4	4.9	0.51	51
I80	88	5.9	4.3	0.50	146
I-C	269	5.2	4.3	0.28	

CAMPANIA					
I61	82	4.5	4.2	0.47	164
I62	40	5.4	4.2	0.71	164
I63	354	4.9	4.4	0.24	124
I64	61	5.6	4.2	0.57	164
I65	136	5.4	4.6	0.41	91
I-D	673	5.0	4.4	0.17	
EMILIA-ROMAGNA					
I33	62	8.6	4.9	0.75	51
I34	83	8.1	4.8	0.67	60
I35	81	7.9	5.3	0.69	31
I36	88	6.0	4.6	0.56	91
I37	195	8.0	4.8	0.41	60
I38	69	6.9	4.3	0.59	146
I39	71	7.7	4.9	0.67	51
I40	89	6.0	3.8	0.42	237
I-E	738	7.3	4.6+	0.20	
FRIULI-VENEZIA GIULIA					
I30	114	8.4	4.8	0.53	60
I31	25	6.5	3.9	0.87	228
I32	56	7.0	3.3	0.58	303
I93	40	5.8	3.7	0.66	252
I-F	235	7.3	4.1	0.32	
LAZIO					
I56	40	6.0	4.3	0.76	146
I57	33	9.1	6.4	1.27	3
I58	590	6.3	4.9++	0.21	51
I59	69	6.7	6.3++	0.77	4
I60	73	6.4	4.6	0.58	91
I-G	805	6.4	5.0++	0.19	
LIGURIA					
I08	31	5.2	2.7--	0.55	341
I09	66	8.4	5.5	0.83	24
I10	225	7.9	4.8	0.38	60
I11	54	8.5	3.9	0.62	228
I-H	376	7.7	4.5	0.28	
LOMBARDIA					
I12	128	6.4	4.9	0.47	51
I13	142	7.3	5.3+	0.48	31
I14	43	9.8	6.9+	1.13	2
I15	724	6.9	5.2++	0.21	38
I16	119	5.4	4.2	0.40	164
I17	165	6.5	5.1+	0.42	43
I18	145	10.7	6.2++	0.62	6
I19	76	8.8	5.6	0.73	21
I20	79	8.1	5.8+	0.78	11
I-I	1621	7.1	5.2++	0.14	
MARCHE					
I41	42	5.1	3.4	0.59	292
I42	83	7.5	4.4	0.55	124
I43	51	6.9	4.4	0.71	124
I44	69	7.7	5.4	0.71	27
I-J	245	6.9	4.4	0.32	
MOLISE					
I70	27	4.5	3.2	0.66	314
I94	20	8.3	5.7	1.37	14
I-K	47	5.6	3.9	0.61	
PIEMONTE					
I01	352	5.8	4.2	0.24	164
I02	77	7.3	4.4	0.61	124
I03	112	8.5	5.2	0.57	38
I04	95	6.9	4.6	0.57	91
I05	51	9.1	5.1	0.86	43
I06	104	8.4	4.8	0.59	60
I-L	791	6.8	4.4	0.18	
PUGLIA					
I71	86	5.0	4.1	0.46	192
I72	172	4.7	4.0	0.32	212
I73	69	4.9	4.2	0.53	164
I74	63	6.4	5.9+	0.76	9
I75	98	5.1	4.1	0.44	192
I-M	488	5.1	4.3	0.20	
SARDEGNA					
I90	56	5.3	4.2	0.60	164
I91	31	4.5	3.6	0.67	269
I92	69	3.9	3.4	0.43	292
I95	16	4.1	2.4--	0.68	350
I-N	172	4.4	3.6-	0.29	
SICILIA					
I81	63	5.9	4.6	0.63	91
I82	138	4.6	3.8	0.34	237
I83	95	5.5	4.4	0.49	124
I84	62	5.2	4.4	0.58	124
I85	18	2.4	2.2--	0.52	351
I86	17	3.3	2.7-	0.70	341
I87	119	4.8	4.1	0.39	192
I88	32	4.7	3.3	0.63	303
I89	46	4.7	4.0	0.61	212
I-O	590	4.8	3.9	0.17	

TOSCANA					
I45	40	7.6	5.5	1.00	24
I46	73	7.3	4.3	0.58	146
I47	44	6.5	4.4	0.79	124
I48	222	7.2	4.2	0.33	164
I49	81	9.2	5.6+	0.73	21
I50	91	9.3	5.5+	0.67	24
I51	59	7.5	4.7	0.72	76
I52	55	8.4	4.4	0.70	124
I53	39	6.9	4.2	0.76	164
I-P	704	7.7	4.7+	0.20	
TRENTINO-ALTO ADIGE					
I21	70	6.4	5.0	0.63	45
I22	57	5.1	3.5	0.52	283
I-Q	127	5.8	4.2	0.41	
UMBRIA					
I54	90	6.2	4.7	0.56	76
I55	32	5.5	3.6	0.71	269
I-R	122	6.0	4.4	0.45	
VALLE D'AOSTA					
I07	9	3.2	1.5--	0.51	354
VENETO					
I23	155	8.0	5.7++	0.51	14
I24	106	5.8	4.4	0.45	124
I25	41	7.0	4.3	0.82	146
I26	125	7.0	4.9	0.48	51
I27	136	6.4	4.8	0.44	60
I28	119	5.8	4.2	0.41	164
I29	46	7.1	4.8	0.77	60
I-T	728	6.6	4.8++	0.19	
I.0	8990	6.3	4.6++	0.05	
IRELAND (1976-80)					
CONNAUGHT					
R07	21	5.2	3.6	0.89	269
R12	2	3.1	2.5	1.86	348
R16	12	4.3	3.0	0.96	326
R20	6	4.7	2.7	1.24	341
R21	9	6.7	4.3	1.62	146
R-A	50	4.9	3.3	0.52	
LEINSTER					
R01	5	5.3	4.0	1.85	212
R06	85	3.3	2.7--	0.31	341
R09	6	2.6	2.5	1.04	348
R10	8	4.8	3.1	1.15	321
R11	4	3.4	2.8	1.49	334
R14	1	1.4	0.4--	0.42	355
R15	10	4.6	4.1	1.34	192
R17	12	5.5	5.2	1.52	38
R19	9	6.5	5.8	2.02	11
R24	8	5.5	3.7	1.42	252
R25	9	3.8	2.8	0.97	334
R26	8	3.8	2.9	1.10	330
R-B	165	3.7	3.0--	0.25	
MUNSTER					
R03	7	3.4	1.9--	0.79	352
R04	59	6.0	4.4	0.62	124
R08	17	5.8	4.4	1.14	124
R13	22	5.6	5.0	1.13	45
R22	19	5.9	4.4	1.08	124
R23	11	5.1	4.2	1.36	164
R-C	135	5.6	4.3	0.39	
ULSTER					
R02	8	6.3	4.5	1.72	110
R05	13	4.4	3.4	0.98	292
R18	8	6.6	5.6	2.11	21
R-D	29	5.3	4.1	0.82	
R.0	379	4.5	3.5--	0.19	
LUXEMBOURG (1971-80)					
LE	19	9.9	7.0	1.85	1
LN	19	7.2	3.6	0.93	269
LS	86	6.4	3.7	0.46	252
L.0	124	6.9	4.0	0.41	
NEDERLAND (1976-80)					
N01	100	7.3	4.3	0.48	146
N02	104	7.3	4.7	0.52	76
N03	54	5.3	3.6	0.53	269
N04	149	6.0	4.3	0.38	146
N05	236	5.6	4.0	0.28	212
N06	157	7.0	5.0	0.43	45
N07	388	6.5	4.2	0.25	164
N08	516	6.6	4.2	0.21	164
N09	53	6.2	4.3	0.67	146
N10	246	4.9	4.1	0.27	192
N11	144	5.4	4.1	0.36	192
N.0	2147	6.1	4.2	0.10	
EEC-9					
EEC	52450	6.5	4.2	0.02	

PUBLICATIONS OF THE INTERNATIONAL AGENCY FOR RESEARCH ON CANCER

Scientific Publications Series

(Available from Oxford University Press through local bookshops)

No. 1 **Liver Cancer**
1971; 176 pages (*out of print*)

No. 2 **Oncogenesis and Herpesviruses**
Edited by P.M. Biggs, G. de-Thé and L.N. Payne
1972; 515 pages (*out of print*)

No. 3 ***N*-Nitroso Compounds: Analysis and Formation**
Edited by P. Bogovski, R. Preussman and E.A. Walker
1972; 140 pages (*out of print*)

No. 4 **Transplacental Carcinogenesis**
Edited by L. Tomatis and U. Mohr
1973; 181 pages (*out of print*)

No. 5/6 **Pathology of Tumours in Laboratory Animals, Volume 1, Tumours of the Rat**
Edited by V.S. Turusov
1973/1976; 533 pages (*out of print*)

No. 7 **Host Environment Interactions in the Etiology of Cancer in Man**
Edited by R. Doll and I. Vodopija
1973; 464 pages (*out of print*)

No. 8 **Biological Effects of Asbestos**
Edited by P. Bogovski, J.C. Gilson, V. Timbrell and J.C. Wagner
1973; 346 pages (*out of print*)

No. 9 ***N*-Nitroso Compounds in the Environment**
Edited by P. Bogovski and E.A. Walker
1974; 243 pages (*out of print*)

No. 10 **Chemical Carcinogenesis Essays**
Edited by R. Montesano and L. Tomatis
1974; 230 pages (*out of print*)

No. 11 **Oncogenesis and Herpesviruses II**
Edited by G. de-Thé, M.A. Epstein and H. zur Hausen
1975; Part I: 511 pages
Part II: 403 pages (*out of print*)

No. 12 **Screening Tests in Chemical Carcinogenesis**
Edited by R. Montesano, H. Bartsch and L. Tomatis
1976; 666 pages (*out of print*)

No. 13 **Environmental Pollution and Carcinogenic Risks**
Edited by C. Rosenfeld and W. Davis
1975; 441 pages (*out of print*)

No. 14 **Environmental *N*-Nitroso Compounds. Analysis and Formation**
Edited by E.A. Walker, P. Bogovski and L. Griciute
1976; 512 pages (*out of print*)

No. 15 **Cancer Incidence in Five Continents, Volume III**
Edited by J.A.H. Waterhouse, C. Muir, P. Correa and J. Powell
1976; 584 pages (*out of print*)

No. 16 **Air Pollution and Cancer in Man**
Edited by U. Mohr, D. Schmähl and L. Tomatis
1977; 328 pages (*out of print*)

No. 17 **Directory of On-going Research in Cancer Epidemiology 1977**
Edited by C.S. Muir and G. Wagner
1977; 599 pages (*out of print*)

No. 18 **Environmental Carcinogens. Selected Methods of Analysis. Volume 1: Analysis of Volatile Nitrosamines in Food**
Editor-in-Chief: H. Egan
1978; 212 pages (*out of print*)

No. 19 **Environmental Aspects of *N*-Nitroso Compounds**
Edited by E.A. Walker, M. Castegnaro, L. Griciute and R.E. Lyle
1978; 561 pages (*out of print*)

No. 20 **Nasopharyngeal Carcinoma: Etiology and Control**
Edited by G. de-Thé and Y. Ito
1978; 606 pages (*out of print*)

No. 21 **Cancer Registration and its Techniques**
Edited by R. MacLennan, C. Muir, R. Steinitz and A. Winkler
1978; 235 pages (*out of print*)

No. 22 **Environmental Carcinogens. Selected Methods of Analysis. Volume 2: Methods for the Measurement of Vinyl Chloride in Poly(vinyl chloride), Air, Water and Foodstuffs**
Editor-in-Chief: H. Egan
1978; 142 pages (*out of print*)

No. 23 **Pathology of Tumours in Laboratory Animals. Volume II: Tumours of the Mouse**
Editor-in-Chief: V.S. Turusov
1979; 669 pages (*out of print*)

No. 24 **Oncogenesis and Herpesviruses III**
Edited by G. de-Thé, W. Henle and F. Rapp
1978; Part I: 580 pages, Part II: 512 pages (*out of print*)

No. 25 **Carcinogenic Risk. Strategies for Intervention**
Edited by W. Davis and C. Rosenfeld
1979; 280 pages (*out of print*)

No. 26 **Directory of On-going Research in Cancer Epidemiology 1978**
Edited by C.S. Muir and G. Wagner
1978; 550 pages (*out of print*)

No. 27 **Molecular and Cellular Aspects of Carcinogen Screening Tests**
Edited by R. Montesano, H. Bartsch and L. Tomatis
1980; 372 pages £29.00

No. 28 **Directory of On-going Research in Cancer Epidemiology 1979**
Edited by C.S. Muir and G. Wagner
1979; 672 pages (*out of print*)

No. 29 **Environmental Carcinogens. Selected Methods of Analysis. Volume 3: Analysis of Polycyclic Aromatic Hydrocarbons in Environmental Samples**
Editor-in-Chief: H. Egan
1979; 240 pages (*out of print*)

No. 30 **Biological Effects of Mineral Fibres**
Editor-in-Chief: J.C. Wagner
1980; **Volume 1:** 494 pages **Volume 2:** 513 pages (*out of print*)

No. 31 ***N*-Nitroso Compounds: Analysis, Formation and Occurrence**
Edited by E.A. Walker, L. Griciute, M. Castegnaro and M. Börzsönyi
1980; 835 pages (*out of print*)

No. 32 **Statistical Methods in Cancer Research. Volume 1. The Analysis of Case-control Studies**
By N.E. Breslow and N.E. Day
1980; 338 pages £25.00

No. 33 **Handling Chemical Carcinogens in the Laboratory**
Edited by R. Montesano *et al.*
1979; 32 pages (*out of print*)

No. 34 **Pathology of Tumours in Laboratory Animals. Volume III. Tumours of the Hamster**
Editor-in-Chief: V.S. Turusov
1982; 461 pages (*out of print*)

No. 35 **Directory of On-going Research in Cancer Epidemiology 1980**
Edited by C.S. Muir and G. Wagner
1980; 660 pages (*out of print*)

Prices, valid for November 1992, are subject to change without notice

No. 36 **Cancer Mortality by Occupation and Social Class 1851-1971**
Edited by W.P.D. Logan
1982; 253 pages (*out of print*)

No. 37 **Laboratory Decontamination and Destruction of Aflatoxins B_1, B_2, G_1, G_2 in Laboratory Wastes**
Edited by M. Castegnaro *et al.*
1980; 56 pages (*out of print*)

No. 38 **Directory of On-going Research in Cancer Epidemiology 1981**
Edited by C.S. Muir and G. Wagner
1981; 696 pages (*out of print*)

No. 39 **Host Factors in Human Carcinogenesis**
Edited by H. Bartsch and B. Armstrong
1982; 583 pages (*out of print*)

No. 40 **Environmental Carcinogens. Selected Methods of Analysis. Volume 4: Some Aromatic Amines and Azo Dyes in the General and Industrial Environment**
Edited by L. Fishbein, M. Castegnaro, I.K. O'Neill and H. Bartsch
1981; 347 pages (*out of print*)

No. 41 ***N*-Nitroso Compounds: Occurrence and Biological Effects**
Edited by H. Bartsch, I.K. O'Neill, M. Castegnaro and M. Okada
1982; 755 pages £50.00

No. 42 **Cancer Incidence in Five Continents, Volume IV**
Edited by J. Waterhouse, C. Muir, K. Shanmugaratnam and J. Powell
1982; 811 pages (*out of print*)

No. 43 **Laboratory Decontamination and Destruction of Carcinogens in Laboratory Wastes: Some *N*-Nitrosamines**
Edited by M. Castegnaro *et al.*
1982; 73 pages £7.50

No. 44 **Environmental Carcinogens. Selected Methods of Analysis. Volume 5: Some Mycotoxins**
Edited by L. Stoloff, M. Castegnaro, P. Scott, I.K. O'Neill and H. Bartsch
1983; 455 pages £32.50

No. 45 **Environmental Carcinogens. Selected Methods of Analysis. Volume 6: *N*-Nitroso Compounds**
Edited by R. Preussmann, I.K. O'Neill, G. Eisenbrand, B. Spiegelhalder and H. Bartsch
1983; 508 pages £32.50

No. 46 **Directory of On-going Research in Cancer Epidemiology 1982**
Edited by C.S. Muir and G. Wagner
1982; 722 pages (*out of print*)

No. 47 **Cancer Incidence in Singapore 1968–1977**
Edited by K. Shanmugaratnam, H.P. Lee and N.E. Day
1983; 171 pages (*out of print*)

No. 48 **Cancer Incidence in the USSR (2nd Revised Edition)**
Edited by N.P. Napalkov, G.F. Tserkovny, V.M. Merabishvili, D.M. Parkin, M. Smans and C.S. Muir
1983; 75 pages (*out of print*)

No. 49 **Laboratory Decontamination and Destruction of Carcinogens in Laboratory Wastes: Some Polycyclic Aromatic Hydrocarbons**
Edited by M. Castegnaro *et al.*
1983; 87 pages (*out of print*)

No. 50 **Directory of On-going Research in Cancer Epidemiology 1983**
Edited by C.S. Muir and G. Wagner
1983; 731 pages (*out of print*)

No. 51 **Modulators of Experimental Carcinogenesis**
Edited by V. Turusov and R. Montesano
1983; 307 pages (*out of print*)

No. 52 **Second Cancers in Relation to Radiation Treatment for Cervical Cancer: Results of a Cancer Registry Collaboration**
Edited by N.E. Day and J.C. Boice, Jr
1984; 207 pages (*out of print*)

No. 53 **Nickel in the Human Environment**
Editor-in-Chief: F.W. Sunderman, Jr
1984; 529 pages (*out of print*)

No. 54 **Laboratory Decontamination and Destruction of Carcinogens in Laboratory Wastes: Some Hydrazines**
Edited by M. Castegnaro *et al.*
1983; 87 pages (*out of print*)

No. 55 **Laboratory Decontamination and Destruction of Carcinogens in Laboratory Wastes: Some *N*-Nitrosamides**
Edited by M. Castegnaro *et al.*
1984; 66 pages (*out of print*)

No. 56 **Models, Mechanisms and Etiology of Tumour Promotion**
Edited by M. Börzsönyi, N.E. Day, K. Lapis and H. Yamasaki
1984; 532 pages (*out of print*)

No. 57 ***N*-Nitroso Compounds: Occurrence, Biological Effects and Relevance to Human Cancer**
Edited by I.K. O'Neill, R.C. von Borstel, C.T. Miller, J. Long and H. Bartsch
1984; 1013 pages (*out of print*)

No. 58 **Age-related Factors in Carcinogenesis**
Edited by A. Likhachev, V. Anisimov and R. Montesano
1985; 288 pages (*out of print*)

No. 59 **Monitoring Human Exposure to Carcinogenic and Mutagenic Agents**
Edited by A. Berlin, M. Draper, K. Hemminki and H. Vainio
1984; 457 pages (*out of print*)

No. 60 **Burkitt's Lymphoma: A Human Cancer Model**
Edited by G. Lenoir, G. O'Conor and C.L.M. Olweny
1985; 484 pages (*out of print*)

No. 61 **Laboratory Decontamination and Destruction of Carcinogens in Laboratory Wastes: Some Haloethers**
Edited by M. Castegnaro *et al.*
1985; 55 pages (*out of print*)

No. 62 **Directory of On-going Research in Cancer Epidemiology 1984**
Edited by C.S. Muir and G. Wagner
1984; 717 pages (*out of print*)

No. 63 **Virus-associated Cancers in Africa**
Edited by A.O. Williams, G.T. O'Conor, G.B. de-Thé and C.A. Johnson
1984; 773 pages (*out of print*)

No. 64 **Laboratory Decontamination and Destruction of Carcinogens in Laboratory Wastes: Some Aromatic Amines and 4-Nitrobiphenyl**
Edited by M. Castegnaro *et al.*
1985; 84 pages (*out of print*)

No. 65 **Interpretation of Negative Epidemiological Evidence for Carcinogenicity**
Edited by N.J. Wald and R. Doll
1985; 232 pages (*out of print*)

No. 66 **The Role of the Registry in Cancer Control**
Edited by D.M. Parkin, G. Wagner and C.S. Muir
1985; 152 pages £10.00

No. 67 **Transformation Assay of Established Cell Lines: Mechanisms and Application**
Edited by T. Kakunaga and H. Yamasaki
1985; 225 pages (*out of print*)

No. 68 **Environmental Carcinogens. Selected Methods of Analysis. Volume 7. Some Volatile Halogenated Hydrocarbons**
Edited by L. Fishbein and I.K. O'Neill
1985; 479 pages (*out of print*)

No. 69 **Directory of On-going Research in Cancer Epidemiology 1985**
Edited by C.S. Muir and G. Wagner
1985; 745 pages (*out of print*)

No. 70 **The Role of Cyclic Nucleic Acid Adducts in Carcinogenesis and Mutagenesis**
Edited by B. Singer and H. Bartsch
1986; 467 pages (*out of print*)

No. 71 **Environmental Carcinogens. Selected Methods of Analysis. Volume 8: Some Metals: As, Be, Cd, Cr, Ni, Pb, Se Zn**
Edited by I.K. O'Neill, P. Schuller and L. Fishbein
1986; 485 pages (*out of print*)

No. 72 **Atlas of Cancer in Scotland, 1975–1980. Incidence and Epidemiological Perspective**
Edited by I. Kemp, P. Boyle, M. Smans and C.S. Muir
1985; 285 pages (*out of print*)

No. 73 **Laboratory Decontamination and Destruction of Carcinogens in Laboratory Wastes: Some Antineoplastic Agents**
Edited by M. Castegnaro *et al.*
1985; 163 pages £12.50

No. 74 **Tobacco: A Major International Health Hazard**
Edited by D. Zaridze and R. Peto
1986; 324 pages £22.50

No. 75 **Cancer Occurrence in Developing Countries**
Edited by D.M. Parkin
1986; 339 pages £22.50

No. 76 **Screening for Cancer of the Uterine Cervix**
Edited by M. Hakama, A.B. Miller and N.E. Day
1986; 315 pages £30.00

No. 77 **Hexachlorobenzene: Proceedings of an International Symposium**
Edited by C.R. Morris and J.R.P. Cabral
1986; 668 pages (*out of print*)

No. 78 **Carcinogenicity of Alkylating Cytostatic Drugs**
Edited by D. Schmähl and J.M. Kaldor
1986; 337 pages (*out of print*)

No. 79 **Statistical Methods in Cancer Research. Volume III: The Design and Analysis of Long-term Animal Experiments**
By J.J. Gart, D. Krewski, P.N. Lee, R.E. Tarone and J. Wahrendorf
1986; 213 pages £22.00

No. 80 **Directory of On-going Research in Cancer Epidemiology 1986**
Edited by C.S. Muir and G. Wagner
1986; 805 pages (*out of print*)

No. 81 **Environmental Carcinogens: Methods of Analysis and Exposure Measurement. Volume 9: Passive Smoking**
Edited by I.K. O'Neill, K.D. Brunnemann, B. Dodet and D. Hoffmann
1987; 383 pages £35.00

No. 82 **Statistical Methods in Cancer Research. Volume II: The Design and Analysis of Cohort Studies**
By N.E. Breslow and N.E. Day
1987; 404 pages £35.00

No. 83 **Long-term and Short-term Assays for Carcinogens: A Critical Appraisal**
Edited by R. Montesano, H. Bartsch, H. Vainio, J. Wilbourn and H. Yamasaki
1986; 575 pages £35.00

No. 84 **The Relevance of *N*-Nitroso Compounds to Human Cancer: Exposure and Mechanisms**
Edited by H. Bartsch, I.K. O'Neill and R. Schulte-Hermann
1987; 671 pages (*out of print*)

No. 85 **Environmental Carcinogens: Methods of Analysis and Exposure Measurement. Volume 10: Benzene and Alkylated Benzenes**
Edited by L. Fishbein and I.K. O'Neill
1988; 327 pages £40.00

No. 86 **Directory of On-going Research in Cancer Epidemiology 1987**
Edited by D.M. Parkin and J. Wahrendorf
1987; 676 pages (*out of print*)

No. 87 **International Incidence of Childhood Cancer**
Edited by D.M. Parkin, C.A. Stiller, C.A. Bieber, G.J. Draper, B. Terracini and J.L. Young
1988; 401 pages £35.00

No. 88 **Cancer Incidence in Five Continents Volume V**
Edited by C. Muir, J. Waterhouse, T. Mack, J. Powell and S. Whelan
1987; 1004 pages £55.00

No. 89 **Method for Detecting DNA Damaging Agents in Humans: Applications in Cancer Epidemiology and Prevention**
Edited by H. Bartsch, K. Hemminki and I.K. O'Neill
1988; 518 pages £50.00

No. 90 **Non-occupational Exposure to Mineral Fibres**
Edited by J. Bignon, J. Peto and R. Saracci
1989; 500 pages £50.00

No. 91 **Trends in Cancer Incidence in Singapore 1968–1982**
Edited by H.P. Lee , N.E. Day and K. Shanmugaratnam
1988; 160 pages (*out of print*)

No. 92 **Cell Differentiation, Genes and Cancer**
Edited by T. Kakunaga, T. Sugimura, L. Tomatis and H. Yamasaki
1988; 204 pages £27.50

No. 93 **Directory of On-going Research in Cancer Epidemiology 1988**
Edited by M. Coleman and J. Wahrendorf
1988; 662 pages (*out of print*)

No. 94 **Human Papillomavirus and Cervical Cancer**
Edited by N. Muñoz, F.X. Bosch and O.M. Jensen
1989; 154 pages £22.50

No. 95 **Cancer Registration: Principles and Methods**
Edited by O.M. Jensen, D.M. Parkin, R. MacLennan, C.S. Muir and R. Skeet
1991; 288 pages £28.00

No. 96 **Perinatal and Multigeneration Carcinogenesis**
Edited by N.P. Napalkov, J.M. Rice, L. Tomatis and H. Yamasaki
1989; 436 pages £50.00

No. 97 **Occupational Exposure to Silica and Cancer Risk**
Edited by L. Simonato, A.C. Fletcher, R. Saracci and T. Thomas
1990; 124 pages £22.50

No. 98 **Cancer Incidence in Jewish Migrants to Israel, 1961–1981**
Edited by R. Steinitz, D.M. Parkin, J.L. Young, C.A. Bieber and L. Katz
1989; 320 pages £35.00

No. 99 **Pathology of Tumours in Laboratory Animals, Second Edition, Volume 1, Tumours of the Rat**
Edited by V.S. Turusov and U. Mohr
740 pages £85.00

No. 100 **Cancer: Causes, Occurrence and Control**
Editor-in-Chief L. Tomatis
1990; 352 pages £24.00

No. 101 **Directory of On-going Research in Cancer Epidemiology 1989/90**
Edited by M. Coleman and J. Wahrendorf
1989; 818 pages £36.00

No. 102 **Patterns of Cancer in Five Continents**
Edited by S.L. Whelan and D.M. Parkin
1990; 162 pages £25.00

No. 103 **Evaluating Effectiveness of Primary Prevention of Cancer**
Edited by M. Hakama, V. Beral, J.W. Cullen and D.M. Parkin
1990; 250 pages £32.00

No. 104 **Complex Mixtures and Cancer Risk**
Edited by H. Vainio, M. Sorsa and A.J. McMichael
1990; 442 pages £38.00

No. 105 **Relevance to Human Cancer of *N*-Nitroso Compounds, Tobacco Smoke and Mycotoxins**
Edited by I.K. O'Neill, J. Chen and H. Bartsch
1991; 614 pages £70.00

No. 106 **Atlas of Cancer Incidence in the Former German Democratic Republic**
Edited by W.H. Mehnert, M. Smans, C.S. Muir, M. Möhner & D. Schön
1992; 384 pages £50.00

No. 107 **Atlas of Cancer Mortality in the European Economic Community**
Edited by M. Smans, C.S. Muir and P. Boyle
1992; 280 pages £35.00

No. 108 **Environmental Carcinogens: Methods of Analysis and Exposure Measurement. Volume 11: Polychlorinated Dioxins and Dibenzofurans**
Edited by C. Rappe, H.R. Buser, B. Dodet and I.K. O'Neill
1991; 426 pages £45.00

No. 109 **Environmental Carcinogens: Methods of Analysis and Exposure Measurement. Volume 12: Indoor Air Contaminants**
Edited by B. Seifert, B. Dodet and I.K. O'Neill
Publ. due 1992; approx. 400 pages £45.00

No. 110 **Directory of On-going Research in Cancer Epidemiology 1991**
Edited by M. Coleman and J. Wahrendorf
1991; 753 pages £38.00

No. 111 **Pathology of Tumours in Laboratory Animals, Second Edition, Volume 2, Tumours of the Mouse**
Edited by V.S. Turusov and U. Mohr
Publ. due 1993; approx. 500 pages

No. 112 **Autopsy in Epidemiology and Medical Research**
Edited by E. Riboli and M. Delendi
1991; 288 pages £25.00

No. 113 **Laboratory Decontamination and Destruction of Carcinogens in Laboratory Wastes: Some Mycotoxins**
Edited by M. Castegnaro, J. Barek, J.-M. Frémy, M. Lafontaine, M. Miraglia, E.B. Sansone and G.M. Telling
1991; 64 pages £11.00

No. 114 **Laboratory Decontamination and Destruction of Carcinogens in Laboratory Wastes: Some Polycyclic Heterocyclic Hydrocarbons**
Edited by M. Castegnaro, J. Barek, J. Jacob, U. Kirso, M. Lafontaine, E.B. Sansone, G.M. Telling and T. Vu Duc
1991; 50 pages £8.00

No. 115 **Mycotoxins, Endemic Nephropathy and Urinary Tract Tumours**
Edited by M. Castegnaro, R. Plestina, G. Dirheimer, I.N. Chernozemsky and H Bartsch
1991; 340 pages £45.00

No. 116 **Mechanisms of Carcinogenesis in Risk Identification**
Edited by H. Vainio, P.N. Magee, D.B. McGregor & A.J. McMichael
1992; 616 pages £65.00

No. 117 **Directory of On-going Research in Cancer Epidemiology 1992**
Edited by M. Coleman, J. Wahrendorf & E. Démaret
1992; 773 pages £42.00

No. 118 **Cadmium in the Human Environment: Toxicity and Carcinogenicity**
Edited by G.F. Nordberg, R.F.M. Herber & L. Alessio
Publ. due 1992; approx. 450 pages

No. 119 **The Epidemiology of Cervical Cancer and Human Papillomavirus**
Edited by N. Muñoz, F.X. Bosch, K.V. Shah & A. Meheus
1992; 288 pages £28.00

No. 120 **Cancer Incidence in Five Continents, Volume VI**
Edited by D.M. Parkin, C.S. Muir, S.L. Whelan, Y.T. Gao, J. Ferlay & J.Powell
1992; 1050 pages £120.00

No. 122 **International Classification of Rodent Tumours.** Part 1. **The Rat**
Editor-in-Chief: U. Möhr
1992/93, 10 fascicles, approx. 600 pages, £120.00

IARC MONOGRAPHS ON THE EVALUATION OF CARCINOGENIC RISKS TO HUMANS

(Available from booksellers through the network of WHO Sales Agents)

Volume 1 **Some Inorganic Substances, Chlorinated Hydrocarbons, Aromatic Amines, *N*-Nitroso Compounds, and Natural Products**
1972; 184 pages (*out of print*)

Volume 2 **Some Inorganic and Organometallic Compounds**
1973; 181 pages (*out of print*)

Volume 3 **Certain Polycyclic Aromatic Hydrocarbons and Heterocyclic Compounds**
1973; 271 pages (*out of print*)

Volume 4 **Some Aromatic Amines, Hydrazine and Related Substances, *N*-Nitroso Compounds and Miscellaneous Alkylating Agents**
1974; 286 pages Sw. fr. 18.

Volume 5 **Some Organochlorine Pesticides**
1974; 241 pages (*out of print*)

Volume 6 **Sex Hormones**
1974; 243 pages (*out of print*)

Volume 7 **Some Anti-Thyroid and Related Substances, Nitrofurans and Industrial Chemicals**
1974; 326 pages (*out of print*)

Volume 8 **Some Aromatic Azo Compounds**
1975; 357 pages Sw. fr. 36.

Volume 9 **Some Aziridines, *N*-, *S*- and *O*-Mustards and Selenium**
1975; 268 pages Sw.fr. 27.

Volume 10 **Some Naturally Occurring Substances**
1976; 353 pages (*out of print*)

Volume 11 **Cadmium, Nickel, Some Epoxides, Miscellaneous Industrial Chemicals and General Considerations on Volatile Anaesthetics**
1976; 306 pages (*out of print*)

Volume 12 **Some Carbamates, Thiocarbamates and Carbazides**
1976; 282 pages Sw. fr. 34.-

Volume 13 **Some Miscellaneous Pharmaceutical Substances**
1977; 255 pages Sw. fr. 30.

Volume 14 **Asbestos**
1977; 106 pages (*out of print*)

Volume 15 **Some Fumigants, The Herbicides 2,4-D and 2,4,5-T, Chlorinated Dibenzodioxins and Miscellaneous Industrial Chemicals**
1977; 354 pages Sw. fr. 50.

Volume 16 **Some Aromatic Amines and Related Nitro Compounds - Hair Dyes, Colouring Agents and Miscellaneous Industrial Chemicals**
1978; 400 pages Sw. fr. 50.

Volume 17 **Some *N*-Nitroso Compounds**
1978; 365 pages Sw. fr. 50.

Volume 18 **Polychlorinated Biphenyls and Polybrominated Biphenyls**
1978; 140 pages Sw. fr. 20.

Volume 19 **Some Monomers, Plastics and Synthetic Elastomers, and Acrolein**
1979; 513 pages (*out of print*)

Volume 20 **Some Halogenated Hydrocarbons**
1979; 609 pages (*out of print*)

Volume 21 **Sex Hormones (II)**
1979; 583 pages Sw. fr. 60.

Volume 22 **Some Non-Nutritive Sweetening Agents**
1980; 208 pages Sw. fr. 25.

Volume 23 **Some Metals and Metallic Compounds**
1980; 438 pages (*out of print*)

Volume 24 **Some Pharmaceutical Drugs**
1980; 337 pages Sw. fr. 40.

Volume 25 **Wood, Leather and Some Associated Industries**
1981; 412 pages Sw. fr. 60

Volume 26 **Some Antineoplastic and Immunosuppressive Agents**
1981; 411 pages Sw. fr. 62.

Volume 27 **Some Aromatic Amines, Anthraquinones and Nitroso Compounds, and Inorganic Fluorides Used in Drinking Water and Dental Preparations**
1982; 341 pages Sw. fr. 40.

Volume 28 **The Rubber Industry**
1982; 486 pages Sw. fr. 70.

Volume 29 **Some Industrial Chemicals and Dyestuffs**
1982; 416 pages Sw. fr. 60.

Volume 30 **Miscellaneous Pesticides**
1983; 424 pages Sw. fr. 60.

Volume 31 **Some Food Additives, Feed Additives and Naturally Occurring Substances**
1983; 314 pages Sw. fr. 60

Volume 32 **Polynuclear Aromatic Compounds, Part 1: Chemical, Environmental and Experimental Data**
1983; 477 pages Sw. fr. 60.

Volume 33 **Polynuclear Aromatic Compounds, Part 2: Carbon Blacks, Mineral Oils and Some Nitroarenes**
1984; 245 pages Sw. fr. 50.

Volume 34 **Polynuclear Aromatic Compounds, Part 3: Industrial Exposures in Aluminium Production, Coal Gasification, Coke Production, and Iron and Steel Founding**
1984; 219 pages Sw. fr. 48.

Volume 35 **Polynuclear Aromatic Compounds, Part 4: Bitumens, Coal-tars and Derived Products, Shale-oils and Soots**
1985; 271 pages Sw. fr. 70.

Volume 36 **Allyl Compounds, Aldehydes, Epoxides and Peroxides**
1985; 369 pages Sw. fr. 70.

Volume 37 **Tobacco Habits Other than Smoking: Betel-quid and Areca-nut Chewing; and some Related Nitrosamines**
1985; 291 pages Sw. fr. 70.

Volume 38 **Tobacco Smoking**
1986; 421 pages Sw. fr. 75.

Volume 39 **Some Chemicals Used in Plastics and Elastomers**
1986; 403 pages Sw. fr. 60.

Volume 40 **Some Naturally Occurring and Synthetic Food Components, Furocoumarins and Ultraviolet Radiation**
1986; 444 pages Sw. fr. 65.

Volume 41 **Some Halogenated Hydrocarbons and Pesticide Exposures**
1986; 434 pages Sw. fr. 65.

Volume 42 **Silica and Some Silicates**
1987; 289 pages Sw. fr. 65.

Volume 43 **Man-Made Mineral Fibres and Radon**
1988; 300 pages Sw. fr. 65.

Volume 44 **Alcohol Drinking**
1988; 416 pages Sw. fr. 65.

Volume 45 **Occupational Exposures in Petroleum Refining; Crude Oil and Major Petroleum Fuels**
1989; 322 pages Sw. fr. 65.

Volume 46 **Diesel and Gasoline Engine Exhausts and Some Nitroarenes**
1989; 458 pages Sw. fr. 65.

Volume 47 **Some Organic Solvents, Resin Monomers and Related Compounds, Pigments and Occupational Exposures in Paint Manufacture and Painting**
1989; 536 pages Sw. fr. 85.

Volume 48 **Some Flame Retardants and Textile Chemicals, and Exposures in the Textile Manufacturing Industry**
1990; 345 pages Sw. fr. 65.

Volume 49 **Chromium, Nickel and Welding**
1990; 677 pages Sw. fr. 95.-

Volume 50 **Pharmaceutical Drugs**
1990; 415 pages Sw. fr. 65.-

Volume 51 **Coffee, Tea, Mate, Methylxanthines and Methylglyoxal**
1991; 513 pages Sw. fr. 80.-

Volume 52 **Chlorinated Drinking-water; Chlorination By-products; Some Other Halogenated Compounds; Cobalt and Cobalt Compounds**
1991; 544 pages Sw. fr. 80.-

Volume 53 **Occupational Exposures in Insecticide Application and some Pesticides**
1991; 612 pages Sw. fr. 95.-

Volume 54 **Occupational Exposures to Mists and Vapours from Strong Inorganic Acids; and Other Industrial Chemicals**
1992; 336 pages Sw. fr. 65.-

Volume 55 **Solar and Ultraviolet Radiation**
1992; 316 pages Sw. fr. 65.-

Supplement No. 1
Chemicals and Industrial Processes Associated with Cancer in Humans (IARC Monographs, Volumes 1 to 20)
1979; 71 pages (*out of print*)

Supplement No. 2
Long-term and Short-term Screening Assays for Carcinogens: A Critical Appraisal
1980; 426 pages Sw. fr. 40.-

Supplement No. 3
Cross Index of Synonyms and Trade Names in Volumes 1 to 26
1982; 199 pages (*out of print*)

Supplement No. 4
Chemicals, Industrial Processes and Industries Associated with Cancer in Humans (IARC Monographs, Volumes 1 to 29)
1982; 292 pages (*out of print*)

Supplement No. 5
Cross Index of Synonyms and Trade Names in Volumes 1 to 36
1985; 259 pages (*out of print*)

Supplement No. 6
Genetic and Related Effects: An Updating of Selected IARC Monographs from Volumes 1 to 42
1987; 729 pages Sw. fr. 80.-

Supplement No. 7
Overall Evaluations of Carcinogenicity: An Updating of IARC Monographs Volumes 1-42
1987; 440 pages Sw. fr. 65.-

Supplement No. 8
Cross Index of Synonyms and Trade Names in Volumes 1 to 46
1990; 346 pages Sw. fr. 60.-

IARC TECHNICAL REPORTS*

No. 1 **Cancer in Costa Rica**
Edited by R. Sierra, R. Barrantes, G. Muñoz Leiva, D.M. Parkin, C.A. Bieber and N. Muñoz Calero
1988; 124 pages Sw. fr. 30.-

No. 2 **SEARCH: A Computer Package to Assist the Statistical Analysis of Case-control Studies**
Edited by G.J. Macfarlane, P. Boyle and P. Maisonneuve
1991; 80 pages (out of print)

No. 3 **Cancer Registration in the European Economic Community**
Edited by M.P. Coleman and E. Démaret
1988; 188 pages Sw. fr. 30.-

No. 4 **Diet, Hormones and Cancer: Methodological Issues for Prospective Studies**
Edited by E. Riboli and R. Saracci
1988; 156 pages Sw. fr. 30.-

No. 5 **Cancer in the Philippines**
Edited by A.V. Laudico, D. Esteban and D.M. Parkin
1989; 186 pages Sw. fr. 30.-

No. 6 **La genèse du Centre International de Recherche sur le Cancer**
Par R. Sohier et A.G.B. Sutherland
1990; 104 pages Sw. fr. 30.-

No. 7 **Epidémiologie du cancer dans les pays de langue latine**
1990; 310 pages Sw. fr. 30.-

No. 8 **Comparative Study of Anti- smoking Legislation in Countries of the European Economic Community**
Edited by A. Sasco, P. Dalla Vorgia and P. Van der Elst
1990; 82 pages Sw. fr. 30.-

No. 9 **Epidemiologie du cancer dans les pays de langue latine**
1991; 346 pages Sw. fr. 30.-

No. 11 **Nitroso Compounds: Biological Mechanisms, Exposures and Cancer Etiology**
Edited by I.K. O'Neill & H. Bartsch
1992; 149 pages Sw. fr. 30.-

No. 12 **Epidémiologie du cancer dans les pays de langue latine**
1992; 375 pages Sw. fr. 30.-

DIRECTORY OF AGENTS BEING TESTED FOR CARCINOGENICITY (Until Vol. 13 Information Bulletin on the Survey of Chemicals Being Tested for Carcinogenicity)*

No. 8 Edited by M.-J. Ghess, H. Bartsch and L. Tomatis
1979; 604 pages Sw. fr. 40.-

No. 9 Edited by M.-J. Ghess, J.D. Wilbourn, H. Bartsch and L. Tomatis
1981; 294 pages Sw. fr. 41.-

No. 10 Edited by M.-J. Ghess, J.D. Wilbourn and H. Bartsch
1982; 362 pages Sw. fr. 42.-

No. 11 Edited by M.-J. Ghess, J.D. Wilbourn, H. Vainio and H. Bartsch
1984; 362 pages Sw. fr. 50.-

No. 12 Edited by M.-J. Ghess, J.D. Wilbourn, A. Tossavainen and H. Vainio
1986; 385 pages Sw. fr. 50.-

No. 13 Edited by M.-J. Ghess, J.D. Wilbourn and A. Aitio 1988; 404 pages Sw. fr. 43.-

No. 14 Edited by M.-J. Ghess, J.D. Wilbourn and H. Vainio
1990; 370 pages Sw. fr. 45.-

No. 15 Edited by M.-J. Ghess, J.D. Wilbourn and H. Vainio
1992; 318 pages Sw. fr. 45.-

NON-SERIAL PUBLICATIONS †

Alcool et Cancer
By A. Tuyns (in French only)
1978; 42 pages Fr. fr. 35.-

Cancer Morbidity and Causes of Death Among Danish Brewery Workers
By O.M. Jensen
1980; 143 pages Fr. fr. 75.-

Directory of Computer Systems Used in Cancer Registries
By H.R. Menck and D.M. Parkin 1986; 236 pages Fr. fr. 50.-

* Available from booksellers through the network of WHO Sales agents.

† Available directly from IARC

Achevé d'imprimer
sur les presses de la SADAG
en janvier 1993
N° d'imprimeur 2094